Vulvar Disease

Jacob Bornstein
Editor

Vulvar Disease

Breaking the Myths

Springer

Editor
Jacob Bornstein
Department of Obstetrics and Gynecology Galilee Medical Center
Bar-Ilan University Faculty of Medicine
Nahariya
Israel

ISBN 978-3-319-61620-9 ISBN 978-3-319-61621-6 (eBook)
https://doi.org/10.1007/978-3-319-61621-6

Library of Congress Control Number: 2018968478

This Springer imprint is published by the registered company Springer Nature Switzerland AG
The registered company address is: Gewerbestrasse 11, 6330 Cham, Switzerland

Foreword

It is a privilege, as President of the International Society for the Study of Vulvovaginal Disease (ISSVD), to write the foreword to Professor Jacob Bornstein's textbook. I have known Professor Bornstein from many years, and he has always been an example of consistency, perseverance, grit and gentleman behavior: his book on vulvar diseases represents him.

Before and after his ISSVD Presidency, Professor Bornstein has dedicated great and combined efforts to clarify the terminology in the field of vulvar diseases. If today the ISSVD terminology is recognized all over the scientific world, it is because the baton has passed from the founding fathers to Professor Bornstein and other ISSVD fellows at present days.

This book on vulvar diseases is an uncommon pearl. It shines like the sweat on the author's forehead, attempting to convey his experience through words and images. It sparkles like the hands under the gloves, delicate in palpating the lesion, its infiltration, and mobility. It shimmers like the images, chosen among thousands to better represent, communicate, remember, and memorize the diseases in our knowledge. It sparkles like the eyes of the reader, who looks with intensity and, as by magic, reconnects all the knowledge of anatomy, physiology, infectivology, and pathology.

The aim to define the clinical morphology for each of the diseases turns out to be less difficult, the list of differential diagnoses decreases, and the ability to determine the most likely diagnosis increases. Indeed the experience transmitted by these pages comes into aid to have a suspicion, an orientation, a diagnosis, and finally a therapy.

"Scientia potentia est" (knowledge is power) is a sentence attributed to a medieval philosopher, and we want to increase, through the pages of this book, our knowledge on vulvar diseases in a more uniform, more expert, more thoughtful mode. It is the best approach to break past misconceptions and myths and to have a modern approach that a simple search on PubMed or on a website can never provide us.

In Prof. Bornstein's textbook, the methodology used represents a continuing intellectual challenge, and it gives the balance between clinical experience and research results: like seed in the ground, this book will remain an updated book for many years.

Good books are like good wines: over time, the taste is better appreciated, and one thinks of the time and the patience that have served to obtain a so good result.

Mario Preti, MD
Department of Obstetrics and Gynecology
University of Torino
Torino, Italy

President, International Society for the
Study of Vulvovaginal Disease (ISSVD)
Waxhaw, NC, USA

President, Italian Interdisciplinary Society
of Vulvology (SIIV)
Torino, Italy

Acknowledgments

Making this book could not have become a reality without my colleagues who contributed their time and mainly their knowledge, experience, and wisdom writing the chapters for this book. This is the opportunity to thank them.

Editing a textbook is a complicated task. I have come to realize that during the months I was reviewing manuscripts, inserting references, and matching figures to texts. Still, it was a rewarding project, and I hope that the result will be liked by you, as it is by me.

I started my interest in vulvar disease in 1985, after graduating from residency in Obstetrics and Gynecology, when I started a 2-year fellowship with Professor Raymond H. Kaufman in Houston, Texas, one of the founding fathers of the study of vulvar disease, a gynecologist and pathologist, and a past president of the International Society for the Study of Vulvovaginal Disease (ISSVD). Since then, the course of matters took me, much because of him and the love to research vulvar disease, to the presidency of the ISSVD and to chairing the terminology committees of both the ISSVD and the International Federation of Cervical Pathology and Colposcopy (IFCPC). Constructing vulvar terminologies actually led to the idea behind this book, as the terminology committees introduced new concepts and novel paradigms by breaking past myths. I wish to thank my fellow members of the ISSVD and IFCPC; from them I have learned so much.

I wish to thank my wife, Jasmin, and my children, Arik and Sandy, for their encouragement and understanding. A special note to my grandchildren—Omer, Zohar, and Shira—I wish that when time comes and you are able to read and comprehend this book, you will remember your grandfather with pride.

And finally, to you, my readers—thank you for reading this book; I hope you will find reading enjoyable and contributory.

Nahariya, Israel Jacob Bornstein

Contents

Abbreviations

AJCC	American Joint Committee on Cancer
AMNGT	Atypical melanocytic nevus of genital type
AN	Acanthosis nigricans
Anti-PDI	Anti-programmed cell death 1
BRAF	Human gene that makes a protein called B-Raf
cKIT	Tyrosine-protein kinase Kit
CTLA4	Cytotoxic T-lymphocyte-associated protein 4
ECOG	Eastern Cooperative Oncology Group
FDA	US Food and Drug Administration
FIGO	International Federation of Gynecology and Obstetrics
HPV	Human papillomavirus
HSV	Herpes simplex virus
KRT5	Keratin5
LEOPARD syndrome	(L)entigines (E)lectrocardiographic conduction defects (O)cular hypertelorism (P)ulmonary stenosis (A)bnormalities of the genitals; (R)etarded growth; and (D)eafness or hearing loss
MRI	Magnetic resonance imaging
MSLT1	Multicenter Selective Lymphadenectomy Trial-I
NRAS	Neuroblastoma RAS viral oncogene homolog
OS	Overall survival
PCOS	Polycystic ovarian syndrome
PET scan	Positron emission tomography scanner
PRKAR1A	Protein kinase CAMP-dependent type I regulatory subunit alpha
PTPN11	Tyrosine-protein phosphatase non-receptor type 11
RAF1	Proto-oncogene, serine/threonine kinase
SLN	Sentinel lymph node
STK11	Serine/threonine kinase 11
vHSIL	Vulvar high-grade squamous intraepithelial lesion

Introduction

1

Jacob Bornstein

The book you are about to read is exceptional, in that instead of presenting only the "how to" diagnose and treat vulvar disease, it also breaks old myths that have been repeatedly discussed in the past, becoming "common knowledge." Instead, you can find here contemporary paradigms of approaching vulvar disease.

In many fields of medicine, despite the fast progress of technology, the medical specialty was slow to adopt and remained conservative. Doctors tend to stick to old axioms and myths, perhaps because they were taught to "primum non nocere" ("first, do no harm") [1].

The study of vulvar disease is no exception. It was frozen for years. Consequently, the approach to vulvar conditions has been an enigma for many clinicians. Another reason for the difficulty in comprehending vulvar diseases was that, although both treat vulvar disease, gynecologists lack the dermatological knowledge that is needed to diagnose and treat vulvar skin diseases, while dermatologists have no experience with vaginal and cervical conditions that may cause or be involved in the development of vulvar disease. Another issue that makes the diagnosis of vulvar disease difficult is that in the vulva, the local warmth and humidity affect the lesion's character. For example, a psoriatic lesion loses the typical scaling while developing on the vulvar skin. The intimate locations of the lesions and the disfiguring potential of vulvar surgery in young patients lead many times to delaying a timely examination of the lesions.

But the main obstacle to the progress of the study of vulvar disease was that every profession of those dealing with vulvar disease developed its own set of concepts and treatments, as well as nomenclatures and working terms. In addition to gynecologists and dermatologists, proctologists and gastroenterologists take care of vulvar conditions. Moreover, physical therapists, psychologists, and sex therapists also provide care to patients affected by diseases of this area. Pathologists have a special role here since in many cases of vulvar disease, the diagnosis may be established only by a tissue sample. Vulvologists spent a lot of time settling the differences between the various approaches and terms [2].

However, recently, some of the concepts that were in discordance between the different disciplines have been discussed, so that consensus has been reached. The editor of this book has been involved, as chair, in a few international committees that set the new terminologies in lower genital tract conditions. Achieving the consensus by these international committees was associated with breaking previous myths and misconceptions. For example, for years, women with dyspareunia—pain during intercourse—were diagnosed as having "vaginismus," a psychosexual dysfunction leading to spasm of the introital muscles.

J. Bornstein (✉)
Department of Obstetrics and Gynecology Galilee Medical Center, Bar-Ilan University Faculty of Medicine, Nahariya, Israel

J. Bornstein (ed.), *Vulvar Disease*, https://doi.org/10.1007/978-3-319-61621-6_1

Even with the introduction of the concept that in most cases they were suffering from a physical condition—vestibulitis—later named "localized provoked vulvodynia (LPV)" or "vestibulodynia," many young women with painful intercourse are still told that the problem is "in their head." This myth has been replaced by the modern concept that LPV is a physical condition and the psychological issues are mainly a result of the disabling nature of vulvar pain and inability to have intercourse [3].

Another myth that was broken recently also had to do with LPV. Edward Friedrich, one of the founding fathers of modern vulvology, in the preface to his book *Vulvar Disease*, cited Goethe, saying: "One only sees what one already knows" [4]. Indeed, women with vulvar pain received a psychological treatment if they initially visited a psychologist. While if they saw a surgeon, they ended up very quickly undergoing surgery. If they were examined by a physical therapist first, they were treated by pelvic rehabilitation therapy, and if they were diagnosed by a pain specialist, their first-line treatment consisted of neuropathic medications. The paradigm has now been changed, and this book is presenting the new paradigm of management of vulvodynia—per the "associated factor"—which is the likely cause of the problem [3].

Myths have also been broken in regard to the approach to vulvar dermatoses, vulvovaginitis, and vulvar intraepithelial neoplasia (VIN). As for VIN, the understanding of the pathogenesis of this precancerous lesion has evolved during the last decade. This was reflected in the repeated alterations of the terminology. In contrast to the cervical intraepithelial neoplasia (CIN), many VIN cases are not caused by HPV. Today it is clear that ignoring the non-HPV associated VIN by the 2012 "Lower Anogenital Squamous Terminology Standardization Project for HPV-Associated Lesions (LAST)" led to disregarding the differentiated type of VIN, resulting in some untoward negligence to treat it. This concept has been changed recently by the terminology committee of the International Society for the Study of Vulvovaginal Disease (ISSVD), headed by the editor of this book, with all variants of vulvar intraepithelial lesions grouped under one terminology [5]. This is explained in detail in the present book.

Another myth that was broken after many discussions was that examination of the vulva should take place with the naked eye and not using the colposcope. That approach had been advocated mainly by dermatologists. However, vulvar conditions are managed in many countries by colposcopists, who are gynecologists experienced with using a colposcope—a magnifying optical tool; they tend to use the colposcope as a magnifying optical tool on all tissues of the lower genital tract [6]. Nonetheless, colposcopists usually receive no specific training in vulvar disease. In addition, the terminology they used for cervical colposcopic pattern recognition is that of the International Federation for Cervical Pathology and Colposcopy (IFCPC) and did not include—until recently—specific vulvar and anal patterns. The editor of the present book also headed a nomenclature committee of the IFCPC that for the first time developed a clinical and colposcopic terminology of lesions in the vagina and vulva (including the anus), in addition to revising the cervix terminology [7]. This 2011 terminology is used in this book as the primary approach to diagnose vulvar lesions, breaking the myth that the colposcope should not be used for the vulva.

One word before you dive into the world of vulvar disease. Many clinicians believe that to diagnose a vulvar disease is extremely difficult and requires years of experience in dermatology, gynecology, and pathology. They also feel that the terminology is hard to understand. This may be the main myth I will break in this book. Using the terminology makes diagnosis and approach to vulvar disease straightforward. After reading this book, you will enjoy making diagnoses and proposing treatment. To conclude, the aim of this book is to provide the clinician with the knowledge needed to diagnose, understand the pathogenesis, and treat vulvar disease and at the same time to teach the new paradigms of the approach to vulvar disease, resulting from breaking old myths.

Welcome to the world of modern vulvology!

Vulvar Disease: Breaking the Myths

- Many clinicians believe that to diagnose a vulvar disease is extremely difficult and that the terminology of vulvar diseases is cumbersome. This is a myth! Using the new terminologies makes diagnosis and treatment of vulvar disease easy and straightforward.
- For years, women with dyspareunia—pain during intercourse—were diagnosed as being "vaginismus," a psychosexual dysfunction leading to spasm of the introital muscles. Many young women with painful intercourse are still told that the problem is "in their head." This myth has been replaced by the modern concept that LPV is a physical condition.
- The vulva is different from the cervix. For example, there is no transformation zone on the vulva, and the CIN 1,2,3 of the cervix do not apply in the vulva. VIN 1,2,3 should not be used. In addition, the "lower anogenital squamous terminology (LAST)" does not cover all vulvar precancers, as not all of them are caused by HPV, and therefore it disregards a lesion with an especially malignant potential—differentiated VIN (dVIN).
- Dermatologists preach that examination of the vulva should take place with the naked eye. However, the colposcope is essential to diagnosing and treatment of HPV and precancerous lesion.
- Many clinicians believe that to diagnose a vulvar disease is extremely difficult. This is the main myth that this book attempts to break: after you read it, diagnosis and approach to vulvar disease will become straightforward.

References

1. The origin of primum non nocere. British Medical Journal electronic responses and commentary, 1 September 2002.
2. Micheletti L, Preti M, Bogliatto F, Lynch PJ. Vulvology. A proposal for a multidisciplinary subspecialty. J Reprod Med. 2002;47:715–7.
3. Bornstein J, Goldstein AT, Stockdale CK, Bergeron S, Pukall C, Zolnoun D, Coady D. 2015 ISSVD, ISSWSH, and IPPS consensus terminology and classification of persistent vulvar pain and vulvodynia. J Low Genit Tract Dis. 2016;20:126–30.
4. Friedrich E. Vulvar diseasc. Saunders; 1976.
5. Bornstein J, Bogliatto F, Haefner HK, Stockdale CK, Preti M, Bohl TG, Reutter J, ISSVD Terminology Committee. The 2015 International Society for the Study of Vulvovaginal Disease (ISSVD) Terminology of Vulvar Squamous Intraepithelial Lesions. J Low Genit Tract Dis. 2016;201:11–4.
6. Micheletti L, Bogliatto F, Lynch PJ. Vulvoscopy: review of a diagnostic approach requiring clarification. J Reprod Med. 2008;53:179–82.
7. Bornstein J, Sideri M, Tatti S, Walker P, Prendiville W, Haefner HK, Nomenclature Committee of International Federation for Cervical Pathology and Colposcopy. 2011 terminology of the vulva of the International Federation for Cervical Pathology and Colposcopy. J Low Genit Tract Dis. 2012;16:290–5.

Part I

The Basics

The Normal Vulva and Vagina

2

Bina Cohen Sacher

2.1 Introduction

The vulva is the term for female external genital organs. It is comprised of the labia majora, labia minora, the vestibule, and the clitoris (Figs. 2.1 and 2.2). The vagina, which is sometimes a misnomer for the vulva, is the muscular tube that passes through the pelvic diaphragm formed by the levator ani muscles and opens into the vestibule.

The vulva is complex in structure and presents different types of skin, and its appearance

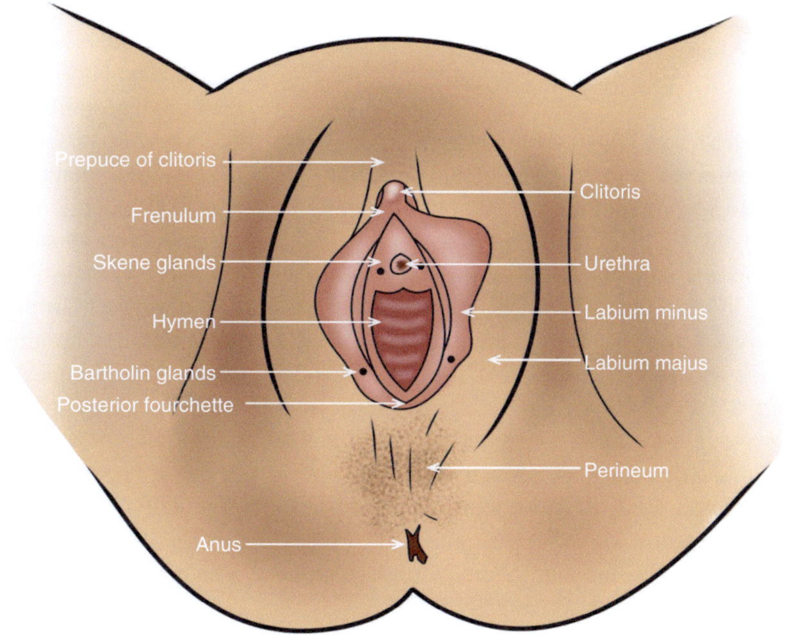

Fig. 2.1 A drawing with annotations of the parts of the vulva, courtesy of Professor Jacob Bornstein

B. Cohen Sacher (✉)
Department of Obstetrics and Gynecology, Helen Schneider Hospital for Women, Rabin Medical Center, Petach Tikva, Israel

J. Bornstein (ed.), *Vulvar Disease*, https://doi.org/10.1007/978-3-319-61621-6_2

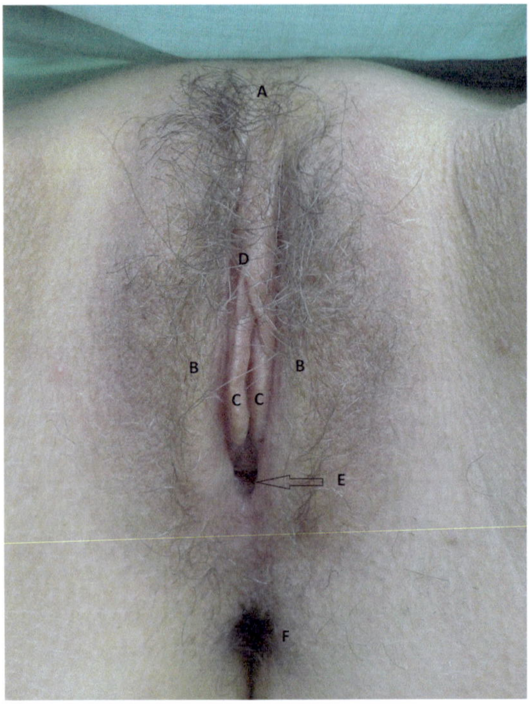

Fig. 2.2 A photograph of the vulva. *A* mons pubis, *B* labia majora, *C* labia minora, *D* clitoral prepuce, *E* vestibule, *F* anus

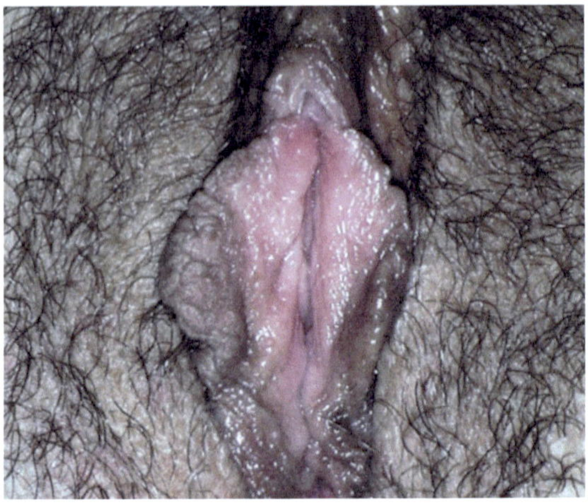

Fig. 2.3 A photograph of the vulva. Courtesy of Professor Jacob Bornstein

changes throughout the woman's life cycle. When we evaluate a woman with vulvar complaints, we should keep in mind her age and hormonal status and judge the findings accordingly.

Normal variants are often mistaken for a disease in the vulva—or rather, an aesthetic problem needing to be fixed—for example, variable shape and forms of the labia minora (Figs. 2.3 and 2.4a–c). Vulvar cosmetic surgeries, once reserved for mending congenital abnormalities or traumatic defects, gain popularity, and its prevalence is on the rise. More than half of US cosmetic surgeons now offer labioplasty [1]. Indeed, most papers dealing with normal vulvar anatomy are cosmetic surgery oriented.

2.2 Embryology

The female lower urogenital tract is the only part of the female body derived from all three embryonic layers—ectoderm, endoderm, and mesoderm. The keratinized skin and its appendages are ectodermal, the vulvar vestibule is of endodermal origin, and the vagina, uterus, and fallopian tubes derive from mesoderm [2].

Until the 8th–9th gestational weeks, the external and internal genitalia can develop to either male or female organs, according to the genetic sex and local hormonal effect, or the lack of it. At the eighth gestational week, the female embryo's gonads start differentiation toward ovaries, but the external genitalia are still indifferent, and both mesonephric (Wolffian) and paramesonephric (mullerian) ducts are present [3–5].

In the female fetus, the mesonephric ducts will degenerate in the next weeks due to lack of anti-mullerian hormone. In the absence of testosterone, the paramesonephric ducts develop and combine partly to a Y-shaped structure: its distal end comes in contact with the posterior wall of the urogenital sinus. The combined ducts will eventually form the upper vagina and uterus, whereas the divided parts will become the fallopian tubes [3, 5].

The lower part of the vagina and the external genitalia originate from the genital tubercle, urogenital folds, and urogenital swellings, which surround the cloacal membrane at the ventral side of the embryo. In the fifth week of embryonic life, a septum divides the cloaca into a ventral portion named the urogenital sinus and a dorsal anorectal canal. Afterward, it begins the differentiation of

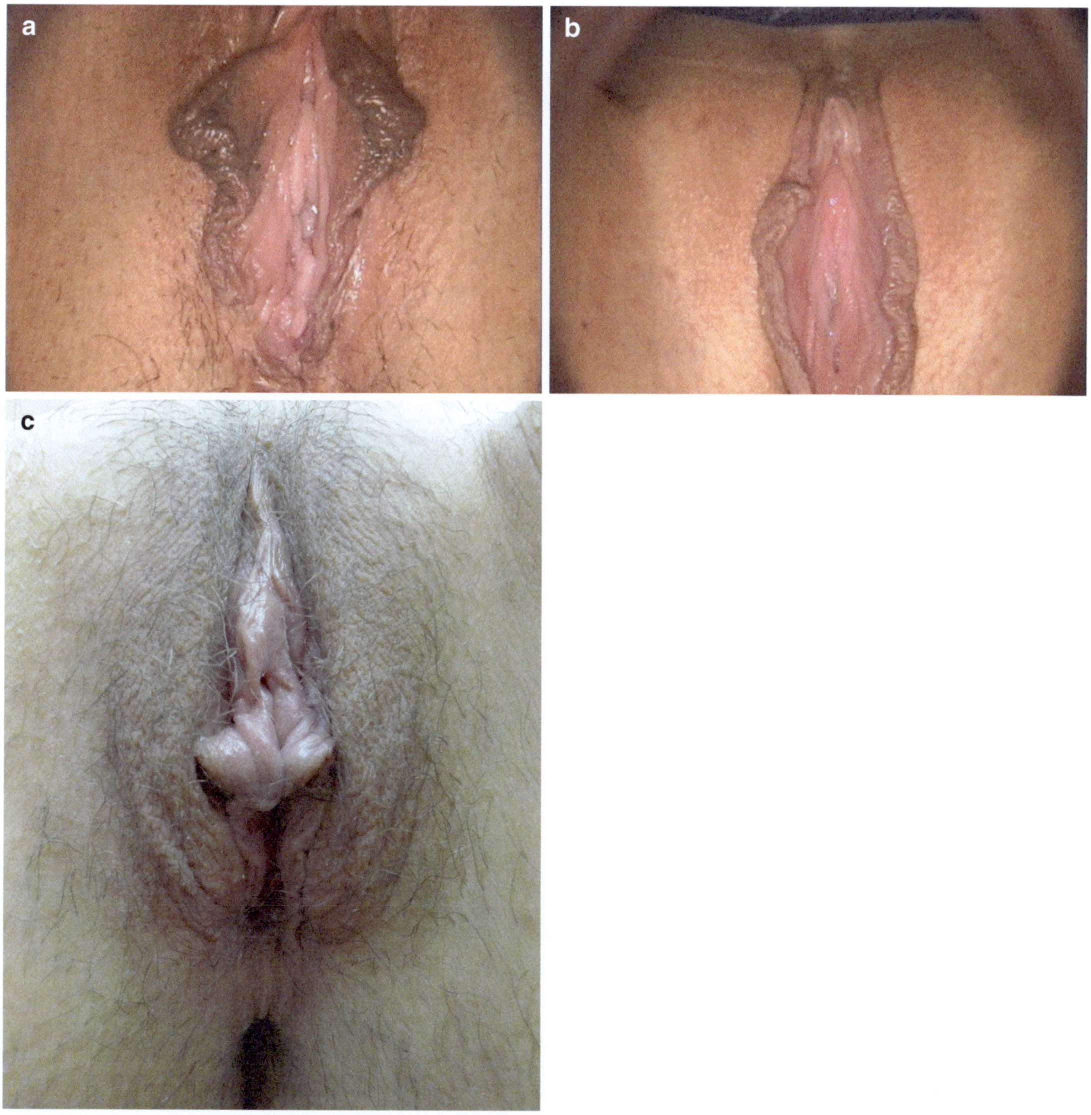

Fig. 2.4 (**a–c**) Photograph of various vulvas. The minor labia are within the "normal" shape and size in all cases. Figures (**a** and **b**) are courtesy of Professor Jacob Bornstein

the external genitalia—in the female, the lack of androgens and the presence of estrogens promote the feminization of the external genitalia, which begins by 11 weeks of gestation. The contact between the combined paramesonephric ducts and the urogenital sinus forms the upper two thirds of the vagina, as the caudal end of the urogenital sinus forms the vestibule. The urogenital folds and swellings remain separated, contrary to the male embryo, and they form the labia majora and minora, respectively. The genital tubercle creates the corpora cavernosa and the glans of the clitoris [5]. The glans is an anatomical separate structure capping the end of the corporal bodies, which are well defined by the tunica albuginea. Large nerve structures are already visible above the tunica albuginea at 17 weeks of gestation. The anatomical structure of the body of the clitoris, erectile tissue within the cavernous body, and clitoral innervation is similar to that of the penis in male fetuses [6].

By 20 weeks of gestation, the female external genitalia are well defined.

2.3 Infancy and Childhood

At birth, the female newborn may show some signs of maternal hormone effect. The breasts may be enlarged, the labia majora are plump, and the labia minora are developed. The vaginal mucosa is rich in glycogen. Physiological white vaginal secretion may be visible. More rarely, hormone withdrawal bleeding may occur [2, 7].

Four weeks after birth, the effect of maternal hormones subsides. The labia majora lose the puffy appearance. The underlying labia minora become thin and small, usually represent only anterior remnants of the clitoral frenulum. The hymen which is a thick elastic membrane at birth becomes thin, frail, and translucent, with several normal variations in its appearance [8, 9]. Vaginal epithelium becomes atrophic, the glycogen diminishes, and vaginal pH becomes neutral or alkaline. The skin over the mons pubis and labia majora becomes thinner as well, and these structures lose some of the subcutaneous fat present at birth. The labia minora are small and due to lack of estrogen may become adherent to each other in early infancy. This situation will usually resolve spontaneously, but if treatment is needed, topical estrogen promotes separation of the labia [7].

Vulvar hair follicles and sebaceous glands are probably present at birth; however, they will mature at puberty when the adrenal glands are activated [2].

2.4 Puberty

Puberty begins between 8 and 11 years of age in general. During this time, the ovaries and adrenal glands increase production of sex hormones. Adrenarche, the maturation of adrenal glands and androgen secretion, begins approximately 2 years before gonadarche—maturation of the pituitary-gonadal axis and production of ovarian steroid hormones. Gonadal maturation occurs during the 2 years preceding menarche [2].

The physical changes observed during these years are accelerated growth, appearance of pubic and axillary hair, breast development, and the onset of menstruation.

In addition to the clearly apparent development of pubic hair, there are more subtle changes influenced by sex hormones occurring in the vulva and vagina. The labia majora and mons pubis become plumper due to increased dermal fat. Increase in pigmentation gives the vulva a slightly darker complexion. The clitoris is more prominent, and the labia minora, vestibule, vagina, and cervix all increase in size. The vestibular and periurethral glands become activated in response to elevated level of the various sex hormones, providing lubrication to the vagina and vestibule. The vaginal epithelium, which contained only basal and parabasal layers of cells in the prepubertal stage, begins proliferating, forming multiple intermediate and superficial layers of cells. The intracellular concentration of glycogen increases, and its metabolism by lactobacilli causes vaginal fluid to become acidic [2, 3, 7, 8].

Menstruation appears about 4 years after these changes begin. The mean age of menarche worldwide is between 12 and 13 years; the differences between races are minor [10].

2.5 Reproductive Years

2.5.1 The Mons Pubis and Labia Majora

The mons pubis in the adult woman is the hair-bearing skin with subcutaneous prominent fat pad overlying the anterior part of the symphysis bone. It is composed mainly of loose adipose tissue overlying fascia, which is a continuation of the Camper's and Scarpa's fascia from the anterior abdominal wall [11]. The labia majora are cutaneous folds originating from the mons pubis anteriorly and posteriorly form the posterior fourchette overlying the perineal body (Fig. 2.1). They are the most lateral structures in the vulva, separated from the inner thighs by the genitocrural folds [1, 3]. The labia majora contain the distal end of the round ligaments, the superficial Camper's fascia with a predominance of fat, and the deeper layer is formed by Colles fascia that corresponds to the Scarpa's fascia in the abdominal wall [1]. An adipose sac, fused with the superior surface of the Colles fascia and connects to the superficial clitoral ligament and round ligament, maintains the labia majora shape [12].

The cutaneous epithelium covering the mons pubis and lateral surface of the labia majora is derived from the embryonic ectoderm. It exhibits a pigmented, keratinized, stratified, squamous structure with sweat gland, sebaceous glands, and hair follicles, whereas the medial part of the labia majora is covered by smooth, fair, and hairless skin [13].

2.5.2 The Labia Minora

The labia minora lie medial to the labia majora and lateral to the vestibule. Anteriorly each separate into two folds that run over and under the glans of the clitoris (Fig. 2.5). The superior folds unite in the midline to form the prepuce;

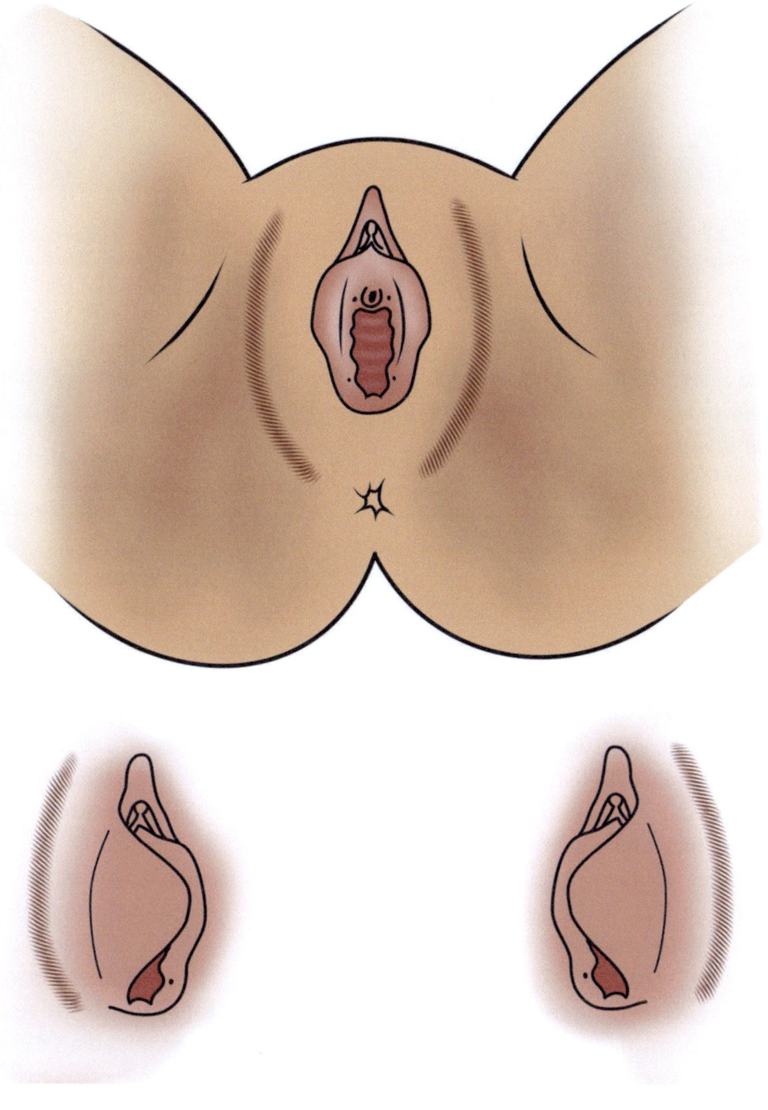

Fig. 2.5 A drawing depicting the labia minora in different aspects. Anteriorly each labium separates into two folds that run over and under the glans of the clitoris. Courtesy of Professor Jacob Bornstein

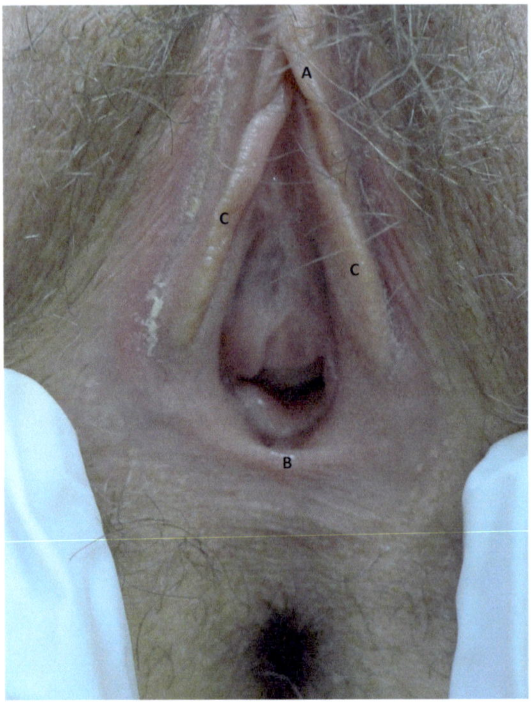

Fig. 2.6 A photograph of the vulva. *A* clitoral prepuce, *B* fourchette, *C* labia minora

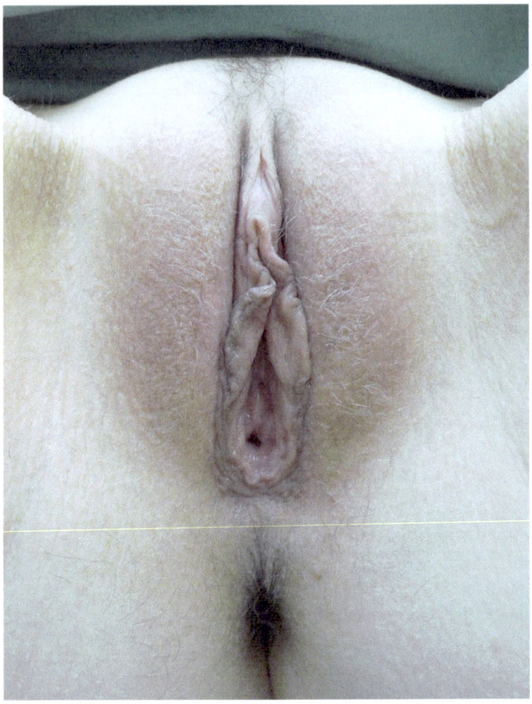

Fig. 2.7 A photograph of the vulva. The labia are within the "normal" size and shape. Courtesy of Professor Jacob Bornstein

the inferior folds insert into the underside of the clitoris to form the frenulum. Posteriorly the labia minora merge with the labia majora in the posterior fourchette (Fig. 2.6) [1, 3]. The labia minora vary in size and morphology (Figs. 2.3, 2.4a–c, and 2.7) and may be asymmetrical or divided.

The labia minora are covered with keratinized skin that contains sebaceous glands but lacks sweat glands or hair follicles. The epidermis is thinner than on the labia majora, and the degree of keratinization diminishes gradually [14]. From the inner third of the labia minora toward the vestibule, the epithelium is nonkeratinized, presenting large, loose, and moderately flattened cells containing glycogen granules [10]. The transition between the keratinized ectodermal-originated epithelium and the nonkeratinized endodermal-derived epithelium is referred to as the Hart line [1]. The labia minora lack subcutaneous fat and contain thick connective tissue rich in elastic fibers and small blood vessels [3, 4]. The arrangement of the blood vessels forms erectile tissue similar to penile corpus spongiosum [1].

2.5.3 The Vestibule

The vestibule extends anteroposterior from the frenulum of the clitoris to the posterior fourchette and laterally from the hymen to the Hart line of the labium minus on each side. The vestibule is covered by endodermal-originated mucosa, as the inner third of the labia minora. It contains no hair follicles, sweat glands, or sebaceous glands [3, 10].

The vestibule surrounds the vaginal orifice and contains the openings of the urethra and several vestibular glands. The area between the frenulum of the clitoris and the urethral meatus is the female corpus spongiosum or pars intermedia. The area between the hymen and posterior fourchette is the fossa navicularis [1].

Surrounding the vaginal opening is a thin membrane of connective tissue, the hymen. The hymen usually has a central opening through which the menstrual blood is secreted. This opening is enlarged with the use of tampons and with intercourse, leaving in time only remnants of the hymen at the edges of the vestibule. There is considerable variation in normal hymeneal appearance. If the hymen is imperforated, it might lead to hematocolpos when menstrual blood accumulates in the vagina.

The glands which open to the vestibule are responsible for secretions that lubricate the vaginal opening and increase during intercourse and with orgasm. The paraurethral (Skene's) ducts open on both sides of the urethra (Fig. 2.8). The Bartholin's glands are located deep in the posterior aspect of the labia majora and are normally not palpable, unless they become enlarged and create a cyst or an abscess. The Bartholin's glands are lobulated structures, containing multiple acini grouped around the termination of each of the many branching ducts. The main duct openings can be seen on the sides of the vaginal opening, usually at 5 and 7 o'clock (Fig. 2.9). Numerous mucous glands, called the minor vestibular glands, open in the vestibule, but these are less obvious to the naked eye [3, 4].

2.5.4 The Clitoris

The clitoris is a highly neurovascular erectile structure. It is embryologically derived from the undifferentiated phallus and therefore considered to be homologous to the male penis [11]. It contains six main components: glans, suspensory ligament, body, root, crura, and vestibular bulbs.

The glans is the tip of the clitoris body, and it is the only external portion of the clitoris. It is covered by the prepuce, which connects to the labia minora bilaterally by the frenulum. It contains specialized genital vascular tissue [1] (Figs. 2.1 and 2.10).

The body of the clitoris contains two corpora cavernosa comprised of erectile tissue. It extends cephalad to the glans and then folds back on itself, bifurcating at the pubic symphysis into two crura. The crura are attached to the pubic rami and covered by the ischiocavernosus muscle [3, 4]. The root is located below the skin of the vestibule. The body and the crura contain the largest amount of erectile tissue but fewer nerves, compared to the glans which is the most innervated part of the clitoris [1].

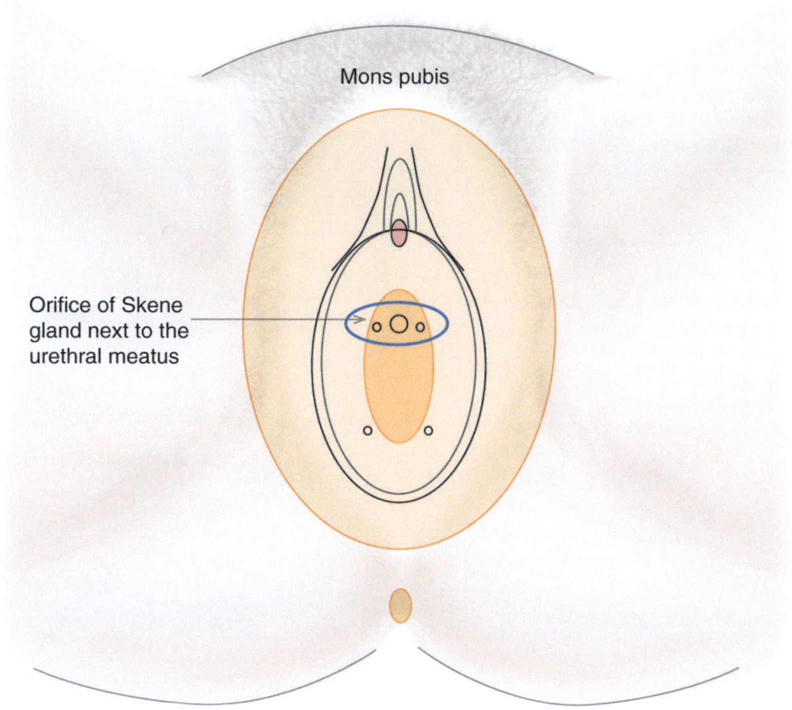

Fig. 2.8 A drawing depicting the openings of the Skene's glands into the vestibule. Anteriorly the Skene's glands lie along the sides of the urethra and open into the vestibule, on both sides of the urethra. Courtesy of Professor Jacob Bornstein

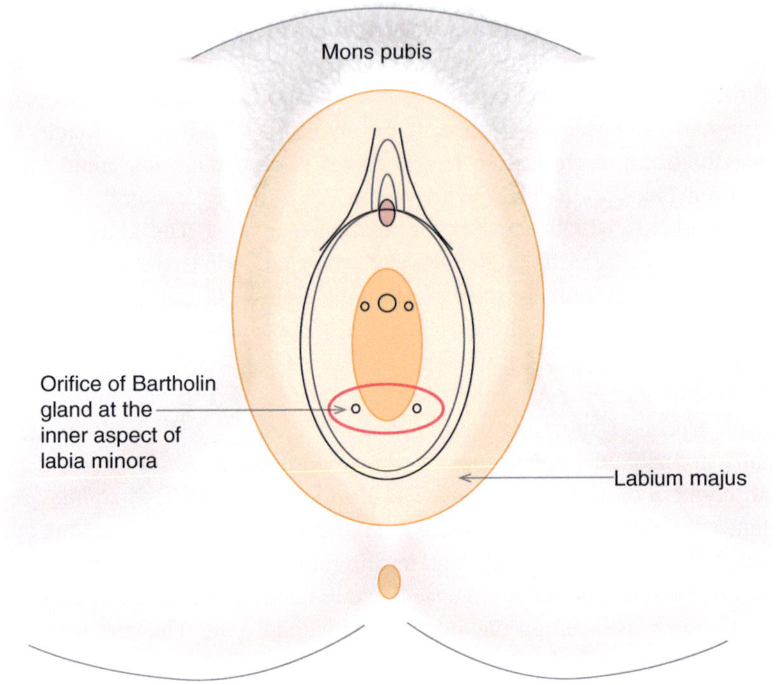

Fig. 2.9 A drawing depicting the vestibule. The Bartholin's glands occupy the posterior parts of both labia majora and open into the posterior vestibule. Courtesy of Professor Jacob Bornstein

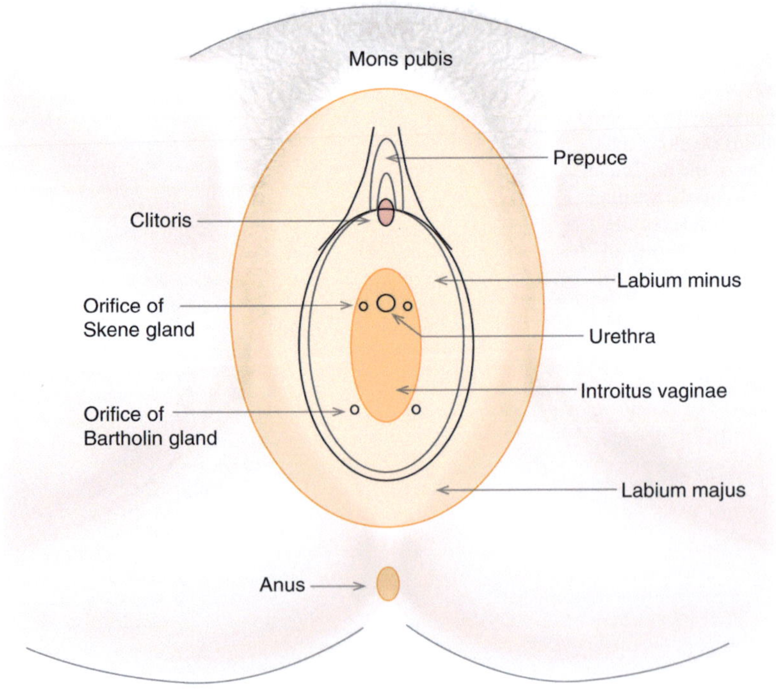

Fig. 2.10 A drawing depicting the relationship between the clitoral prepuce to the labia minora and other parts of the vulva. Courtesy of Professor Jacob Bornstein

The bulbs are two erectile organs contiguous with the glans and body of the clitoris. The bulbs lay beneath the labia majora. They become engorged with arousal and add to lubrication and stability of vaginal walls.

The suspensory ligaments of the clitoris arise from the deep fascia of the mons pubis and converge onto the body of the clitoris, which is covered by the tunica albuginea. It extends down into the medial aspect of the labia majora. It is hypothesized to support and restrict the movement of the body of the clitoris [1].

2.5.5 The Vagina

The vagina extends from the vestibule toward the uterine cervix, shaped as a 7–10-cm-long fibromuscular cylinder, in approximation to the urine bladder and urethra anteriorly, to the levator ani muscle and endopelvic fascia laterally, and to the rectum posteriorly [3, 11].

The walls of the vagina are collapsed and in contact except the upper end where the cervix keeps them separated. The folds that surround the vaginal portion of the cervix are termed fornices, referred to as anterior, posterior, and two lateral fornices by their position. They are, however, continuous with each other. The posterior fornix is the deepest and is closely related to the rectouterine pouch [3, 11].

Histologically, vaginal walls consist of three layers. The lining mucosal layer consists of nonkeratinized squamous epithelium, which appears folded to many small rugae due to its thickness. Underneath the epithelium there's a loose vascular connective tissue, the lamina propria. The middle vascular layer is comprised of smooth muscle fibers intermingled with striated muscle fibers from the pelvic floor, and the adventitial layer contains collagen and elastin, with neurovascular bundle and lymphatics. There are no glands in vaginal walls, and lubrication is provided by transudation from vessels, the cervical glands, and Bartholin's and Skene's glands [11].

Vaginal mucosa is rich in glycogen granules. In the reproductive years, the normal vaginal pH is below 4.5, due to metabolism of glycogen by lactobacilli bacteria [7].

Vaginal support incudes the uterosacral cardinal complex suspending the upper portion of the vagina. The walls of the vagina are attached to the arcus tendineus fascia pelvis anteriorly and the levator ani fascia posteriorly. The terminal 2–3 cm of the vagina is attached to the surrounding structures: urethra and perineal membrane anteriorly, levator ani laterally, and the perineum and perineal body posteriorly [11].

2.6 Pregnancy

During pregnancy, pigmentation changes further deepen the coloration of the vulva. Blood flow through the pelvic circulation is increased two- to fivefold. Focal hyperplasia of cutaneous blood vessels may manifest as spider telangiectasia, and other vascular lesions as hemangiomas may appear [2, 3]. The vaginal mucosa becomes violaceous, and the cervix becomes more vascular and soft [12]. The connective tissue of the vulva, vagina, and perineum relax, and the muscle fibers of the vaginal wall increase in size. Varicose veins may appear on the vulva [2, 3, 7].

2.7 Menopause

Menstruation ceases at a median age of 50 years in the western industrialized societies, following a few years of perimenopause. The postmenopausal changes in the genital and urinary tracts are in part the result of decreased estrogen levels. Pubic hair becomes gray and sparse, the labia majora lose subcutaneous fat, and the labia minora decrease in size. The vaginal epithelial layers are reduced in number, making it thin and pale. The typical rugae disappear, and the vaginal lining losses its elasticity. Secretions decrease, and the vaginal mucosa becomes dry and more irritable. Lack of estrogen depletes vaginal intracellular glycogen, resulting in reduced lactobacilli bacteria, causing increased vaginal pH. Loss of muscle tone may cause pelvic organ prolapse and urinary incontinence [2, 3, 7]. These changes may lead to genitourinary syndrome of menopause (GSM), which is the combination of vulvovaginal atrophy and symptoms such as vaginal dryness, burning, and irritation, lack of lubrication, dyspareunia, dysuria, and urinary urgency [15]. Women with GSM were found to have 2.5 times higher prevalence of vaginal infections [16].

2.8 Innervation

The pudendal nerve (S2–4) is the main sensory and motor nerve of the perineum. It runs underneath the piriformis muscle, exits through the greater sciatic foramen, passes behind the ischial spine, and reenters the pelvis through the lesser sciatic foramen. The pudendal nerve runs in the Alcock's canal in the obturator fascia ventral to the sacrotuberous ligament. As it enters the perineum, the pudendal nerve lies on the lateral wall of the ischiorectal fossa and divides into three branches: the inferior rectal, the perineal, and the dorsal nerve of the clitoris.

The dorsal nerve of the clitoris supplies the skin of the clitoris, while the erectile tissue is innervated by visceral fibers via the cavernous nerves. The perineal nerve divides into several branches and supplies the skin of the medial portion of the labia majora, the labia minora, and the vestibule. It also innervates the external urethral sphincter, pelvic floor muscles bulbocavernosus and ischiocavernosus, and the superficial perineal muscles. The inferior rectal nerve supplies the perianal skin and the external anal sphincter.

Additional innervation is supplied by the cutaneous branch of the ilioinguinal nerve, the genital branch of the genitofemoral nerve, and the perineal branch of the posterior femoral cutaneous nerve [1, 11].

The upper two thirds of the vagina have visceral innervation derived from the uterovaginal plexus. The vagina's lower one third is innervated by branches of the pudendal nerve [11].

2.9 Vascular Supply

The vulva derives its vascular supply primarily from the internal pudendal arteries, branches of the internal iliac arteries, and external pudendal arteries, branches of the femoral arteries. The veins drain subsequently into the internal iliac veins.

The internal pudendal arteries on each side follow the course of the pudendal nerve and supply the superficial perineal muscles and external genitalia via different branches: the inferior rectal artery supplies the anal canal, the perineal artery supplies the superficial perineal muscles, and other branches supply their corresponding structures—posterior labial branch, artery to the bulb of the vestibule, dorsal and deep arteries of the clitoris, and the urethral artery.

The superficial and deep external pudendal arteries distribute into the labia majora and anastomose with branches of the internal pudendal artery. There is a network of anastomosis between branches of these arteries throughout the female external genitalia [1, 11].

Vascular supply to the vagina is through the descending branch of the uterine artery, vaginal artery, and internal pudendal artery. The veins form vaginal venous plexuses that ultimately drain into the uterine vein and the internal iliac veins [11].

2.10 What Is a "Normal" Vulva?

More cosmetic procedures are done on the vulva nowadays than in past years. This increase may be driven by women's distorted perception of a normal vulva, which is derived from books, consultations with their physicians, and pornography [17]. However, normality is an elusive concept. People come in different shapes and sizes, and the female genitalia are no exception. This variety is often overlooked in medical textbooks [18, 19] or even by physicians [20].

Several papers published in the last decade tried to set normal measurements for the different vulvar parts. Lloyd et al. examined 50 premenopausal women [21]. Basaran et al. examined 100 pre- and postmenopausal women [22]. Their results are shown in Table 2.1. Akbiyik et al. examined 205 girls ages 1 month to 10 years old and generated equations to estimate the expected

Table 2.1 Vulvar measurements in pre- and postmenopausal women in recent literature

		Lloyd et al. [21]	Basaran et al. [22]	
			Premenopause	Postmenopause
Clitoral length (mm)	Mean (SD)	19.1 (8.7)	17.7 (10.6)	17.2 (8.4)
	Range	5–35	2–39	3–33
Clitoral width (mm)	Mean (SD)	5.5 (1.7)	10.2 (5.2)	10.3 (6.5)
	Range	3–10	3–27	3–32
Clitoris-urethra distance (mm)	Mean (SD)	28.5 (7.1)	29.2 (8)	28.7 (8.6)
	Range	16–45	15–45	12–52
Labia minora length (mm)	Mean (SD)	60.6 (17.2)	55.7 (11.9)	51.9 (11.4)
	Range	20–100	34–74	26–73.5
Labia minora width (mm)	Mean (SD)	21.8 (9.4)	17.9 (4.1)	15.4 (4.7)
	Range	7–50	11–30	8–27
Labia majora length (mm)	Mean (SD)	93 (13)	87.4 (11.9)	84.3 (11.3)
	Range	70–120	34–74	55.5–104.5
Vaginal length (mm)	Mean (SD)	96 (15)	90.3 (14.8)	82.3 (11.2)
	Range	65–125	70–132	62–113
Perineal length (mm)	Mean (SD)	31.1 (8.5)	30.1 (9.9)	31.3 (10)
	Range	15–55	12–53	15–53

Table 2.2 Akbiyik et al. [23] equations for vulvar measurements in prepubertal girls

Genital structure	Equation
Clitoris length	7.710 mm + (1.087 × yrs age)
Clitoris width	4.624 mm + (0.135 × yrs age)
Labia majora length	13.477 mm + (0.492 × kg body wt) + (0.147 × cm ht)
Labia minora length	6.198 mm + (0.231 × kg body wt)
Labia minora width	3.2 mm + (0.089 × kg body wt)
Perineal distance	10.314 mm + (0.230 × kg body wt)

Yrs years, *wt* weight, *ht* height

Table 2.3 Chalmers et al. [24] vulvar measurements in prepubertal girls, in millimeters

Age (years)	<2	2–5	5–11	>11
Clitoris length (SD)	3.7 (0.8)	5.4 (1.4)	5.3 (1.6)	7.6 (2.5)
Clitoris width (SD)	3.6 (1.8)	3.7 (1.0)	3.9 (1.5)	4.0 (1.7)
Clitoris to urethra (SD)	8.8 (3.5)	11.5 (3.5)	15.8 (4.7)	24.6 (12.9)
Clitoris to anus (SD)	40.7 (7.1)	46.6 (6.9)	57.6 (11.9)	82.0 (24.4)
Clitoris to posterior fourchette (SD)	15.6 (6.7)	21.4 (9.4)	28.1 (7.6)	52.0 (13.0)
Posterior fourchette (SD)	5.1 (0.8)	6.9 (2.6)	8.2 (2.0)	15.6 (6.0)

external genitalia dimensions in girls according to their age, weight, and height (Table 2.2) [23]. Chalmers et al. examined and measured the genitalia of 56 Tanner stage 1 girls in several age groups (Table 2.3) [24]. These papers show that diversity is greater than previously documented, both in women [20] and premenarchal girls of the same age group [22, 24]. No differences were found related to parity, ethnicity, hormonal use, or sexual activity. In postmenopausal women, vaginal length was significantly shorter and labia minora narrower, when compared to premenopausal women [21].

When dealing with cosmetic procedures, the decision for cosmetic surgery should take into consideration the woman's distress relating to her vulvar appearance, may it be physical or emotional, and whether this distress is expected to be solved by surgery.

2.11 Summary

Caregivers who treat patients with vulvovaginal complaints should be familiar with the normal appearance of the vulva in the different stages of the woman's life. It is important to acknowledge the wide range of normal appearance of the vulva and identify nonpathologic variants. Once the examiner is knowledgeable of the normal anatomy, identifying an abnormality becomes explicit.

The Normal Vulva and Vagina: Breaking the Myths

- The vulva does not remain the same throughout the woman's life cycle. Therefore, vulvar complaints should be evaluated according to age and hormonal status.
- Currently, most papers dealing with normal vulvar anatomy are cosmetic surgery oriented.
- The female lower urogenital tract is the only part of the female body derived from all three embryonic layers—ectoderm, endoderm, and mesoderm.
- The female external genitalia are slow to develop. They are well defined only by 20 weeks of gestation.
- More cosmetic procedures are done on the vulva nowadays than in past years. This increase may be driven by our distorted perception of a normal vulva, ignoring that normal female genitalia come in different shapes and sizes.

Disclosure None.

References

1. Yeung J, Pauls RN. Anatomy of the vulva and the female sexual response. Obstet Gynecol Clin N Am. 2016;43:27–44.
2. Farage M, Maibach HI. Lifetime changes in the vulva and vagina. Arch Gynecol Obstet. 2006;273:195–202.
3. Neill SM, Lewis FM. Basics of vulval embryology, anatomy and physiology. In: Neill SM, Lewis FM, editors. Ridley's the vulva. 3rd ed. Hoboken: Wiley; 2009. p. 1–33.
4. Puppo V. Embryology and anatomy of the vulva: the female orgasm and women's sexual health. Eur J Obstet Gynecol Rerod Biol. 2011;154:3–8.
5. Sajjad Y. Development of the genital ducts and external genitalia in the early human embryo. J Obstet Gynecol Res. 2010;36(5):929–37.
6. Baskin LS, Erol A, Li YW, Liu WH, et al. Anatomical studies of the human clitoris. J Urol. 1999;162:1015–20.
7. Farage MA, Maibach HI. Morphology and physiological changes of genital skin and mucosa. Curr Probl Dermatol. 2011;40:9–19.
8. Wingo Colvin C, Abdullatif H. Anatomy of female puberty: the clinical relevance of developmental changes in the reproductive system. Clin Anat. 2013;26:115–29.
9. Edwards L. Genital anatomy. In: Edwards L, Lynch P, editors. Genital dermatology atlas. 2nd ed. Philadelphia: Lippincott Williams and Wilkins; 2011. p. 1–10.
10. Yermachenko A, Dvornyk V. Nongenetic determinants of age at menarch: a systematic review. Biomed Res Int. 2014;2014:371583.
11. Yavagal S, de Faria TF, Medina CA, et al. Normal vulvovaginal, perineal and pelvic anatomy with reconstructive considerations. Semin Plast Surg. 2011;25:121–9.
12. Ramos-e-Silva M, Martins NR, Kroumpouzos G. Oral and vulvovaginal changes I pregnancy. Clin Dermatol. 2016;34:353–8.
13. Ostrzenski A, Krajewski P, Davis K. Anatomy and histology of the newly discovered adipose sac structure within the labia majora: international original research. Arch Gynecol Obstet. 2016;294:549–54.
14. Farage M, Maibach HI. The vulvar epithelium differs from the skin: implications for cutaneous testing to address topical vulvar exposures. Contact Dermatitis. 2004;51:201–9.
15. Portman DJ, Gass MI. Vulvovaginal atrophy terminology consensus conference panel. Genitourinary syndrome of menopause: new terminology for vulvovaginal atrophy from the International Society for the Study of Women's Sexual Health and the North American Menopause Society. Maturitas. 2014;79:349–54.
16. Palma F, Volpe A, Villa P, et al. Vaginal atrophy of women in postmenopause. Results from a multicentric observational study: the AGATA study. Maturitas. 2016;83:40–4.
17. Yurteri-Kaplan LA, Antosh DD, Sokol AI, et al. Interest in cosmetic vulvar surgery and perception of vulvar appearance. Am J Obstet Gynecol. 2012;207:428.e1–7.
18. Andrikopoulou M, Michala L, Creighton SM, et al. The normal vulva in medical textbooks. J Obstet Gynecol. 2013;33:648–50.
19. Howarth H, Sommer V, Jordan FM. Visual depictions of female genitalia differ depending on source. Med Humanit. 2010;36:75–9.
20. Michala L, Koliantzaki S, Antsaklis A. Protruding labia minora: abnormal or just uncool? J Psychosom Obstet Gynecol. 2011;32(3):154–6.

21. Lloyd J, Crouch NS, Minto CL, et al. Female genital appearance: 'normality' unfolds. BJOG. 2005;112:643–6.
22. Basaran M, Kosif R, Bayar U, et al. Characteristics of external genitalia in pre- and postmenopausal women. Climacteric. 2008;11:416–21.
23. Akbiyik F, Kutlu AO. External genital proportions in prepubertal girls: a morphometric reference form female genitoplasty. J Urol. 2010;184:1476–81.
24. Chalmers DJ, O'Donnell CI, Casperson KJ, et al. Normal anatomic relationship in prepubescent female external genitalia. J Pediatr Urol. 2014;10:1117–21.

3 Cytology and Pathology of the Vulva

Debra S. Heller

3.1 What the Pathologist Wants the Clinician to Know About Vulvar Pathology

The pathologist is an integral part of the patient's team, and a pathology report is a consultation, not an automated test like a blood count. As such, clinicians can maximize the utility of the report for themselves by keeping a few things in mind. First, a thorough relevant clinical history should always be provided, including the appearance of a lesion, symptoms, and any prior treatment, which may be significant in that it changes the histology of the lesion, or allows the pathologist to compare the tissue to prior biopsies or excisions on the patient. There is often not a single answer in pathology, as in clinical medicine, and the information the clinician provides is used in developing a differential diagnosis.

The clinician might find it helpful to understand some of the workings of a pathology laboratory. Briefly, after confirmation of identification of the specimen, the specimen is measured, weighed when appropriate, and described grossly, and the tissue is submitted for processing. The gross description becomes part of the final pathology report. Also in the gross description is whether the specimen was entirely submitted to make the slides, as in a biopsy, or if representative sections were submitted, as in a larger excision. These larger specimens are kept for a period of time after the case is signed out and can be gone back to if additional sampling is warranted. The tissue that will be made into slides is placed into a plastic tissue cassette, which goes through a processor that takes it through several steps of dehydration. This is usually on a computerized timer, and tissue is processed in batches. Hence a specimen labeled "rush" may derail the schedule for other patients by altering the timing of the processing run, and this request should be used with discretion. After processing, the tissue is embedded in paraffin on the outside of the tissue cassette, and slices are cut off this tissue block with a microtome, producing very thin (4–5 micron) sections that can be placed on slides and stained. Many sequential sections can be made from the same block. The remainder of the block is maintained on file for many years, according to local regulations. As such, duplicate slides can be produced. Recuts are the next section that comes off the block and are often used for creating slides to send out for second opinions or for special staining. Levels go deeper into the tissue block, and as such can be used to evaluate more of a tiny area, such as when assessing for superficial invasion. During the gross examination of a specimen, ink may be applied when marginal status is important, so that the ink shows on the slides. This allows for determination of whether or not a lesion is completely excised. If there is no tumor at the ink, the margins are clear.

D. S. Heller (✉)
Department of Pathology, Immunology, and Laboratory Medicine, Rutgers New Jersey Medical School, Newark, NJ, USA
e-mail: hellerds@njms.rutgers.edu

J. Bornstein (ed.), *Vulvar Disease*, https://doi.org/10.1007/978-3-319-61621-6_3

There are some caveats applicable to vulvar pathology that are important to note and relate to the adequacy of a biopsy or excision or use of appropriate fixation or solution for a specimen to be diagnostic. For exophytic lesions, it is important to get a deep enough biopsy. As an example, in verrucous carcinoma, the features that identify it as a malignant neoplasm are at the deepest point of the lesim, and hence this must be sampled. For some lesions, the tumor extends beyond what is grossly visible to the clinician. This is not a rare occurrence with Paget's disease of the vulva. Intraoperative consultation with frozen section is sometimes utilized to make sure the margins are clear when excisions are performed. Vesiculobullous diseases may require immunofluorescence, and these specimens should not be put in formalin, as the tissue needs to be frozen in the laboratory for testing. Specimens for immunofluorescence can be submitted fresh on a saline-moistened gauze if transport time is short or in specific media if longer. Contacting your laboratory in advance regarding special needs specimens will avoid problems and assure that the correct fixative or solution is available.

The clinician wants a report from the pathologist that is prompt and interpretable and explains what is seen clinically. Providing the appropriate information to the pathologist will help achieve that result. Pathology is an art as well as a science. Not everything is a black and white diagnosis. Communication is critical between the members of the patient's healthcare team to achieve the goal of optimal patient care. If practice circumstances permit, establishing a relationship with the pathologist will aid in this goal, and a quick phone call is often very helpful to both parties.

3.2 Cytology of the Vulva

Cytology of the vulva is not in widespread use, but it can be helpful at times in reaching a diagnosis. In a study of methodology, Dennerstein [1] compared utilizing a spatula, a swab, and a scalpel blade scraping for evaluation of vulvar cytology and found that only the scalpel scraping produced reliable results, when evaluating intraepithelial neoplasia, condyloma, basal cell carcinoma, and Paget's disease. However, other authors have not found cytology helpful in evaluating vulvar neoplasia [2]. The disappointing results from vulvar cytology may relate to the scant cellularity usually obtained. A pilot study utilizing a vulvar brush [3] reported feasibility evaluating normal vulva, lichen sclerosus, usual or differentiated VIN, or squamous cell carcinoma, and the authors suggested it may be useful as an instrument of triage.

While the cytology of Paget's disease has been described [4], only histology will demonstrate whether or not a lesion is invasive [5], but cytology may be useful in surveillance [4]. Smears of unroofed blisters may show the characteristic inclusions of herpesvirus (Fig. 3.1). Fine needle aspiration of inguinal nodes may

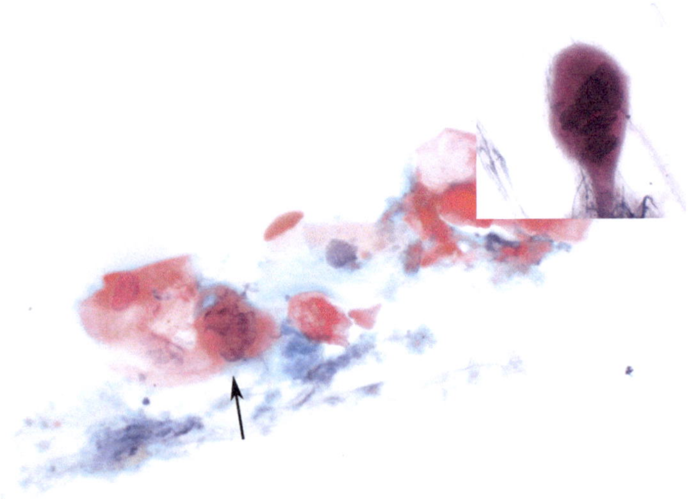

Fig. 3.1 Herpes simplex cytology—smears of an unroofed vesicle may show multinucleation with molding and a glassy appearance (Papanicolaou stain, arrow; inset, Giemsa stain)

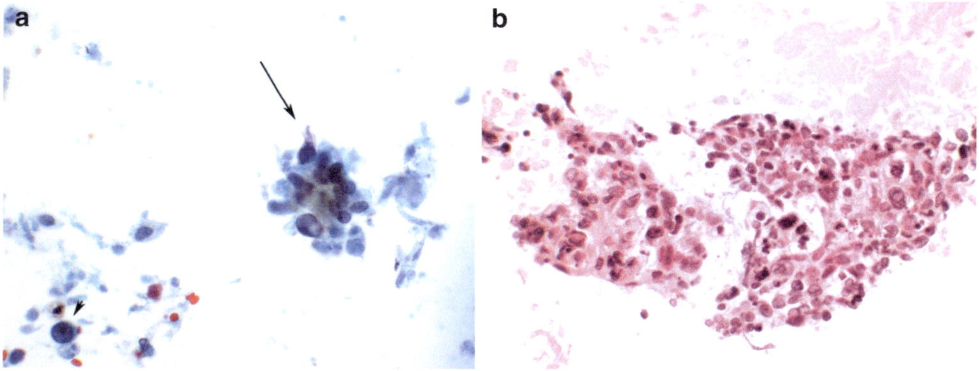

Fig. 3.2 Squamous cell carcinoma on FNA—this fine needle aspiration (FNA) specimen shows a cluster of malignant cells (arrow) and a single malignant cell in the left lower corner (arrowhead), with features consistent with squamous cell carcinoma (**a**). If enough material is available, it can be spun down and a cell block, similar to a tissue block created, which may resemble histology (**b**)

identify metastases from a vulvar squamous cell carcinoma (Fig. 3.2). Fine needle aspiration may occasionally be helpful in solid lesions such as aggressive angiomyxoma [6]. Aspiration of cystic lesions may be therapeutic, but does not usually provide cells from the cyst lining, and thus is often nondiagnostic.

3.3 Pathology of the Vulva

The International Society for the Study of Vulvovaginal Disease (ISSVD) has produced terminologies to assist with diagnosis and treatment of vulvovaginal disease. The terminologies relating to pathology are discussed below.

3.3.1 Vulvar Dermatoses

The ISSVD has two complementary classifications for vulvar dermatoses. The more recent clinical terminology [7] is aimed at assisting the clinician in evaluating the lesion by its appearance when examining the patient. The pathologic terminology [8] (Table 3.1) is not replaced by the newer clinical terminology, but is complementary, and was devised to assist clinicians with interpretation of pathology reports. The pathology terminology is based on histopathologic patterns of disease. Dermatopathologic diagnosis is based on specific histologic patterns that are

Table 3.1 ISSVD classification for vulvar dermatoses

Spongiotic pattern
Atopic dermatitis
Allergic contact dermatitis
Irritant contact dermatitis
Acanthotic pattern (formerly squamous cell hyperplasia)
Psoriasis
Lichen simplex chronicus
Primary (idiopathic)
Secondary (superimposed on lichen sclerosus, lichen planus, or other vulvar disease)
Lichenoid pattern
Lichen sclerosus
Lichen planus
Dermal homogenization/sclerosis pattern
Lichen sclerosus
Vesiculobullous pattern
Pemphigoid, cicatricial type
Linear IgA disease
Acantholytic pattern
Hailey–Hailey disease
Darier disease
Papular genitocrural acantholysis
Granulomatous pattern
Crohn disease
Melkersson–Rosenthal syndrome
Vasculopathic pattern
Aphthous ulcers
Behçet's disease
Plasma cell vulvitis

ISSVD International Society for the Study of Vulvovaginal Disease, *IgA* immunoglobulin A

Lynch, PJ. 2006 International Society for the Study of Vulvovaginal Disease Classification of Vulvar Dermatoses: A Synopsis. J Low Gen Tract Dis 2007;11(1):1-2 used to categorize lesions when developing a differential diagnosis. These patterns are often not diagnostic of a specific disease entity and can represent many conditions. Additional histologic features, as well as clinical features, are utilized in arriving at a more definitive diagnosis. This is why supplying a good clinical history is critical. Adjunctive studies may be helpful in some cases as well. Individual entities will be discussed elsewhere, but an overview of the patterns follows.

3.3.1.1 Spongiotic Pattern

Spongiosis is the presence of intercellular edema seen in the epidermis. An example is allergic contact dermatitis (Fig. 3.3), where there is space seen between the cells due to edema fluid. This can be severe enough to manifest as blisters. Other features help establish the specific diagnosis, including clinical exposure history, and different types of inflammatory cells may be seen within spongiotic foci in the different processes. In this case, the presence of eosinophils is helpful in arriving at the diagnosis of allergy.

3.3.1.2 Acanthotic Pattern

Acanthosis is the deepening and broadening of the rete pegs, which can fuse. It is seen in psoriasis, which has other characteristic features, as well as in lichen simplex chronicus (Fig. 3.4). Lichen simplex chronicus may be idiopathic, or

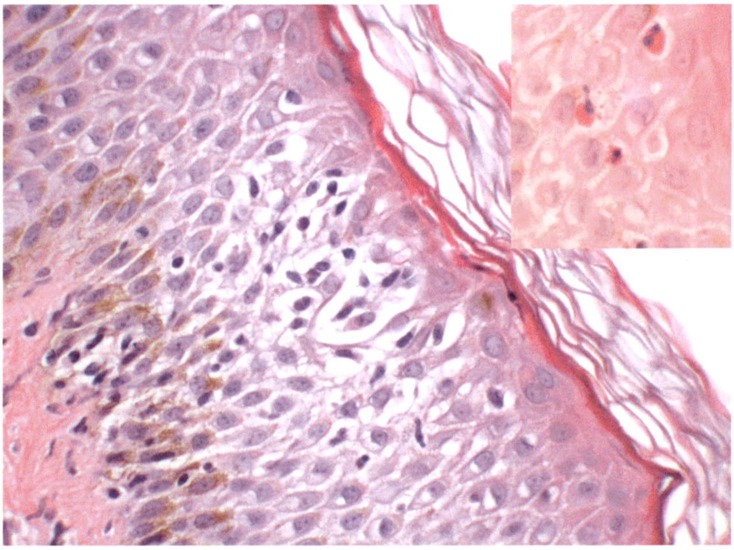

Fig. 3.3 Allergic contact dermatitis—spongiosis (intraepithelial edema) is forming spaces between the keratinocytes. The presence of eosinophils (inset) was useful in ascribing the etiology to allergy

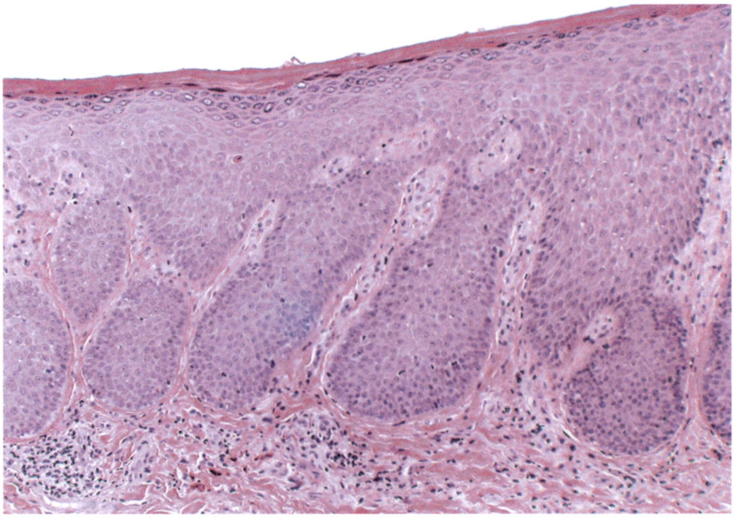

Fig. 3.4 Lichen simplex chronicus—the main feature demonstrated here is acanthosis, with elongation and broadening of the rete pegs

superimposed on another process, and is due to an uninterrupted itch-scratch cycle, which leads to exaggeration of skin markings grossly, and corresponding development of epithelial hyperplasia, manifested as hyperkeratosis, acanthosis, and variable chronic inflammation in the dermis.

3.3.1.3 Lichenoid Pattern

The lichenoid pattern is one that resembles lichen planus (Figs. 3.5 and 3.6). The characteristic features are a band-like (lichenoid) chronic inflammatory infiltrate in the dermis composed mainly of lymphocytes, best appreciated at low power (Fig. 3.5), as well as vacuolar degeneration of the basal keratinocytes, associated sometimes with "sawtooth" acanthosis, as the rete pegs become narrow and pointed at the bottom (Fig. 3.6). Lichen sclerosus may also have a band-like (lichenoid) infiltrate of chronic inflammatory cells but has other distinguishing features.

3.3.1.4 Dermal Homogenization/ Sclerosis Pattern

Lichen sclerosus has variable degrees of chronic inflammation in the dermis, which can be band-like at times (lichenoid), and also shows epidermal thinning with loss of rete pegs. A prominent feature is the dermal change, where the dermis develops a uniform appearance that may be glassy (homogenization) or more fibrotic (sclerosis) with loss of usual dermal appendages (Fig. 3.7).

3.3.1.5 Vesiculobullous Pattern

Vesicles (blisters) and larger (>0.5 cm) bullae may arise within or below the epidermis and tend to be characteristic of the specific disorder. For example, pemphigus is intraepidermal, and pemphigoid is subepidermal. Vesicles and bullae contain fluid and possibly inflammatory cells. Some of the conditions are immune-related and will require immunofluorescence studies, such as pemphigoid, cicatricial type (Fig. 3.8), which can be associated with scarring, hence the name, and linear IgA disease, both of which can occur on the vulva.

3.3.1.6 Acantholytic Pattern

Acantholysis is the loss of cohesion between keratinocytes due to loss of intercellular bridges

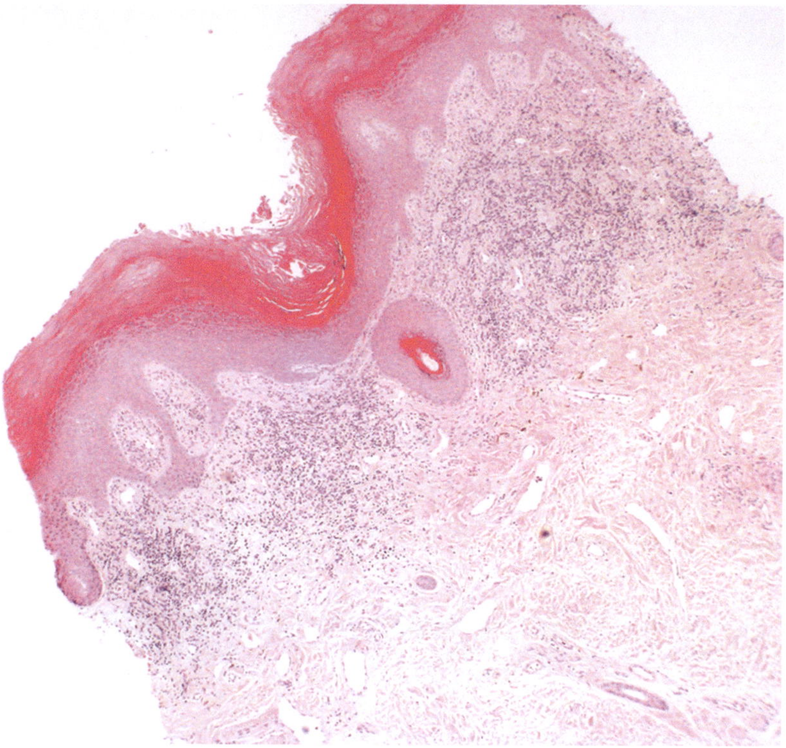

Fig. 3.5 Lichen planus—low-power view of lichen planus demonstrates the band-like dermal infiltrate of lymphocytes

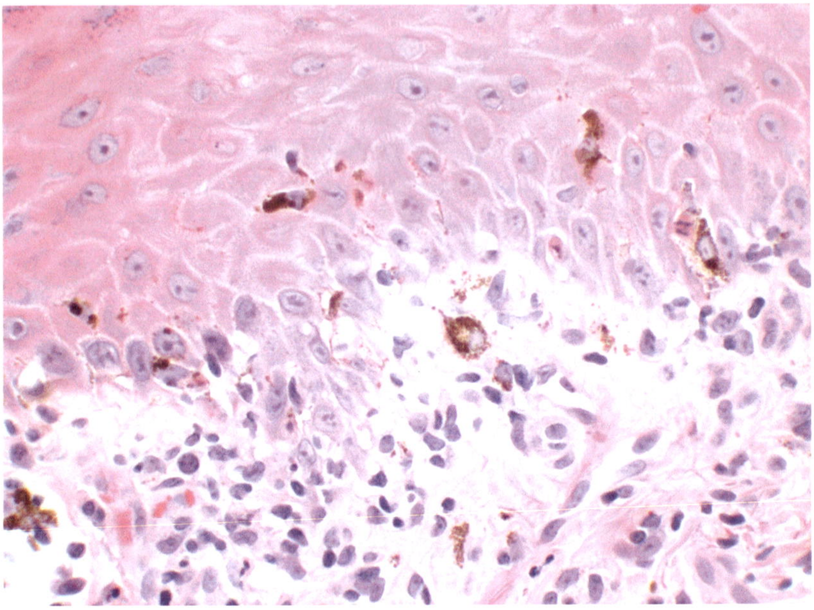

Fig. 3.6 On higher power, vacuolar degeneration of the basal layer of keratinocytes can be seen at the interface with the dermis in this case of lichen planus

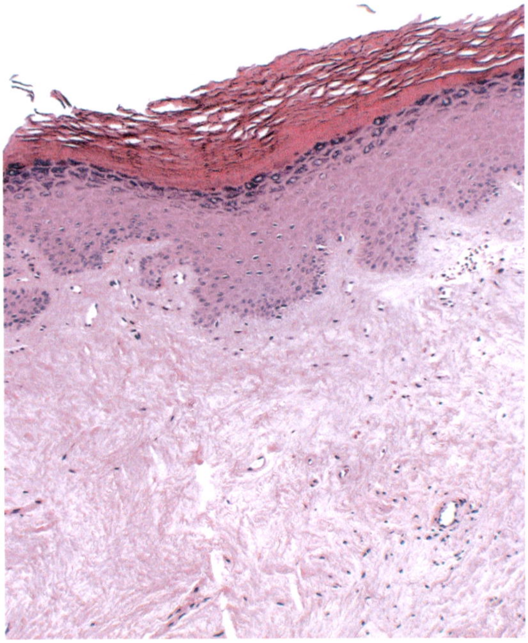

Fig. 3.7 Lichen sclerosus—the dermis in this case of lichen sclerosis shows homogenization, with a glassy appearance and loss of dermal appendages. There is overlying hyperkeratosis as well and thinning, but not total loss, of rete pegs

and can be seen in a variety of diseases. An example affecting the vulva is Hailey–Hailey disease, also known as benign familial pemphigus, where separation of the keratinocytes can be seen within the epidermis (suprabasilar) (Fig. 3.9). While pemphigus vulgaris may appear similar histologically, there are distinguishing features, and immunofluorescence may be helpful in the distinction.

3.3.1.7 Granulomatous Pattern

Granulomas are seen in granulomatous inflammation. There are various types of inflammation. For the clinician, acute inflammation and chronic inflammation are more time-related. For the pathologist, acute inflammation means neutrophils, while chronic inflammation includes a variety of cells including lymphocytes, plasma cells, and macrophages. These patterns correspond somewhat to the temporally related determinations. A specific type of chronic inflammation is granulomatous, where multinucleated giant cells are seen within aggregates of epithelioid histiocytes and other chronic inflammatory cells. Granulomas may be necrotizing, as in tuberculosis, or non-necrotizing, as in sarcoid or Crohn's disease. Crohn's disease affecting the

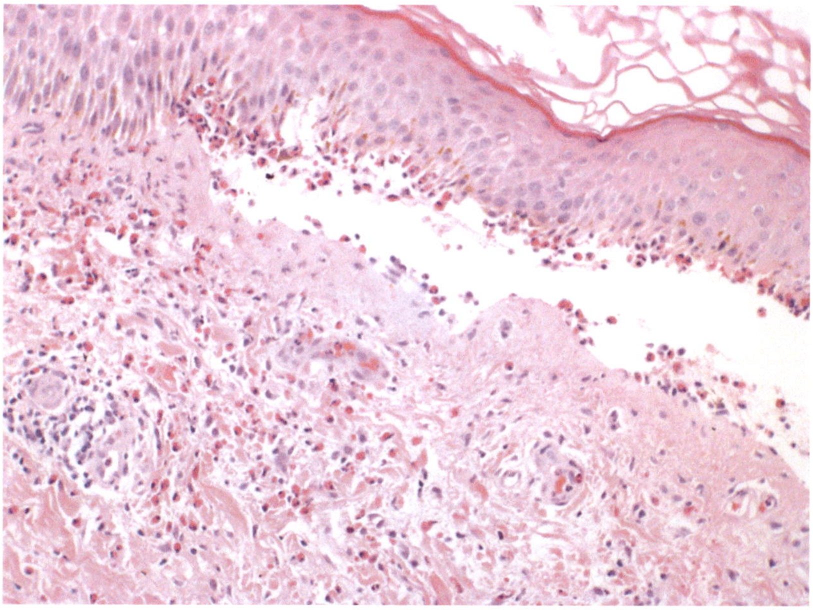

Fig. 3.8 Cicatricial pemphigoid—there is subepidermal bullous formation

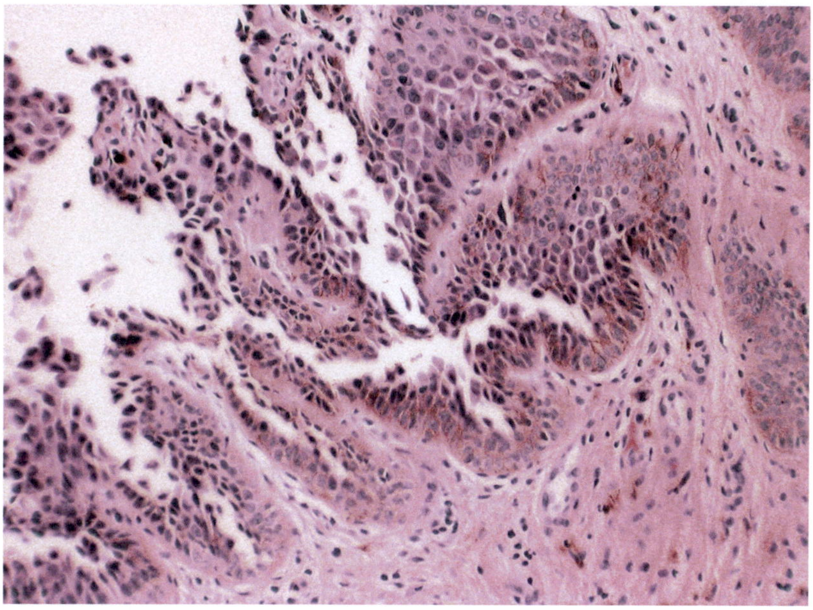

Fig. 3.9 Hailey–Hailey disease—there is acantholysis, leading to a splitting of the epidermis, with the formation of "villous" structures

vulva may present with fistulas. Histology of the vulvar lesions can show the characteristic non-necrotizing granulomas (Fig. 3.10).

3.3.1.8 Vasculopathic Pattern

The list of diseases associated with a vasculopathic pattern, i.e., inflammation around vessels (vasculitis), is large. Caliber of vessels involved location of vessels, type of inflammatory cells, as well as clinical presentation factor into determining the correct diagnosis. Behçet's disease is an example of a vasculitis that can affect the vulva, where there can be ulceration and vasculitis (Fig. 3.11).

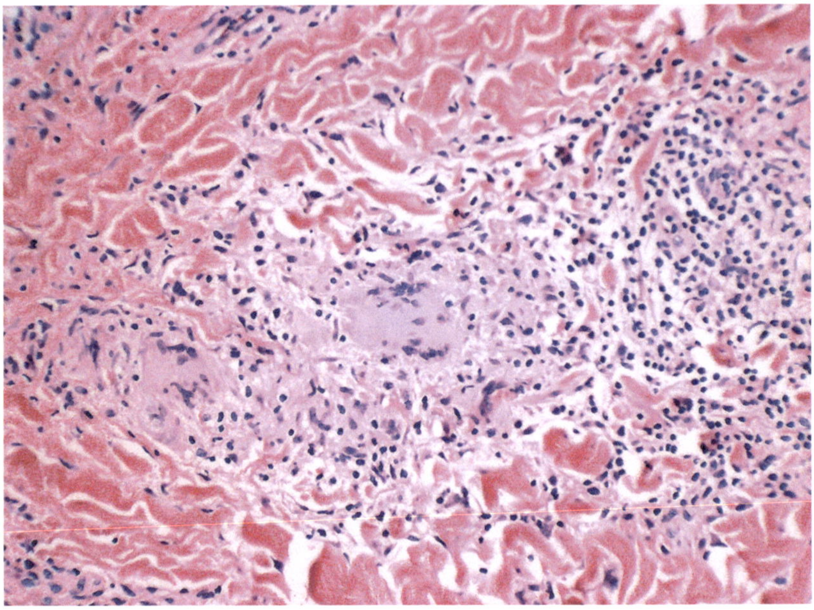

Fig. 3.10 Crohn's disease—this high-power view shows a non-necrotizing granuloma containing several multinucleated giant cells

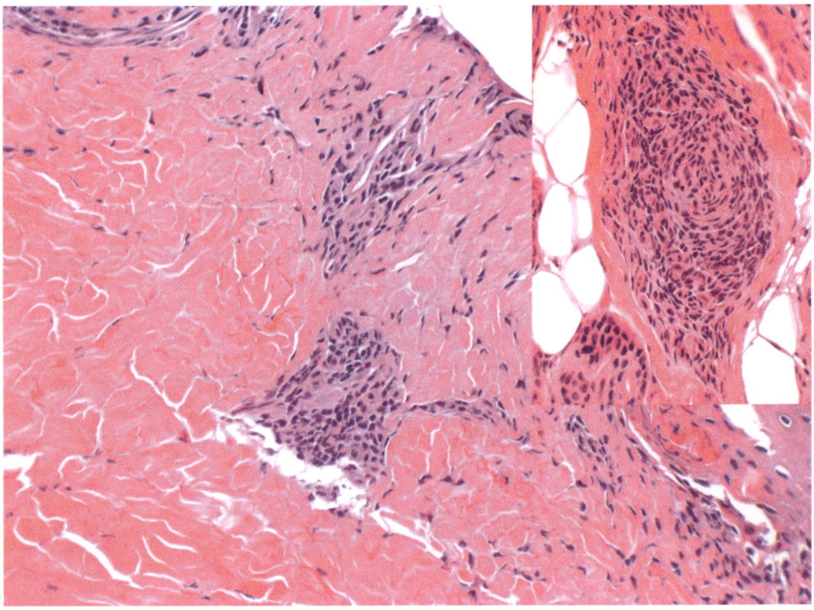

Fig. 3.11 Behçet's disease—the characteristic finding of vasculitis, inflammation around vessels, is shown here and at higher power in inset

3.3.2 Vulvar SILS (Squamous Intraepithelial Lesions)

The ISSVD has provided terminology for vulvar squamous intraepithelial lesions (SILS). Intraepithelial neoplasia may be squamous or non-squamous. Intraepithelial means that the lesion has not broken through the basement membrane and hence cannot metastasize. For all intents and purposes, the high-grade squamous intraepithelial lesions are analogous to a "carcinoma in situ"; however, this term is no longer used. The ISSVD has developed terminology for the squamous intraepithelial lesions (Table 3.2), which convey the Society's views, while in step with the World Health Organization (WHO) terminology, as well as the Lower Anogenital Squamous Terminology (LAST), which the ISSVD participated in developing. The ISSVD terminology emphasizes two important points. One is that there is HPV-related intraepithelial neoplasia, low grade and high grade (LSIL, HSIL) (Figs. 3.12 and 3.13) which need to be distinguished from non-HPV-related differentiated vulvar intraepithelial neoplasia (DVIN) (Fig. 3.14), a lesion of different histology and biology. DVIN is thought to be more likely than HPV-related ("usual") VIN to develop into invasive carcinoma. Carcinomas arising in conjunction with DVIN are the non-HPV-related squamous cell carcinomas. The other significant view of the ISSVD is that LSIL represents an HPV-related lesion, basically a condyloma, and overtreatment is not warranted for a lesion with essentially no malignant potential.

Table 3.2 The 2015 International Society for the Study of Vulvovaginal Disease (ISSVD) terminology of vulvar squamous intraepithelial lesions

• LSIL of the vulva (vulvar LSIL, flat condyloma, or HPV effect)
• HSIL of the vulva (vulvar HSIL, VIN usual type)
• DVIN

SIL squamous intraepithelial lesion, *LSIL* low-grade SIL, *HPV* human papillomavirus, *HSIL* high-grade SIL, *VIN* vulvar intraepithelial neoplasia, *DVIN* differentiated-type VIN
Bornstein J, Bogliatto F, Haefner HK, Stockdale CK, Preti M, Bohl TG, Reutter J; ISSVD Terminology Committee. J Low Genit Tract Dis. 2016;20(1):11-4

The ISSVD terminology for SILs does not include other non-squamous "in situ" lesions that can affect the vulva, which include Paget's disease, when noninvasive, as well as melanoma in situ.

3.3.3 Other Vulvar Lesions That May Result in a Pathology Specimen

A variety of specimen types may come to the pathology laboratory. Biopsies may be performed to establish a diagnosis, monitor a condition, or rule out malignancy. These specimens are usually rapidly diagnosed, unless special adjunctive studies are needed. Excisions are meant to be curative and may require additional fixation of larger tissue, evaluation of the margins to demonstrate total excision, as well as diagnosis of the process itself and hence may take longer to report. The list of possible lesions is quite large and beyond the scope of this chap-

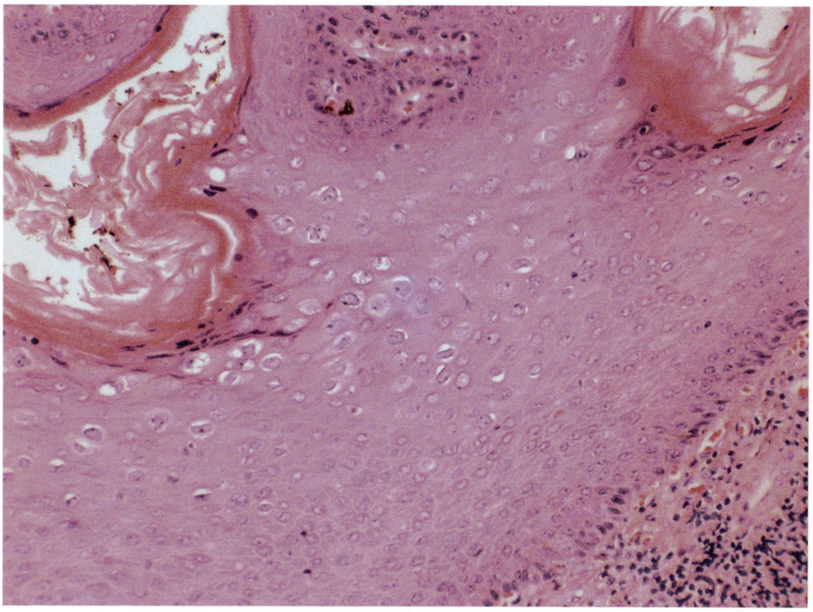

Fig. 3.12 LSIL—there is koilocytosis with atypical nuclei with perinuclear halos; however there is maturation present

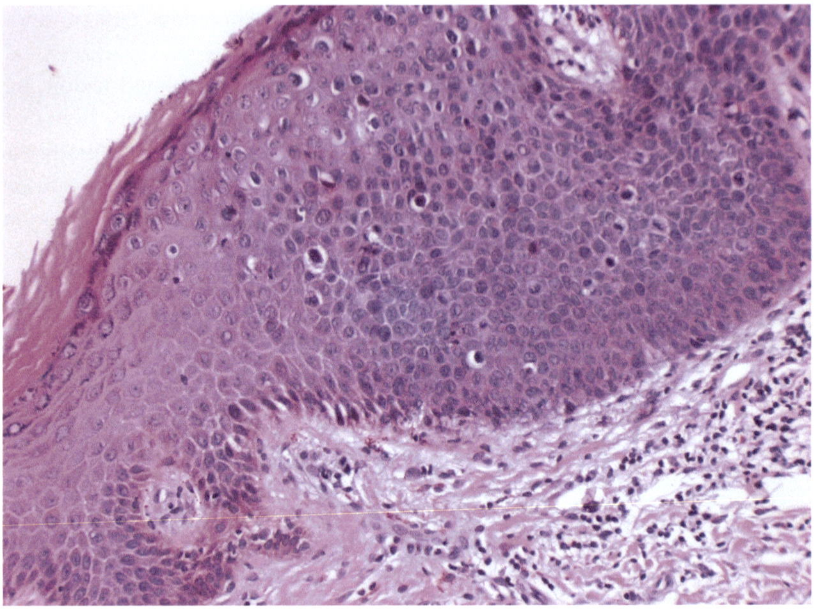

Fig. 3.13 HSIL—in high-grade SIL, there is loss of maturation that extends above the lower portion of the epithelium, seen on the right. Adjacent on the left is normal maturation, with an abrupt transition to HSIL

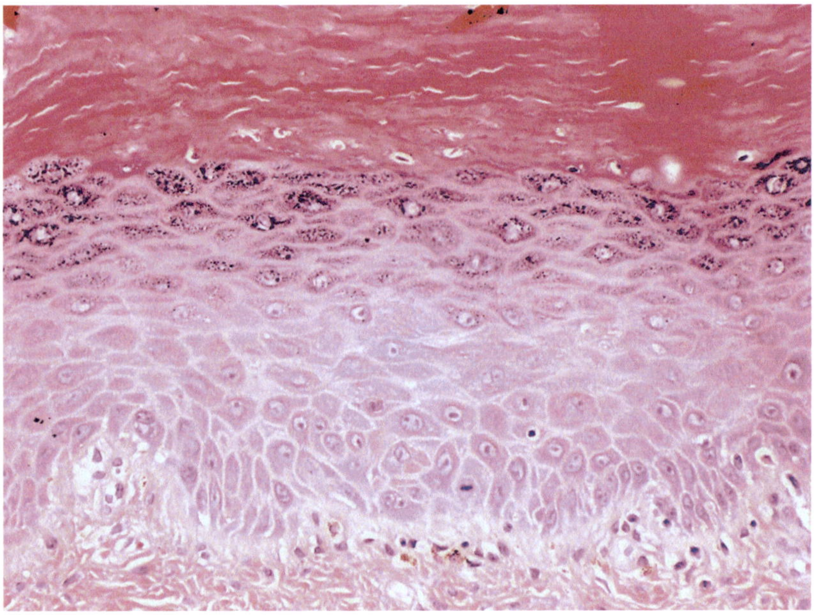

Fig. 3.14 Differentiated VIN—differentiated VIN shows maturation, and so is deceptively bland appearing, but has basal atypia and prominent nucleoli. A deep enough biopsy is necessary to establish this diagnosis

ter. The reader is referred to a pathology text for specific details of various entities [9].

3.4 Summary

Communication between the clinician and the pathologist is essential in optimal patient outcomes. These interactions between professionals are useful both for the individual patient and for patients in general, as the process is educational for both specialties. The goal of terminology is to communicate, and utilization of appropriate terminologies will provide the most comprehensible pathology report.

Cytology and Pathology of the Vulva: Breaking the Myths

- The pathology report is not an automated test like a blood count but rather a consultation by a team member.
- Not all biopsies should be treated the same! Vesiculobullous diseases may require immunofluorescence, and these specimens should not be put in formalin. Call the laboratory for specific instructions.

References

1. Dennerstein G. Cytology of the vulva. J Reprod Med. 1988;33:703–4.
2. Bae-Jump VL, Bauer M, Van Le L. Cytological evaluation correlates poorly with histological diagnosis of vulvar neoplasias. J Low Genit Tract Dis. 2007;11(1):8–11.
3. van den Einden L, Grefte J, van der Avoort I, et al. Cytology of the vulva: feasibility and preliminary results of a new brush. Br J Cancer. 2012;106:269–73.
4. Gilliland K, Knapik J, Wilkinson EJ. Cytology of vulvar/vaginal paget disease: report of a case and review of the literature. J Lower Gen Tract Dis. 2013;4:e26–30.
5. Klapsinou E, Terzakis E, Arnogiannaki N, Daskalopoulou D. Paget's disease of the vulva detected in vulvar and vaginal brushing smears: case report. Acta Cytol. 2010;54(5 suppl):898–902.
6. Nalini G, Duggal R, Neelam A, Vanita S, Arvind R. Fine needle aspiration cytology in a case of recurrent aggressive angiomyxoma of the vulva. Cytopathology. 2010;21:207–8.
7. Lynch PJ, Moyal-Barracco M, Scurry J, Stockdale C. 2011 ISSVD terminology and classification of vulvar dermatological disorders: an approach to clinical diagnosis. J Low Genit Tract Dis. 2012;16:339–44.
8. Lynch PJ. 2006 International Society for the Study of Vulvovaginal Disease classification of vulvar dermatoses: a synopsis. J Low Genit Tract Dis. 2007;11(1):1–2.
9. Hoang MP, Selim MA. Vulvar pathology. New York: Springer; 2015.

4 Terminology

Jacob Bornstein

4.1 Introduction

Over the years, several terminologies and classifications have been developed for vulvar lesions and disorders [1–4], reflecting the input of the various disciplines that take care of vulvar disease. Members of each discipline, i.e., gynecologists, dermatologists, pathologists, and physical therapists, created different sets of terms. Only during recent years, with the establishment of the international societies dealing with vulvar disease, consensus terminologies were established [5–11]. In this chapter we present the contemporary terminologies regarding classification of vulvar lesions that were accepted by the relevant international societies and are being used throughout the book:

- The clinical terminology of the International Federation of Cervical Pathology and Colposcopy (IFCPC) which provides basic definitions of the normal and abnormal vulva [9]
- The classification of the International Society for the Study of Vulvovaginal Disease (ISSVD) which provides the differential diagnosis of vulvar dermatological disorders [10]
- The ISSVD terminology of eczematous and lichenified diseases [8]

These terminologies are pertinent to the diagnostic process of a vulvar lesion. It is recommended to define the pattern of the lesion by using the IFCPC clinical terminology of the vulva and then looking in the ISSVD terminology for further characterization of that pattern. This book is organized according to this recommendation. Hence, the reader can use this book as a guide to diagnosis.

4.2 The IFCPC Terminology of the Vulva [9]

Many women affected by diseases of the vulva are being referred for care to gynecologists working in colposcopy clinics rather than to expert vulva specialists, who are rare in certain regions. However, most colposcopists have not been trained in genital dermatology, but rather in the use of the colposcope to identify pathological cervical transformation zone in women with abnormal cervical Papanicolaou (Pap) smears. Although colposcopists are experienced in diagnosing and treating human papillomavirus (HPV) related diseases and intraepithelial neoplasia of the whole lower genital tract, they usually have no training in benign vulvar disease.

This is the reason why the Nomenclature Committee of the International Federation of Colposcopy and Cervical Pathology (IFCPC), headed by the author of this book, created a comprehensive, "total" lower genital tract col-

J. Bornstein (✉)
Department of Obstetrics and Gynecology Galilee Medical Center, Bar-Ilan University Faculty of Medicine, Nahariya, Israel

J. Bornstein (ed.), *Vulvar Disease*, https://doi.org/10.1007/978-3-319-61621-6_4

poscopic terminology, not only of cervical and colposcopy findings [12] but also of the vagina and vulva including the anus [9].

However, the introduction of the IFCPC "total" terminology uncovered a debate between dermatologists and colposcopists. The debate was about the question if there was a requirement to use the colposcope in examining vulvar lesions and weather a colposcopic terminology of the vulva is needed. The final vulvar terminology, as approved by the IFCPC general assembly in 2011, solved this debate, as it uses colposcopic terms in a specialized section, but the overall terminology is "clinical," not "colposcopic" [9].

Indeed, the IFCPC terminology of the vulva (Table 4.1) is composed of several sections: The first part is "Basic Definitions." It describes the various structures of the vulva and anus and their composition—skin or mucosa. Although some conditions affect both skin and mucosa, many diseases are unique to the skin alone or to the mucosa alone. The significance of introducing the basic definitions is further underlined by the division of the vulvar skin into "hairy" (e.g., labia majora) and "non-hairy" (e.g., clitoris). Again, there is a clinical application to this differentiation; hairy skin harbors skin appendages, which may become involved with a variety of diseases, such as vulvar intraepithelial neoplasia (VIN). This involvement is the reason for the recommendation to excise hair-bearing areas affected by VIN, while superficial CO_2 laser vaporization is preferred for the treatment of VIN in non-hair-bearing areas, where VIN is limited to the superficial 1–2 mm.

Normal findings in the vulva that are mentioned in the terminology include, among others, micropapillomatosis (Fig. 4.1), sebaceous glands (Fordyce spots), and vestibular redness. The inclusion of these terms has an "educational" purpose, as each of these findings was, in the past, considered an abnormal condition and was a cause for treatment, CO_2 laser ablation and antibiotics for presumed infection or excision, respectively. Today, these findings are considered normal and should be left alone.

Table 4.1 2011 IFCPC clinical/colposcopic terminology of the vulva (including the anus) [9]

Section	Pattern		
Basic definitions	*Various structures* Urethra, Skene's duct openings, clitoris, prepuce, frenulum, pubis, labia majora, labia minora, interlabial sulci, vestibule, vestibular duct openings, Bartholin's duct openings, hymen, fourchette, perineum, anus, anal squamocolumnar junction (dentate line)		
	Composition Squamous epithelium: hairy/non-hairy, mucosa		
Normal findings	Micropapillomatosis, sebaceous glands (Fordyce spots), vestibular redness		
Abnormal findings	General principles: size in centimeters, location		
	Lesion type • Macule • Patch • Papule • Plaque • Nodule • Cyst • Vesicle • Bulla • Pustule	*Lesion color* • Skin-colored • Red • White • Dark	*Secondary morphology* • Eczema • Lichenification • Excoriation • Purpura • Scarring • Ulcer • Erosion • Fissure • Warty
Miscellaneous findings	• Trauma • Malformation		
Suspicion of malignancy	Gross neoplasm, ulceration, necrosis, bleeding, exophytic lesion, hyperkeratosis With or without white, gray, red, or brown discoloration		
Abnormal colposcopic/other magnification findings	Acetowhite epithelium, punctation, atypical vessels, surface irregularities		
	Abnormal anal squamocolumnar junction (note location in regard to dentate line)		

Abnormal findings are sorted in the terminology according to five characteristics: type, color, secondary morphology, size, and location. Recognition of the lesion's characteristics enables reaching a differential diagnosis. The terms used for the abnormal findings description are detailed below (Tables 4.2 and 4.3, Figs. 4.1, 4.2 and 4.3). These include *lesion type* (macule, patch (Fig. 4.2), papule, plaque (Fig. 4.3), nodule, cyst, vesicle, bulla, pustule), *lesion color* (skin-colored, red, white, dark), and *secondary morphology* (eczema, lichenification, excoriation, purpura, scarring, ulcer, erosion, fissure (Fig. 4.4), warty).

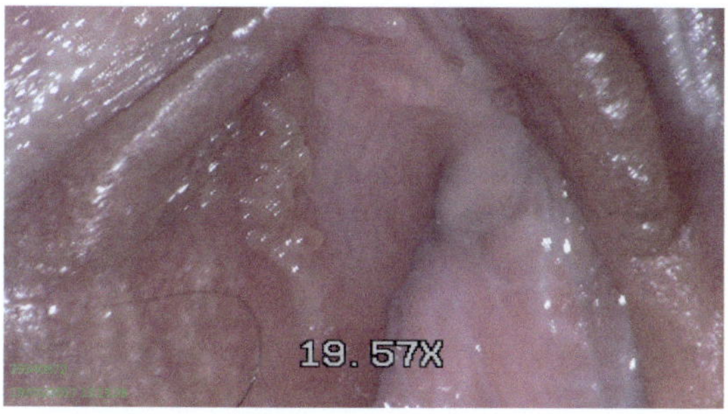

Fig. 4.1 Micropapillomatosis. These vesicles are a normal variant of the vestibule and need no treatment. In the past they were suspected to be condylomata acuminata

Table 4.2 Definitions of primary lesion types [9]

Term	Definition
Macule	Small (<1.5 cm) area of color change; no elevation and no substance on palpation
Patch	Large (>1.5 cm) area of color change; no elevation and no substance on palpation
Papule	Small (<1.5 cm), elevated, and palpable lesion
Plaque	Large (>1.5 cm), elevated, palpable, and flat-topped lesion
Nodule	A large papule (>1.5 cm); often hemispherical or poorly marginated; may be located on the surface, within or below the skin; nodules may be cystic or solid
Vesicle	Small (<0.5 cm) fluid-filled blister; the fluid is clear (blister, a compartmentalized, fluid-filled elevation of the skin or mucosa)
Bulla	A large (>0.5 cm) fluid-filled blister; the fluid is clear
Pustule	Pus-filled blister; the fluid is white or yellow

The terminology includes miscellaneous findings such as traumatic insults to the vulva, for example, hematoma. "Suspicion of malignancy" contains patterns that indicate the presence of malignancy: gross neoplasm, ulceration, necrosis, bleeding, exophytic lesion, and hyperkeratosis with or without white, gray, red, or brown discoloration.

Table 4.3 Definitions of secondary morphology presentation [9]

Term	Definition
Eczema	A group of inflammatory diseases that are clinically characterized by the presence of itchy, poorly marginated red plaques with minor evidence of microvesiculation and/or, more frequently, subsequent surface disruption
Lichenification	Thickening of the tissue and increased prominence of skin markings. Scale may or may not be detectable in vulvar lichenification. Lichenification may be bright red, dusky red, white, or skin colored in appearance
Excoriation	Surface disruption (notably excoriations) occurring as a result of the "itch-scratch cycle"
Erosion	A shallow defect in the skin surface; absence of some, or all, of the epidermis down to the basement membrane; the dermis is intact
Fissure	A thin, linear erosion of the skin surface
Ulcer	Deeper defect; absence of the epidermis and some, or all, of the dermis

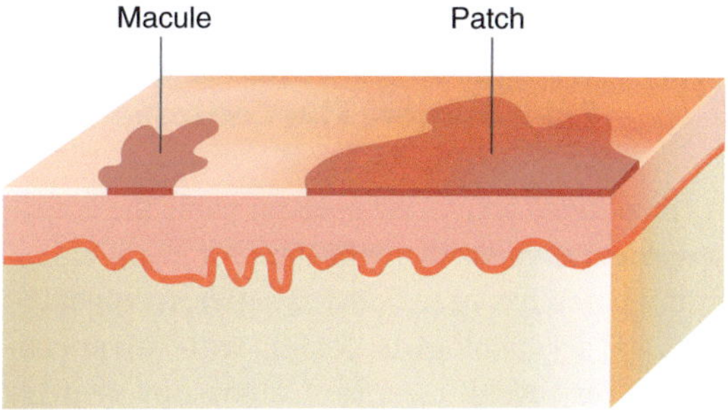

Fig. 4.2 *Macule* (small [<1.5 cm] area of color change; no elevation and no substance on palpation) and *patch* (large [>1.5 cm] area of color change; no elevation and no substance on palpation)

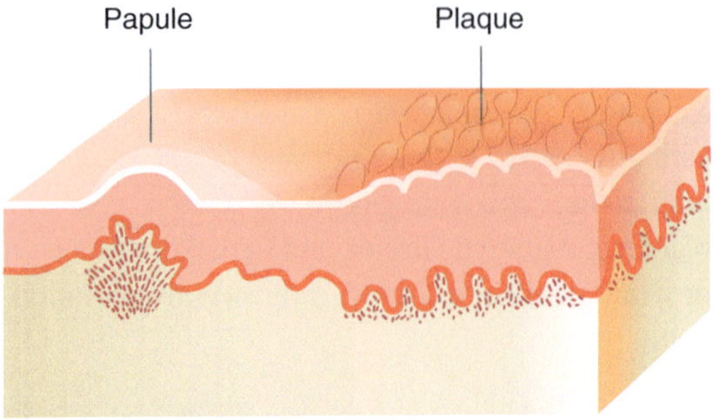

Fig. 4.3 *Papule* (small [<1.5 cm] elevated and palpable lesion) and *plaque* (large [>1.5 cm] elevated, palpable, and flat-topped lesion)

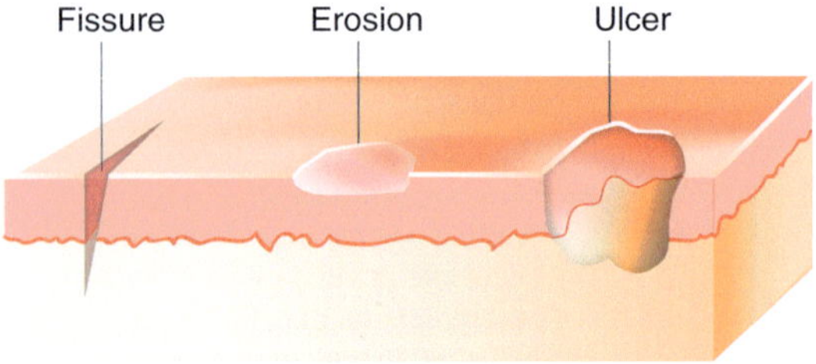

Fig. 4.4 *Fissure* (a thin, linear erosion of the skin surface), *erosion* (a shallow defect in the skin surface; absence of some, or all, of the epidermis down to the basement membrane; the dermis is intact), and *ulcer* (deeper defect; absence of the epidermis and some, or all, of the dermis)

Lastly, terms to describe the findings of vulvar and anal colposcopy are listed, such as acetowhite epithelium, punctation, atypical vessels, surface irregularities, and abnormal anal squamocolumnar junction.

4.2.1 Using a Colposcope for Vulvar Examination: The Controversy

As mentioned above, the need for using the colposcope and acetic acid application for every vulvar examination has been debated between colposcopists and dermatologists, dealing with vulvar conditions for several reasons: Colposcopy primary aim is to examine the cervix with magnification, after staining it with 3–5% acetic acid. This is done to detect HPV lesions and intraepithelial neoplasia. On the cervix, colposcopy evaluates a small area, the transformation zone, which may be abnormal when a patient is referred for having had a pathological Pap smear. However, the vulva has an anatomical structure different from the cervix, as it is composed of skin and mucosa and lacks a transformation zone [13]. Whitening of the tissue by acetic acid is significant for abnormal tissue in the cervix. However, on the vulva, acetowhitening may occur in normal tissue [14]. Hence the critics of using colposcopy for every vulvar lesion warn that vulvar colposcopy might lead to overdiagnosis and unnecessary vulvar biopsies and treatment. It must be noted, though, that practitioners who object to the use of colposcopy for the vulva may themselves use a magnifying glass and "dermoscopy," which is an optical magnifying tool to better diagnose pigmented skin lesions [4]. So, while colposcopy of the vulva is very different from colposcopy of the cervix, magnification is very helpful for many vulvar lesions.

The supporters of applying colposcopy to the vulva claim that many physicians that take care of vulvar conditions are in fact colposcopists that have used the IFCPC cervical terminologies for years and requested that the terminology be extended to include the vulvar conditions. Colposcopists have experience with examining vulvar lesions, since as a part of evaluating patients with cervical intraepithelial lesions, they are taught to look for vulvar intraepithelial neoplasia (VIN), perianal intraepithelial neoplasia (PAIN), and anal intraepithelial neoplasia (AIN). The colposcopic examination after the application of acetic acid ("vulvoscopy," "anoscopy") helps to delineate an HPV lesion or intraepithelial neoplasia and choose the biopsy site. Also, the term "vulvoscopy" is in widespread use and refers to an examination of the vulva by a colposcope. Several texts and papers have been published on the use of vulvoscopy to diagnose vulvar lesions [15–19]. However, because of the past absence of terminology dedicated to the vulva, the description of vulvar findings has been inconsistent. In addition, in locations where vulvar experts are rare, patients with various vulvar symptoms, such as pruritus or pain, are being evaluated by colposcopists.

Therefore, the IFCPC accepted the terminology of vulvar examination, including the section with colposcopy terms.

4.3 The ISSVD Clinical Classification [10]

The "2011 ISSVD clinical classification of vulvar dermatological disorders" (Table 4.4) is complimentary to the IFCPC terminology. Once the examiner characterizes the vulvar lesion according the IFCPC terminology, he or she looks for the differential diagnosis of that morphologic abnormality in the ISSVD terminology. The diseases are listed in eight morphological groups: skin-colored lesions, red lesions: patches and plaques, red lesions: papules and nodules, white lesions, dark-colored (brown, blue, gray or black) lesions, blisters, erosions and ulcers, edema. They are subdivided into about 50 of the most commonly encountered disorders along with a few uncommon important conditions, such as melanoma. This terminology does not include symptoms such as pruritus and pain, which are encountered in routine clinical care.

Some skin diseases contain several patterns. For instance, the lesions of vulvar intraepithelial neoplasia may appear as white, red, or skin-colored papules, ulcers, or fissures. To allow for correct recognition of disorders that are polymorphous in appearance, their various presentations are listed in more than one place in this classification. In this book, however, they are described only once, according to their most frequent presentation.

4.4 The ISSVD Pathological Terminology [8]

A different, specific histological classification of vulvar dermatoses has also been developed by the ISSVD terminology committee: "The ISSVD terminology of eczematous and lichenified diseases" (Table 4.5) [8]. While the previously described terminologies are clinical, this classification is based

Table 4.4 The 2011 ISSVD clinical classification of vulvar dermatological disorders [10]

(1) Skin-colored lesions
A. Skin-colored papules and nodules
1. Papillomatosis of the vestibule and medial labia minora (a normal finding; not a disease)
2. Molluscum contagiosum
3. Warts (HPV infection)
4. Scar
5. Vulvar intraepithelial neoplasia
6. Skin tag (acrochordon, fibroepithelial polyp)
7. Nevus (intradermal type)
8. Mucinous cysts of the vestibule and medial labia minora (may have yellow hue)
9. Epidermal cyst (syn. epidermoid cyst; epithelial cyst)
10. Mammary-like gland tumor (hidradenoma papilliferum)
11. Bartholin's gland cyst and tumor
12. Syringoma
13. Basal cell carcinoma
B. Skin-colored plaques
1. Lichen simplex chronicus and other lichenified diseases (see definitions in discussion of terms related to eczematous and lichenified diseases)
2. Vulvar intraepithelial neoplasia
(2) Red lesions: patches and plaques
A. Eczematous and lichenified diseases (see definitions in discussion of terms related to eczematous and lichenified diseases)
1. Allergic contact dermatitis
2. Irritant contact dermatitis
3. Atopic dermatitis (rarely seen as a vulvar presentation)
4. Eczematous changes superimposed on other vulvar disorders
5. Diseases clinically mimicking eczematous disease (candidiasis, Hailey-Hailey disease, and extramammary Paget disease)
6. Lichen simplex chronicus (lichenification with no preceding skin lesions)
7. Lichenification superimposed on an underlying preceding pruritic disease
B. Red patches and plaques (no epithelial disruption)
1. Candidiasis
2. Psoriasis
3. Vulvar intraepithelial neoplasia
4. Lichen planus
5. Plasma cell (Zoon's) vulvitis
6. Bacterial soft tissue infection (cellulitis and early necrotizing fasciitis)
7. Extramammary Paget disease
(3) Red lesions: papules and nodules

(continued)

Table 4.4 (continued)

A. Red papules
1. Folliculitis
2. Wart (HPV infection)
3. Angiokeratoma
4. Molluscum contagiosum (inflamed)
5. Hidradenitis suppurativa (early lesions)
6. Hailey-Hailey disease
B. Red nodules
1. Furuncles ("boils")
2. Wart (HPV infection)
3. Prurigo nodularis
4. Vulvar intraepithelial neoplasia
5. M. contagiosum (inflamed)
6. Urethral caruncle and prolapse
7. Hidradenitis suppurativa
8. Mammary-like gland adenoma (hidradenoma papilliferum)
9. Inflamed epidermal cyst
10. Bartholin's duct abscess
11. Squamous cell carcinoma
12. Melanoma (amelanotic type)
(4) White lesions
A. White papules and nodules
1. Fordyce spots (a normal finding; may sometimes have a yellow hue)
2. M. contagiosum
3. Wart
4. Scar
5. Vulvar intraepithelial neoplasia
6. Squamous cell carcinoma
7. Milium (pl. milia)
8. Epidermal cyst
9. Hailey-Hailey disease
B. White patches and plaques
1. Vitiligo
2. Lichen sclerosus
3. Postinflammatory hypopigmentation
4. Lichenified diseases (when the surface is moist see definitions in discussion of terms related to eczematous and lichenified diseases)
5. Lichen planus
6. Vulvar intraepithelial neoplasia
7. Squamous cell carcinoma
(5) Dark-colored (brown, blue, gray, or black) lesions
A. Dark-colored patches
1. Melanocytic nevus
2. Vulvar melanosis (vulvar lentiginosis)
3. Postinflammatory hyperpigmentation
4. Lichen planus
5. Acanthosis nigricans
6. Melanoma in situ
B. Dark-colored papules and nodules
1. Melanocytic nevus (includes those with clinical and/or histological atypia)
2. Warts (HPV infection)
3. Vulvar intraepithelial neoplasia
4. Seborrheic keratosis
5. Angiokeratoma (capillary angioma, cherry angioma)
6. Mammary-like gland adenoma (hidradenoma papilliferum)
7. Melanoma
(6) Blisters
A. Vesicles and bullae
1. Herpesvirus infections (herpes simplex, herpes zoster)
2. Acute eczema (see definitions in discussion of terms related to eczematous and lichenified diseases)
3. Bullous lichen sclerosus
4. Lymphangioma circumscriptum (lymphangiectasia)
5. Immune blistering disorders (cicatricial pemphigoid, fixed drug eruption, Steven-Johnson syndrome, pemphigus)
B. Pustules
1. Candidiasis (candidosis)
2. Folliculitis
(7) Erosions and ulcers
A. Erosions
1. Excoriations (see the disorders in group 2A)
2. Erosive lichen planus
3. Fissures arising on normal tissue (idiopathic, intercourse related)
4. Fissures arising on abnormal tissue (candidiasis, lichen simplex chronicus, psoriasis, Crohn's disease, etc.)
5. Vulvar intraepithelial neoplasia, eroded variant
6. Ruptured vesicles, bullae, and pustules (see all of the disorders listed in group 6 "blisters")
7. Extramammary Paget disease
B. Ulcers
1. Excoriations (related to eczema, lichen simplex chronicus)
2. Aphthous ulcers (syn. aphthous minor), aphthous major, Lipschutz ulcer (occurring either as an idiopathic process or secondary to other diseases such as Crohn's, Behcet's, and various viral infections)
3. Crohn's disease
4. Herpesvirus infection (particularly in patients who are immunosuppressed)
5. Ulcerated squamous cell carcinoma
6. Primary syphilis (chancre)
(8) Edema (diffuse genital swelling)
A. Skin-colored edema
1. Crohn's disease

Table 4.4 (continued)

2. Idiopathic lymphatic abnormality (congenital Milroy's disease)
3. Postradiation and postsurgical lymphatic obstruction
4. Postinfectious edema (especially staphylococcal and streptococcal cellulitis)
5. Postinflammatory edema (especially hidradenitis suppurativa)
B. Pink or red edema
1. Venous obstruction (e.g., pregnancy and parturition)
2. Cellulitis (primary or superimposed on already existing edema)
3. Inflamed Bartholin's duct cyst/abscess
4. Crohn's disease
5. Mild vulvar edema may occur with any inflammatory vulvar disease

Table 4.5 2006 histological classification of vulvar dermatoses pathological subsets and their clinical correlates [8]

Pattern	Subset
Spongiotic pattern	Atopic dermatitis Allergic contact dermatitis irritant contact dermatitis
Acanthotic pattern (formerly squamous cell hyperplasia)	Psoriasis Lichen simplex chronicus Primary (idiopathic) Secondary (superimposed on lichen sclerosus, lichen planus, or other vulvar diseases)
Lichenoid pattern	Lichen sclerosus Lichen planus
Dermal homogenization/sclerosis pattern	Lichen sclerosus
Vesiculobullous pattern	Pemphigoid, cicatricial type Linear IgA disease
Acantholytic pattern	Hailey-Hailey disease Darier disease Papular genitocrural acantholysis
Granulomatous pattern	Crohn's disease Melkersson-Rosenthal syndrome
Vasculopathic pattern	Aphthous ulcers Behcet's disease Plasma cell vulvitis

on histopathology. It divided the lesions presented with eczema and lichenification into those with spongiotic, acanthotic, lichenoid, dermal homogenization/sclerosis, vesiculobullous, acantholytic, granulomatous, or vasculopathic patterns.

Dictionary: several dermatologic terms are commonly used:

Eczema: refers to a group of pruritic inflammatory diseases that are clinically characterized by red plaques with an indistinct margin. There is microvesiculation leading to surface disruption. Histologically, a "spongiotic pattern" is pathognomonic of this condition [1]. In chronic forms scaling and lichenification develop. The term dermatitis is used as a synonym for eczema (e.g., atopic dermatitis and atopic eczema).

Surface Disruption: weeping, crusting, microvesiculation, fissuring in the folds, and erosions most often occurring as a result of excoriation.

Lichenification: lichenification develops as a result of chronic scratching and/or rubbing (the "itch-scratch cycle"); it presents as a palpable thickening of the tissue with increased prominence of skin markings. Scale may or may not be detectable in vulvar lichenification. Lichenification may be bright red, dusky red, white, or skin colored in appearance; the white color occurs as a result of moisture retention in the thickened outer layer of the epidermis. Excoriations may, or may not, be present. Histologically, lichenification is characterized by an "acanthotic pattern" [1]. Lichenification may arise from a normal-appearing skin ("lichen simplex chronicus") or may be superimposed on some other underlying dermatological disorders such as psoriasis, lichen sclerosus, lichen planus, etc.

4.5 Lichen Simplex Chronicus

The term lichen simplex chronicus is used when the lichenification develops on skin that had been previously normal.

4.6 Atopic Dermatitis (Atopic Eczema)

Atopic dermatitis is a pruritic, chronic inflammatory disease that arises in previously normal-appearing skin. It is composed of red plaques with evidence of surface disruption (mainly excoriations).

Terminology: Breaking the Myths

- How to make a diagnosis of a vulvar lesion? The lack of a thorough experience in vulvar disease should not discourage the clinician. With the three terminologies presented in this chapter, the approach became straightforward:
  - Start by defining the pattern of the lesion by using the 2011 IFCPC clinical terminology of the vulva.
  - Review the differential diagnosis of that pattern, and match it to the most appropriate vulvar lesion, in the 2011 ISSVD clinical classification of vulvar dermatological disorders and, if needed, in the 2006 ISSVD pathological terminology of eczematous and lichenified diseases.

References

1. Michalany J. Vulva leukoplakia. Incongruency of concept and nomenclature and its identification with various dermatologic lesions, mainly scleroatrophic lichen. AMB Rev Assoc Med Bras. 1975;21:174–80.
2. Kaufman RH, Woodruff JD. Vulvar dystrophies, atypias, carcinomata in situ: an invitational symposium. Historical background in developmental stages of the new nomenclature. J Reprod Med. 1976;17:132–6.
3. Weström L, Mårdh PA. Definitions of infectious and infectious-like conditions in the lower genital tract of the female. Scand J Infect Dis Suppl. 1983;40:65–70.
4. Lallas A, Kyrgidis A, Tzellos TG, Apalla Z, Karakyriou E, Karatolias A, Lefaki I, Sotiriou E, Ioannides D, Argenziano G, Zalaudek I. Accuracy of dermoscopic criteria for the diagnosis of psoriasis, dermatitis, lichen planus and pityriasis rosea. Br J Dermatol. 2012;166:1198–205.
5. Micheletti L, Preti M, Bogliatto F, Lynch PJ. Vulvology. A proposal for a multidisciplinary subspecialty. J Reprod Med. 2002;47:715–7.
6. Friedrich EG. Report of the committee on terminology. New nomenclature for vulvar disease. Obstet Gynecol. 1976;47:122–4.
7. Wilkinson EJ, Kneale B, Lynch PJ. Report of the ISSVD terminology committee. J Reprod Med. 1986;31:973–4.
8. Lynch PJ, Moyal-Barracco M, Bogliatto F, Micheletti L, Scurry J. 2006 ISSVD classification of vulvar dermatoses: pathologic subsets and their clinical correlates. J Reprod Med. 2007;52:3–9.
9. Bornstein J, Sideri M, Tatti S, Walker P, Prendiville W, Haefner HK, Nomenclature Committee of International Federation for Cervical Pathology and Colposcopy. 2011 terminology of the vulva of the International Federation for Cervical Pathology and Colposcopy. J Low Genit Tract Dis. 2012;16:290–5.
10. Lynch PJ, Moyal-Barracco M, Scurry J, Stockdale C. 2011 ISSVD terminology and classification of vulvar dermatological disorders: an approach to clinical diagnosis. J Low Genit Tract Dis. 2012;16(4):339–44.
11. Bornstein J, Bogliatto F, Haefner HK, Stockdale CK, Preti M, Bohl TG, Reutter J, ISSVD Terminology Committee. The 2015 International Society for the Study of Vulvovaginal Disease (ISSVD) terminology of vulvar squamous intraepithelial lesions. J Low Genit Tract Dis. 2016;201:11–4.
12. Bornstein J, Bentley J, Bösze P, Girardi F, Haefner H, Menton M, Perrotta M, Prendiville W, Russell P, Sideri M, Strander B, Tatti S, Torne A, Walker P. 2011 colposcopic terminology of the international Federation for Cervical Pathology and Colposcopy. Obstet Gynecol. 2012 Jul;120(1):166–72.
13. Micheletti L, Bogliatto F, Lynch PJ. Vulvoscopy: review of a diagnostic approach requiring clarification. J Reprod Med. 2008;53:179–82.
14. Van Beurden M, van de Vange N, de Craen AJ, Tjong-A-Hung SP, ten Kate FJ, ter Schegget J, Lammes FB. Normal findings in vulvar examination and vulvoscopy. Br J Obstet Gynaecol. 1997;104:320–4.
15. Wright VC, Chapman WB. Colposcopy of intraepithelial neoplasia of the vulva and adjacent sites. Obstet Gynecol North Am. 1993;20:231–55.
16. Hatch K. Colposcopy of vaginal and vulvar human papillomavirus and adjacent sites. Obstet Gynecol Clin North Am. 1993;20:203–15.
17. Ritter J, Baladuf JJ, Philippe E, Dreyfus M, Dillmann JC. Colposcopy of the vulva. J Gynecol Obstet Biol Reprod (Paris). 1991;20:511–8.
18. Sener AB, Kuscu E, Seckin NC, Gokmen O, Taner D, Cobanoglu O, Zorlu G. Postmenopausal vulvar pruritus – colposcopic diagnosis and treatment. J Pak Med Assoc. 1995;45:315–7.
19. Gagné HM. Colposcopy of the vagina and vulva. Obstet Gynecol Clin North Am. 2008;35:659–69.

Principles of Diagnosis

5

Bina Cohen Sacher

5.1 Introduction

Vulvovaginal complaints are one of the most common reasons for ob-gyn consultations and visits. Evaluation of these symptoms requires meticulous examination and utilization of some simple tools [1]. Unfortunately, it is too common for practitioners to perform only some of the recommended methods to obtain a diagnosis. In a retrospective study checking the evaluation of patients complaining of vaginitis, Wiesenfeld and Macio found that pH measure and whiff test were not done in >90% of the visits, microscopy was not done by 42% of physicians, and cultures were not taken in 83% of the visits [2]. Since the signs and symptoms of vulvovaginal diseases are not specific and often overlap, it is important to use these simple office diagnostic testing in order to achieve the correct diagnosis. A methodological exam of the vulva and vagina could save the patient discomfort and suffering.

5.2 Medical History

Evaluation of a woman with vulvovaginal complaints should include obtaining of a focused history about the entire spectrum of her symptoms: itching, pain, irritation, burning, appearance of swelling or lesions, discharge, and dyspareunia. The patient should be asked about the location of the symptoms, the duration, whether a treatment was given (either prescribed or not prescribed), and what was the response. A thorough investigation of any products that came in contact with the vulva and vagina should take place, as well as the patient's hygienic habits and sexual history.

Notably, the medical history is important, mainly chronic illnesses, medication, and known allergies. Some systemic diseases may cause vulvar or vaginal symptoms, occasionally being the first manifestation of the disease. Therefore, questions should be asked as relevant to the case.

5.3 Vulvar Observation

The examination of the vulva starts with observation. A systemic approach should be utilized, to make sure all vulvar parts are included in the examination. The examiner should pay attention to skin texture, color, and the presence of lesions, ulcers, cysts, excoriations, and anything else that catches the eye as unusual. Hair distribution, the skin of the mons pubis, labia majora, and minora

Disclosure: None.

B. Cohen Sacher (✉)
Department of Obstetrics and Gynecology,
Helen Schneider Hospital for Women,
Rabin Medical Center, Petach Tikva, Israel

J. Bornstein (ed.), *Vulvar Disease*, https://doi.org/10.1007/978-3-319-61621-6_5

should be looked at. When examining the clitoris, it is important to make sure the prepuce can easily be retracted, exposing the clitoris. The position of the urethral meatus, glands' openings in the vestibule, the perineal body, and anus should also be inspected.

Palpation may be indicated to evaluate lesions such as cysts or nodules. Palpation of inguinal lymph node may indicate certain infectious etiologies.

There are some common normal variants which may be mistaken for pathology. Enlarged sebaceous glands, called Fordyce spots, present as multiple small yellow patches along the inner aspects of the labia minora. They can coalesce into cobblestone appearance, but have no clinical significance [3, 4].

Another common normal variant is vulvar papillomatosis, which is found in 8–48% of women in the reproductive age group. These are filiform soft projections often found in the vestibule. They can be mistaken for condylomas: however, individual papules are separated at the base in contrary to filiform warts which tend to fuse at the base. Also, papillomatosis is usually confined to the vestibule and the inner aspect of labia minora, whereas condylomas are more prevalent on vulvar keratinized skin [3–5].

5.4 Vulvoscopy

The role of vulvoscopy in evaluating vulvar complaints is controversial. Although some papers indicated the benefits of the high power magnification, particularly in diagnosing premalignant lesions [6, 7], others concluded there is no evidence that vulvoscopy is effective as a screening tool for evaluating vulvar diseases [8, 9]. Lower power magnification, as handheld magnifying glass, low-power eyeglass loupes, and so forth, is sufficient in most of cases for evaluating vulvar skin lesions. Full discussion on this issue can be found in section "Terminology" in this book.

The application of acetic acid for the detection of high-grade intraepithelial neoplasia has proven itself in evaluating the cervix but is controversial when dealing with vulvar lesions. Studies show wide range of sensitivity, but most agree that the specificity is low and that some acetowhite lesions on the vulva are not dysplastic and may even have normal histology [10–12]. The prediction of HPV-related lesions is also low [10, 11]. This method has good negative predictive value, with the risk of performing unnecessary biopsies due to its low specificity [12].

5.5 Q-Tip Test

After observation of the vulva is complete, preferably with the least contacting possible, it is advisable to perform the Q-tip or "swab" test. The Q-tip test is a principle method of evaluating possible vulvodynia, which is suspected when a patient complains of pain or burning, especially but not exclusively with intercourse. The Q-tip test is performed by touching gently with a cotton swab at the different vulva parts, from the labia majora gradually toward the introitus, where the pain is expected to be worse. Ask the patient to indicate if the touch elicits pain, burning, itch, or other discomfort and to what degree. This helps in differentiating generalized and localized pain, assessing the degree of pain in the different vulvar parts, and will be beneficial in assessing improvement in subsequent examinations [13]. This test will be further explained later in this book, in the chapter on vulvar pain.

5.6 Vaginal Examination

Evaluation of the vulvar area cannot be complete without evaluation of the vagina, as symptoms originating from vulvar or vaginal conditions often overlap. A speculum should be used for the inspection of the vagina and cervix—the color and rugae of the vaginal walls, vaginal discharge, and signs of cervicitis can all be assessed at this point. If present, a discharge is collected with a cotton swab from the midportion of lateral vaginal walls for the purpose of checking the pH and performing microscopy examination [14, 15]. Vaginal cultures can be taken as well during speculum examination for diagnosis of infectious vaginitis.

5.7 pH Measurement

Normal vaginal pH for women in the reproductive age is 3.5–4.5. It is higher for premenarchal girls and postmenopausal women with vaginal atrophy. Measuring vaginal pH is a good way to rule out several conditions, such as bacterial vaginosis and trichomoniasis, which elevate the pH above 4.5.

The most suitable pH test strips are those which measure a limited spectrum. pH can be tested using a swab, by obtaining a sample from the lateral vaginal wall or by placing the strip directly against the vaginal wall in the middle third of the vagina. Make sure not to sample the cervix, as its secretion is normally of higher pH [15].

Vaginal pH is not diagnostic on its own and the general specificity reported is low [14]. Others have found it to be correlated with wet mount findings, but not to symptoms [16]. According to ACOG recommendations, when the wet mount microscopy is without abnormal findings, and no infectious cause is found, an elevated vaginal pH in itself is of no clinical importance [1].

5.8 Wet Mount Microscopy

An essential diagnostic tool is wet mount microscopy. It is considered by ACOG as the first line in diagnosing vaginal candidiasis and trichomoniasis [1]; it is utilized in Amsel's criteria for the diagnosis of bacterial vaginosis [17], superior to PCR and Nugent scoring [18], and an important part of evaluating desquamative inflammatory vaginitis [19]. In a retrospective meta-analysis, Anderson et al. found microscopy to have a wide range of reported sensitivity values for diagnosing candidiasis (between 38 and 83%) and a high positive predictive value for diagnosing *Trichomonas vaginalis* [14]. In another study, Nathan et al. found wet mount microscopy to be inferior compared to four other diagnosing methods for *Trichomonas* [20].

Wet mount microscopy is performed by smearing vaginal fluid collected by a cotton swab onto two slides. A drop of normal saline is mixed with the discharge on one slide and a drop of 10% potassium hydroxide on the second slide. Methylene blue may be used instead of saline, to accentuate cells and bacteria. The fluid on the slides is covered by a cover slip and examined under the microscope at X100 and X400 power [21].

The wet mount evaluation includes identifying epithelial cells, white blood cells, bacteria, and, if present, certain pathogens such as yeast and *Trichomonas vaginalis*. The addition of potassium hydroxide dissolves the epithelial cells and accentuates the presence of yeast.

In women at the reproductive age, or menopausal women that use estrogen replacement therapy, the wet mount will normally present the epithelial cells of the superficial layers, large cells with high cytoplasm:nucleus ratio. The margins are usually regular. The vaginal flora consists mainly of lactobacilli rods, with few white blood cells, not more than 1:3 ratio to the epithelial cells (Fig. 5.1).

The lack of estrogen in premenarchal or postmenopausal women causes the depletion of glycogen-containing cells of the intermediate layer, leading to a loss of substrate for lactobacilli. The wet mount of an atrophic vagina will show para-

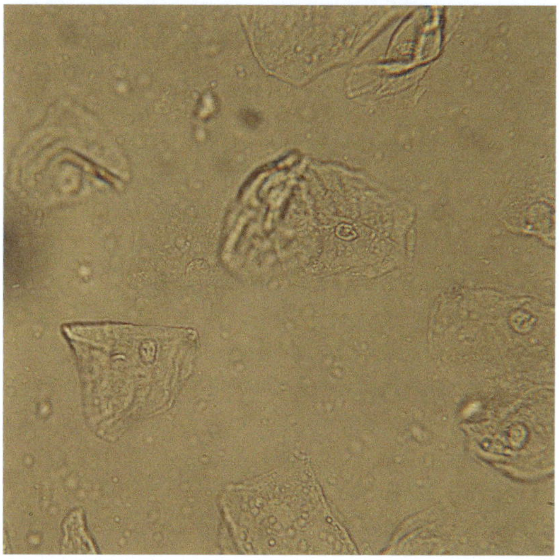

Fig. 5.1 A wet mount smear of a woman at the reproductive age, showing superficial layer epithelial cells. Large cells are seen, with pyknotic nuclei, and a high cytoplasm:nucleus ratio. The margins of the cells are usually regular. Many lactobacilli rods are seen. The ratio of white blood cells to epithelial cells is not more than 1:3

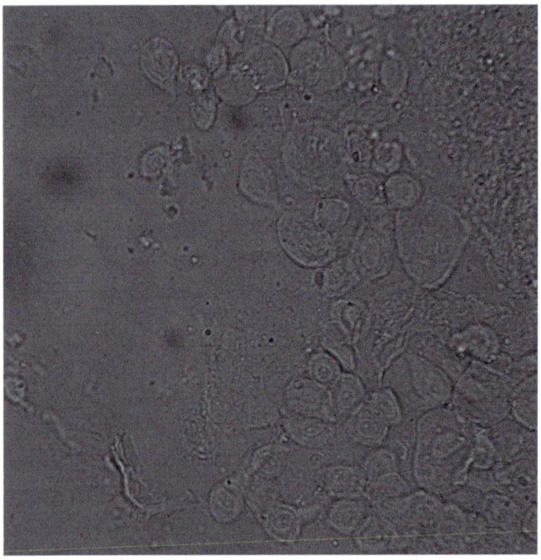

Fig. 5.2 A wet mount of an atrophic vagina: Many parabasal cells are seen. These epithelial cells are round, with low cytoplasm:nucleus ratio. No lactobaccili-like rods are present but rather coccoid bacteria

basal cells—epithelial cells adjacent to the basal layer of the epithelium. These cells are smaller and round, with small cytoplasm/nucleus ratio (Fig. 5.2). No lactobacilli-like rods are present but rather coccoid bacteria, and vaginal pH is expected to be between 4.2 and 6.0 and even higher [22].

Vulvovaginal candidiasis (Fig. 5.3) is usually present in the well-estrogenized vagina. In the case of the more prevalent *Candida albicans*, the wet mount will present hyphae, with or without yeast buds. In cases of *non-albicans* candidiasis, only yeast buds are seen. Usually, there will be no elevated number of white blood cells.

Bacterial vaginosis is characterized by the presence of clue cells—large epithelial cells with granular appearance borders obscured by bacteria [17]. However, other findings in wet mount may point to the diagnosis, such as the lack of lactobacilli-like rods, the presence of numerous mixed-type bacteria, and paucity of white blood cells [15].

In other forms of vaginitis, abnormal wet mount may suggest an infection, but final diagnosis requires a positive culture [22]. When suspecting *Neisseria gonorrhoeae* or *Chlamydia trachomatis* infection, for example, wet mount would be of no benefit [23].

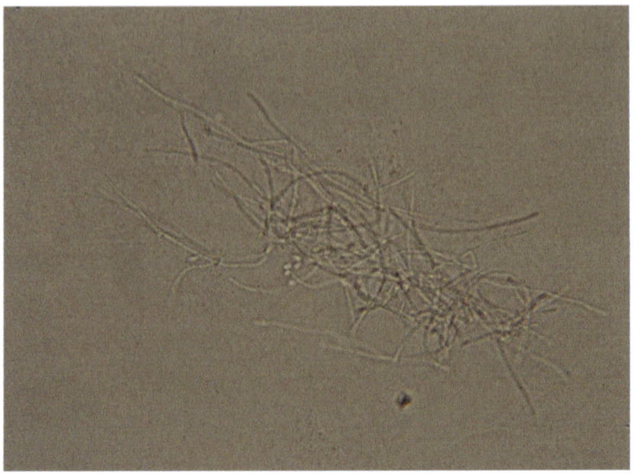

Fig. 5.3 A wet mount of a patient with vulvovaginal candidiasis. Hyphae are present and yeast buds

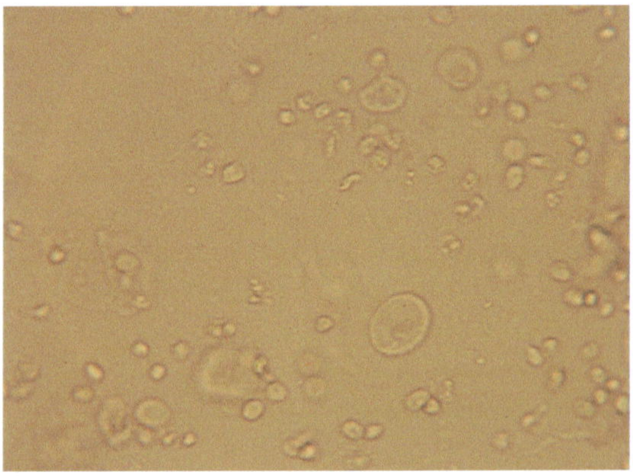

Fig. 5.4 A wet mount typical of desquamative inflammatory vaginitis. Large amount of white blood cells are seen, with over 1:1 ratio to epithelial cells

The presence of large amount of white blood cells, over 1:1 ratio to epithelial cells, or at least 25 in high-power field, together with increase of parabasal cells, is typical to desquamative inflammatory vaginitis (Fig. 5.4) [15, 19].

5.9 Whiff Test

In their paper on "nonspecific vaginitis," Amsel et al. introduced the diagnostic criteria that have since been used worldwide for the clinical diagnosis of bacterial vaginosis. These criteria included at least three of the following: vaginal pH above 4.5, characteristic thin homogenous discharge, positive potassium hydroxide odor ("whiff test"), and clue cells found on saline wet mount [17].

Adding a drop of 10% potassium hydroxide to vaginal discharge, on a slide or cotton tip, may cause alkalinization of the discharge and volatilize abnormal amines present in the discharge of women suffering from bacterial vaginosis. The result is an offensive "fishy" odor. Positive whiff test can be found in trichomoniasis as well in bacterial vaginosis [14].

5.10 Microbiology Testing

Although microscopy is an important tool for evaluating vulvovaginal diseases, its sensitivity for diagnosing vaginal infections is limited. Yeast cultures should be obtained in cases of symptomatic women with negative microscopy results or recurrent complaints after treatment.

DNA testing or cultures for *Trichomonas vaginalis*, *Chlamydia trachomatis*, and *Neisseria gonorrhoeae* should be taken when appropriate. Rapid point-of-care tests for trichomonas antigen are available for the diagnosis of *Trichomonas vaginalis* in some countries, with reliable results available within 10 min.

Bacterial cultures have no use in diagnosing bacterial vaginosis due to its bacterial heterogeneity. However, rare forms of bacterial vaginitis, such as *group A Streptococcus*, may be identified by bacterial cultures [1]. *Group A Streptococcus* may also cause vulvitis and cellulitis of the nearby skin as the perineum, glutei, and thighs [24].

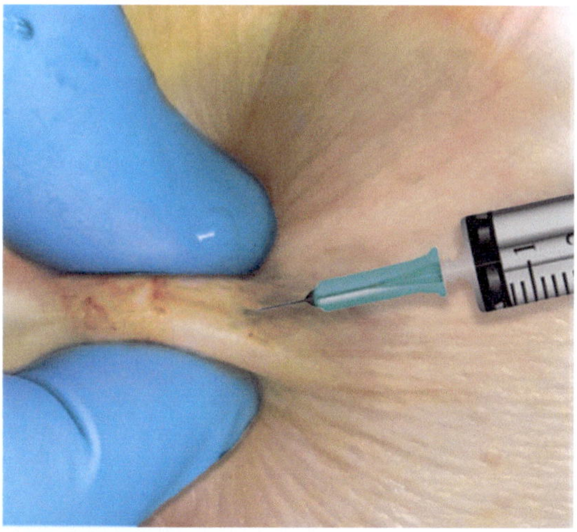

Fig. 5.5 Before a vulvar biopsy is done, an intralesional anesthesia is injected through a #30-gauge needle. Courtesy of Professor Jacob Bornstein

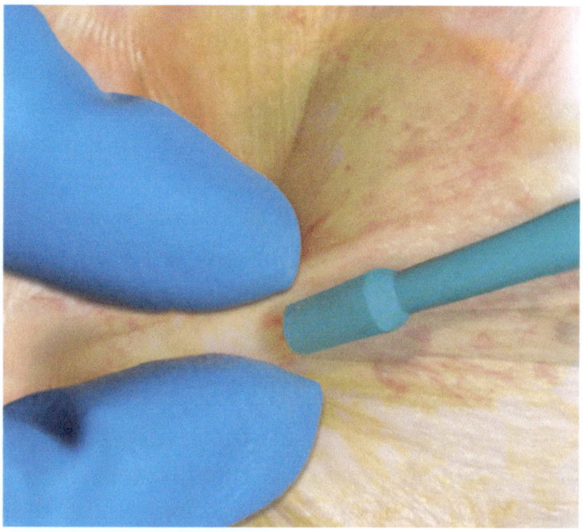

Fig. 5.6 The Keyes biopter is twisted into the skin, taking a representative sample from the lesion. Courtesy of Professor Jacob Bornstein

5.11 Vulvar Biopsy

When needed, a vulvar biopsy should be taken. The main reasons for taking a biopsy are ruling out premalignancy or malignancy or establishing a diagnosis of nonmalignant skin conditions.

The technique of obtaining a vulvar biopsy is depicted in Figs. 5.5, 5.6, and 5.7.Topical anesthesia is strongly advised prior to taking the biopsy (Fig. 5.5). A designated skin Keyes biopter is preferable, as it does not squeeze the tissue (Fig. 5.6); however a cervical biopter is also acceptable. Then the incised piece of skin is held by pickup forceps, the base is cut by scissors, and the specimen removed (Fig. 5.7). Bleeding can be controlled by applying topically Monsell's solution or pressure with an argentum nitrate stick.

The biopsy should be taken from a representative part of the lesion, preferably from its edge, containing normal skin as well.

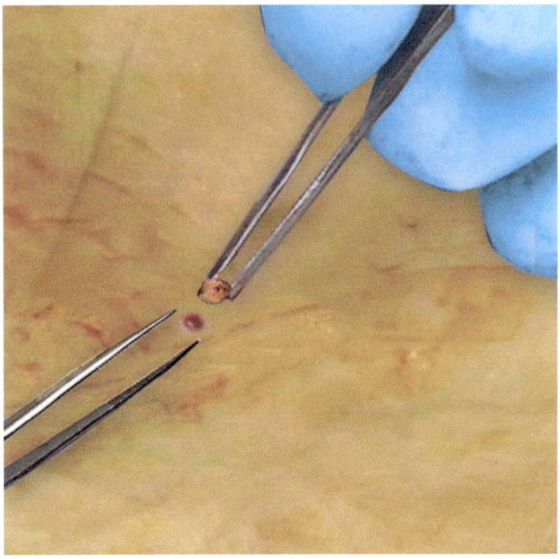

Fig. 5.7 The incised piece of skin is held by pickup forceps. Courtesy of Professor Jacob Bornstein

Sometimes, the pathologist will not define a specific diagnosis but rather describe a pathological pattern. The ISSVD classification for pathological patterns can come in handy [25]. It is also important to look at the pathologist's report in conjunction with the clinical setting. When necessary, a repeat biopsy is acceptable [26].

5.12 Patch Tests

Last but not the least, when suspecting the presence of allergic contact dermatitis, the role of patch tests for allergy cannot be underestimated. Vulvar skin is more permeable than skin in other body parts. It is thinner, moister, and covered by clothes most of the time, making it more vulnerable to irritative and allergenic products [27]. Studies report various positive patch testing, ranging from 16 to 78% [27–31]. This wide range is explained partially by different populations tested, either patients suffering from general vulvar pruritus, specific dermatoses, or highly suspected of contact dermatitis and whether the reaction measured was relevant to the clinical presentation. The rate of allergic and irritant contact dermatitis among patients suffering from vulvar symptoms is unclear, but not insignificant, and it can be superimposed on other established vulvar conditions [27, 29]. Patients suffering from vulvar-vaginal symptoms tend to treat themselves with various over-the-counter topical medicaments and add a plethora of prescribed medications from the many doctors they see in their search for a solution. These products may be irritating, allergenic, or both, further complicating their condition and making diagnosis a real challenge [29].

When the reaction to treatment is less than expected, or when a sudden deterioration occurs after initial improvement, patch testing should be considered. Patch tests are used to identify the cause of allergic contact dermatitis. The test involved the application of allergens to the skin of the upper aspect of the back, under occlusion, for a period of 2 days. Commercially patch test allergen kits are available. The first reading is performed after 48 h, grading the severity of the reaction from negative to extreme positive reaction, based on appearance and severity of erythema, edema, vesicles, and bullae. A classification system for grading patch test results was suggested by the International Contact Dermatitis Research Group. A second reading should be performed no sooner than 72 h after the allergens were initially applied. This reading is important to distinguish true allergic response from irritation and to identify delayed allergic response. Once allergens have been identified, their relevance to the clinical scenario must be determined—current or past exposure of the patient to the allergen, in correlation with the appearance of symptoms [32].

5.13 Summary

The most important evaluation tools one needs to make a diagnosis of a vulvar condition are the eyes and ears. In many cases, one can reach a diagnosis, or at least narrow the differential diagnosis to a minimum, by listening to what your patient tells you. The examination includes a careful observation, with the use of simple diagnostic tools.

Vulvar and Vaginal Examination and Evaluation Tools: Breaking the Myths

- Diagnosing a vulvar or vaginal condition may be complicated, as signs and symptoms are not specific and often overlap. Therefore, adjuncts to diagnosis, such as using pH measure, whiff test, and microscopy, are important. However, in 83–90% of the cases, these tests are not carried out!
- Vulvar papillomatosis is not an HPV lesion. It is a normal finding in 8–48% of women in the reproductive age group. These are filiform soft projections often found in the vestibule. In contrast to condylomata that are separate lesions, vulvar papillomatosis fuse at the base.
- pH determination is helpful for evaluation of vaginal discharge However, it is not diagnostic on its own. When the wet mount microscopy is normal, an elevated vaginal pH is of no clinical importance.
- In the past, routine vaginal cultures were obtained from women suspected to suffer from bacterial vaginosis. Today, cultures are regarded as unnecessary, due to BV bacterial heterogeneity. However, rare forms of bacterial vaginitis, such as group A *Streptococcus*, are significant and may be identified by bacterial cultures.
- A rarely used test is patch testing for allergy. When suspecting the presence of contact dermatitis, its role cannot be underestimated.

References

1. ACOG Committee on Practice Bulletins – Gynecology. ACOG practice bulletin. Clinical management guidelines for obstetrician-gynecologists, number 72, May 2006: vaginitis. Obstet Gynecol. 2006;107(5):1195–206.
2. Wiesenfeld HC, Macio I. The infrequent use of office-based diagnostic tests for vaginitis. Am J Obstet Gynecol. 1999;181:39–41.
3. Margesson LI. Vulvar disease pearls. Dermatol Clin. 2006;24:145–55.
4. Edwards L. Dermatologic therapy of chronic genital disease. Dermatol Ther. 2004;17:1–7.
5. Wollina U, Verma S. Vulvar vestibular papillomatosis. Indian J Dermatol Venereol Leprol. 2010;76(3):270–2.
6. Reid R, Greenberg MD, Daoud Y, Husain M, et al. Colposcopic findings in women with vulvar pain syndromes. A preliminary report. J Reprod Med. 1988;33(6):523–32.
7. MacLean AB, Reid WM. Benign and premalignant diseases of the vulva. Br J Obstet Gynaecol. 1995;102(5):359–63.
8. Eva LI. Screening and follow up of vulval skin disorders. Best Pract Res Clin Obstet Gynaecol. 2012;26(2):175–88.
9. Micheletti L, Bogliatto F, Lynch PJ. Vulvoscopy: review of a diagnostic approach requiring clarification. J Reprod Med. 2008;53(3):179–82.
10. Jonsson M, Karlsson R, Evander M, et al. Acetowhitening of the cervix and vulva as a predictor of subclinical human papillomavirus infection: sensitivity and specificity in a population-based study. Obstet Gynecol. 1997;90:744–7.
11. Van Beurden M, Van der Vange N, de Craen AJ, et al. Normal findings in vulvar examination and vulvoscopy. Br J Obstet Gynecol. 1997;104(3):320–4.
12. Santoso JT, Likes W. Colposcopic acetowhitening of vulvar lesion: a validity study. Arch Gynecol Obstet. 2015;292:387–90.
13. Stockdale CK, Lawson HW. 2013 vulvodynia guideline update. J Low Genit Tract Dis. 2014;18(2):93–100.
14. Anderson MR, Klink K, Cohrssen A. Evaluation of vaginal complaints. JAMA. 2004;291(11):1368–79.
15. Frobenius W, Bogdan C. Diagnostic value of vaginal discharge, wet mount and vaginal pH – an update on the basics of gynecologic infectiology. Geburshilfe Frauenheilkd. 2015;75(4):355–66.
16. Pavletic AJ, Hawes SE, Geske JA, et al. Experience with routine vaginal pH testing in a family practice setting. Infect Dis Obstet Gynecol. 2004;12:63–8.
17. Amsel R, Totlen PA, Spiegel CA, et al. Nonspecific vaginitis. Diagnostic criteria and microbial and epidemiologic associations. Am J Med. 1983;74(1):14–22.
18. Rumyantseva Tatiana A, Gert B, Romanuk Tatiana N, et al. Utility of microscopic techniques and quantitative real time polymerase chain reaction for the diagnosis of veginal microflora alterations. J Low Genit Tract Dis. 2015;19(2):124–8.
19. Reichman O, Sobel J. Desquamative inflammatory vaginitis. Best Pract Res Clin Obstet Gynecol. 2014;28(7):1042–50.
20. Nathan B, Appiah J, Saunders P, et al. Microscopy outperformed in a comparison of five methods for detecting Trichomonas vaginalis in symptomatic women. Int J STD AIDS. 2014;26(4):251–6.
21. Kottmel A, Peterson EE. Vaginal wet mount. J Sex Med. 2013;10:2616–9.
22. Mylonas I, Bergauer F. Diagnosis of vaginal discharge by wet mount microscopy: a simple and underrated method. Obstet Gynecol Surv. 2011;66:359–68.
23. Stampler KM, Lieberman A, Fraga M, et al. Vaginal wet mounts on asymptomatic adolescent females:

are they beneficial? J Pediatr Adolesc Gynecol. 2008;21:227–30.
24. Verstraelen H, Verhelst R, Vaneechoutte M, et al. Group A streptococcal vaginitis: an unrecognized cause of vaginal symptoms in adult women. Arch Gynecol Obstet. 2011;284:95–8.
25. Lynch PJ, Moyal-Barracco M, Bogliatto F, et al. 2006 ISSVD classification of vulvar dermatoses, pathological subsets and their clinical correlates. J Reprod Med. 2007;52:3–9.
26. Lynch PJ, Moyal-Barracco M, Scurry J, et al. 2011 ISSVD terminology and classification of vulvar dermatological disorders: an approach to clinical diagnosis. J Low Genit Tract Dis. 2012;16(4):339–44.
27. Utas S, Ferahbas A, Yildiz S. Patients with vulvar pruritus: patch test results. Contact Dermatitis. 2008;58(5):296–8.
28. Bauer A, Oehme S, Geier J. Contact sensitization in the anal and genital area. Curr Probl Dermatol. 2011;40:133–41.
29. Margesson LI. Contact dermatitis of the vulva. Dermatol Ther. 2004;17:20–7.
30. O'Gorman SM, Torgerson RR. Allergic contact dermatitis of the vulva. Dermatitis. 2013;24(2):64–72.
31. Haverhoek E, Reid C, Gordon L, et al. Prospective study of patch testing in patients with vulval pruritus. Aust J Dermatol. 2008;49:80–5.
32. Mowad CM, Anderson B, Scheinman P, et al. Allergic contact dermatitis. Patient diagnosis and evaluation. J Am Acad Dermatol. 2016;74(6):1029–40.

6 Principles of Medical Treatment

Candace S. Brown, Candi C. Bachour, and Gloria A. Bachmann

6.1 Introduction

Vulvar conditions are common in women at every stage of their adult life cycle. However, depending on the age of the woman, there are more common ones seen at different points in the age spectrum. For reproductive-aged women, infections such as vulvar herpes and candida will often be seen. In the menopausal women, the genitourinary syndrome of menopause (formerly referred to as vulvovaginal atrophy) is typically the presenting complaint when there are vulvar complaints. In the postmenopausal age group, vulvar intraepithelial neoplasia increases in prevalence. Vulvodynia, a chronic pain condition, is a vulvar condition that occurs throughout the life cycle of the female. Unfortunately, this pain condition continues to be elusive in regard to both etiology and treatment. Treatment of infection, atrophy, and dysplasia usually follows evidence-based interventions that effectively treat the vulvar condition. On the other hand, clinicians caring for women with vulvodynia have utilized several pharmacologic interventions for management with varying degrees of efficacy and safety. This chapter presents an update on the medical treatment of vulvar disease, with an emphasis on the pharmacologic interventions for vulvodynia, since this is the one area that there remain many unanswered questions.

6.2 Vulvar Infections

Candidiasis is the most common vulvovaginal infection, affecting 75% of all women with at least one episode during their lifetimes [1]. It typically presents with patient symptoms of vulvar pruritus, irritation, dysuria, and dyspareunia. Women may also report redness of the vulvar area and a white, curd-like discharge at the introital area. Although candida is the most common agent for vulvar infection, other sexually transmitted diseases that affect the vulva are also seen. The Center for Disease Control (CDC) classification for vulvovaginal infections is shown in Table 6.1 [2].

6.3 Genitourinary Syndrome of Menopause

With the loss of estrogen due to ovarian follicular depletion, a frequent condition in menopausal women that affects the vulva in addition to the vagina and lower genital tract is the genitouri-

C. S. Brown (✉) · C. C. Bachour
University of Tennessee Health Science Center, Memphis, TN, USA
e-mail: csbrown@uthsc.edu; cbachour@uthsc.edu

G. A. Bachmann
Rutgers-Robert Wood Johnson Medical School, New Brunswick, NJ, USA
e-mail: bachmaga@rwjms.rutgers.edu

J. Bornstein (ed.), *Vulvar Disease*, https://doi.org/10.1007/978-3-319-61621-6_6

Table 6.1 CDC classifications for vulvar and/or vaginal infections

A. Sexually transmitted diseases
• HIV infection
• Diseases characterized by genital, anal, or perianal ulcers
– Chancroid, genital HSV infections, granuloma inguinale (donovanosis, lymphogranuloma venereum (LGV)
• Syphilis
• Chlamydial infections
• Gonococcal infections
• Diseases characterized by vaginal discharge
– Bacterial vaginosis
– Trichomoniasis
– Vulvovaginal candidiasis
• Pelvic inflammatory disease (PID)
• Human papillomavirus (HPV)
– HPV-associated cancers and precancers
• Anogenital warts
• Viral hepatitis
• Ectoparasitic infections

Source: 2015 Sexually Transmitted Disease Treatment Guidelines (CDC)

Table 6.2 Diagnostic classification of menopause and related disorders

A. Menopause
B. Midlife body changes
• Vulvovaginal changes
– Estrogen loss and aging (irritation, burning, itching, vaginal discharge, postcoital bleeding, and dyspareunia)
– Genitourinary syndrome of menopause (GSM)
Vulvovaginal atrophy (VVA)
– Vulvovaginitis (candida, bacterial vaginosis, trichomoniasis)
– Vulvar dystrophies (dermatoses) (lichen sclerosis, lichen planus, and squamous cell hyperplasia/lichen simplex chronicus)
– Vulvar dysplasia/vulvar cancer
C. Clinical issues
• Decline in fertility
• Uterine bleeding
• Vasomotor symptoms
• Genitourinary syndrome of menopause/ symptomatic vulvovaginal atrophy (GSM/VVA)
• Urinary incontinence
• Sexual function
• Sexually transmitted infections (HPV, HIV, hepatitis C, gonorrhea, and chlamydia)
D. Disease risk (endometrial, cervical, ovarian, and colorectal cancer)

Source: North American Menopause Society (NAMS) Recommendations for Clinical Care of Midlife Women

nary syndrome of menopause (GSM). Formerly referred to as vulvovaginal atrophy, GSM nomenclature was recently adopted since this condition includes adverse changes to not only the vulva and vagina but also the urethra, bladder, and lower pelvis [3]. Vulvar symptoms include genital dryness, burning, entry dyspareunia, and irritation, as well as decreased lubrication, pain with intercourse, urinary urgency, dysuria, and recurring urinary tract infection.

6.4 Vulvar Dermatoses

Chronic vulvar dermatoses, although occurring in all age groups, are most frequently seen in postmenopausal women. However, dermatoses in menopausal women occur less frequently than GSM. Of the vulvar dermatoses, lichen sclerosus (LS) is the one most commonly seen. LS is characterized by vulvar scarring, loss of the normal architecture, and whitish, crinkled vulvar skin. Dyspareunia can result from vulvar fissures, erosions, scarring, and introital narrowing associated with LS dermatologic changes [4]. Lichen planus (LP), another vulvar dystrophy, can, unlike LS, involve both the vulva and vagina. Due to changes in vulvar and vaginal integrity, dyspareunia also may result, although the prevalence with LP is lower as compared to LS. Lichen simplex chronicus, or squamous cell hyperplasia, is not as prevalent as LS or LP but when present usually occurs in the older age group. The diagnostic classification of menopause and related disorders developed by the North American Menopause Society is shown in Table 6.2 [5].

6.5 Vulvar Pain

Pain often accompanies vulvar infection, dermatoses, estrogen loss, and allergic/contact dermatitis etiologies. After eliminating recognizable causes of vulvar pain, the diagnosis of vulvodynia can be made, as this pain condition is a diagnosis of exclusion. Women with vulvodynia may complain of mild vulvar discomfort to searing vulvar pain. Clinicians must rule out specific infectious, inflammatory, neoplastic, or neurologic disorders before treating the woman for this condition.

6.6 Vulvodynia

In 2014, the International Society for the Study of Vulvovaginal Disease (ISSVD), the International Society for the Study of Women's Sexual Health (ISSWSH), and the International Pelvic Pain Society (IPPS) revised the terminology of vulvar pain, on the basis of the significant increase in high-quality etiologic studies published in the last decade (Table 6.3) [6]. The table below describes those vulvar pain conditions, for which a cause can be clearly identified, and vulvodynia, where there is no clear identifiable cause.

By the age of 40 years, 7–8% of women report vulvar pain consistent with vulvodynia [7]. Despite the high prevalence of this pain condition, the number of clinical trials testing the effectiveness of pharmacologic interventions is relatively sparse. Below are several that are in common use.

Table 6.3 ISSVD terminology and classification of vulvar pain

A. Vulvar pain caused by a specific disorder[a]
• Infectious (e.g., recurrent candidiasis, herpes)
• Inflammatory (e.g., lichen sclerosus, lichen planus, immunobullous disorders)
• Neoplastic (e.g., Paget's disease, squamous cell carcinoma)
• Neurologic (e.g., postherpetic neuralgia, nerve compression or injury, neuroma)
• Trauma (e.g., female genital cutting, obstetrical)
• Iatrogenic (e.g., postoperative, chemotherapy, radiation)
• Hormonal deficiencies (e.g., genitourinary syndrome of menopause [vulvovaginal atrophy], lactational amenorrhea)
B. Vulvodynia—vulvar pain of at least 3 months duration without clear identifiable cause, which may have potential associated factors

Source: 2015 ISSVD, ISSWSH, and IPPS Consensus Terminology and Classification of Persistent Vulvar Pain and Vulvodynia

[a]Women may have both a specific disorder and vulvodynia

6.7 Tricyclic Antidepressant (TCA)

TCAs, both topical and oral formulations, are commonly used as first-line treatments for vulvodynia. Two RCTs and two case series have been published with oral treatment and one prospective and one retrospective study with topical therapy. Data suggest that TCAs alter nociceptive processing by prolonging synaptic activity of norepinephrine and serotonin, thereby enhancing descending inhibitory action in the spinal cord [8].

One double-blind placebo-controlled RCT compared (1) oral desipramine 25 mg with placebo cream, (2) lidocaine 5% cream and oral desipramine, (3) lidocaine 5% cream with placebo tablets, and (4) placebo cream and tablets in 133 women with localized provoked vulvodynia (LPV) [9]. Reduction of pain, the primary endpoint as measured by the tampon test, was similar for all treatment arms at 12 weeks: 24% for desipramine-placebo, 36% for lidocaine-desipramine, 33% for placebo-placebo, and 20% for lidocaine cream-placebo. Similarly, no differences were observed between the treatment arms in self-reported daily pain and intercourse pain.

The second RCT also found negative findings when low-dose amitriptyline, 10–20 mg amitriptyline plus topical steroid, and a self-management program (consisting of cognitive behavioral therapy (CBT), education, and physical and sex therapy) were compared in 53 women with provoked, unprovoked, or mixed vulvodynia with symptoms [10]. Therapy continued for 12 weeks and was evaluated on the basis of change from baseline for pain scores on the McGill Pain Questionnaire (MPQ). No significant difference was found in reduction of pain scores among the three groups, but significant within-group reduction in pain was seen in the self-management group only.

In contrast, Reed et al. presented a prospective case series of 209 women with mixed vulvodynia types (generalized and localized) receiving amitriptyline or desipramine (at a starting dose of 25 mg and titrated up weekly) and found the antidepressant-treated patients showed greater improvement than the control group [11]. Similarly, a retrospective case series by Munday et al. included 33 women with mixed vulvodynia types (generalized and localized) and reported that amitriptyline or desipramine resulted in a complete response in 47% of women [12]. However, in a retrospective case series conducted by McKay et al., there was no improvement in pain with 40–60 mg/day of amitriptyline in 20 women with generalized vulvodynia [12]. Pain measures were not identified in either the Munday et al. or the McKay et al. studies.

Pagano and Wong conducted a prospective study in 150 women with LPV using topical amitriptyline cream [13]. They found that 10% had excellent improvement, 29% had moderate improvement, 17% had slight improvement, and 44% had no response as measured by questionnaires. In a retrospective study, Nyirjesy et al. treated 38 women with LPV with a combination of 2% amitriptyline and 2% baclofen cream and reported that 53% were very much improved, 18% moderately improved, and 29% had little or no improvement in the frequency of intercourse, VAS scores, and on an interview survey [14].

TCAs are frequently used to treat vulvodynia, but controlled trials demonstrate limited efficacy. Moreover, side effects, such as drowsiness, constipation, nausea, dizziness, and sexual dysfunction, may occur. Although extremely rare, cardiac arrhythmias and conduction disturbances have been reported. Currently, TCAs are not recommended for vulvodynia treatment.

6.8 Anticonvulsants

Gabapentin, the most commonly used anticonvulsant to treat vulvodynia, acts by binding to alpha2delta-1 subunits of calcium channels in the central nervous system [15]. A retrospective case series by Boardman et al. examined topical gabapentin cream (2–6%) in a study that included 51 women with LPV and generalized vulvodynia [16]. In this study, 80% of subjects showed greater than 50% improvement using visual analogue scores.

Only two retrospective case series with oral gabapentin therapy have been conducted. Harris et al. reported that among 601 women with generalized unprovoked vulvodynia, 64% had adequate resolution, but a high percentage of subjects had comorbidities, and rating scales were not used [12]. Ben David found significant improvement of symptoms when rated on a visual analogue scale (VAS) in 73 women with vulvodynia (unspecified type). Although the quality of evidence is low, data suggests that gabapentin may be effective and can be offered to women with vulvodynia; however, it is unclear which subgroups may respond. Currently, a multicenter double-blind RCT is underway to determine its efficacy in the treatment of women with LPV [17]. These findings may provide data on its efficacy and safety in this group of women.

In addition to gabapentin, lamotrigine also has been investigated. By inhibiting voltage-sensitive sodium channels and the release of the excitatory amino acid glutamate, lamotrigine may suppress pathways involved in central neuronal hyperexcitability and persisting pain [15]. Although 1 open label study evaluated oral lamotrigine in 43 women with LPV and found significant reductions in the MPQ and VAS rating scales, there are not enough data to recommend routine use [12].

6.9 Antinociceptive Agents

Lidocaine exerts its analgesic effect via blockade of sodium channels on peripheral nociceptors and by blocking transmission of discharges from peripheral sensory nerves [18]. Sensitization of the peripheral vestibular nerves has been suggested as a possible mechanism of the pain in vestibulodynia. Therefore the theory behind the use of local anesthetics is to achieve long-lasting desensitization of the vestibular nerves.

The efficacy of topical lidocaine has been investigated in three trials and injectable lidocaine in five studies. The majority have shown little to no effect, with the exception of overnight use and concomitant corticosteroid therapy.

Zolnoun reported that 54% of women had at least a 50% reduction in dyspareunia following overnight use of topical 5% lidocaine ointment in a case series of 69 subjects [19]. In contrast, Danielsson found no difference between topical 5% lidocaine ointment and electromyographic (EMG) feedback in 46 women with LPV in an RCT using a vulvar algesiometer or in quality of life or sexual functioning [20]. Similarly, Bohm-Starke compared EMG to topical lidocaine in a case-control study of 35 women with LPV and found no differences between treatments using pressure pain thresholds and questionnaires [12].

In a case series of 27 women with LPV, Rapkin et al. reported that 46% improved on the McGill Pain Questionnaire (MPQ), 57% by self-report, and 41% on algesiometer following administration of epidural, pudendal, and vulvar injections of ropivacaine and bupivacaine [21]. McDonald and Rapkin also reported in a case series a significant decrease in pain on the MPQ, but not intercourse pain, using the same anesthetics and methods of administration in 32 women with vulvodynia [22].

The efficacy of submucosal infiltrations of lidocaine combined with corticosteroids also has been investigated. In a prospective case series of 22 women with LPV, Murina et al. found 68% showed some improvement with a combination of lidocaine and methylprednisolone, and 32% had complete improvement [23]. Both Dede and Segal reported case studies where women with LPV had complete remission following lidocaine and betamethasone submucosal infiltrations [12].

Considering a 30% placebo rate in women with vulvodynia, the improvement reported with lidocaine alone or with combined therapy, regardless of route of administration, is modest. However, given the ease of topical administration, its low cost, and safety when used as directed, it provides a useful option for the treatment of this condition. In select patients, lidocaine injections are an alternative approach.

The rationale for the use of capsaicin in the treatment of vulvodynia is based on increased vanilloid receptor (VR1) innervation found in this disorder and the agonist effects of capsaicin on vanilloid receptors located in the peripheral terminals of nociceptors [24]. After hyperesthesia to the initial exposure, capsaicin produces a long-lasting desensitization to burning and pain.

One prospective and one retrospective case series have evaluated the efficacy of capsaicin cream in LPV. In the prospective study of 33 women receiving 0.05% capsaicin cream, 59% improved and 41% showed no improvement in dyspareunia [25]. Steinberg conducted a retrospective case series of 52 women with LPV and found that application of 0.025% capsaicin cream resulted in significant improvement on the touch test and Marinoff dyspareunia scale but provided no absolute numbers [12]. However, in both studies, lidocaine was given preceding the capsaicin to prevent irritation/burning on administration, so it is impossible to isolate the effect of capsaicin. Because of the potential for significant adverse events, such as serious application site burns, and limited data on efficacy, capsaicin is not recommended as a standard treatment for vulvodynia.

Botulinum (Botox®) (BTA) inhibits the release of glutamate and substance P from nociceptive neurons [26]. Current hypotheses suggest that the inhibition of these nociceptors may reduce peripheral and central sensitization associated with vulvodynia. The efficacy of BTA has been evaluated in one double-blind placebo-controlled RCT and three case series. The controlled study found no difference between BTA (100u) and placebo in level of pain on a VAS scale, quality of life, and sexual function in 64 women with LPV [27].

In contrast, a prospective case series of 20 women with LPV reported that 80% of women had an improvement in pain, and 72% were able to have sexual intercourse following 100 U of BTA [28]. Quality of life and sexual function also improved. In another prospective case series of 39 women with LPV, Bertolasi et al. reported that 63% recovered completely from vaginismus secondary to LPV, and 15% needed reinjections with BTA (a mean dose of 25 U was used per treatment session) [12]. However, in this study recovery was not defined. Similarly, lower doses (35–50 U) were found to significantly decrease pain using a VAS scale, decreased medication use, and improved quality of life in a retrospective study of 19 women with LPV [12].

Given that the RCT showed no improvement with BTA as compared to placebo, and because of the expense, complexity of the medical procedure, and potential for serious side effects, BTA is not recommended as first-line treatment for vulvodynia.

6.10 Anti-inflammatory Agents

Because tissue levels of interleukin (IL-β) have been reported to be significantly higher in the hymen region of the vestibule of women with LPV [29], corticosteroids also have been used to treat vulvodynia symptoms. As inhibitors of IL-1 production, corticosteroids should be a potential treatment option [30].

Three RCTS have been conducted evaluating the efficacy of topical corticosteroids in the treatment of vulvodynia. Munday compared a super high potency (clobetasol 0.05%) to a low potency (hydrocortisone 0.5%, "placebo") corticosteroid in a crossover study of 22 women with LPV [31]. Seventy-three percent of women improved on clobetasol, while 60% improved with hydrocortisone cream. Desrochers et al. found significant improvement in pain and sexual function with both a 1% corticosteroid cream (type unreported) and cognitive behavioral therapy (CBT) in 111 women with LPV [32]. In a three-treatment arm study, Brown et al. found no difference between groups receiving amitriptyline vs. amitriptyline and 0.1% triamcinolone cream (medium potency) vs. self-management in 53 women with vulvodynia (mixed symptoms) [10]. These data suggest that topical corticosteroids are minimally effective in treating LPV. The lowest potency creams, such as hydrocortisone (1.0–2.5%), triamcinolone (0.025%), desonide (0.05%), or fluocinolone (0.01), can be prescribed for short 1- to 2-week intervals. It is unclear whether submucosal infiltrations of lidocaine combined with corticosteroids are effective, as no RCTs have been conducted to date.

Interferon (INF) is approved for the treatment of condylomata acuminate. It downregulates the expression of proinflammatory cytokines [33] and is theorized to be effective in LPV because tissue levels of cytokines have been reported to be significantly higher in the hymen region of the vestibule of LPV patients [29]. One RCT, three case series, and one case study have examined the efficacy of INF in LPV. Bornstein compared total perineoplasty to subtotal perineoplasty plus INF-α2b infiltration in 19 women with LPV and found that 67% of those undergoing total perineoplasty had a complete response compared to 70% of those having subtotal perineoplasty + INF-α [34]. In a prospective case series of 55 women, 49% of women treated with INF-α had substantial or partial improvement in coital pain and vestibular tenderness [35]. Of the 19 who elected to have surgery, 84% had a substantial improvement, and 11% had partial improvement in symptoms. Complete remission was reported in the majority of subjects in two small retrospective studies and one case study[12]. Further studies are necessary to determine if INF alone, or combined with surgery, is an effective treatment for LPV.

In a double-blind, placebo-controlled RCT of 34 women with LPV, Nyirjesy found that 54% of women receiving cromolyn cream, a mast cell stabilizer, compared to 38% of those receiving placebo cream had at least a 50% improvement in dyspareunia and vestibular tenderness [36]. In another double-blind, placebo-controlled RCT of 40 women with LPV, Donders found that fibroblast lysate cream, containing a variety of anti-inflammatory cytokines, produced a significant, although modest reduction in vestibular sensitivity and intercourse pain compared to placebo [37]. Another intervention, montelukast, reduces inflammation by inhibiting cysteinyl leukotriene receptors. A case-control study with montelukast was conducted in 47 women with LPV and found 52% were improved compared to 15% improvement with controls [38]. At this time, cromolyn cream, lysate cream, or montelukast is not recommended for use in the treatment of LPV.

6.11 Novel Agent

A double-blind study of enoxaparin, a low-molecular-weight heparin with anti-heparanase properties, was recently conducted in 40 women with LPV, based on findings of increased anti-heparanase in the vestibule of women with vulvodynia [39]. Compared to placebo, self-administration of enoxaparin (40 mg daily for 90 days) produced a significant, although modest, reduction in dyspareunia and vestibular sensitivity to a Q-tip exam. Decreased vestibular sensitivity was correlated with a reduction in intraepithelial-free nerve fibers in the enoxaparin group, but not in the placebo group, suggesting that enoxaparin may reduce neuroproliferation and penetration of nerve fibers in the epithelium.

6.12 Summary

Medical management of vulvar conditions depends on evidence-based guidance from various governmental agencies and professional societies. Those for vulvar infection, atrophy, and dystrophies are updated on a regular basis. However, for vulvodynia, there is a lack of significant efficacy in most pharmacologic interventions used. With vulvodynia, the patient, with her clinician, should decide if the risk profile is worth the limited efficacy of the treatment.

Medical Treatment: Breaking a Myth

- Although tricyclic antidepressants are frequently used to treat vulvodynia, controlled trials demonstrated limited efficacy. Currently, they are not recommended for vulvodynia treatment

References

1. American College of Obstetricians and Gynecologists. Vulvar disorders. ACOG clinical updates in women's health care. VIII ed. Washington, DC: ACOG; 2010. p. 36.
2. Centers for Disease Control and Prevention. Sexually transmitted diseases treatment guidelines, 2015. MMWR Recomm Rep. 2015;64(RR-3):1–137.
3. Portman DJ, Gass ML, Vulvovaginal Atrophy Terminology Consensus Conference Panel. Genitourinary syndrome of menopause: new terminology for vulvovaginal atrophy from the International Society for the Study of a Women's sexual health and the North American Menopause Society. Menopause. 2014;10:1063–8.
4. Danby CS, Margesson LJ. Approach to the diagnosis and treatment of vulvar pain. Dermatol Ther. 2010;23:485–504.
5. Shifren JL, Gass ML. The North American Menopause Society recommendations for clinical care of midlife women. Menopause. 2014;21(10):1038–62.
6. Bornstein J, Goldstein AT, Stockdale CK, et al. 2015 ISSVD, ISSWSH and IPPS consensus terminology and classification of persistent vulvar pain and Vulvodynia. Obstet Gynecol. 2016;127(4):745–51.
7. Harlow BL, Kunitz CG, Nguyen RHN, Rydell SA, Turner RM, MacLehose RF. Prevalence of symptoms consistent with a diagnosis of vulvodynia: population-based estimates from 2 geographic regions. Am J Obstet Gynecol. 2014;210:40.e1–8.
8. Jasmin L, Tien D, Janni G, et al. Is noradrenaline a significant factor in the analgesic effect of antidepressants? Pain. 2003;106:3–8.
9. Foster DC, Kotok MB, Huang L, et al. Oral desipramine and topical lidocaine for vulvodynia: a randomized controlled trial. Obstet Gynecol. 2010;116:583–93.
10. Brown CS, Wan J, Bachmann G, et al. Self-management, amitriptyline, and amitriptyline plus triamcinolone in the management of vulvodynia. J Women's Health. 2009;18:163–9.
11. Reed BD, Caron AM, Gorenflo DW, et al. Treatment of vulvodynia with tricyclic antidepressants: efficacy and associated factors. J Low Genit Tract Dis. 2006;10:245–51.
12. De Andres J, Sanchis-Lopez N, Asensio-Samper JM, et al. Vulvodynia—an evidence-based literature review and proposed treatment algorithm. Pain Pract. 2015;16(2):204–36.
13. Pagano R, Wong S. Use of amitriptyline cream in the management of entry dyspareunia due to provoked vestibulodynia. J Low Genit Tract Dis. 2012;16:394–7.
14. Nyirjesy P, Lev-Sagie A, Mathew L, Culhane JF. Topical amitriptyline-baclofen cream for the treatment of provoked vestibulodynia. J Low Genit Tract Dis. 2009;13:230–6.
15. Rogawski MA, Loscher W. The neurobiology of antiepileptic drugs for the treatment of nonepileptic conditions. Nat Med. 2004;10:685–92.
16. Boardman LA, Cooper AS, Blais LR, Raker CA. Topical gabapentin in the treatment of localized and generalized vulvodynia. Obstet Gynecol. 2008;112:579–85.
17. Brown CS, Foster DC, Wan JY, Rawlinson L, Bachmann GA, GABA Study Group. Rationale and design of a multicenter randomized clinical trial of extended release gabapentin in provoked vestibulodynia and biological correlates of response. Contemp Clin Trials. 2013;36:154–65.
18. Cummins TR. Setting up for the block: the mechanism underlying lidocaine's use-dependent inhibition of sodium channels. J Physiol. 2007;582(Pt 1):11.

19. Zolnoun DA, Hartmann KE, Steege JF. Overnight 5% lidocaine ointment for treatment of vulvar vestibulitis. Obstet Gynecol. 2003;102:84–7.
20. Danielsson I, Torstensson T, Brodda-Jansen G, Bohm-Starke N. EMG biofeedback versus topical lidocaine gel: a randomized study for the treatment of women with vulvar vestibulitis. Acta Obstet Gynecol Scan. 2006;85:1360–7.
21. Rapkin AJ, McDonald JS, Morgan M. Multilevel local anesthetic nerve blockade for the treatment of vulvar vestibulitis syndrome. Amer J Obstet Gynecol. 2008;198:41.e1–5.
22. McDonald JS, Rapkin AJ. Multilevel local anesthetic nerve blockade for the treatment of generalized vulvodynia: a pilot study. J Sex Med. 2012;9:2919–26.
23. Murina F, Tassan P, Roberti P, Bianco V. Treatment of vulvar vestibulitis with submucous infiltrations of methylprednisolone and lidocaine: an alternative approach. J Reprod Med. 2001;46:713–6.
24. Tympanidis P, Casula MA, Yiangou Y, Terenghi G, Dowd P, Anand P. Increased vanilloid receptor VR1 innervation in vulvodynia. Eur J Pain. 2004;8:129–33.
25. Murina F, Radici G, Bianco V. Capsaicin and the treatment of vulvar vestibulitis syndrome: a valuable alternative? Med Gen Med. 2004;6:48.
26. Cui M, Khanijou S, Rubino J, Aoki KR. Subcutaneous administration of botulinum toxin a reduces formalin-induced pain. Pain. 2004;107:125–33.
27. Petersen CD, Giraldi A, Lundvall L, Kristensen E. Botulinum toxin type A—a novel treatment for provoked vestibulodynia? Results from a randomized, placebo controlled, double blinded study. J Sex Med. 2009;6:2523–37.
28. Pelletier F, Parratte B, Penze S, Moreno JP, Aubin F, Humbert P. Efficacy of high doses of botulinum toxin a for treating provoked vestibulodynia. Brit J Dermatol. 2011;164:617–22.
29. Foster DC, Hadsday JD. Elevated tissue levels of interleukin-1 beta and tumor necrosis factor-alpha in vulvar vestibulitis. Obstet Gynecol. 1997;89:291–6.
30. Snyder DS, Unanue ER. Corticosteroids inhibit murine macrophage 1a expression and interleukin 1 production. J Immunol. 1982;129:1803–5.
31. Munday PE. Treatment of vulval vestibulitis with a potent topical steroid. Sex Transm Infect. 2004;80:154–5.
32. Desrochers G, Bergeron S, Khalife S, Dupuis M-J, Jodoin M. Provoked vestibulodynia: psychological predictors of topical and cognitive-behavioral treatment outcome. Behav Res Ther. 2010;48:106–15.
33. Kieseier BC. The mechanism of action of interferon-β in relapsing multiple sclerosis. CNS Drugs. 2011;25:491–502.
34. Bornstein J, Abramovici H. Combination of subtotal perineoplasty and interferon for the treatment of vulvar vestibulitis. Gynecol Obstet Investig. 1997;44:53–6.
35. Marinoff SC, Turner ML, Hirsch RP, Richard G. Intralesional alpha interferon: cost effective therapy for vulvar vestibulitis syndrome. J Reprod Med. 1993;38:19–24.
36. Nyirjesy P, Sobel JD, Weitz MV, Leaman DJ, Small MJ, Gelone SP. Cromolyn cream for recalcitrant idiopathic vulvar vestibulitis: results of a placebo-controlled study. Sex Transm Inf. 2001;77:53–7.
37. Donders GG, Bellen G. Cream with cutaneous fibroblast lysate for the treatment of provoked vestibulodynia: a double-blind randomized placebo-controlled crossover study. J Lower Genital Tract Dis. 2012;16:427–36.
38. Kamdar N, Fisher L, MacNeill C. Improvement in vulvar vestibulitis with montelukast. J Reprod Med. 2007;52:912–6.
39. Farajun Y, Zarfati D, Abramov L, Livoff A, Bornstein J. Enoxaparin treatment of vulvodynia. A randomized controlled trial. Obstet Gynecol. 2012;120:565–73.

7 Vulvar Pruritus

Nicholas Lawrance and Jennifer Yell

7.1 Introduction

Vulvar pruritus (itching) is common, affecting about 10% of women during their lifetime [1–3]. If persistent, significant morbidity can result in secondary skin thickening (lichen simplex), sleep disturbance and sexual and psychological difficulty. A systematic history and clinical examination will usually identify the cause. In those women with normal skin, pruritus may be due to an underlying medical cause.

Table 7.1 Classification of pruritus [4]

Classification	Explanation
Pruritoceptive	Cutaneous, e.g. scabies, urticaria
Neuropathic	Due to lesions of afferent pathways of the nervous system, e.g. peripheral neuritis, nerve entrapment, brain tumours
Neurogenic	Due to centrally acting mediators which do not damage the central nervous system, e.g. morphine, opioid peptides of cholestasis
Psychogenic	For example, delusional parasitosis

7.2 Pathophysiology of Pruritus

Pruritus (itching, pruritus vulvae) is a poorly localized, unpleasant sensation which results in scratching. Pruritus and pain (vulvodynia) are different. Pruritus causes scratching. Pain causes withdrawal. Multiple neural pathways and molecular mechanisms are responsible for the sensation of pruritus. The precise relationship between pruritus and pain remains controversial, although there is evidence for separate pathways for pruritus and pain: a class of C-fibres, mechanically insensitive, slowly conducting and histamine responsive, support the theory of a separate pruritus pathway peripherally, along with a feline study showing a separate central pathway for pruritus, in which mechanically insensitive feline spinothalamic tract (STT) neurons were activated by histamine [4, 5].

Patients' description of pruritus varies from burning, through pricking, to sensations of insects crawling over the skin. Vulvar pruritus, pain and/or burning can co-exist.

Pruritus has been formally classified as per Table 7.1. In formal studies clear measurement methods are required as per Table 7.2. The factors affecting pruritus are listed in Table 7.3.

7.3 Causes of Pruritus

The common causes of vulvar pruritus are listed in Table 7.4. In chronic pruritus [17], 1/3 of patients with generalized pruritus have an underlying systemic disease (see Table 7.5), 2/3 have skin disease-associated pruritus (which can include failure of the skin to retain water with age

N. Lawrance (✉) · J. Yell
British Society for the Study of Vulval Disease, Manchester, UK

J. Bornstein (ed.), *Vulvar Disease*, https://doi.org/10.1007/978-3-319-61621-6_7

[18] and atopy), and about 7% are idiopathic (including psychogenic factors, such as anxiety and parasitophobia). Dermatology clinic review of 141 women with chronic vulvar symptoms identified eczema as the commonest reason for referral (54%), followed by lichen sclerosus (13%), chronic vulvovaginal candidiasis (10%), dysaesthetic vulvodynia (generalized spontaneous vulvodynia) (9%) and psoriasis (5%) [14]. Eczema was found to be the commonest cause of pruritus among patients presenting to gynecologists in the USA too [19]. Apart from atopy, other eczema causes include contact irritant (incontinence of urine/faeces, due to detergents, over cleaning or sanitary pads) or contact allergic (common sensitizers include preservatives in moist wipes and perfumes and can be identified with patch testing). The physiological causes of pruritus are shown in Table 7.6.

Table 7.2 Measurement of pruritus

Purpose of measurement	Method of measurement
Clinical outcome measure	Visual analogue scales [5]
Clinical trials	Symtrack computerized continuous pruritus-rating system [6]
Clinical trials	Piezoelectric device attached to the middle fingernail [7]

7.4 History

As cause determines successful treatment, a systematic history followed by examination is required. Important points to cover in the history include:

1. Pruritus versus pain.
2. Duration: acute pruritus—infection.
3. Timing: very severe nocturnal pruritus causing wakening suggests lichen sclerosus, or lichen simplex commonly, or threadworms (especially with perianal pruritus).
4. Associated symptoms:
   (a) Dyspareunia due to splitting: if pruritus is associated with superficial dyspareu-

Table 7.3 Factors affecting pruritus

Mediator	Receptor(s) involved in pruritus	Function in pruritus	Treatments
Histamine [8]	H_1; possibly H_4	Urticaria Atopic eczema	Sedating H_1 systemic antihistamines [9]
Acetylcholine	Muscarinic acetylcholine receptors	Sweating in atopic dermatitis	
Substance P	Neurokinin (NK)	Prime mast cells for histamine release	Topical capsaicin [10]
Calcitonin gene-related peptide (CGRP)	CGRP receptors	Sensitization of pruritus-receptive neurones	
Opioid peptides	μ-Opioid receptors	Central pruritus, cholestasis	Naloxone
Proteases	Proteinase-activated receptor-2 (PAR-2)	Release of substance P	
Neurotrophins	Trk a, b, c; NT3, NT4	Atopic eczema, sensitizes pruritus-receptive neurons	
Cytokines	Receptor mediated	Indirect via other mediators?	Cyclosporine (IL-2T inhibitor) atopic dermatitis [11]
Prostaglandin E	PGE receptors	Sensitize pruritus receptors to histamine	Topical (not systemic) aspirin, (prostaglandin synthetase inhibitor) good in localized pruritus [12, 13]

Table 7.4 The common causes of vulvar pruritus [14, 15]

1. Skin disease part of a generalized endogenous skin disorder (eczema, psoriasis)
2. Vulvar-specific skin disease: lichen sclerosus, lichen planus
3. Infections and infestations:
(a) Candida can be a cause of napkin dermatitis in babies. Candida is the commonest infection postpubertal. Postmenopausal women are unlikely to have *Candida albicans* infection, unless they are diabetic and they are treated with oestrogen or antibiotics
(b) Pinworms can cause pruritus when they exit at night
4. Neoplastic conditions: although often asymptomatic, they may cause pruritus, especially squamous intraepithelial lesions (SIL, also known as vulvar intraepithelial neoplasia or VIN) and extramammary Paget's disease (Fig. 7.5)
5. Neuropathy: this usually causes pain/vulvodynia but may lead to pruritus
6. Hormonal changes
(a) Prepubertal: streptococcal vaginitis or lichen sclerosus commonest
(b) Menstruating: consider any of the above causes
(c) Postmenopausal: lichen sclerosus commonest
(d) Breastfeeding elevates prolactin, dropping oestrogen levels, with vaginal dryness and pruritus
(e) Pregnancy causes vulvar engorgement, increased vaginal discharge and an increased incidence of candidal vulvovaginitis
7. Systemic causes: see Table 7.5
8. Most skin diseases and infections and infestations, when they affect the vulvar skin, may cause pruritus. These less common causes are covered in the chapters dealing with these specific entities, for example, scabies, trichomoniasis, benign tumours of the vulvar (seborrhoeic warts, syringomas), etc.

Table 7.5 Pruritus associated with systemic or internal disease (neurogenic pruritus) [16]

Cause	Specific diseases
Uraemia	
Liver disease	Cholestasis
Haematological disease	Iron deficiency Polycythaemia vera
Malignant disease	Solid tumours Lymphomas
Endocrine disease	Thyroid disease Diabetes
HIV infection	
Adverse drug reaction	Morphine, aspirin, codeine

nia and splitting, think of a local skin cause, for example, lichen planus or psoriasis.
(b) Vaginal discharge: infection (candida commonest, bacterial vaginosis or trichomoniasis).
(c) Hygiene practices: overwashing and perfumed detergents can result in irritant contact dermatitis.
(d) Contraception: allergy to spermicides or natural rubber latex (condoms and diaphragms).
(e) Hormones: personal or family history of atopy (asthma, eczema, hay fever) or psoriasis.
(f) Markers for diabetes mellitus or systemic illness.

5. Psychosexual assessment.

7.5 Examination

The principles of a general skin examination performed with empathy and adequate time, are the baseline. When trying to diagnose a skin condition based on the appearance (morphology), try and identify the primary morphology for a correct diagnosis of cause, rather than the secondary morphology (namely, that due to scratching, e.g. lichenification, hyperpigmentation, linear excoriations) (see Fig. 7.1), which may occur in any cause of pruritus.

Specific vulvar examination for the symptom of pruritus:

Determine the precise location of the symptoms and ask the patient to show you. Pruritus often only affects one area of the vulva.

Skin groin/mons pubis (see Fig. 7.2): If pink, lichenified, consider endogenous skin disease (eczema or psoriasis), irritant contact dermatitis due to urinary incontinence (symmetrical) or rarely, allergic contact dermatitis (asymmetrical) or nonspecific or candidal intertrigo.

Labia majora: See Fig. 7.3a, endogenous skin disease (eczema or psoriasis), lichen simplex.

Table 7.6 Physiological causes of pruritus

Cause	Pathogenesis	Clinical findings	Treatment
Senescence	Failure of the skin to retain water [20] Dystrophic changes in afferent nerve terminals [21, 22]	Skin dryness and fine cracking	Emollients multiple, e.g. soft white paraffin improve barrier function [23]
Psychogenic	Anxiety [18]		Doxepin 10–20 mg
	Parasitophobia		Olanzapine Paroxetine (selective serotonin reuptake inhibitor) [24]
Female hormonal changes (see text for all life stages) postmenopausal	Oestrogen deficiency, associations: candidiasis, diabetes	Hot flushes. nocturnal	Hormone therapy [25]
Atopic dermatitis	Pruritoceptive neurogenic, psychogenic	Nocturnal pruritus worse with wool, sweat, spicy foods, alcohol	Emollients topical immunosuppressants (glucocorticosteroids, calcineurin inhibitors) second-line treatments: narrowband UVB phototherapy, cyclosporine, azathioprine, methotrexate

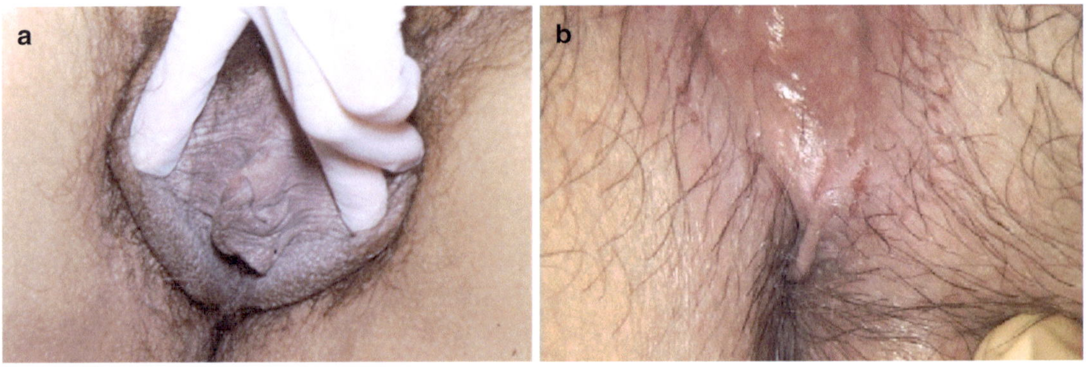

Fig. 7.1 (**a**) Chronic scratching resulting in lichenification and hyperpigmentation of the vulva in a patient (the end result of a pruritus-scratch cycle) with Fitzpatrick skin type 4. In this case her pruritus was due to anaemia. (**b**) Fissures resulting from excoriations in a patient with chronic pruritus

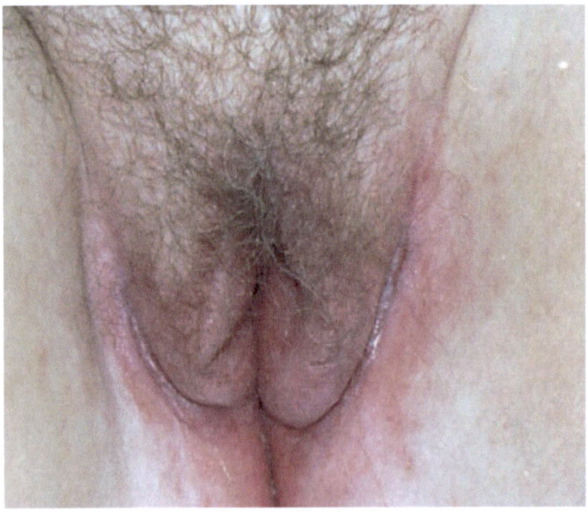

Fig. 7.2 Eczema is the commonest cause of pruritus presenting to specific vulval clinics

Part labia majora/check interlabial sulci (splitting suggests seborrhoeic eczema/psoriasis; see Fig. 7.3b).

Clitoris and hood: if adhesions are present—either red shiny patches or white areas— consider vulvar-specific dermatosis (lichen planus or lichen sclerosus).

Labia minora: lichen sclerosus, lichen planus.

Vagina: if discharge exists, consider infection, particularly thrush (see Fig. 7.4).

Introitus/perineum: if there are red shiny patches or white areas, consider vulvar-specific dermatosis (lichen planus or lichen sclerosus), splitting with eczema and psoriasis)

Examination of the *perianal area*: if figure of eight whiteness/cigarette paper atrophy is seen, con-

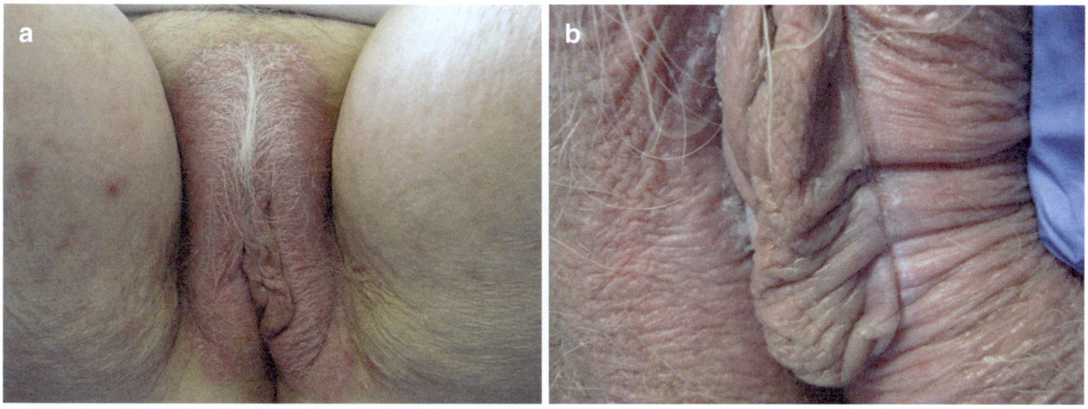

Fig. 7.3 (**a**) Flexural psoriasis presents with symmetrical well-demarcated pink plaques, without scale. Psoriasis is a common cause of interlabial and natal cleft splits. (**b**) Same patient on close inspection with interlabial splitting

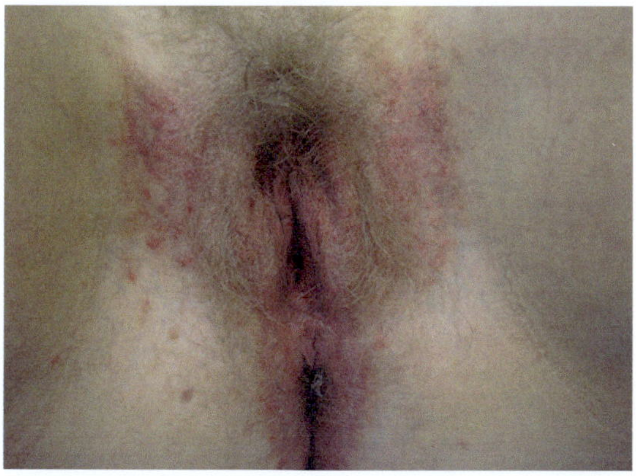

Fig. 7.4 Extensive prolonged candidiasis untreated for 1 year. Candidiasis—erythema, oedema and satellite lesions. The typical discharge and swelling of acute candidiasis may be absent in recurrent vulvovaginal candidiasis, where skin fissuring and pruritus may be the presentation

sider lichen sclerosus; if pink or red, particularly if extending up natal cleft with splitting, consider seborrhoeic eczema/psoriasis.

Any site: neoplasia.

7.5.1 Examination Notes

If no skin disease can be detected in a woman with vulvar pruritus, then consider that infection may be the cause of the pruritus. If swabs and cultures do not yield an infective microorganism, consider that the pruritus is due to systemic causes. If after a clear history and systematic examination diagnostic doubt persists, then further investigations may be required; see list below.

7.6 Specific Investigations for Vulvar Pruritus

1. Take a swab for infective agent in all pubertal women (in a few cases, chronic vulvovaginal candidiasis may be of little or no discharge).
2. Biopsy if skin disease is present and diagnosis is in doubt or if any possibility of malignancy exists. Spongiosis may be detected in the biopsy. This is one of the pathological features of eczema, but in the vulva, this may be the only feature present in psoriasis too.
3. Perform a patch test if contact allergic dermatitis is a possibility.
4. If eczema is present, check for iron deficiency anaemia and hypothyroidism.
5. Test for blood glucose level.

7.7 Treatment

Underlying causes should be managed. The aim of treatment is to relieve pruritus, reduce scratching, and break the pruritus-scratch cycle using the stepwise approach outlined below.

Treatment fundamentals for endogenous skin disease (eczema or psoriasis) [26]:

1. Emollients as soap and moisturizer.
2. Moderate topical glucocorticosteroid twice daily for 2 weeks, steroid to active skin disease first, followed by a moisturizer/emollient.
3. Review. If improved, drop treatment to twice daily weekends only (tolerance to topical steroids develops with long-term use). If relapsing rapidly, consider introduction of calcineurin inhibitor twice daily Monday to Friday (Pimecrolimus cream).
4. Referral to a dermatologist is indicated if the cause is unclear and symptoms persist, to consider: further investigation for cause of eczema, for example, patch testing, introduction of Vit D3 analogues for ongoing maintenance in psoriasis or escalation to second-line systemic treatments, for example, methotrexate.
5. Urgent referral (within 2 weeks) to a gynaeoncologist is indicated if vulvar carcinoma is suspected (e.g. an unexplained vulvar lump or ulcer) (Fig. 7.5) [26].

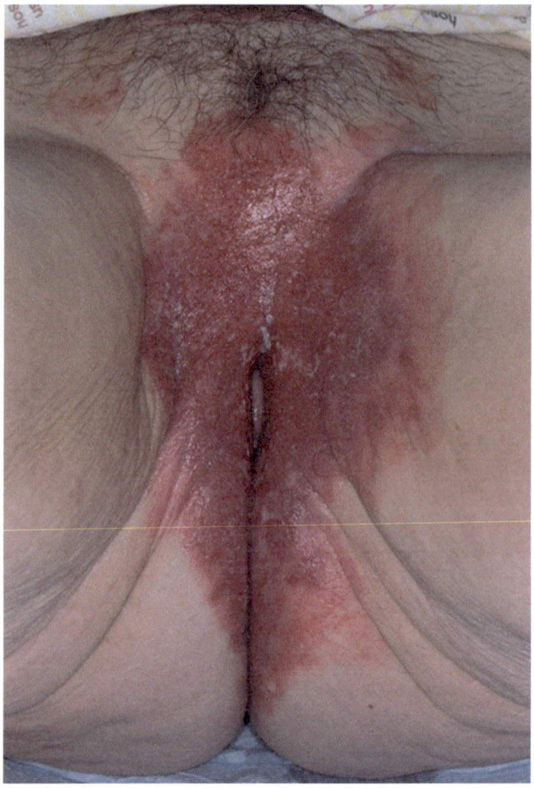

Fig. 7.5 Paget's disease. Consider malignancy with an irregularly outlined and coloured plaque, firm to touch and/or ulcerated and bleeding

In women with pregnancy induced pruritus, treat the cause. The following are deemed the least unsafe measures in the pruritic pregnant patient:

1. Topical: 1–2% menthol cream or lotion
2. 5% urea cream (for dry skin)
3. Benzyl benzoate application (for scabies)
4. Topical steroids (low–moderate potency only)
5. Systemic—chlorpheniramine, diphenhydramine, hydroxyzine
6. Others—UVB phototherapy

For treatment of vulvar-specific skin disease, see the relevant chapters in this textbook.

The treatments outlined in the list below are regularly used for idiopathic pruritus.

Systemic treatments of proven effectiveness for pruritus of unknown cause not confined to the vulva:

1. Antihistamines [27]
2. Systemic tricyclic antidepressants (doxepin 10–25 mg nocte) [28]
3. Transcutaneous nerve stimulation [29]
4. Acupuncture [30]
5. Opioid μ-receptor antagonists (naloxone) [31]
6. Paroxetine (selective serotonin reuptake inhibitor) [32]
7. Mirtazapine, a dual serotonergic and noradrenergic antidepressant [33, 34]
8. Gabapentin [35]
9. Broadband or narrowband ultraviolet B phototherapy (UVB) for [36]

Vulvar Pruritus: Breaking the Myths

- Vulvovaginal candidiasis is not the main cause of vulvar pruritus, eczema is, followed by lichen sclerosus, chronic vulvovaginal candidiasis and psoriasis.

- Physical examination in cases of vulvar pruritus is not always contributory.
  - However, if no skin disease can be detected in a woman with vulvar pruritus, then consider that infection may be the cause of the pruritus.
  - If swabs and cultures do not yield an infective microorganism, consider that the pruritus is due to systemic causes.

References

1. Harlow BL, Wise LA, Stewart EG. Prevalence and predictors of chronic lower genital tract discomfort. Am J Obstet Gynecol. 2001;185:545–50. https://doi.org/10.1067/mob.2001.116748.
2. Doxanakis A, Fairley CK, Bradshaw C. Vulval itch: all that itches is not thrush. Med Today. 2004;5:54–64.
3. Bohl TG. Overview of vulvar pruritus through the life cycle. Clin Obstet Gynecol. 2005;48:786–807.
4. Twycross R, Greaves MW, Handwerker H, et al. Itch: scratching more than the surface. QJM. 2003;96:7–26.
5. Ebata T, Iwasaki S, Kamide R, Niimura M. Use of a wrist activity monitor for the measurement of nocturnal scratching in patients with atopic dermatitis. Br J Dermatol. 2001;144:305–9.
6. Hägermark O, Wahlgren CF. Some methods for evaluating clinical itch and their application for studying pathophysiological mechanisms. J Dermatol Sci. 1992;4:55–62.
7. Molenaar HA, Oosting J, Jones EA. Improved device for measuring scratching activity in patients with pruritus. Med Biol Eng Comput. 1998;36:220–4.
8. Akiyama T, Carstens E. Neural processing of itch. Neuroscience. 2013;250:697–714. https://doi.org/10.1016/j.neuroscience.2013.07.035.
9. Krause L, Shuster S. Mechanism of action of antipruritic drugs. Br Med J. 1983;287:1199–200.
10. Lynn B. Capsaicin: actions on C fibre afferents that may be involved in itch. Skin Pharmacol. 1992;5:9–13.
11. Wahlgren CF, Scheynius A, Hägermark O. Antipruritic effect of oral cyclosporin A in atopic dermatitis. Acta Derm Venereol. 1990;70:323–9.
12. Yosipovitch G, Sugeng MW, Chan YH, et al. The effect of topically applied aspirin on localized circumscribed neurodermatitis. J Am Acad Dermatol. 2001;45:910–3. https://doi.org/10.1067/mjd.2001.117399.
13. Colbert S, O'Hanlon DM, Galvin S, et al. The effect of rectal diclofenac on pruritus in patients receiving intrathecal morphine. Anaesthesia. 1999;54:948–52.
14. Fischer GO. The commonest causes of symptomatic vulvar disease: a dermatologist's perspective. Australas J Dermatol. 1996;37:12–8.
15. Stewart K. Vulvar dermatoses: a practical approach to evaluation and management. JCOM. 2012;19:205–20.
16. Archer CB. Skin and systemic diseases. In: Warell D, Cox T, Firth J, editors. Oxford textbook medicine. 5th ed. Oxford: Oxford University Press; 2010.
17. Weisshaar E, Apfelbacher C, Jäger G, et al. Pruritus as a leading symptom: clinical characteristics and quality of life in German and Ugandan patients. Br J Dermatol. 2006;155:957–64. https://doi.org/10.1111/j.1365-2133.2006.07430.x.
18. Thaipisuttikul Y. Pruritic skin diseases in the elderly. J Dermatol. 1998;25:153–7.
19. ACOG Practice Bulletin No. 93: diagnosis and management of vulvar skin disorders. Obstet Gynecol. 2008;111:1243–53. https://doi.org/10.1097/AOG.0b013e31817578ba.
20. Hara M, Kikuchi K. Senile xerosis, functional morphological and biochemical studies. J Geriatr Dermatol. 1993;1:111–20.
21. Nusbaum NJ. Aging and sensory senescence. South Med J. 1999;92:267–75.
22. Ward JR, Bernhard JD. Willan's itch and other causes of pruritus in the elderly. Int J Dermatol. 2005;44:267–73. https://doi.org/10.1111/j.1365-4632.2004.02553.x.
23. Ghadially R, Halkier-Sorensen L, Elias PM. Effects of petrolatum on stratum corneum structure and function. J Am Acad Dermatol. 1992;26:387–96.
24. Biondi M, Arcangeli T, Petrucci RM. Paroxetine in a case of psychogenic pruritus and neurotic excoriations. Psychother Psychosom. 2000;69:165–6.
25. Tzingounis VA, Aksu MF, Greenblatt RB. Estriol in the management of the menopause. JAMA. 1978;239:1638–41.
26. NICE. Pruritus vulvae—NICE CKS. 2016. http://cks.nice.org.uk/pruritus-vulvae. Accessed 27 Oct 2016.
27. Epstein E, Pinski JB. A blind study. Arch Dermatol. 1964;89:548–9.
28. Tennyson H, Levine N. Neurotropic and psychotropic drugs in dermatology. Dermatol Clin. 2001;19:179–97.
29. Ekblom A, Fjellner B, Hansson P. The influence of mechanical vibratory stimulation and transcutaneous electrical nerve stimulation on experimental pruritus induced by histamine. Acta Physiol Scand. 1984;122:361–7. https://doi.org/10.1111/j.1748-1716.1984.tb07520.x.
30. Lundeberg T, Bondesson L, Thomas M. Effect of acupuncture on experimentally induced itch. Br J Dermatol. 1987;117:771–7.
31. Taddese A, Nah SY, McCleskey EW. Selective opioid inhibition of small nociceptive neurons. Science. 1995;270:1366–9.
32. Zylicz Z, Krajnik M, van Sorge AA, Costantini M. Paroxetine in the treatment of severe non-

dermatological pruritus: a randomized, controlled trial. J Pain Symptom Manag. 2003;26:1105–12.
33. Hundley JL, Yosipovitch G. Mirtazapine for reducing nocturnal itch in patients with chronic pruritus: a pilot study. J Am Acad Dermatol. 2004;50:889–91. https://doi.org/10.1016/j.jaad.2004.01.045.
34. Demierre M-F, Taverna J. Mirtazapine and gabapentin for reducing pruritus in cutaneous T-cell lymphoma. J Am Acad Dermatol. 2006;55:543–4. https://doi.org/10.1016/j.jaad.2006.04.025.
35. Yesudian PD, Wilson NJE. Efficacy of gabapentin in the management of pruritus of unknown origin. Arch Dermatol. 2005;141:1507–9. https://doi.org/10.1001/archderm.141.12.1507.
36. Rivard J, Lim HW. Ultraviolet phototherapy for pruritus. Dermatol Ther. 2005;18:344–54. https://doi.org/10.1111/j.1529-8019.2005.00032.x.

The Vulva During Childhood

8

Adriadna Caussade

8.1 Anatomy of the Vulva in Girls

The transient effect of maternal estrogen fades within the first 6 months of the infant's life. Consequently, before puberty, the anatomy of a girl's vulva differs significantly from the adult woman's. Contrary to the adult vulva, the girl's is hairless and has very little subcutaneous fat, both in the labia majora and the mons pubis. This makes girls more prone to deep bruising and injuries when they are exposed to trauma, so frequent in childhood. The labia minora look atrophic and are barely noticeable; consequently, the introitus opens widely, and the vagina is more readily exposed to injuries; in addition, the very short distance from the anus to the introitus favors local inflammation and infections [1, 2].

The apocrine glands of the labia majora, prepuce, *vestibulum vaginae*, and perineal body are not activated until puberty; as a result, the conditions associated with these structures are rare in childhood. However, the sweat glands do function before puberty, and their obstruction may cause sudamen, a condition frequently seen in neonates [1]. During childhood, the hymen is a vascularized mucous membrane that separates the vagina from the introitus. It may vary in size, thickness, and shape. The normal diameter is about 1 cm, and its compliance is quite limited until estrogen begins to act in puberty. The most common shapes observed tend to be annular, in crescents, or fimbriated. In some cases, a small slit observed at 6 o'clock may be a remnant of hymenal septae, and not necessarily a sign of abuse. However, the presence of clefts at three or nine would suggest that possibility. There are some developmental or permeabilization abnormalities, including cribriform, septate [2], or even imperforate hymens, which can lead to primary amenorrhea and hematometra, which is corrected by making an incision in the hymen and thus releasing any accumulated vaginal and uterine discharge.

8.2 Physical Examination of the Girl

For a satisfactory examination, it is important to achieve a good rapport between the doctor and parents or caregivers but especially between the doctor and the child [3]. The examining doctor should be affectionate but not fawning. If the physical examination is impossible at the first visit, it should be left for the second, and if it continues to be difficult, or if the case is urgent and really warrants anesthesia, then this latter procedure should not be spared [4].

The physical examination of the girl is done by placing her in a frog position, her legs falling sideways, and gently pulling them to the side, to allow a partial view of the vagina (Fig. 8.1). The Valsalva

A. Caussade (✉)
Clínica de Tracto Genital Inferior,
Montevideo, Uruguay

J. Bornstein (ed.), *Vulvar Disease*, https://doi.org/10.1007/978-3-319-61621-6_8

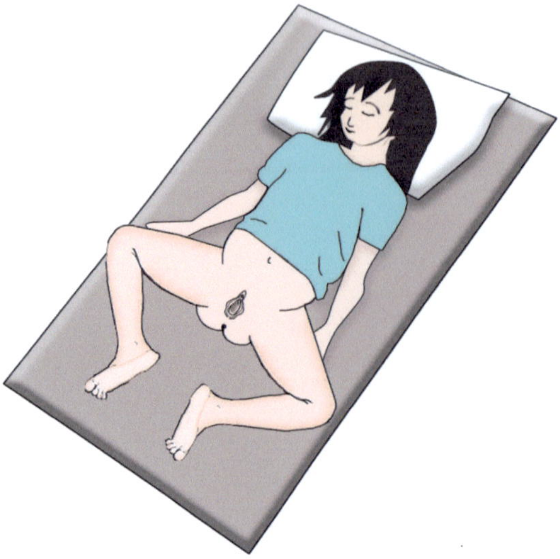

Fig. 8.1 Examination of the genitalia in a child. The girl is placed in a frog position, possible on her mother's lap, with the girl's legs falling sideways, to allow a partial view of the vagina. Having the girl push (a Valsalva maneuver) may provide sight of the vagina. Courtesy of Professor Jacob Bornstein

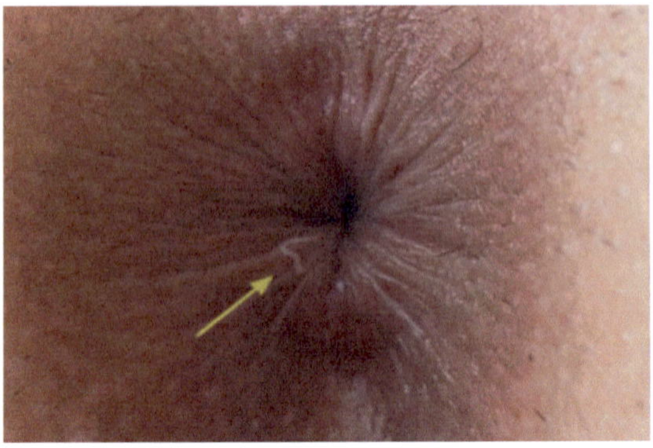

Fig. 8.2 Direct visualization of a worm at the perianal area. Pinworms cause pruritus. Courtesy of Professor Jacob Bornstein

maneuver may even provide a nonaggressive and noninvasive sight of almost the entire vagina. In the little girl, mucous membranes are red, well vascularized, and very thin, unlike the adult's. This examination is also an excellent opportunity to assess the girl's hygiene [5].

8.3 Vulvovaginitis

Vulvovaginitis is one of the most common problems among girls [6] accounting for 80–90% of the gynecologic visits. In the pediatric population, vulvitis and vaginitis may occur together or separately. Signs and symptoms of vulvitis include vulvar itching, burning, pain, dysuria, and erythema. The presence of discharge suggests the association with vaginitis. Girls presenting with these symptoms frequently have other underlying diseases, including dermatitis, psoriasis, or lichen sclerosus.

The most common infectious vulvovaginitis in girls is caused by group A beta-hemolytic *Streptococcus*; in premenarchal girls, however, nonspecific vulvovaginitis accounts for 50–75% of the cases. In the absence of estrogen, the vaginal lining is thin and frail, and the absence of lactobacilli makes it more prone to infections. Prior to menarche, specific vulvovaginitis is often secondary to respiratory or digestive infections and less frequently do they occur as a result of abuse [7]. Organisms originated in the respiratory tract are transferred from the nose and mouth because of poor hygiene habits. The most common agents are group A *Streptococcus*, *Staphylococcus aureus*, *Haemophilus influenzae*, *Streptococcus pneumoniae*, and *Neisseria meningitidis*; enteric organisms include *Shigella* and *Yersinia*.

It is suggested that if the discharge is abundant and the inflammatory changes significant, a vaginal smear (wet mount) should be obtained for microbiological testing. The transparent tape test may be used to detect pinworms at the anus (Figs. 8.2 and 8.3), while the ova and parasite (O&P) exams should be performed to detect lower GIT parasitic infections. Chlamydia or gonorrhea should only be sought if sexual abuse is suspected [8]. Many girls with pinworms (*Enterobius vermicularis*) may be asymptomatic, but recurrent and predominantly nocturnal itching and perianal erythema should suggest their presence. Secondary *E. coli* infection may also develop, with the spread of pinworms from the anus to the vagina.

Although tinea may occur sporadically in some girls, once the little girl overgrows the diapers, candidiasis does not occur if immunity is

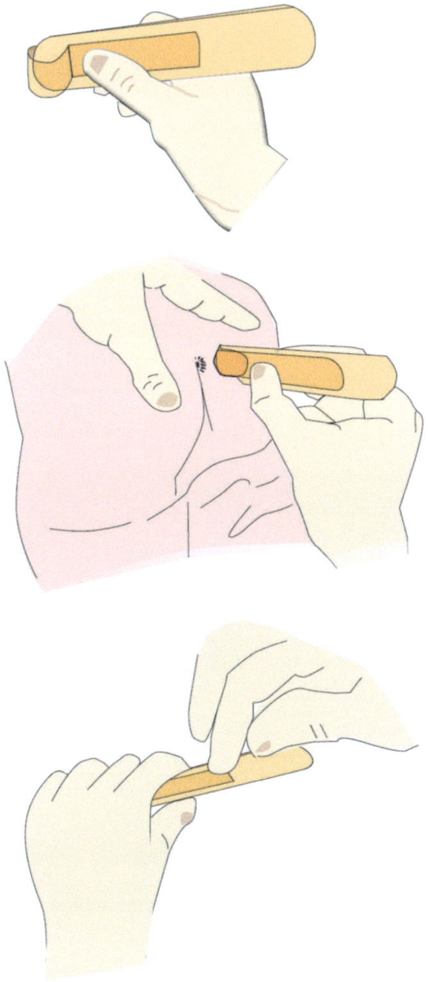

Fig. 8.3 The tape test. In cases where a pinworm infection is suspected, a transparent tape should be put on the perianal area, removed and put on a glass, and examined for ova and parasites under the microscope. Courtesy of Professor Jacob Bornstein

well preserved, because it is a hypoestrogenic mucosa [9–11].

Candidiasis is a common misdiagnosis in girls presenting with either dermatitis, psoriasis, or other skin diseases, and the antifungal creams prescribed just worsen the underlying condition.

8.3.1 Therapy

As in many cases, the cause of vulvovaginitis is nonspecific; therapy will be based on correcting hygiene conditions. If specific bacteria are detected, the treatment will also include antibiotics. If the specific antibiotic treatment fails after two episodes, examination under anesthesia should be considered, in search of foreign bodies [8].

8.4 Condylomatosis in the Girl

Girls with a potential HPV infection should be examined and managed delicately and with extreme care, to minimize any psychological trauma [12].

The diagnosis of human papillomavirus (HPV) infection in girls usually suggests a sexually transmitted disease and, therefore, sexual abuse. However, the sexual route is not the only pathway for infection in girls. New forms of transmission continue to be reported [13], and HPV may be transmitted in different ways, including sexual abuse, vertical transmission, horizontal transmission, and autoinoculation [12]. Hence, it is very difficult—and inappropriate—to rule out or to confirm abuse simply on the basis of the absence or presence of genital warts. Viral typing will not provide much information either in that regard, since some viral types, such as HPV 1 and 2, may be transmitted through the hands, and they may come from adult caregivers that carry the virus on their hands, or from sexual abuse by manipulation of the child's genitals. Although the confirmation of viral types such as HPV 6, 11, and even 16 might suggest abuse, in fact they may have been autoinoculated, since they are very common virus types in the oral mucosa [14].

More certain signs of abuse are hymen tears or sexually transmitted diseases such as gonorrhea or syphilis. The presence of sperm and/or pregnancy can be considered conclusive, but local congestion, erosions, vaginal discharge, or even the hymen polyps are nonspecific for diagnosis.

In utero mother-to-child transmission is known as vertical transmission. It would be the cause of HPV infections in many virgins and girls that raise so many doubts in treating physicians. Indeed, many authors have recently published comprehensive studies showing that the mother-to-child route is not at all negligible [15, 16].

Horizontal transmission is due to skin contact between the girl and her mother or caregiver. Autoinoculation may occur by way of scratching and passage from one area to another. It is very common to find the same types of virus in mucous membranes and hand skin, for instance. Thus, when a girl "bites" or nibbles the genital warts on her hands, the virus may be inoculated into the mucosa and later appear on her lips; the type found in these lesions is type 2 [17]. Given the fragility of the girl's skin and mucosa, there is no ideal treatment for girls; hence, the treatment of condyloma will vary according to the site and size of the lesions, as well as to their persistence.

Five percent imiquimod cream has shown to be a good alternative when treating large areas. Being for topical use, it can be applied by the patient herself, or, if the girl is too young, it could be applied by her mother or caregiver. It is important to mention that there may be side effects, including local irritation and abrasions; if they occur, therapy should not be discontinued, but the drug should be administered less frequently. Treatment should start by applying a small amount of cream on the condyloma three times a week. The recurrence rate is low—approximately 13%.

The application of trichloroacetic acid at low concentrations by the physician may be another option, with weekly or biweekly applications, depending on the clinical response. Podophyllin is not recommended, and cryotherapy could be painful for the girl.

Surgical treatment, radiofrequency, and laser are reserved for lesions that are either very large or very resistant to the above therapies and should always be performed under general anesthesia. The high rate of recurrence should not be surprising.

8.5 Dermatitis

At least 30% of the girls with vulvar itching suffer from dermatitis [9].

It is important to investigate the use of diapers, not only in infants; some older girls with a history of chronic diarrhea, enuresis, or nocturnal incontinence may wear diapers and may therefore present the complications inherent to their use, such as contact dermatitis. However, the most common causes of contact dermatitis are scented soaps, foam, and pool chlorine. The labia are the most commonly involved area (Fig. 8.4). The lesion usually presents as a diffuse scaly erythema, rough skin, and some swelling and flaking of the labia minora. The flakes may soil the underwear and be mistaken for discharge; in some cases, there may even be bloody spots caused by skin erosions. Diaper rash begins by impairing the integrity of the stratum corneum. Once the barrier has been damaged, chemical or mechanical irritants cause inflammation. Continuous exposure to irritating agents generates edema, rash, and excoriation (Fig. 8.5).

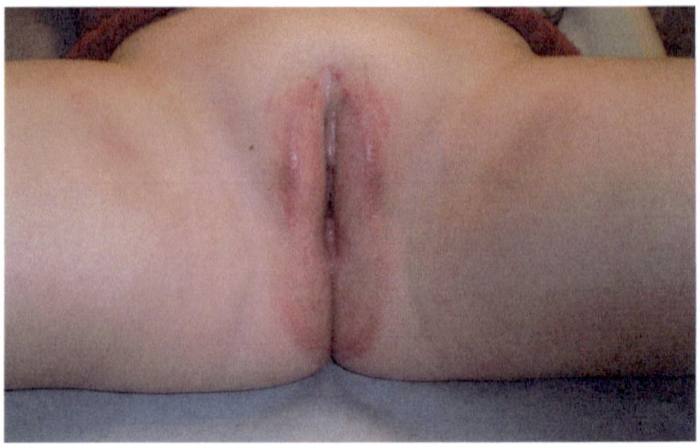

Fig. 8.4 Vulvar dermatitis in an infant, provoked by soaps

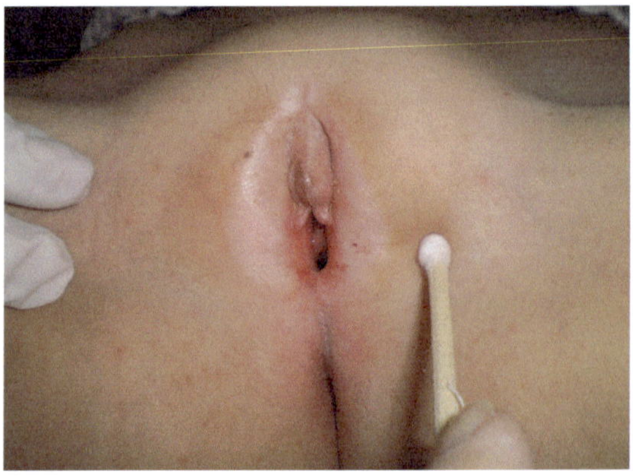

Fig. 8.5 Lichen sclerosus in an infant, with a white vulvar lesion and subepithelial bruising

8.5.1 Therapy

In essence, therapy consists of reducing contact with moisture and local irritants [18]. An important mainstay of treatment is to apply a semipermeable film on the damaged skin to stimulate repair. Many cases of dermatitis initially respond to the use of 1% hydrocortisone. Prefer the ointment than the cream, since the latter can cause local burning. In more severe cases, 0.05% desonide can reverse symptoms until there is a better response, after which the patient is maintained on hydrocortisone. Bacterial infections require antibiotics.

The differential diagnoses of genital dermatitis include all the conditions that present with erythema and scaling, such as psoriasis, tinea, perianal streptococcal dermatitis, pinworm infection, and even some cases of lichen sclerosus.

8.6 Lichen Sclerosus

Lichen sclerosus (LS) is a dermatosis of unknown origin and one of the most common vulvar ailments in girls. Its prevalence in childhood is about 1 in 900 [19]. LS was the second most frequent (18%) diagnosis in a series of 130 prepubescent girls who consulted for various vulvar symptoms [11]. Regardless, it has been found that from 5 to 15% of the cases of LS are diagnosed during childhood [20, 21]. While LS can occur at any age, it clearly predominates in premenarchal and postmenopausal women. Despite that remark, the association between estrogen metabolism and LS is not well understood [22].

8.7 Diagnosis and Clinical Characteristics

The average age of onset of LS symptoms is 5.0 years (ranging from 1 to 12), and the mean age at diagnosis is 6.7 (ranging from 3 to 14) [23]. The gap between the age of onset of symptoms and diagnosis is probably due to the lack of early diagnosis.

The most common symptom in girls is intractable pruritus. Other common presenting signs and symptoms are dysuria, subepithelial bruising, abrasions, and blisters that ultimately rupture and end up as with genital bleeding (Fig. 8.5) [7]. Dyschezia is one of the most common symptoms to be born in mind. It tends to be misdiagnosed as simple constipation, and as such, it is usually treated with laxatives and diet. Sclerosis of the perianal mucosa is important, causing an intensely painful defecation, as a result of the lack of compliance of the mucosa and the frequent fissures that occur in the area. Dysuria is also due to similar causes, since the cracks may burn at voiding.

These signs and symptoms differ from those observed in the adult, where there is predominance of pruritus and dyspareunia [24].

Clinically, LS is very similar in girls and adults, with a white lesion surrounding the vulva, perineum, and the perianal area [5] (Fig. 8.6). The skin should be scrutinized, since there may be small plaques of leukoplakia, or simply pale mucous membranes, cracks, bruising, telangiectasia, erosions, and more rarely, blood vesicles or blisters. Occasionally, signs of LS in girls can lead to misdiagnosis of sexual abuse. At any rate, we must not forget that unfortunately, these two situations may coexist [25].

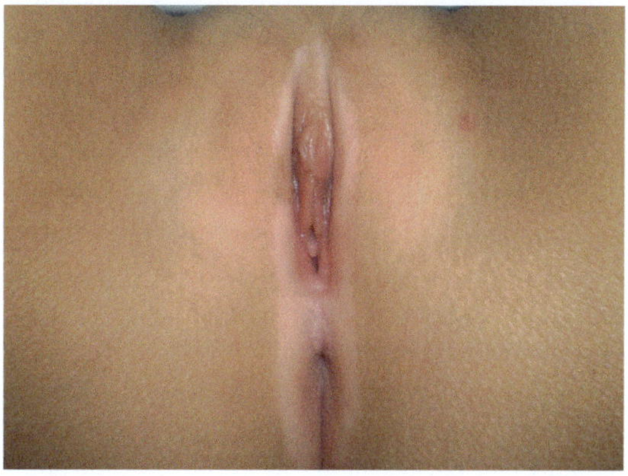

Fig. 8.6 Lichen sclerosus in an infant—a white lesion surrounding the vulva, perineum, and the perianal area

8.8 Course and Prognosis

In the past, it was believed that approximately two thirds of the cases of LS regress before or around menarche [26]. This has not been proven. Girls that do not show involution or regression of their LS may present with atrophy of the clitoris, with coalescence and fusion of the labia minora over the clitoris, which leads to the narrowing of the introitus. The reason why LS remits in some girls and progresses in others is unknown. After monitoring several girls, Powell and Wojnarowska concluded that actually LS only gets better in puberty, but without fully going away [19]. Although the risk of progression to malignancy in childhood is unknown, there are reports in adults claiming that the risk of turning into a squamous cell carcinoma ranges from 4% to 6% [27].

8.8.1 Therapy

There are various opinions concerning the treatment of LS, but as in adults, it is undisputed that ultra-powerful corticosteroids are the treatment of choice. The indicated corticosteroid is 0.05% clobetasol propionate.

Low or medium power corticosteroids reduce the symptoms, but the skin changes do not reverse [28, 29].

In the past, the therapy consisted of milder corticosteroid creams or even progesterone ointments. The clobetasol ointment causes the rapid reversion of symptoms, improving the hyperkeratosis, ecchymoses, and white plaques on the skin. This powerful corticosteroid should be kept from 2 weeks to 6 months, but it is suggested not to administer them daily beyond 3 months. Therapy can be started with two daily applications; the dosage is then tapered depending on the case. The ointment is always better tolerated on the skin, especially in childhood. To illustrate the amount of ointment to be applied each time, patients can be instructed to apply a small pearl the size of their fingertips. The treatment should often be extended to prolong the duration of the remission of LS [30]. No therapy protocols have been developed yet for girls, indicating the duration of long-term treatments; therefore, the duration should be guided by the clinical response and the family setting.

Some severe cases of LS that fail to respond to conventional treatments show a good response to low-dose (0.03%) tacrolimus ointment [31]. However, local discomfort has been observed in some cases, and the long-term treatment has not been substantiated for girls [32]. Finally, since the treatment of LS should be seen as long term at all ages, it is essential to establish an excellent relationship based on trust with both the child and her family—a relationship that should hopefully last at least until puberty.

8.9 Coalescence of the Labia Minora

This is a genital skin condition seen in girls, where the two labia minora get fused in different degrees (Fig. 8.7). Although some call it synechia or fusion of the labia minora, this term should be avoided, because the coalescence is a transient and reversible defect. In a recent study, Leung et al. report a peak incidence between the girl's 13th and 23rd months of age [33]. Overall it is asymptomatic and can be diagnosed by the girl's parents or by her physician during routine examination [34]. The incidence reported ranges from 0.6% to 3.0%, although the figures have

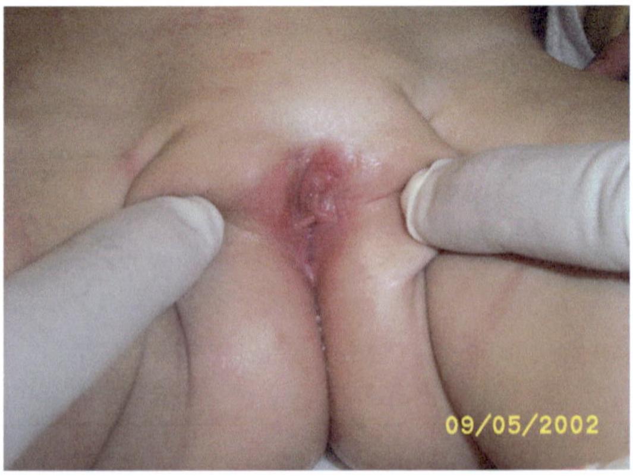

Fig. 8.7 The labia minora appear almost completely attached

been recently adjusted between 1.8% and 3.3% [33, 35]. Even when the etiology is unknown, it is a fact that it is favored by low estrogen levels, associated with local irritants. Thus, chronic irritation of the girl's vulva favors erosion; subsequently, during the healing process, epithelial bridges get formed, favoring the adhesion of the labia minora. This condition is not observed in newborn girls, as they are under the influence of their mothers' hormones. When untreated girls reach puberty, the increase in their natural estrogens leads to the spontaneous reversion of coalescence in 80% of the cases.

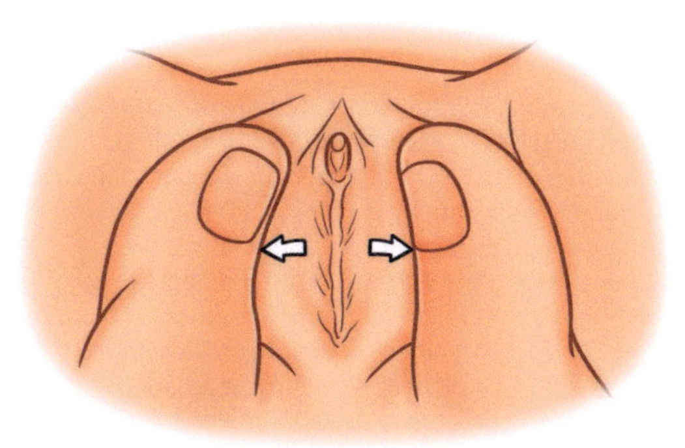

Fig. 8.8 Separating labial coalescence, under anesthesia, in cases where conservative therapy failed. Courtesy of Professor Jacob Bornstein

8.10 Diagnosis

Some patients may report difficulty urinating, or they may even be seen using Valsalva maneuvers to empty urine from the vagina. This creates discomfort, as reported by the patients themselves. Others may present leakage of urine by the genitalia, trickling out. It has been difficult to determine if this favors the occurrence of urinary tract infections. In addition, pelvic ultrasound examination should be done to rule out androgen insensitivity (testicular feminization syndrome) and urologic renal malformations.

8.10.1 Therapy

Topical estrogens would be indicated if during the follow-up the resolution failed to occur spontaneously at the expected time or if the girl's parents pressed to find a solution to the issue. Treatment consists of the topical application of estrogens in the mid raphe of the coalescence. Parents should be instructed to apply estriol or estradiol cream with a cotton swab twice a day, exerting a gentle pressure. While therapy should start with two applications a day, as treatment can be long, it will require a monthly check to establish the dosage, reducing the number of applications, depending on the response. Although some side effects may appear, such as irritation or pigmentation of the vulva, they disappear once the treatment is discontinued. If the pediatrician is not very happy about the results of the topical hormone therapy, separating the labia in the operating theater under anesthesia is the last resort (Fig. 8.8).

The Vulva in Childhood: Breaking the Myths

- Although in childhood the vulva is not usually exposed to intimate sexual relationships, it is more frequently bruised and injured because the girl's vulva is hairless and has very little subcutaneous fat.
- A lithotomy position is not required for the vulvar examination of a girl. Rather, a frog position, with the legs falling sideways and to the side, allows a view of the vulva and a part of the vagina. The addition of a Valsalva maneuver provides a nonaggressive and noninvasive sight of almost the entire vagina.
- Although regarded as an adult woman common condition, vulvovaginitis is one of the most common problems among girls, accounting for 80–90% of the gynecologic visits.
- Although candidiasis is common in adult women, it is very rare in girls. Furthermore, antifungal creams just worsen the underlying condition.
- HPV infections in many virgin girls are usually caused by in utero mother-to-child transmission.
- Leakage of urine is not always a sign of bladder condition. It may be caused by coalescence of the labia minora.

References

1. Kurman RJ. Blaustein's. Pathology of the female genital tract. 5th ed. New York: Springer; 2002.
2. Sanfillipo J, Muram D, Lee P, Dewhurst JC. Pediatric and adolescent gynecology. Philadelphia: WB Saunders; 2001. p. 187–9.
3. Yung-Weng W, Ying-Ju C. A preliminary study of bottom care effects on premature infants' heart rate and oxygen saturation. J Nurs Res. 2004;12(2):161–8.
4. Barclay L. Guidelines issued for gynecologic examination for adolescents in the pediatric office setting. Medscape medical news; 2010.
5. Caussade A. La patología vulvar en las niñas. Vulva y vagina. Diagnóstico y tratamiento. Montevideo: Bibliomédica ediciones; 2015. p. 319–39.
6. Singleton AF. Vaginal discharge in children and adolescents. Evolution and management: a review. Clin Pediatr. 1980;19:799–804.
7. Smith SD, Fischer GD. Childhood onset vulval lichen sclerosus does not resolve at puberty: a prospective case series. Pediatr Dermatol. 2009;26:725–9.
8. Krapf JM. Vulvovaginitis. Emedicine. Updated: Jan 19, 2018. https://emedicine.medscape.com/article/2188931-overview. Last accessed: 15 October 2018.
9. Fischer GO. Vulval disease in pre-pubertal girls. Australas J Dermatol. 2001;42:225–36.
10. Fischer G, Rogers M. Vulvar diseases in children: a clinical audit of 130 cases. Pediatr Dermatol. 2000;17:1–6.
11. Fischer G, Rogers M. Paediatric vulvovaginitis. In: Proceedings of the 3rd symposium on diseases of the vulva and vagina. Melbourne: Melbourne University; 1997. p. 26–9.
12. Caussade A. Condilomatosis vulvar en la niña. Vulva y vagina. Diagnóstico y tratamiento. Montevideo: Bibliomédica ediciones; 2015. p. 341–46.
13. Antonsson A, Karanfilovska S, Lindqvist PG, Hansson BG. General acquisition of human papillomavirus infections of skin occurs in early infancy. J Clin Microbiol. 2003;41:2509–14.
14. Syrjanen S. Current concepts on human papillomavirus infections in children. APMIS. 2010;118:494–509.
15. Medeiros LR, Ethur AB, Hilgert JB, Zanini RR, Berwanger O. Bozzetti MCl, et al. vertical transmission of the human papillomavirus: a systematic quantitative review. Cad Saude Publica. 2005;21:1006–15.
16. Rintala MA, Grenman SE, Puranen MH, Isolauri E, Ekblad U, Kero PO, et al. Transmission of high-risk human papillomavirus (HPV) between parents and infant: a prospective study of HPV in families in Finland. J Clin Microbiol. 2005;43:376–81.
17. Syrjanen S. HPV infections in children. Invited review. Papillomavirus Rep. 2003;14:93–110.
18. Atherton DJ. The aetiology and management of irritant diaper dermatitis. J Eur Acad Dermatol Venereol. 2001;15(Suppl. 1):1–4.
19. Powell JJ, Wojnarowska F. Childhood vulvar lichen sclerosus: an increasingly common problem. J Am Acad Dermatol. 2001;44:803–6.
20. Berth-Jones J, Graham-Brown RAC, Burns DA. Lichen sclerosus et atrophicus: a review of 15 cases in young girls. Clin Exp Dermatol. 1991;16:14–7.
21. Meyrick Thomas RH, Ridley CM, McGibbon DH, Black MM. Anogenital lichen sclerosus in women. J R Soc Med. 1996;89:694–8.
22. Funaro D. Lichen sclerosus: a review and practical approach. Dermatol Ther. 2004;17:28–37.
23. Poindexter G, Morrell D. Anogenital pruritus: lichen sclerosus in children. Pediatr Ann. 2007;36:785–91.
24. Maronn ML, Esterly NB. Constipation as a feature of anogenital lichen sclerosus in children. Pediatrics. 2005;115:230–2.
25. Priestley BL, Bleehen SS. Lichen sclerosus et atrophicus in children misdiagnosed as sexual abuse. Br Med J. 1987;295:211.
26. Goodfield MJD, Jones SK, Veale DJ. The connective tissue diseases. In: Burns T, Breathnach S, Cox N, Griffiths C, editors. Rook's textbook of dermatology. 7th ed. Massachusetts: Blacwell Publishing Company; 2004. p. 56.119–25.
27. Heymann WR. Lichen sclerosus. J Am Acad Dermatol. 2007;56:683–4.
28. Serrano G, Millan F, Fortea JM, Grau M, Aliaga A. Topical progesterone as a treatment of choice in genital lichen sclerosus et atrophicus in children. Pediatr Dermatol. 1993;10:201.
29. Torok E, Orley J, Goracz G, Daroczy J. Lichen sclerosus et atrophicus in children: clinical and pathological analysis of 33 cases. Mod Probl Paediatr. 1975;17:262–71.
30. Bradford J, Fischer G. Long-term management of vulval lichen sclerosus in adult women. Aust N Z J Obstet Gynecol. 2010;50(2):148–52.
31. Matsumoto Y, Yamamoto T, Isobe T, Kusunoki T, Tsuboi R. Successful treatment of vulvar lichen sclerosus in a child with low-concentration topical tacrolimus ointment. J Dermatol. 2007;34:114–6.
32. Assmann T, Becker-Wegerich P, Grewe M, Megahed M, Ruzicka T. Tacrolimus ointment for the treatment of vulvar lichen sclerosus. J Am Acad Dermatol. 2003;48:935–7.
33. Leung AK, Robson WL, Tay-Uyboco J. The incidence of labial fusion in children. J Paediatr Child Health. 1993;29:235–6.
34. Gaudens DA, Moh-Ello N, Fiogbe M, et al. Labial fusion in the paediatric surgery department of Yopougon University hospital (cote d'Ivoire): 108 cases. Sante. 2008;18(1):35–8.
35. Capraro VJ, Greenberg H. Adhesions of the labia minora. Obstet Gynecol. 1972;39:65–9.

9 The Vulva in Pregnancy and Delivery

Maya Wolf

The pregnant woman undergoes profound anatomic and physiologic changes in almost every organ system. These adaptations to the pregnant state begin just after conception and evolve through delivery, after which they almost completely revert back to the nonpregnant state over a period of weeks. Pregnancy may be associated with changes resulting in many common symptoms and signs of pregnancy. The changes include general symptoms such as amenorrhea, weight gain, sleep alterations, fatigue, and other changes that are more specific to various physiologic systems/organs [1]. These symptoms are usually self-limited and can be treated to provide relief.

Skin changes may include linea nigra, stretch marks, chloasma, and various vascular changes [2]. It may also include hyperpigmentation—darkening of linea alba (linea nigra), axillae, areola, perineum, and inner thighs due to melanocytic stimulation by estrogen and progesterone [3].

Pruritus in pregnant women may be physiologic, related to a flare of disorder present prior to conception, or related to pregnancy-specific dermatoses. Pruritus without any underlying pathologic process affects up to 20% of pregnant woman. Common pruritic locations are the scalp, anus, vulva, and, during the third trimester, the abdominal skin. Patients with more generalized pruritus should be evaluated for intrahepatic cholestasis of pregnancy [2].

Skin vascular changes attributed to physiologic changes in estrogen and increased blood volume include spider telangiectasias, palmar erythema, and non-pitting edema. Vulvar, saphenous, or hemorrhoidal varicosities are reported in about 40% of pregnant women.

9.1 Vulvar Varicose Veins (Figs. 9.1 and 9.2)

Reported incidence is 8% of pregnant women and up to 23% of pregnant women with varicose veins. Although rare in nonpregnant women, in pregnancy it may appear as lobulated, purplish-colored lesions involving the labia majora. Symptoms include tenderness and discomfort during sexual intercourse. The etiology is partly hemodynamic, due to increased blood volume and venous pressure in femoral and pelvic vessels from the enlarging uterus. Genetic predisposition also plays a role. Vulvar varicose veins may persist or worsen in subsequent pregnancies and cannot be prevented [4]. Jacquemier's sign refers to venous distention in the vestibule and vagina and is associated with vulvar varicosities, which are particularly difficult to treat [5]. They usually regress, at least partially, postpartum. During pregnancy, they are managed conservatively by vulvar support and compression and by avoiding prolonged standing.

M. Wolf (✉)
Maternal-Fetal Unit, Department of Obstetrics and Gynecology, Galilee Medical Center, Azrieli Faculty of Medicine, Bar-Ilan University, Nahariya, Israel
e-mail: MayaW@gmc.gov.il

J. Bornstein (ed.), *Vulvar Disease*, https://doi.org/10.1007/978-3-319-61621-6_9

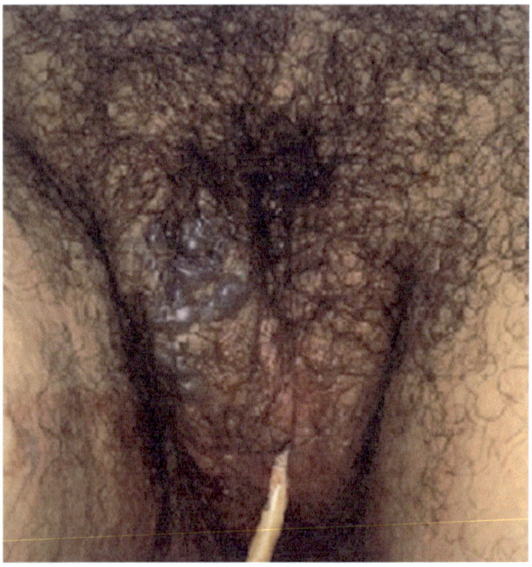

Fig. 9.1 Vulvar large varicosities during pregnancy covering the labia majora, spreading to the thighs (Courtesy of Professor Jacob Bornstein)

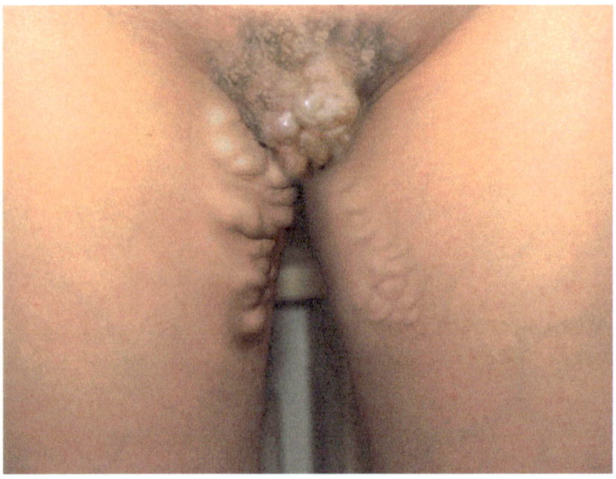

Fig. 9.2 Vulvar varicose veins postpartum, covering the mons pubis and labia majora

9.1.1 Pelvic Symptoms and Signs

1. Congestion and bluish discoloration of the vagina (Chadwick sign) in early first trimester due to increased blood flow [3] and bluish discoloration of the cervix (Goodell sign) [3] and softening of cervix (Hegar sign).
2. Round ligament pain, sharp groin pains caused by spasm of the round ligament associated with movement, is common in pregnancy; incidence increases as pregnancy progresses. The clinical presentation may be diverse from pelvic and low back pain, mostly on the right side, to severe sharp pain with ligament spasms or debilitating pain that affects daily living activities [5]. Modification of activity with gradual rising and sitting down and avoidance of sudden movement will decrease this type of pain.
3. Pelvic girdle pain refers to pregnancy-related pain in the lumbosacral, sacroiliac, and symphysis pubis joints; reported prevalence is 22% with 5% reporting severe symptoms and disability [6]. Pelvic girdle pain resolves in 99% of pregnancies by 12 weeks after delivery regardless of treatment.
4. Symphysis pubis diastasis, separation of the pubic symphysis that may have long-term consequences, usually occurs late in pregnancy or during delivery [7]. Radiographic signs of pubic symphysis separation of above 10–13 mm represent a subdislocation, and separation of above >14 mm indicates damage to the sacroiliac joint [8].
5. In general, pelvic pain may be managed by some lifestyle modifications such as bed rest during painful periods or by exercise and acetaminophen and nonsteroidal anti-inflammatory drugs (NSAIDs) (avoid during third trimester, since chronic use may lead to oligohydramnios and constriction of the fetal ductus arteriosus) [8].

9.2 Genital Herpes in Pregnancy (See Also Chap. 42)

Herpes genitalis is one of the most common sexually transmitted diseases. HSV is a member of the *Herpesviridae* family of viruses. It contains a double-stranded linear deoxyribonucleic acid (DNA) genome [9] and an envelope. Like all *Herpesviridae* viruses, HSV shares the biological properties of latency and reactivation, which causes recurrent infections in the host. HSV enters the human host through inoculation of oral, genital, or conjunctival mucosa or breaks in the skin, infects the sensory nerve endings, and then transports via retrograde axonal flow to the dorsal root ganglia, where it remains for the life of the host. The fetus may be infected through retrograde spread through ruptured or even seemingly intact membranes and rarely transplacentally [9]. Latent virus is not susceptible to antiviral drugs, and infection (even after antiviral therapy) is lifelong. Clinical findings are similar in pregnant and nonpregnant women. The classical presentation of primary herpes simplex virus (HSV)-1 or HSV-2 genital infection is characterized by bilateral clusters of erythematous papules and vesicles on external genitalia (Fig. 9.3), usually 2–14 days after sexual exposure, after which they rupture and become ulcers (Fig. 9.4). Although primary infection can be severe, with painful genital ulcers, pruritus, dysuria, urinary retention, fever, and tender inguinal lymphadenopathy, most patients have only mild symptoms or remain asymptomatic. Cases of recurrence vary in frequency and intensity; usually there are mild symptoms and few lesions or no symptoms at all. In patients who develop lesions, prodromal symptoms (pruritus, burning, or pain) may occur before the lesions are visible. Clinical diagnosis should be confirmed with laboratory tests. Swab from the base of the genital lesion can be tested by viral culture, HSV antigen detection, and polymerase chain reaction (PCR) of HSV DNA. During pregnancy, the major concern of maternal HSV infection is transmission to the fetus, as neonatal infection can result in serious morbidity and mortality and leaves many survivors with permanent sequelae [10, 11]. Transmission of herpes simplex virus (HSV) to neonates usually occurs during labor and delivery as a result of direct contact with virus shed from infected sites (vulva, vagina, cervix, perianal area). Viral shedding can occur when maternal symptoms and lesions are absent [12]. The concentration and duration of viral shedding are higher with primary versus nonprimary disease and in HSV-2 versus HSV-1 infection [12]. Therapy should always be offered to patients with primary or first-episode genital nonprimary infection and may be indicated for recurrent infection for symptomatic relief [13]. Treatment decreases the risks of severe or prolonged symptoms and a complicated infection in the mother. In addition, prophylactic acyclovir therapy decreases the incidence of HSV shedding and reduces the number of cesarean deliveries; therefore it should be added at ≥36 weeks of gestation to women with active recurrent genital herpes during pregnancy [14]. A systematic review of

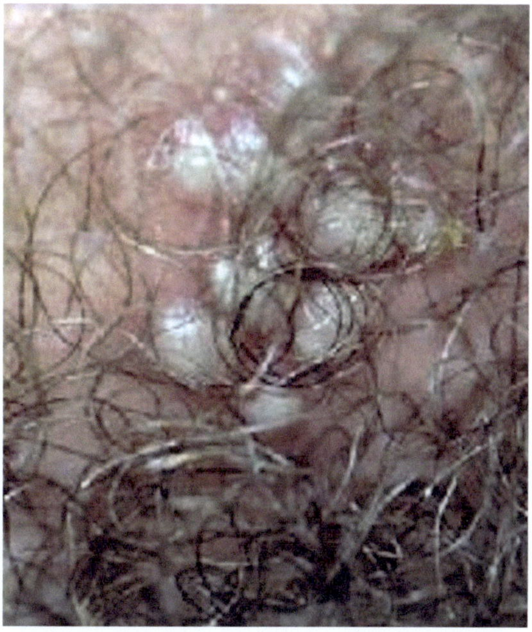

Fig. 9.3 Primary herpes genitalis in pregnancy: vesicles covering the mons pubis (Courtesy of Professor Jacob Bornstein)

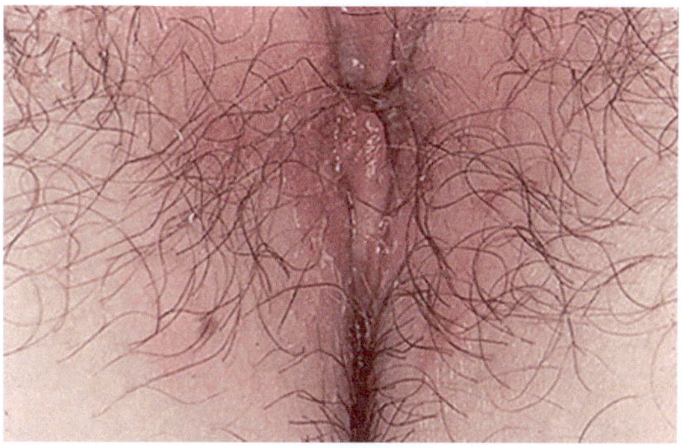

Fig. 9.4 Recurrent herpes genitalis during pregnancy: the erosive lesions are hardly depicted and usually mistaken for vulvovaginal candidiasis (Courtesy of Professor Jacob Bornstein)

randomized controlled trials assessed the effectiveness of acyclovir suppression therapy. The risk of recurrence at delivery was reduced by 75%, and the rate of cesarean delivery for recurrent genital herpes was reduced by 40% for women who received suppression therapy after 36 weeks of gestation [14]. The CDC recommendation for suppression therapy with acyclovir is 400 mg orally, three times daily from 36 weeks of estimated gestational age until delivery. Cesarean delivery for herpes simplex virus (HSV) is indicated only for women with a history of HSV infection with active genital lesions, or prodromal symptoms, such as vulvar pain or burning at delivery [15].

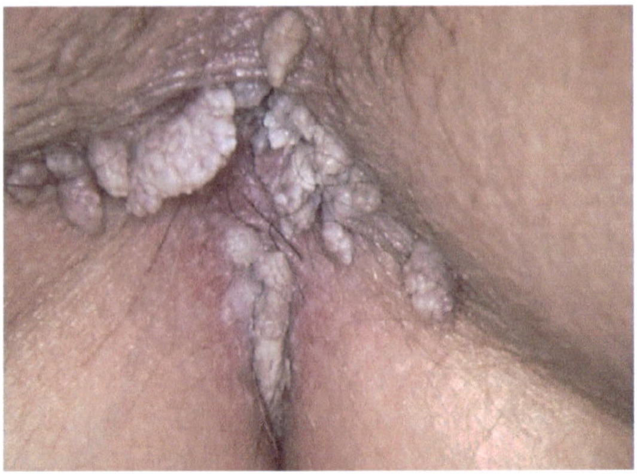

Fig. 9.5 Condylomata acuminata in pregnancy—lesions spread quickly and cover the perineum (Courtesy of Professor Jacob Bornstein)

9.3 Condylomata Acuminata (Anogenital Warts)

Condyloma acuminatum, commonly referred to as anogenital warts, is a proliferation of anogenital skin and mucosa in response to infection by human papillomavirus (HPV). An estimated 500,000 to 1 million new cases of genital warts are reported in the United States annually, and about 80% of cases are reported to occur in patients aged 17–33 years [16].

The types of HPV that cause genital warts are different from those that cause anogenital cancers. HPV-6/11 are low malignant risk subtypes and cause 90% of genital warts [17]. Lesions are usually located within the epithelium of the anogenital tract on the external genitalia [18] (Fig. 9.5). Although treatment can eradicate the warts, disease recurrence is common and occurs in 20–30% of patients overall. Lesions are usually asymptomatic, often characterized by large clusters of lesions on external genitalia, usually 2–3 months after initial exposure.

The diagnosis is usually made by history and visual inspection of characteristic skin lesions during clinical exam without any need for testing.

In pregnant women rapid worsening of anogenital warts was reported presumably due to pregnancy-associated decreased cell-mediated immunity, which may cause worsening of viral infection.

Indications for treatment of anogenital warts in pregnant women are similar to those for nonpregnant women: symptoms like pruritus, burning, vaginal discharge, pain, bleeding, obstruction of the vagina, dyspareunia, or psychologic distress [18, 19]. Treatment options are limited in pregnancy because podophyllin, podophyllotoxin, interferon, and 5-FU are all contraindicated because of potential fetal harm. Trichloroacetic acid has no systemic absorption and no known fetal effects [20]. Laser ablation in pregnancy for bulky or obstructive lesions has been described, with good success rates [21]. HPV and anogenital warts in pregnancy have been linked with juvenile-onset respiratory papillomatosis with an estimated rate of transmission of 7 per 1000 affected women [22]. A few reports that elective cesarean delivery failed to prevent transmission of HPV made the past indication for elective cesarean section in that indication controversial [23]. In addition, lesions that potentially obstruct the birth canal (vagina and perineum) should be treated to avoid complications during vaginal birth although treatment may not reduce the risk of vertical transmission [23]. Therefore, cesarean delivery is indicated if vulvar or vaginal warts obstruct the birth canal, as the lesions may hemorrhage or cause dystocia during an attempted vaginal delivery.

9.4 Episiotomy and Perineal Laceration

Perineal lacerations, either spontaneous or with episiotomy, are the most common complication of vaginal deliveries. Episiotomy is usually performed when the perineum is distended, just prior to the crowning of the fetal head in purpose to increase the diameter of pelvic outlet, facilitating delivery, and reduce the time for expulsion of the infant. The mediolateral episiotomy is more commonly employed in Europe. The incision is initiated at the fourchette and cut at an angle almost perpendicular to the midline (80–90°) (Fig. 9.6). The median episiotomy is the more commonly used technique in the United States. A vertical incision is begun at the fourchette and extended caudally in the midline. The anatomical structures involved in the incision include the vaginal epithelium, perineal body, and the junction of the perineal body with the bulbocavernosus muscle in the perineum. It is typically easier to repair than a mediolateral episiotomy or a spontaneous vaginal/perineal laceration and yields a better cosmetic result [24]. The prevalence of episiotomy varies by geographic region. In the United States, changing trends in obstetrical practice have influenced the decision to perform an episiotomy and resulted in a continued drop in episiotomy rates from 61% in 1979 to 12% in 2012 [25]. A first-degree tear/laceration is defined as a superficial tear confined to the epithelial layer of the perineum and vaginal epithelium only. The perineal muscles remain intact. It may or may not need to be repaired depending on the amount of bleeding. Second-degree laceration extends into the perineal body: fascia and the deep and superficial transverse perineal muscles and fibers of the pubococcygeus and bulbocavernosus muscles. Third-degree laceration involves superficial or deep injury to the external anal sphincter, and it is subdivided to the following: (a) <50% of external anal sphincter thickness is torn, (b) >50% of external anal sphincter thickness is torn, and (c) complete rupture of the external anal sphincter and in addition the internal anal sphincter is torn, whereas a fourth-degree tear extends completely through the sphincter and the rectal mucosa [26]. Routine mediolateral episiotomy in primigravida is associated with a higher prevalence of obstetrical anal sphincter injuries [27]. The most common complications of episiotomy are bleeding, infection, dehiscence, and extension. Bleeding can usually be controlled with pressure or sutures, although a hematoma may occasionally develop.

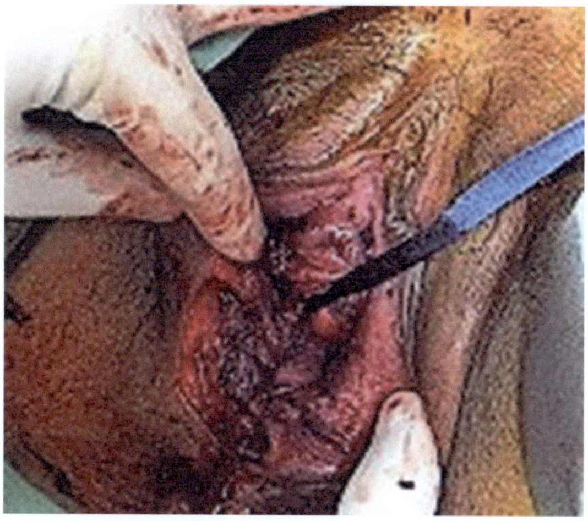

Fig. 9.6 Mediolateral episiotomy incision

Guidelines and surgical technique for episiotomy repair (Figs. 9.5, 9.6, and 9.7):

- Good exposure by a retractor or vaginal pack (to prevent uterine bleeding in the surgical field).
- Third- or fourth-degree tears should be repaired first in order to restore the continuity of the external and internal anal sphincters and to obtain an anatomically and functionally correct anal canal. The repair consists of a multilayer closure.
- The repair begins at the apex of the vaginal laceration and ends just above the level of the posterior fourchette.
- There is no clear evidence favoring overlap technique over end-to-end sphincter repair technique.
- The vagina, perineal muscles, and skin are sutured by continuous non-locking suture techniques.

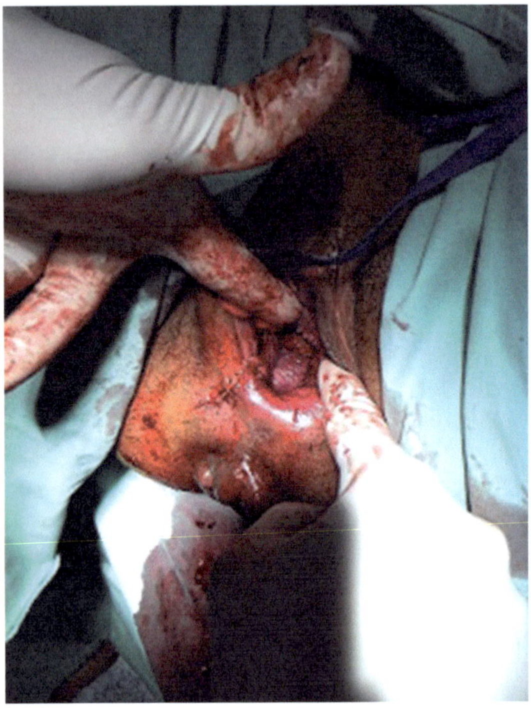

Fig. 9.7 Repair of mediolateral episiotomy

The Vulva in Pregnancy: Episiotomy, Breaking the Myths

- Although performing routine mediolateral episiotomy in primigravida was thought to protect the perineum from rupture and future pelvic floor dysfunction, it is actually associated with a higher prevalence of obstetrical anal sphincter injuries.
- The overlap technique for repairing anal sphincter rupture was considered to have better outcome. However, there is no clear evidence favoring it over the end-to-end sphincter repair technique.

References

1. Facco FL, Kramer J, Ho KH, Zee PC, Grobman WA. Sleep disturbances in pregnancy. Obstet Gynecol. 2010;115(1):77–83.
2. Rimoin LP, Kwatra SG, Yosipovitch G. Female-specific pruritus from childhood to postmenopause: clinical features, hormonal factors, and treatment considerations. Dermatol Ther. 2013;26(2):157–67.
3. Tunzi M, Gray GR. Common skin conditions during pregnancy. Am Fam Physician. 2007;75(2):211–8.
4. Verma SB. Varicosities of vulva (vulvar varices): a seldom seen entity in dermatologic practice. Int J Dermatol. 2012;51(1):123.
5. Martin AG, Leal-Khouri S. Physiologic skin changes associated with pregnancy. Int J Dermatol. 1992;31:375.
6. Huancahuari N. Emergencies in early pregnancy. Emerg Med Clin North Am. 2012;30(4):837.
7. Keriakos R, Bhatta SR, Morris F, Mason S, Buckley S. Pelvic girdle pain during pregnancy and puerperium. J Obstet Gynaecol. 2011;31(7):572.
8. Henry L. Chiropractic management of postpartum pubic symphysis diastasis: a case report. J Can Chiropr Assoc. 2015;59(1):30.
9. Kimberlin DW. Neonatal herpes simplex infection. Clin Microbiol Rev. 2004;17:1.
10. Roberts S. Herpes simplex virus: incidence of neonatal herpes simplex virus, maternal screening, management during pregnancy, and HIV. Curr Opin Obstet Gynecol. 2009;21:124.
11. Mahnert N, Roberts SW, Laibl VR, et al. The incidence of neonatal herpes infection. Am J Obstet Gynecol. 2007;196:e55.
12. Wald A, Zeh J, Selke S, et al. Reactivation of genital herpes simplex virus type 2 infection in asymptomatic seropositive persons. N Engl J Med. 2000;342:844.
13. http://www.cdc.gov/std/treatment/2010/. Accessed 28 Feb 2013.
14. ACOG Committee on Practice Bulletins. ACOG Practice Bulletin. Clinical management guidelines for obstetrician-gynecologists. No. 82 June 2007. Management of herpes in pregnancy. Obstet Gynecol. 2007;109:1489.
15. Workowski KA, Bolan GA, Centers for Disease Control and Prevention. Sexually transmitted diseases treatment guidelines. MMWR Recomm Rep. 2015;64:1.
16. Patel H, Wagner M, Singhal P, Kothari S. Systematic review of the incidence and prevalence of genital warts. BMC Infect Dis. 2013;13(1):39.
17. Aubin F, Prétet JL, Jacquard AC, et al. Human papillomavirus genotype distribution in external acuminata condylomata: a Large French National Study (EDiTH IV). Clin Infect Dis. 2008;47:610.
18. Steben M, LaBelle D. Genital warts: Canadians' perception, health-related behaviors, and treatment preferences. J Low Genit Tract Dis. 2012;16:409.
19. Manhart LE, Koutsky LA. Do condoms prevent genital HPV infection, external genital warts, or cervical neoplasia ? A meta-analysis. Sex Transm Dis. 2002;29:725.
20. Ferenczy A. HPV-associated lesions in pregnancy and their clinical implications. Clin Obstet Gynecol. 1989;32:191.
21. Arena S, Marconi M, Frega A, Villani C. Pregnancy and condyloma. Evaluation about therapeutic effec-

tiveness of laser CO_2 on 115 pregnant women. Minerva Ginecol. 2001;53:389.
22. Silverberg MJ, Thorsen P, Lindeberg H, et al. Condyloma in pregnancy is strongly predictive of juvenile-onset recurrent respiratory papillomatosis. Obstet Gynecol. 2003;101:645.
23. Patsner B, Baker DA, Orr JW Jr. Human papillomavirus genital tract infections during pregnancy. Clin Obstet Gynecol. 1990;33:258.
24. Coats PM, Chan KK, Wilkins M, Beard RJ. A comparison between midline and mediolateral episiotomies. Br J Obstet Gynaecol. 1980;87:408.
25. Friedman AM, Ananth CV, Prendergast E, et al. Variation in and factors associated with use of episiotomy. JAMA. 2015;313:197.
26. Gabbe SG, Niebyl JR, Simpson JL, Landon MB, Galan HL, Jauniaux ERM, Driscoll DA. Obstetrics—normal and problem pregnancies. 6th ed. Philadelphia: Elsevier; 2012.
27. Sulaiman AS, Ahmad S, Ismail NA, Rahman RA, Jamil MA, Mohd Dali AZ. A randomized control trial evaluating the prevalence of obstetrical anal sphincter injuries in primigravida in routine versus selective mediolateral episiotomy. Saudi Med J. 2013;34(8):819–23.

10 Vulvar Cosmetics

Claudia Marchitelli

10.1 Introduction

Over the past decade, there has been a great surge in aesthetic vulvovaginal surgery [1]. Publicity and media coverage [2] have placed these procedures in the public eye. This massive influx of information has led to several developments; on one hand, women have begun to observe their genitals in detail and compare them to those of other women, either through online searches or magazines, raising consciousness. On the other hand, this awareness has also given way to a misleading belief, which is that there is such thing as an "adequate vaginal design" or the "perfect vulva or vagina" [3]. This erroneous concept has encouraged many women to consult their gynecologist in search of a solution for a technically inexistent problem.

One controversial issue regarding these practices is the standardization of their names and indications. This is important, because many physicians around the world use different names for these procedures, frequently based more on marketing than science, which makes them appear novel, when in fact they are traditional gynecologic procedures which should *not* be labeled as new cosmetic practices. The creation of registered trademarks and a business model based on this area of gynecologic practice not only interferes with medical knowledge but is also ethically quite questionable and leads to a generalized understatement of the techniques, which following the correct indication and with adequate patient information are a very useful tool in the gynecologist or plastic surgeon's practice.

Another issue that leads to great discussion is whether or not these practices increase sexual pleasure. This erroneous belief arises from the way that some practitioners publicize vulvar and vaginal aesthetic surgery, which lead women to associating the procedures with better orgasms or greater sexual pleasure. However, there is no scientific, evidence-based proof to support the use of these surgeries to that end. These surgeries are strictly anatomical and are not oriented toward vulvar physiology and therefore do not guarantee sexual improvement. However, it must be taken into consideration that for some women, a change in the vulvar or vaginal anatomy may lead to improvement of self-confidence, increasing comfort and self-acceptance. This may impact psychologically on the patient, allowing her to enjoy sexual intercourse from a different viewpoint, free from embarrassment, inhibitions, and self-consciousness.

C. Marchitelli (✉)
Unit of Vulvar Diseases, Hospital Italiano de Buenos Aires, Buenos Aires, Argentina

School of Medicine, Instituto Universitario, Hospital Italiano of Buenos Aires, Buenos Aires, Argentina

ISSVD (International Society for the Study of Vulvovaginal Diseases), Waxhaw, NC, USA

J. Bornstein (ed.), *Vulvar Disease*, https://doi.org/10.1007/978-3-319-61621-6_10

It is because of all of these reasons, it is highly recommended that all patients have a thorough preoperative consult, oriented toward the issues that motivate the surgery. If the problem is functional (anorgasm, lack of sexual pleasure, partner discomfort, etc.), it is important not to perform the surgery and to focus instead on working with the patient on her sexuality, by a professional who specializes in the area. There is no such thing as a "standard vulva" [4], and there is no definition for "beauty" when referring to the vulvovaginal area, since there are many variations in vulvar anatomy. Because of this, it is essential for the surgeon to clearly explain to the patient the extent and expected goals of the surgery, and these should be documented clearly in the informed consent form.

10.2 Aesthetic Vulvovaginal Surgeries

10.2.1 Labia Minora Labiaplasty (Labia Minora Reduction Surgery)

This surgery is indicated in cases of hypertrophy of the labia minora (Fig. 10.1a–f). It is difficult to define when a patient has hypertrophic labia, since there is no standard vulvar size nor accepted proportions between vulvar components predefined. There are many variations of vulvar anatomy [4].

In addition, women are being misled or are confused about what is normal. They must know that there is not a "one-size" normal vulva, that

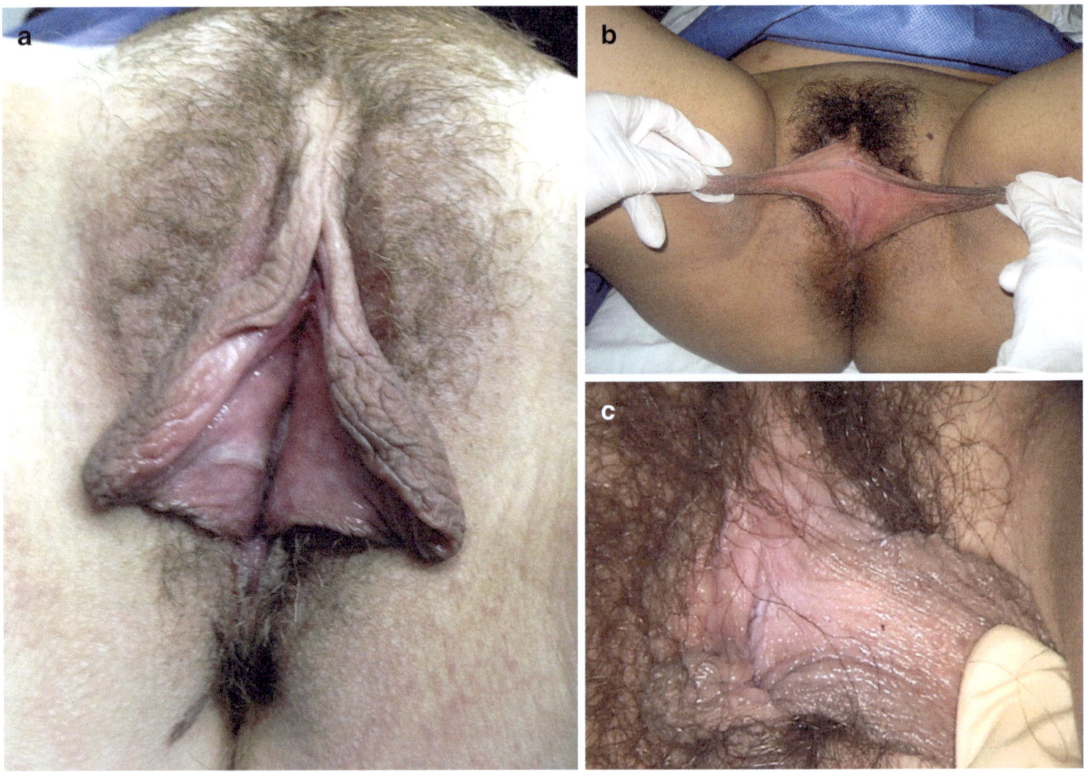

Fig. 10.1 (**a**) A 30-year-old patient with hypertrophic labia minora. (**b**) A 22-year-old patient with hypertrophic labia minora. (**c**) A 25-year-old patient with asymmetry due to unilateral hypertrophic labia minora. (**d**) A 21-year-old patient with asymmetry due to unilateral hypertrophic labia minora. (**e**) A 28-year-old patient with asymmetry due to unilateral atrophic labium minor. (**f**) A 31-year-old patient with hypertrophic labia minora

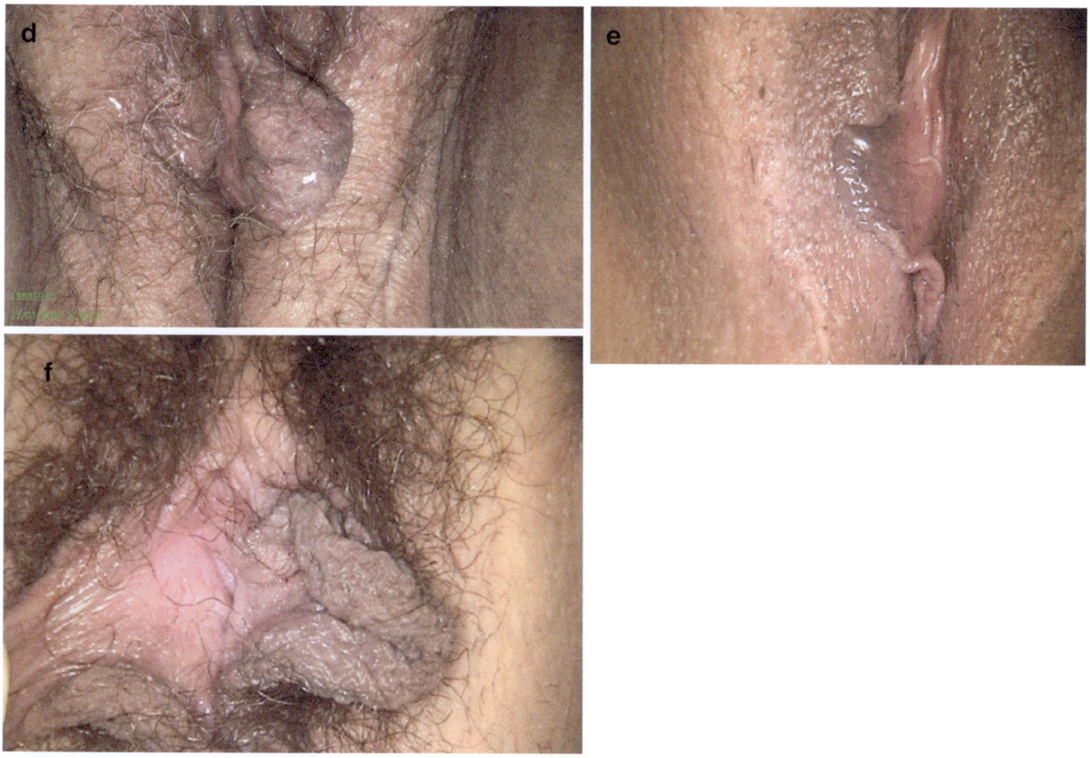

Fig. 10.1 (continued)

there is a great variety in appearance among women, and that there is no evidence that a certain size or shape is better than another.

Several studies have shown the extent to which the exposure to images of the so-called perfect vulva/vagina may lead to the development of unrealistic concepts of "normal genitalia" based on the uniform morphology.

10.2.1.1 Labiaplasty Surgical Techniques

Labiaplasty is usually an outpatient procedure. There is currently no consensus regarding which is the best technique to perform this surgery.

Free Edge Resection Technique (Fig. 10.2)
In this technique, the free edges of both labia minora are excised by an elliptic incision, always attempting to maintain and respect the vulvar anatomy. It is most useful in those patients who do not desire to keep the hyperpigmented labial edge (Fig. 10.3a, b).

Wedge Resection and Reconstruction from the Remaining Flaps (Fig. 10.4)
The original technique, described by Alter [5], consists of a wedge-shaped resection of the inferior half of the labia and reconstruction with the remaining superior segment. The point of this technique is to hide the incisions and preserve the labia's natural pigmented border (Fig. 10.5a, b).

Inferior Pedicle Resection and Reconstruction with Superior Pedicle Flap (Fig. 10.4)
Rouzer et al. [6] proposed a modified version of the previous technique. They describe a "v"-shaped resection of the inferior part of the labia. As in the previous surgery, the color of the labia's free edge is preserved (Fig. 10.6a, b).

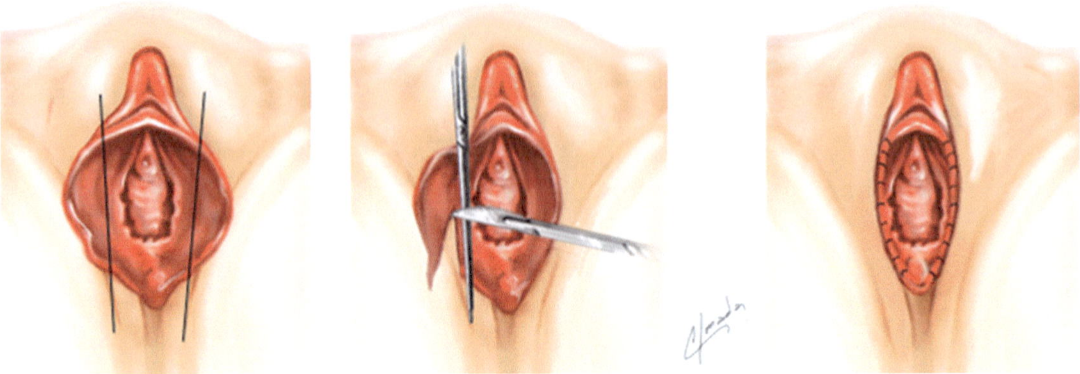

Fig. 10.2 Free edge resection technique of hypertrophic labia minora

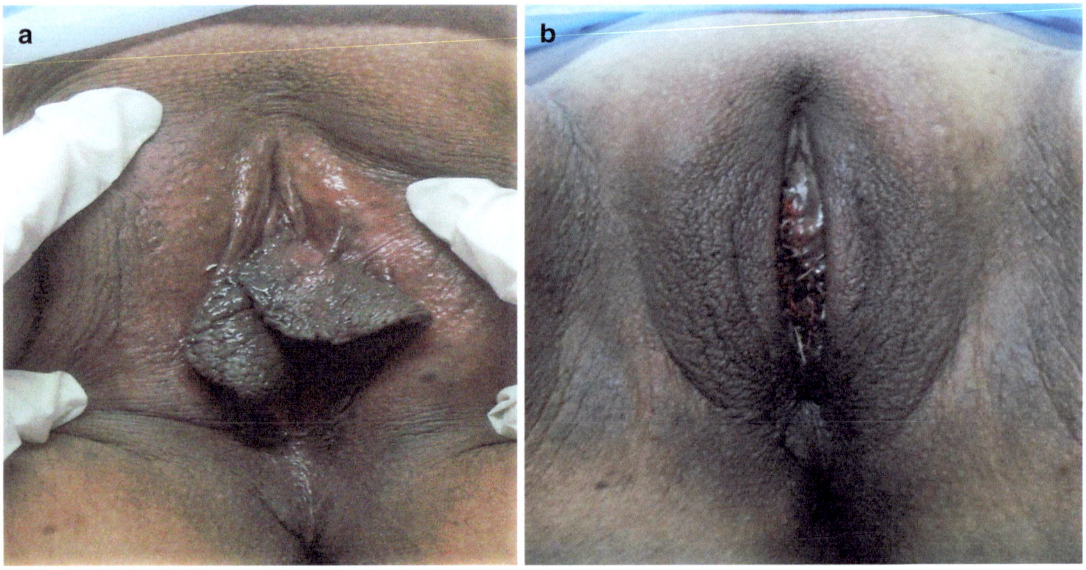

Fig. 10.3 (**a**) Free edge resection technique of hypertrophic labia minora—before surgery. (**b**) Hypertrophic labia minora immediately post-op. Resection of the free border. The longitudinal suture can be seen following the length of the labia minora

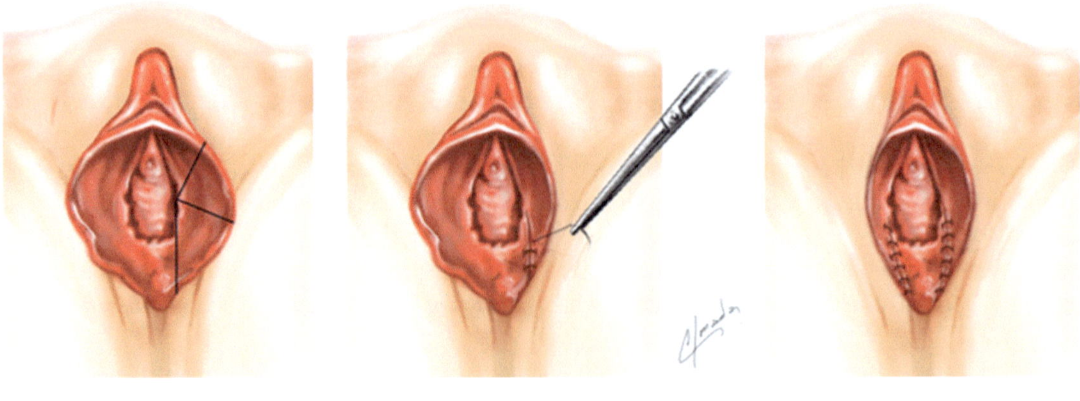

Fig. 10.4 Wedge resection technique of hypertrophic labia minora and inferior pedicle and reconstruction with superior pedicle flap technique

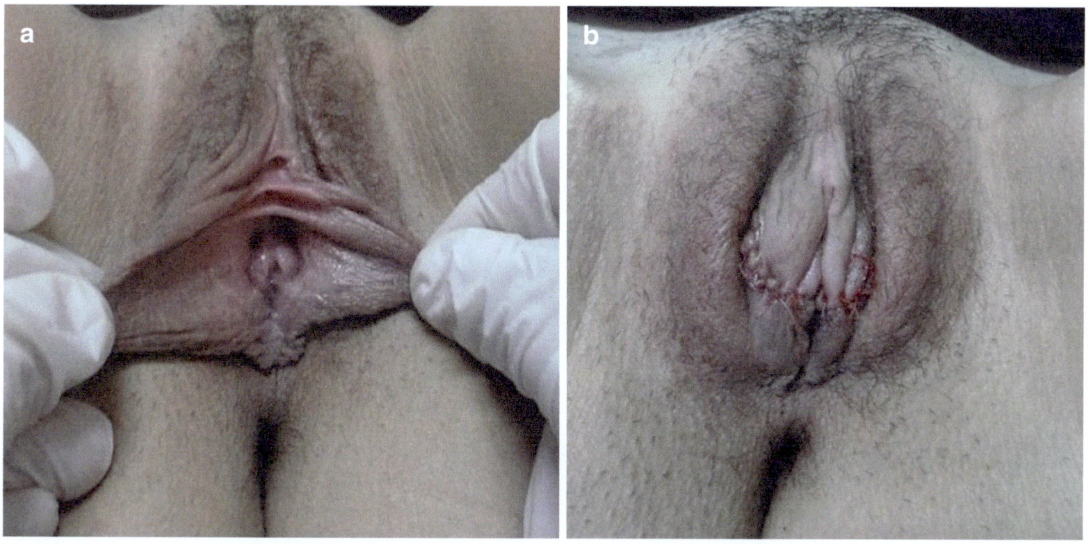

Fig. 10.5 (**a**) Wedge resection technique of hypertrophic labia minora before surgery. (**b**) Hypertrophic labia minora -immediate post-op. The horizontal suture can be appreciated through the midsection of each labia, conserving the free edge

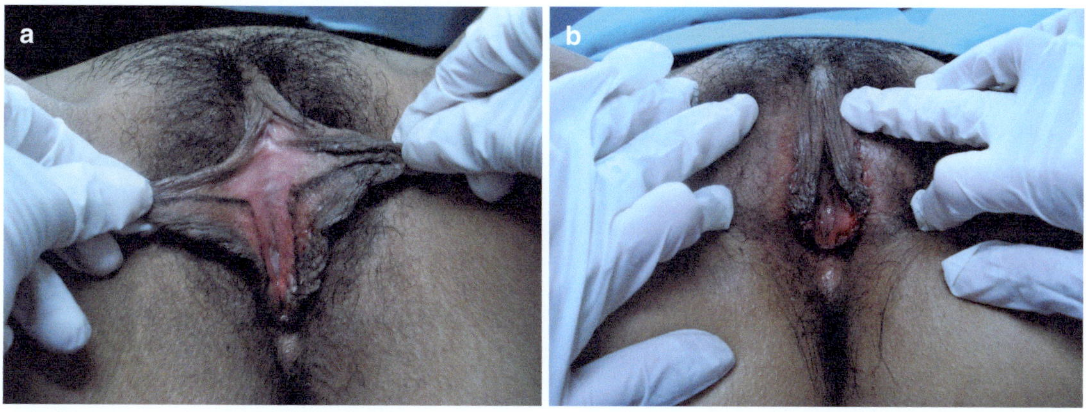

Fig. 10.6 (**a**) Hypertrophic labia minora surgery—inferior pedicle and reconstruction with superior pedicle flap technique. Before surgery. Demarcation of the area that will be incised. (**b**) Immediate post-op of hypertrophic labia minora surgery. Sutured pedicle. The free border of the labia minora is conserved

Central Wedge Resection Technique with 90° Z-Plasty (Fig. 10.7)

Two 90° Z-plasties are drawn facing each other on the internal and external surface of the labia minora. These "Z"s converge from the free edge of the midsection of the labia to a common origin at the base of each labia (pointing toward the ventral zone of the introital meatus). This outlines the irregular shape of the wedge, which is then removed. Finally the edges of the resection are sutured directly with interrupted stitches with 4.0 Vicryl® [7].

CO_2 Laser Technique

Any of the aforementioned techniques can be performed with a carbon dioxide laser. In this case the laser must be set at scalpel mode to incise at the same time that it coagulates.

10.2.1.2 Complications (Table 10.1)

Possible complications of these surgeries are hematomas, wound dehiscence or infection, vulvar edema, necrosis, sensory alterations, and dyspareunia.

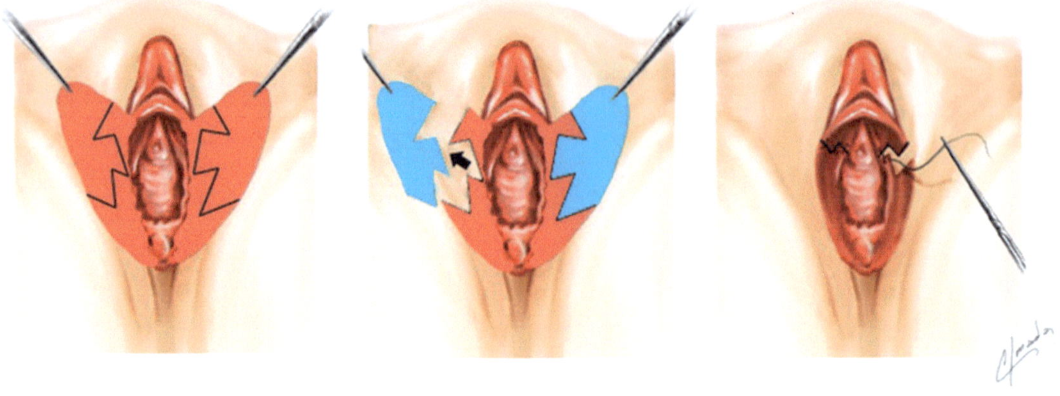

Fig. 10.7 90° Z-plasty technique of hypertrophic labia minora

Table 10.1 Labia minora reduction surgery: patients, follow-up, technique, and complications

Study	*N*	Follow-up (months)	Technique	Complications				
				Necrosis	Infection	Dehiscence	Hematoma	Pain
Alter [5]	4	–	Central wedge resection	0	0	0	0	0
	13	72	Lateral W resection	0	0	1 (7.6)	1 (7.6)	13 (100)
Rouzier et al. [6]	163	30	Inferior V resection	–	–	11 (6.7)	–	104 (64)
	6	–	Central deepithelization	0	0	0	0	0
Giraldo et al. [7]	15	30	90° Z-plasty	0	0	2 (13.3)	6 (40)	0
	55	–	Laser labiaplasty	0	0	3 (5.4)	0	2 (3.6)
	21	46	Inferior wedge resection and reconstruction with superior pedicle	1 (4.7)	1 (4.7)	2 (9.5)	1 (4.7)	0
Marchitelli et al. [8]	42	19	Combined techniques	0	0	3 (7.4)	3 (7.4)	–

10.2.2 Labia Majora Labiaplasty

This surgery consists of the removal of excessive skin along with the adjacent subcutaneous fatty tissue. It is indicated in cases of flaccidity of the labia majora. The most frequently used technique is the elliptic excision of the skin and subcutaneous tissue, which is later repaired with absorbable sutures, with either a continuous intradermic stitch or interrupted stitches.

10.2.3 Reduction Vaginoplasty

This surgery is sometimes also referred to as "vaginal rejuvenation." The term "reduction vaginoplasty" is preferred to "colpoperineoplasty" in cases of reconstruction of the perineal body, not associated with pelvic organ prolapse or urinary incontinence. This surgery is reserved for the few cases in which the size of the vagina results in uncomfortable sexual intercourse or allowing

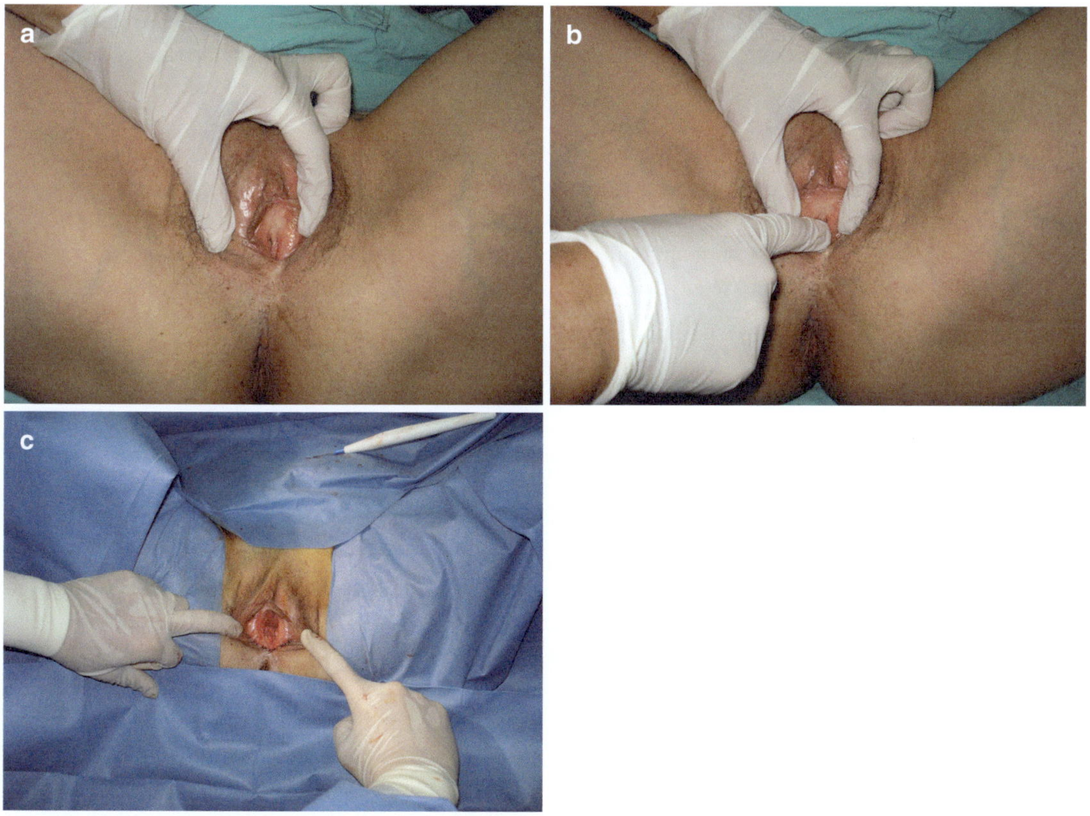

Fig. 10.8 (**a**, **b**) Introital stenosis after "vaginal rejuvenation" procedure. (**c**) Vaginoplasty

incontinence of vaginal gas. It must be taken into account that in most cases, vaginal volume does not interfere with the female orgasm nor prevent a satisfactory sex life, which is why this surgery is not indicated in these cases.

The patient must be fully informed and educated about female sexuality [8]. The main complication of this kind of surgery is dyspareunia and inability of vaginal penetration (Fig. 10.8a, b). Those patients will need an additional surgery to widen the introitus (Fig. 10.8c).

10.3 Practices Not Recommended

10.3.1 G-Spot Amplification

G-spot amplification with collagen, fatty tissue, or hyaluronic acid has become quite popular and is offered by some physicians who perform aesthetic gynecologic procedures. Nonetheless, controversy is surrounding its actual existence. So far, the "G-spot," named after the first German doctor who described it in 1944, Dr. Ernst Grafenberg, has not yet been scientifically proven. The technique and results of practice-spot amplification have not been published in the medical literature, and the reports of performance are merely anecdotal. ACOG affirms that there is no evidence allowing an association between this surgical technique and increased sexual gratification [8]. An ISSVD expert panel declared that there was no indication at all for procedures like the G-spot amplification.

10.3.2 Vulvar and/or Anal Bleaching

In vulvar and anal bleaching, the most common practice is the abrasion of the superficial layer of the epidermis with fractional laser or pulsed light. This stimulates the regeneration of the epithelium, which in theory restores the vulva to its "pink juvenile shade." There are no studies to support this practice, and its use is discouraged due to the fact that it can produce vulvodynia. The vulva gets pigmented again requiring more procedures leading to vulvar pain. Our team believes this practice to be inefficient and iatrogenic.

10.3.3 Reduction Vaginoplasty

Not recommended for sexual issues [8].

ISSVD cosmetic committee recommends that there is no indication at all for procedures like G-spot amplification, vaginal rejuvenation (including surgical and laser approaches), "revirgination," and vulvar bleaching.

10.4 New Procedures

10.4.1 Fractionated Laser

Genitourinary syndrome of menopause (GSM) has been accepted as a consensus new terminology for vulvovaginal atrophy and defined as a collection of symptoms and signs associated with a decrease in estrogen and other sex steroids syndrome, including but not limited to genital symptoms of dryness, burning, and irritation; sexual symptoms of lack of lubrication, discomfort or pain, and impaired function; and urinary symptoms of urgency, dysuria, and recurrent urinary tract infections [9]. The goals of GSM management are to alleviate symptoms and to reverse atrophic anatomic changes. Local estrogen preparations in the form of tablets, rings, or creams are often prescribed as they are perceived to have a low systemic absorption and have been shown to result in significant symptomatic benefit [10]. Local estrogen treatments have a high recurrence rate once they are discontinued, and patients are increasingly expressing high concern over cancer-related consequences. This is the reason why in recent times, new treatments that work on the long term and also on the level of connective tissue and vascularization are being developed. Thermal laser treatment is one of the newer procedures.

Depending on the laser energy delivered and the time during which it is delivered, the tissue effect ranges from a more destructive one (e.g., tissue ablation) to a thermal only effect (e.g., coagulation, photochemical reactions). Thermal energy from the laser source enhances the collagen component and the vascularization [11] improving GSM symptoms.

Lasers have become a very expensive option for the treatment of symptomatic GSM, without a single trial comparing active laser treatment to placebo. There is insufficient evidence on the long-term effects including safety. An important limitation of these short-term studies is that the potential risks of long-term complications, such as scarring, were not addressed.

Although FDA cleared laser technology and it is being marketed extensively to healthcare practitioners and directly to consumers, there is an urgent need for large, long-term, randomized, placebo-controlled, and drug-controlled studies to further evaluate the safety and efficacy of this procedure. Until these studies are not available, it is not advisable to be recommended for use in the clinical practice [12].

10.5 Conclusions

Performing aesthetic gynecological practices ethically is possible, by giving our patients adequate information about the procedures and possible complications and offering sexual counseling when necessary, based on the recommendations of the ACOG [1].

We must always take into consideration that surgeries which produce sexual problems, changes in function, or pain should not be performed, regardless of the patient's request. Scientific societies should elaborate consensus opinions defining the indications and contraindications of these procedures. Also, marketing-based deceiving practices should be prohibited and eradicated.

Creating medical terminology based on an economic model that attempts to control clinical and scientific knowledge is clearly unethical.

Before performing these procedures, we must inform our patients about the lack of data regarding the efficacy and potential long-term complications possibly associated with the surgery.

The indication of vulvoplasties and vaginoplasties should not be based solely on the surgical outcome but also on the satisfaction of those patients who choose not to go through with the procedures after receiving complete counseling during their consult.

However, there is no doubt that prospective, randomized studies with long-term follow-up that evaluate the safety and efficacy of these procedures are clearly necessary.

Vulvar Cosmetics: Breaking the Myths

- In contrast to a common belief, vulvar and vaginal cosmetic surgery does not increase sexual pleasure.
- There is no such thing as a "standard vulva," and there is no definition for "beauty" when referring to the vulvovaginal area, since there are many variations in vulvar anatomy.
- Although fractionated lasers have been cleared by FDA, there is no large, long-term, randomized, placebo-controlled study to evaluate the safety and efficacy of this procedure.
- Fractionated lasers have become an expensive option for the treatment of symptomatic vaginal atrophy.

References

1. American College of Obstetricians and Gynecologists. Vaginal rejuvenation and cosmetic vaginal procedures. ACOG Committee Opinion. Obstet Gynecol. 2007;110:737–8.
2. Bramwell R, et al. Expectations and experience of labial reduction: a qualitative study. BJOG. 2007;114:1493–9.
3. Renganathan A. Gynecological cosmetic surgery. Expert Rev Obstet Gynecol. 2009;4(2):101–4.
4. Likes WM, et al. Aesthetic practice of labial reduction. J Lower Genital Tract Dis. 2008;12(3):210–6.
5. Alter GJ. A new technique for aesthetic labia minora reduction. Ann Plast Surg. 1998;40(3):287–90.
6. Rouzier R, Louis-Sylvestre C, Paniel B, Haddad B. Hypertrophy of labia minora: experience with 163 reductions. Am J Obst Gynecol. 2000;182:35–40.
7. Giraldo F, González C, de Haro F. Central wedge nymphectomy with a 90-degree Z plasty for aesthetic reduction of the labia minora. Plast Reconst Surg. 2004;113(6):1820–5.
8. Marchitelli CE, Sluga MC, Perrotta M, Testa R. Initial experience in a vulvovaginal aesthetic surgery unit within a general gynecology department. J Lower Genit Tract Dis. 2010;14(4):295–300.
9. Portman DJ, Gass ML, Vulvovaginal Atrophy Terminology Consensus Conference Panel. Genitourinary syndrome of menopause: new terminology for vulvovaginal atrophy from the International Society for the Study of Women's Sexual Health and the North American Menopause Society. Menopause. 2014;21(10):1063–8.
10. North American Menopause Society. Management of symptomatic vulvovaginal atrophy: 2013 position statement of The North American Menopause Society. Menopause. 2013;20(9):888–902. quiz 903–904.
11. Salvatore S, Leone Roberti Maggiore U, Athanasiou S, Origoni M, Candiani M, Calligaro A, Zerbinati N. Histological study on the effects of microablative fractional CO_2 laser on atrophic vaginal tissue: an ex vivo study. Menopause. 2015;22(8):845–9.
12. Arunkalaivanan A, Kaur H, Onuma O. Laser therapy as a treatment modality for genitourinary syndrome of menopause: a critical appraisal of evidence. Int Urogynecol J. 2017;28(5):681–5.

Part II

Vulvar Lesions: Skin-Colored Papules and Nodules

11 Skin-Colored Papules and Nodules: Introduction

David Nunns and Rosalind Simpson

11.1 Introduction

In the following chapters and throughout the book, a number of causes of papules and nodules that may clinically present the same color as the patient's skin are presented. An outline of the classification of the different conditions is given in Table 11.1.

Table 11.1 Summary of causes of skin-colored papules and nodules

Cysts	Solid lesions
Mucinous cysts Epidermoid cysts Cyst of the canal of nuck Pilonidal cysts Bartholin gland cyst	Skin tag (acrochordon, fibroepithelial polyp) Scars Benign tumors • Syringoma • Mammary-like gland tumor (hidradenoma papilliferum) Malignant tumors • Squamous cell carcinoma • Basal cell carcinoma Infection • Human papilloma virus infection • Molluscum contagiosum

Skin Coloured Papules and Nodules: Breaking the Myths

- Papillae on the vestibule and medial vulva minora usually do not represent HPV infection. They are papillomatosis (micropapillomatosis)—a normal finding.
- Usually, tumors do not cause pruritus. An exception is syringoma—multiple, confluent white or skin-colored papules on the labia majora, associated with pruritus.

D. Nunns (✉)
Department of Gynaecological Oncology, Nottingham University Hospital, Nottingham, UK

R. Simpson
Centre of Evidence Based Dermatology, University of Nottingham, Nottingham, UK
e-mail: Rosalind.Simpson@nottingham.ac.uk

J. Bornstein (ed.), *Vulvar Disease*, https://doi.org/10.1007/978-3-319-61621-6_11

Papillae, Skin Tags, and Scars

12

David Nunns and Rosalind Simpson

12.1 Papillomatosis of the Vestibule and Medial Labia Minora

Vestibular papillae (also known as vestibular papillomatosis) are a common, normal finding in women [1].

They have no distinctive histopathological appearances and, in the past, were mistaken for HPV infection [2].

They are asymptomatic and present as small soft papillae, variable in number, and located in the vestibule and medial labia minora (Fig. 12.1).

They can vary in size with some being up to 6 mm in length and 1–2 mm wide. They are skin colored and can occur in isolation or can cover the vestibule.

No investigation is needed, and they can be diagnosed clinically. As they are a normal finding, no treatment is required, and patients can be reassured.

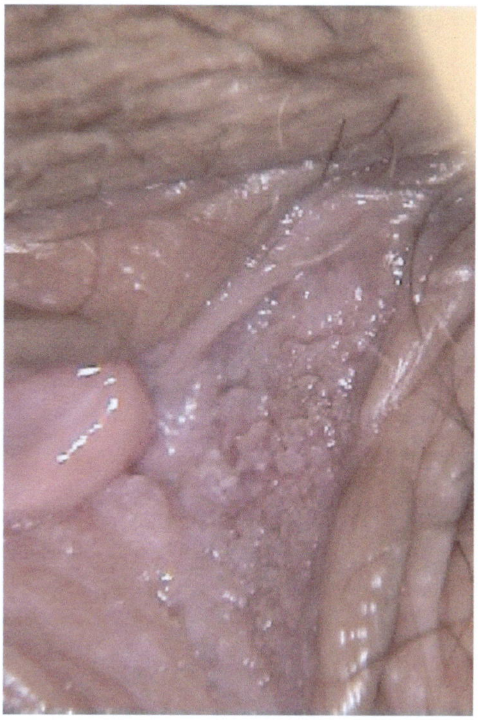

Fig. 12.1 Vestibular papillae (vestibular papillomatosis)—soft papillae in the medial labia minora. Courtesy of Professor Jacob Bornstein

12.2 Skin Tags (Acrochordon, Fibroepithelial Polyp)

These are benign, very common skin tags often found on the neck, groin, and anogenital

D. Nunns (✉)
Department of Gynaecological Oncology, Nottingham University Hospital, Nottingham, UK

R. Simpson
Centre of Evidence Based Dermatology, University of Nottingham, Nottingham, UK
e-mail: Rosalind.Simpson@nottingham.ac.uk

J. Bornstein (ed.), *Vulvar Disease*, https://doi.org/10.1007/978-3-319-61621-6_12

area. On the vulva, they can involve the labia majora.

They are associated with obesity and diabetes.

Histologically, the features are bland with normal epidermis covering connective tissue.

Clinically, they are skin-colored, soft, painless tags that can range in size from a few millimeters to several centimeters.

They are usually asymptomatic; therefore, patients should be reassured.

Removal may be indicated if patients have concerns, or they are associated with dyspareunia. Methods of excision include excision under local anesthetic or cryotherapy.

12.3 Vulvar Scar

Scar tissue is common on the vulva especially among women who have undergone vulvovaginal surgery such as episiotomy or prolapse repair.

Histologically there is usually bland fibrous tissue, but scars are usually evident from a history and clinical examination.

No treatment is necessary if the patient is symptom-free. Surgical excision of scar tissue has a limited place in management as this can cause more scar tissue and may not reduce symptoms or improve function. However, symptomatic vulvar scarring, such as that causing dyspareunia or pain when at the posterior fourchette, may require adjusting using techniques such as Z-plasty [3].

Papillae, Skin Tags and Scars: Breaking the Myths

- Vestibular papillae (also known as vestibular papillomatosis) were mistaken for HPV infection and treated. However, they are a common, normal finding in women and need no treatment.
- Skin tags are benign and common. However, they may be associated with obesity and diabetes.
- Vulvar scarring rarely requires surgical excision as surgery can cause more scar tissue and may not reduce symptoms or improve function.

References

1. van Beurden M, van der Vange N, de Craen AJ, Tjong-A-Hung SP, ten Kate FJ, ter Schegget J, Lammes FB. Normal findings in vulvar examination and vulvoscopy. Br J Obstet Gynaecol. 1997;104(3):320–4.
2. Moyal-Barracco M, Leibowitch M, Orth G. Vestibular papillae of the vulva. Lack of evidence for human papillomavirus etiology. Arch Dermatol. 1990;126(12):1594–8.
3. Wilkinson EJ. Introital stenosis and z-plasty. Obstet Gynecol. 1971;38(4):638–40.

13 Cysts

David Nunns and Rosalind Simpson

13.1 Mucinous Cysts of the Vestibule and Medial Labia Minora

These are common, usually asymptomatic subepithelial cysts occurring in the vestibule [1].

They are of variable sizes and usually solitary lesions that are skin colored, red, and yellow or occasionally have a bluish tinge.

The cysts are lined histologically by mucinous epithelium and are of interest as they are derived from the urogenital sinus embryologically [2] (Fig. 13.1).

No treatment is needed, and patients can be reassured, unless they become big or located in the clitoris area (Figs. 13.2, 13.3, 13.4, and 13.5).

13.2 Epidermal Cyst (Epidermoid Cyst; Epithelial Cyst)

These are the commonest skin cysts occurring on vulva and usually develop in hair-bearing areas (Figs. 13.6, 13.7, 13.8, and 13.9).

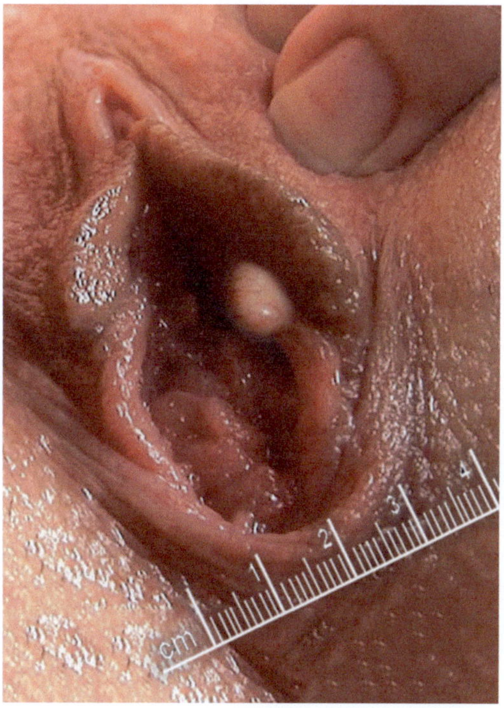

Fig. 13.1 Mucinous cyst of the vestibule. Courtesy of Professor Jacob Bornstein

The cause is unknown but may be iatrogenic following surgery or blockage of the pilosebaceous unit. Histologically, epidermoid cysts are lined by stratified squamous epithelium and are filled with keratin to produce lesions that clinically contain a white content.

D. Nunns (✉)
Department of Gynaecological Oncology, Nottingham University Hospital, Nottingham, UK

R. Simpson
Centre of Evidence Based Dermatology, University of Nottingham, Nottingham, UK
e-mail: Rosalind.Simpson@nottingham.ac.uk

J. Bornstein (ed.), *Vulvar Disease*, https://doi.org/10.1007/978-3-319-61621-6_13

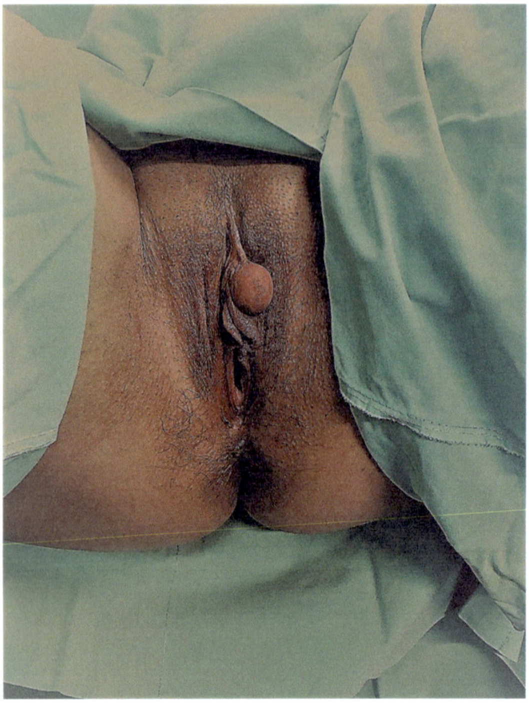

Fig. 13.2 Mucinous cyst in the clitorial area. Courtesy of Professor Jacob Bornstein

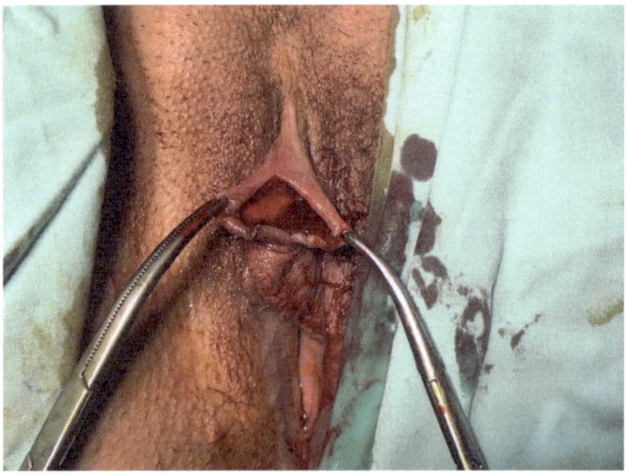

Fig. 13.3 Excision of the clitorial cyst. Courtesy of Professor Jacob Bornstein

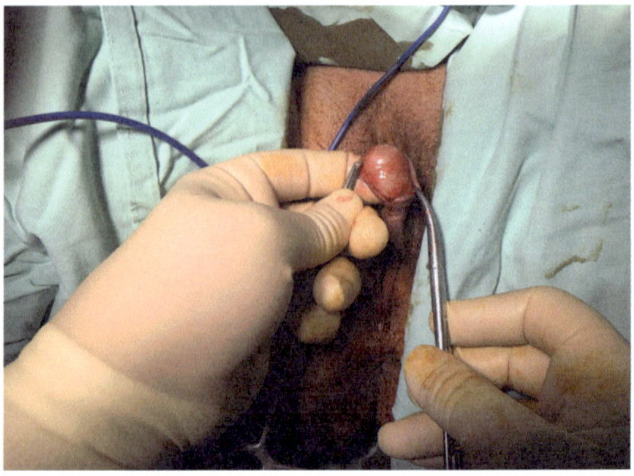

Fig. 13.4 Excision of the clitorial cyst. Courtesy of Professor Jacob Bornstein

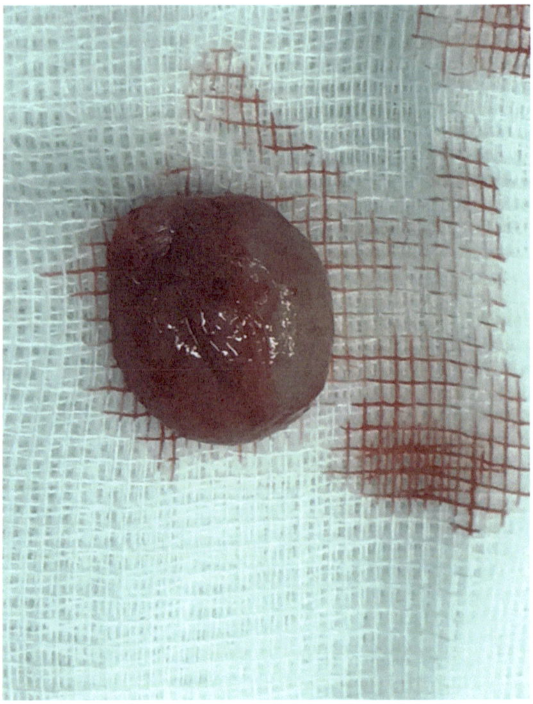

Fig. 13.5 The cyst enucleated from the clitoris. Courtesy of Professor Jacob Bornstein

They are usually asymptomatic, but some patients may complain that they are unsightly or irritating. Some reported cases have involved the clitoral hood to give the impression of clitoromegaly [3]. Infected cysts are painful and can discharge pus.

They can vary in size from 1–2 mm (often called milia) to several cm and also color (skin colored to clinically obvious yellow nodules).

A biopsy is not usually necessary, and management depends on symptoms. Asymptomatic

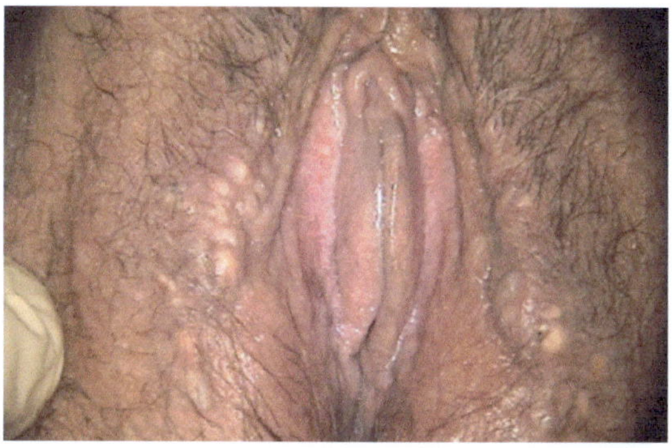

Fig. 13.6 Epidermal cysts: skin colored nodules. Courtesy of Professor Jacob Bornstein

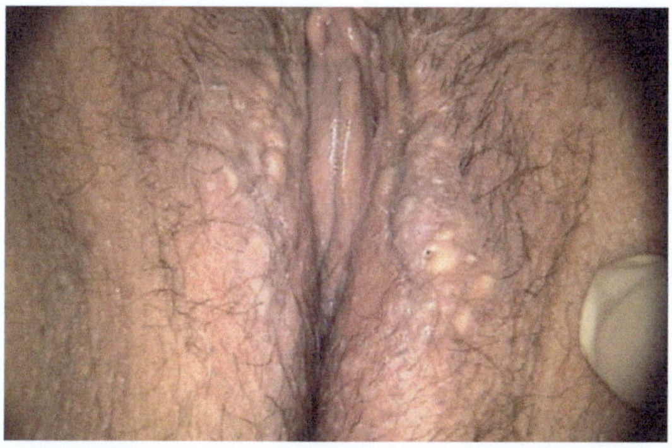

Fig. 13.7 Epidermal cysts: skin colored nodules. Courtesy of Professor Jacob Bornstein

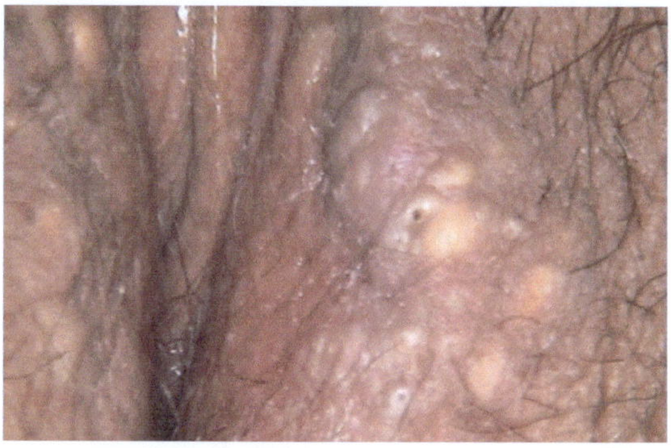

Fig. 13.8 Epidermal cysts: skin colored nodules. Courtesy of Professor Jacob Bornstein

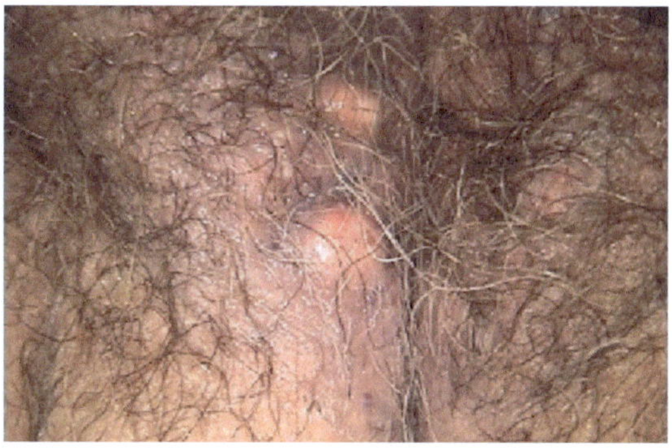

Fig. 13.9 Epidermal cysts: skin colored nodules. Courtesy of Professor Jacob Bornstein

lesions can be managed expectantly, while other lesions can be locally excised.

13.3 Bartholin Gland Cyst, Abscess, and Tumor

There are two Bartholin glands situated within the labia majora on both sides, with their ducts open to the vestibule at 4 and 8 o'clock. They have the function of producing mucous for lubrication during intercourse. They are unusual in that they have a long duct from the main body of the gland which may become blocked to produce a deep-seated cystic swelling region of the gland that histologically is lined by mucinous epithelium.

Bartholin gland cyst is diagnosed clinically. Small cysts are often asymptomatic and can be managed conservatively. A few become infected and form an abscess. Some patients may complain of the feeling of a lump or pain during intercourse. Traditionally, symptomatic cysts are managed surgically with marsupialization during which the cyst wall is incised and the edge sutured so there is a continuous surface from the interior to the exterior enabling the interior to drain. This procedure has a high cure

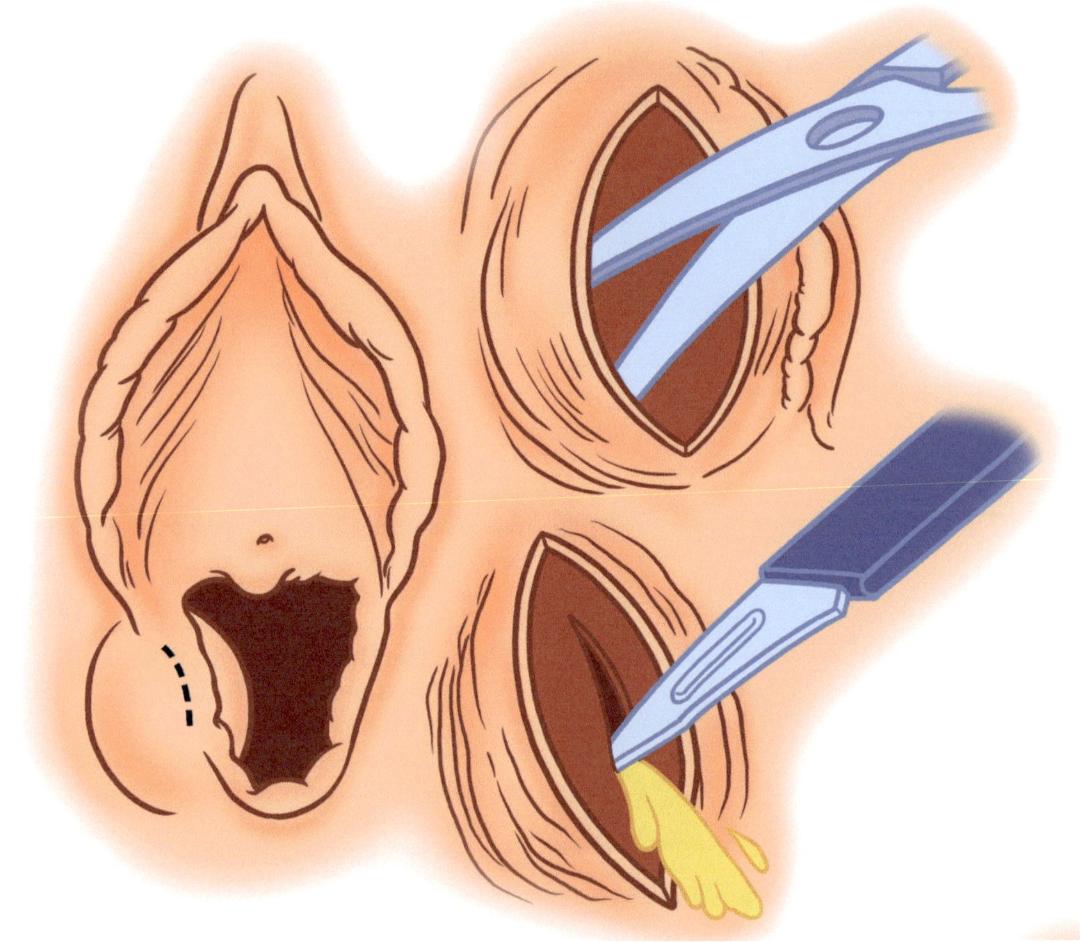

Fig. 13.10 Bartholin cyst. On the left, the cyst presents as a bulge in the right vestibule; top, enucleation of the cyst; bottom, incision and drainage of the cyst. Courtesy of Professor Jacob Bornstein

rate (Fig. 13.10). Another option which involves inserting a Word catheter into the cyst has been advocated and can be carried out in the outpatient setting [4]: Under local anesthesia, a small balloon with an inflatable distal end is inserted into the cyst cavity. The aim of the balloon catheter insertion is to create an epithelialized fistula or sinus tract to allow drainage. The catheter has a stem (3 cm long) and an inflatable balloon tip to hold saline, which allows the catheter to remain in the cyst cavity. There is no good clinical evidence to support either technique. Other techniques that have been suggested include the use of silver nitrate gland ablation, sclerotherapy, and CO_2 ablation; however, a systematic review of the different clinical practices failed to show any one as a superior treatment [5].

Cysts may become infected, creating a Bartholin gland abscess with *Escherichia coli* being the single most common pathogen [6]. The management of Bartholin gland abscess is incision and drainage of the abscess usually with an incision on the inner side of the vestibule. The use of the Word catheter is an alternative. If an abscess spontaneously discharges, then there is less value in incision and drainage, and the abscess should slowly resolve. Routine antibiotics are not usually necessary.

Bartholin's gland carcinoma is a rare tumor, and it is often initially misdiagnosed as Bartholin's gland cyst. Many cases present as a cyst that, however, when the latter does not respond to standard conservative therapy [7]. The malignant tumor is often long-standing and presents with a painless vulvar mass [8]. Most tumors are squamous cell carcinomas or adenocarcinomas. The current evidence base is insufficient to suggest different management from vulvar squamous cell carcinoma [9]. The lesions are often deep-seated or likely to be associated with metastatic disease. The proximity to the anal sphincter may necessitate partial resection with reconstruction. In a case series of 36 patients, the 5-year survival rate was 84% [10]. It is estimated that patients with lymph node metastases have an overall survival of 40–50% which is lowered to 18% if 2 or more nodes are involved [11].

Epidermal Cyst: Breaking the Myths

- Of all vulvar cysts, epidermal cysts are the commonest.
- Biopsy is not usually necessary for this cyst.

References

1. Newland JR, Fusaro RM. Mucinous cysts of the vulva. Nebr Med J. 1991;76(9):307–10.
2. Wechter ME, Wu JM, Robboy SJ, Ross JS, Prat J, Keh PC, Welch WR. Urogenital sinus origin of mucinous and ciliated cysts of the vulva. Obstet Gynecol. 1978;51(3):347–51.
3. Anderson-Mueller BE, Laudenschlager MD, Hansen KA. Epidermoid cyst of the clitoris: an unusual cause of clitoromegaly in a patient without history of previous female circumcision. J Pediatr Adolesc Gynecol. 2009;22(5):e130–2.
4. Haider Z, Condous G, Kirk E, et al. The simple outpatient management of Bartholin's abscess using the word catheter: a preliminary study. Aust N Z J Obstet Gynaecol. 2007;47:137–40.
5. Marzano D, Haefner H. Management of Bartholin duct cysts and abscesses: a systematic review. Obstet Gynecol Surv. 2009;64(6):395–404.
6. Kessous R, Aricha-Tamir B, Sheizaf B, Steiner N, Moran-Gilad J, Weintraub AY. Clinical and microbiological characteristics of Bartholin gland abscesses. Obstet Gynecol. 2013;122(4):794–9.
7. Cardosi RJ, Speights A, Fiorica JV, Grendys EC Jr, Hakam A, Hoffman MS. Bartholin's gland carcinoma: a 15-year experience. Gynecol Oncol. 2001;82(2):247–51.
8. RCOG guidance on the management of vulval cancer, May 2014. https://www.rcog.org.uk/globalassets/documents/guidelines/vulvalcancerguideline.pdf.
9. Copeland LJ, Sneige N, Gershenson DM, McGuffee VB, Abdul-Karim F, Rutledge FN. Bartholin gland carcinoma. Obstet Gynecol. 1986;67(6):794–801.
10. Sonnex C, Schofield JH, Kocjan G, et al. Anal human papillomavirus infection in heterosexuals with genital warts: prevalence and relation with sexual behaviour. BMJ. 1991;303:1243.
11. Leuchter RS, Hacker NF, Voet RL, Berek JS, Townsend DE, Lagasse LD. Primary carcinoma of the Bartholin gland: a report of 14 cases and review of the literature. Obstet Gynecol. 1982;60:361–8.

14 Benign and Malignant Tumors

David Nunns and Rosalind Simpson

14.1 Syringoma

This is a benign tumor of the eccrine sweat glands and ducts that tends to occur in young women. The cause remains unknown, but there are reported series of familial cases [1].

Histologically the features include dilated ductal structures with characteristic "comma-like" tails within a sclerotic dermis. The nests have a characteristic tadpole-like morphology.

They are common on the face but uncommon on the vulva where they can be associated with pruritus. On the vulva they usually occur on the labia majora as multiple, confluent white or skin-colored papules, usually 1–4 mm diameter, but they may measure up to 2 cm (Fig. 14.1).

Patients may also have synchronous lesions elsewhere.

A biopsy can usually confirm the diagnosis. As these are benign skin tumors, a conservative approach is possible with symptomatic management of any associated pruritus. Symptomatic

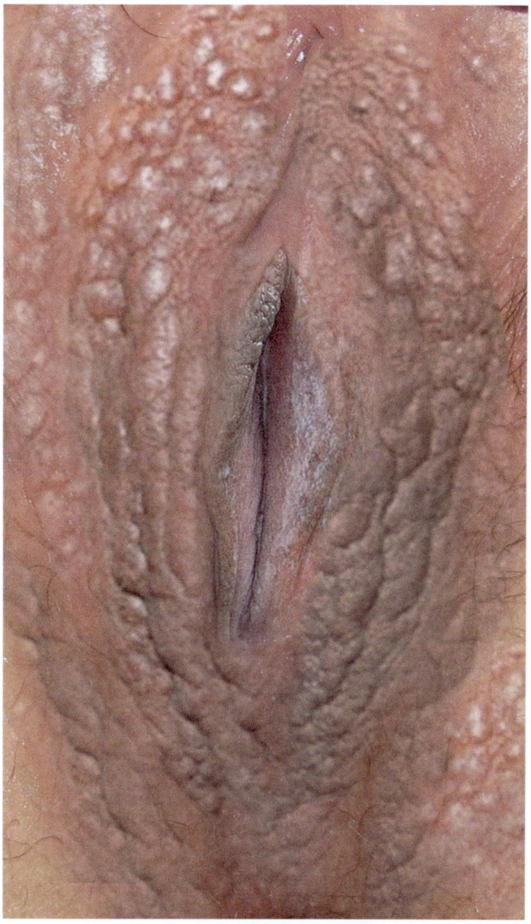

Fig. 14.1 Syringoma. Patient complains of intense pruritus. The labia majora contains multiple, confluent skin-colored papules. Courtesy of Professor Jacob Bornstein

D. Nunns (✉)
Department of Gynaecological Oncology, Nottingham University Hospital, Nottingham, UK

R. Simpson
Centre of Evidence Based Dermatology, University of Nottingham, Nottingham, UK
e-mail: Rosalind.Simpson@nottingham.ac.uk

J. Bornstein (ed.), *Vulvar Disease*, https://doi.org/10.1007/978-3-319-61621-6_14

patients may be treated with CO_2 laser treatment as an alternative [2].

14.2 Basal Cell Carcinoma

Basal cell carcinomas (BCC) are the commonest skin cancer on non-vulval skin, but on the vulva they are less common and account for only 5% of vulval skin cancers. They tend to occur in women with average age at diagnosis being 70 years [3].

BCC usually present with a solitary vulval nodule, papule, or ulcer on the labia majora and rarely affect the mucosal surfaces [4]. They are usually around 1–2 cm in diameter but can vary in size from a few mm to several cm giving rise to symptoms of pain or itch. Bleeding occurs if the tumor is ulcerated.

Histological features are the same as those seen elsewhere and classically include proliferation of nests of small basal cells with high nuclear-to-cytoplasmic ratio, peripheral palisading, mitotic figures, apoptosis, and retraction artifact. A wide variety of histologic types have been described including the following patterns: nodular, infiltrating, and morpheaform [3]. The presence of perineural invasion can predict local recurrence. The cause remains unknown, but chronic irritation, immunosuppression, and genetic predisposition have been suggested. Sun exposure is a risk factor for non-vulvar areas, but this is not believed to be a risk for vulvar disease.

Diagnosis is usually made by an incisional biopsy rather than excision a piece of the lesion for biopsy. Incisional biopsies can enable accurate surgical planning once the diagnosis is confirmed. In principle diagnostic excisional biopsies of suspicious vulvar lesions are to be avoided as surgical margins may be incomplete and re-excision may be required which might compromise function and cause scarring.

Management is usually by removal of the tumor with at least 4 mm margin which should achieve clearance of the lesion [4]. Recurrence occurs in 10–20% of lesions when the tumor is present at the margins. Metastases are rare, but BCC can cause local destruction if left untreated. If the tumor is close to a sphincter, surgical excision may lead to involved margins. In these cases, radiotherapy to the vulvar skin is an acceptable alternative to preserve function. The use of topical treatments for BCC has not gained popularity on the vulva because of the side effects of irritancy, so surgery remains the preferred treatment.

Benign and Malignant Tumors: Breaking the Myths

- Although basal cell carcinomas (BCC) are the commonest skin cancer on non-vulval skin, on the vulva they are less common and account for only 5% of vulval skin cancers.
- Incisional biopsy is preferred over diagnostic excisional biopsies, in case of suspicious vulvar lesions. With biopsies the surgical margins may be incomplete, and re-excision may be required which might compromise function and cause scarring.
- Management of BCC is usually by removal of the tumor with at least 4 mm margin.

References

1. Dereli T, Turk BG, Kazandi AC. Syringomas of the vulva. Int J Gynaecol Obstet. 2007;99(1):65–6.
2. Huang YH, Chuang YH, Kuo TT, Yang LC, Hong HS. Vulvar syringoma: a clinicopathologic and immunohistologic study of 18 patients and results of treatment. J Am Acad Dermatol. 2003;48(5):735–9.
3. Gibson GE, Ahmed I. Perianal and genital basal cell carcinoma: a clinicopathologic review of 51 cases. J Am Acad Dermatol. 2001;45(1):68–71.
4. Telfer NR, Colver GB, Morton CA, British Association of Dermatologists. Guidelines for the management of basal cell carcinoma. Br J Dermatol. 2008;159(1):35–48.

15 Molluscum Contagiosum

David Nunns and Rosalind Simpson

Molluscum contagiosum (MC) is caused by a DNA poxvirus. MC may occur in adults but is much more common in childhood. Most infections are asymptomatic, and serological evidence of infection is present in up to 14% of adults [1]. The mode of transmission is through skin-to-skin contact, so in adults the mode of transmission of the virus is often through sexual contact, but some patients with skin disease treated with topical steroids may develop lesions. Immunosuppression is also a risk factor [2].

The common skin surfaces to be affected include the face, limbs, and trunk. When the genital area is infected, there are usually multiple skin-colored papular lesions involving the mons pubis, labia majora, and inner thigh (Fig. 15.1a, b). The lesions are characteristically discrete, pearly, umbilicated papular lesions of varying size, ranging from 2 to 3 mm to over 1 cm. A specific variant, "giant" molluscum, may mimic a large genital wart if it occurs on the vulva.

Diagnosis is made clinically in the majority of cases. Where diagnostic doubt exists, biopsy can be taken. Histology shows classical features of viral intracytoplasmic inclusion bodies that contain MCV copies. These viruses may be shed and spread infection.

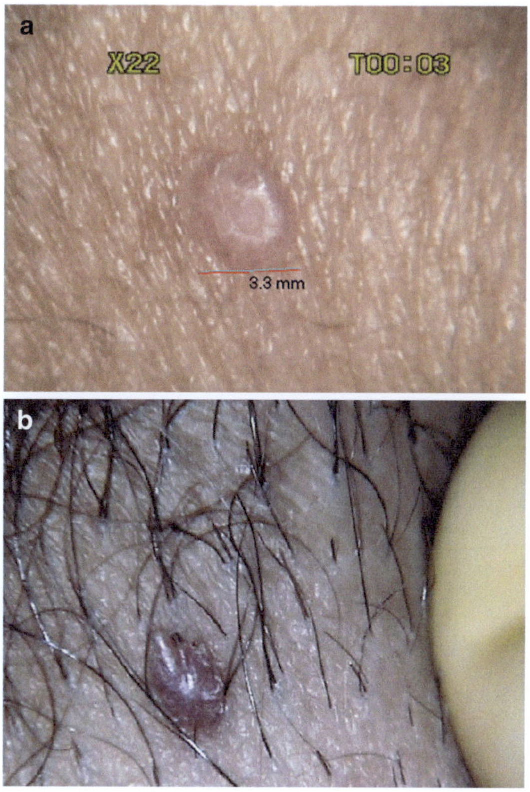

Fig. 15.1 (**a**, **b**) Molluscum contagiosum—the lesions are discrete, pearly, umbilicated papular lesions of 2–3 mm. Courtesy of Professor Jacob Bornstein

D. Nunns (✉)
Department of Gynaecological Oncology, Nottingham University Hospital, Nottingham, UK

R. Simpson
Centre of Evidence Based Dermatology, University of Nottingham, Nottingham, UK
e-mail: Rosalind.Simpson@nottingham.ac.uk

J. Bornstein (ed.), *Vulvar Disease*, https://doi.org/10.1007/978-3-319-61621-6_15

Molluscum Contagiosum: Breaking the Myth

- Molluscum contagiosum (MC) should be considered in the differential diagnosis of vulvar condyloma acuminatum.
- While in childhood, molluscum contagiosum (MC) is a common face contagious infection, in adults it is often transmitted through sexual contact.
- In addition, immunosuppression should be ruled out.

There are no long-term health implications from this infection. The condition usually resolves spontaneously over months to years in an immunocompetent patient, and no treatment is required. Treatment may be considered in adults with unsightly lesions, and the ideal method of treatment remains unknown in the absence of robust clinical trials [3]. Cryotherapy, curettage, and topical application of imiquimod or cantharidin are all options.

References

1. Sherwani S, Farleigh L, Agarwal N, Loveless S, Robertson N, Hadaschik E, Schnitzler P, Bugert JJ. Seroprevalence of Molluscum contagiosum virus in German and UK populations. PLoS One. 2014;9(2):e88734. https://doi.org/10.1371/journal.pone.0088734.eCollection2014.
2. Gur I. The epidemiology of Molluscum contagiosum in HIV-seropositive patients: a unique entity or insignificant finding? Int J STD AIDS. 2008;19(8):503–6. https://doi.org/10.1258/ijsa.2008.008186.
3. van der Wouden JC, van der Sande R, van Suijlekom-Smit LW, Berger M, Butler CC, Koning S. Interventions for cutaneous molluscum contagiosum. Cochrane Database Syst Rev. 2009;7(4):CD004767. https://doi.org/10.1002/14651858.CD004767.pub3. Review.

16 Genital Condyloma (HPV Infection)

Eduardo Schejter

16.1 Epidemiology

Genital warts (condyloma acuminata) are one of the most common benign vulvar diseases. It is mostly caused by the human papilloma virus (HPV) types 6 and 11 (90% of cases), although many more types of HPV may be associated with it. It is transmitted through sexual contact (genital, orogenital, manual-genital, and non-penetrative genital contact), with a transmission rate of 60% between partners [1].

At least 40 identified HPV types infect the genital tract. If a college female student has at least one different partner per year for 4 years, the probability is greater than 85% that she will leave college with an HPV infection. Condoms do not completely protect from acquiring the virus because the areas around the genitals, including the inner thigh, are obviously not protected, thus exposing them to the infected partner's skin. Sharing of contaminated objects may transmit HPV, but nonsexual transmission is less common. Finger-genital contact is also a possible way of transmission, but it is unlikely to be a significant source [2–4].

It has been estimated that about 1% of the sexually active adult population in the Western world suffers from clinical warts during their lifetime. The peak prevalence is between 20 and 24 years of age (6.2/1000 person years) in women and 25 and 29 years of age (5.0/1000 person years) in men [1, 4], and this incidence has increased significantly during the last three decades [5, 6]. It is estimated that around 30 million persons suffer from genital warts worldwide [7]. Many healthcare providers have stressed the importance of raising awareness of the risks of contracting sexually transmitted diseases in young populations; however, there has been a further dramatic increase in sexually transmitted diseases in the 30- to 45-year age range as well. It is estimated that this increase in infection stems from what is known as the "second chapter" in life, following divorce, and that the increase in casual sex increases the risks of contracting sexually transmitted diseases in mature individuals [8, 9].

The prevalence of condyloma acuminata seems to be similar for men and women. A study from one sexually transmitted disease (STD) clinic found that 13% of men and 9% of women had condylomata acuminata [10]. One of the long-held beliefs is that intercourse using a condom is safe, but the virus may be transmitted by contact of uncovered skin in the genital area, making the protection for HPV infection partial at best. The facts that the virus is highly prevalent, and that it is latent without any external manifestations, significantly increase the risk of infection.

E. Schejter (✉)
Women's Health Center, Maccabi Healthcare Services, Tel Aviv, Israel
e-mail: schejter_a@mac.org.il

J. Bornstein (ed.), *Vulvar Disease*, https://doi.org/10.1007/978-3-319-61621-6_16

In addition, unlike the level of awareness of risks of HIV infection, knowledge about diseases that are transmitted by sexual contact in spite of the use of condoms is very low among sexually active young people and adults [11].

Genital warts are more common among smokers, but there is no evidence that cessation of smoking improves treatment outcome [12, 13].

16.2 Natural Course

The HPV types that cause genital warts do not cause cancerous changes [14]. Most of the infections are transient, and 90% of them disappear spontaneously after 2 years, with a median duration of 8 months. The infection persists in 10% of the patients, however, and it may also produce late recurrences, especially in states of immune deficiency [11]. In low-grade infections (HPV 6 and 11), the genome is present as an episome (circular, non-integrated DNA architecture), while in high-risk infection (HPV 16 and 18), it may become integrated into host DNA; this integration usually occurs within the open reading frame of the E2 gene and results in the loss of E2 repressive action, leading to higher levels of E6 and E7 expression (i.e., the oncogenes responsible for the neoplastic effect of the virus) [15]. The average incubation period is 3 months (range, 3 weeks to 8 months), followed by the clinical appearance of warts that may recur, depending on the immune response of the patient. For example, HIV-positive patients have a much higher risk for condyloma (5.6%) than HIV-negative patients (0.8%) [16].

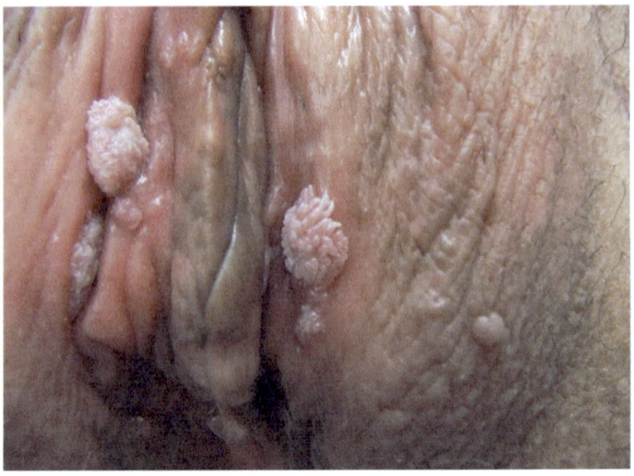

Fig. 16.1 Condylomata acuminata—the lesions look like cauliflower and are spread on the labia majora, labia minora, and clitoris

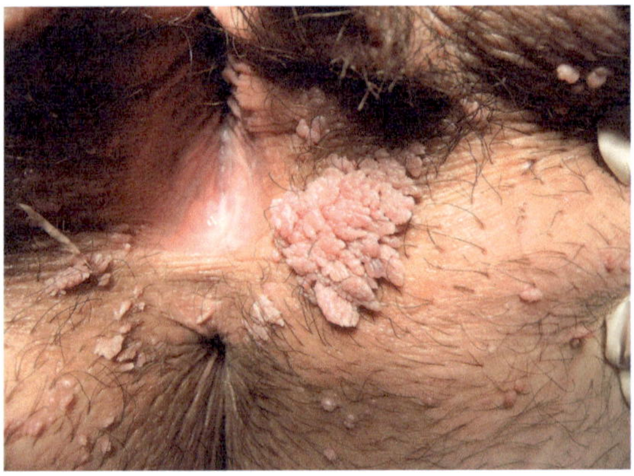

Fig. 16.2 Condylomata acuminata spread on the vulva and perianal area

16.3 Clinical Manifestation

Genital warts are usually asymptomatic, but they may occasionally cause pain or pruritus. The disease classically manifests itself as skin lesions that look like cauliflower florets and sometimes as flat, papular, or pedunculated growths on the genital mucosa, mainly the vulvar labia (Figs. 16.1 and 16.2). It can occur at multiple sites in the anogenital area, including the clitoris (Fig. 16.3), the perineum (Fig. 16.4), vagina, and cervix (Fig. 16.5). Intra-anal condylomas are commonly observed in patients who have had receptive anal intercourse, although it can also occur in men and women without a history of anal sexual contact. They are infecting and may be found on the male penis (Figs. 16.6 and 16.7). Classical genital warts can be diagnosed by clinical inspection, and biopsy is rarely indicated. The indications for biopsy are treatment failure to standard therapy, atypical warts, ulcerated pigmented lesions, and in immunocompromised patients.

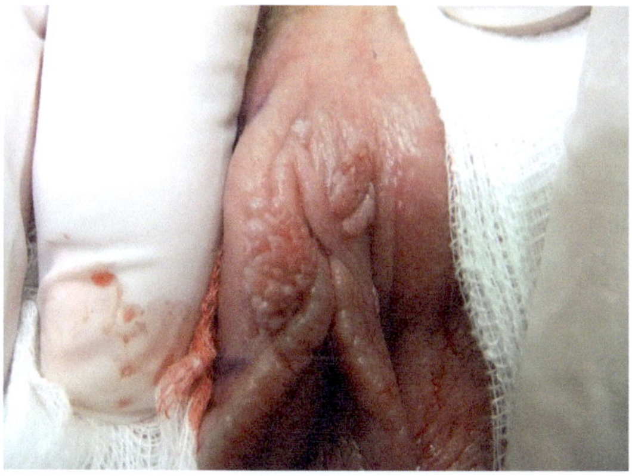

Fig. 16.3 Periclitoral condylomata acuminata

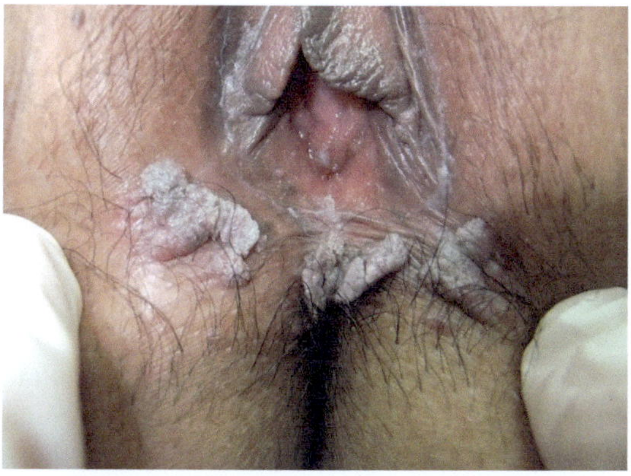

Fig. 16.4 Perineal condylomata acuminata—bilateral "kissing" lesions

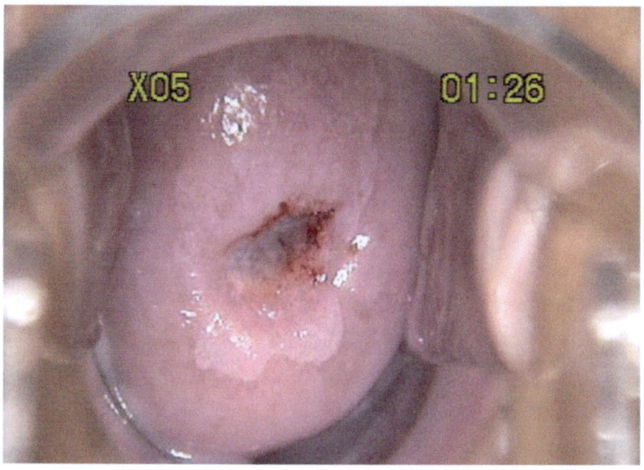

Fig. 16.5 Flat condyloma on the cervix, colposcopic examination after application of 5% acetic acid. Courtesy of Professor Jacob Bornstein

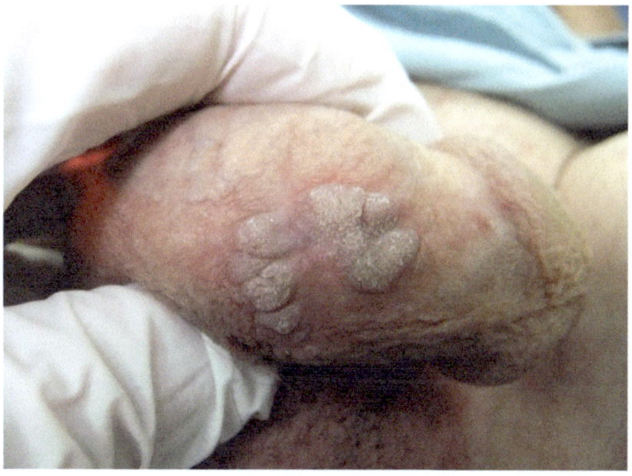

Fig. 16.6 Hyperkeratosis on the penis, suspicious for condyloma. In this case a histological confirmation is mandatory

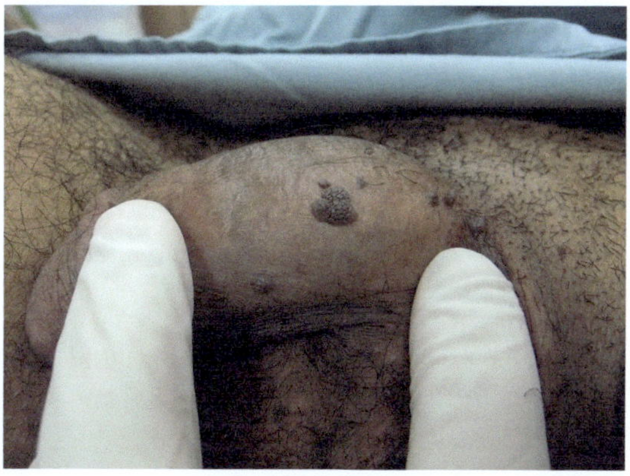

Fig. 16.7 Pigmented penile condylomata

HPV DNA testing of genital warts is unnecessary and has no clinical relevance, and the application of acetic acid 3–5% is non-specific [17]. The preputial cavity (glans penis, coronal sulcus, frenulum, inner aspect of the foreskin) is most commonly affected in uncircumcised men, while the shaft of the penis is often involved in circumcised men. Warts in men may also occur at the urethral meatus, pubis, scrotum, groin, perineum, perianal area, and anal canal, while lesions in women occur at the fourchette, labia minora, labia majora, pubis, clitoris, urethral meatus, perineum, perianal region, anal canal, introitus, vagina, and ectocervix [18–20].

A giant condyloma or Buschke-Lowenstein tumor is a rare variant of HPV 6 and 11 disease. It is controversial if it is the same as verrucous carcinoma. The latter is characterized by local infiltration into dermal structures. The treatment is radical surgical extirpation and oncologic counseling [21].

16.4 Effect on Quality of Life

Pain and discomfort are reported in ~50% of the cases. They are caused by secondary infection. In addition, 60% of the patients report to have associated emotional consequences of genital warts, including anxiety, decrease in self-image, and declined libido [22]. The disease disrupts the daily life of the patient, causing physical problems, such as itching and pain, as well as difficulties in intimate relationships. Both men and women are often ashamed to disclose their condition and sometimes avoid seeking and receiving appropriate treatment.

On the quality-adjusted life-year scale, the utility weight of genital warts (0.91) is higher (indicating a better state of well-being) than that of uncomplicated type II diabetes (0.81) and similar to that of well-controlled asthma and CIN 1 lesions (0.92) [8].

16.5 Genital Warts and Pregnancy

Higher HPV infection rates have been reported in pregnant women compared to nonpregnant women, due, in part, to suppression of immunity during pregnancy and hormonal changes [23]. Development of condylomas among pregnant women is also relatively rapid.

It is important to treat genital warts during pregnancy because of the risk of transmission of infection to the newborn and the appearance of warts in its respiratory system in the future. HPV types 6 and 11 can cause recurrent respiratory papillomatosis (RRP) in infants and children, although the route of transmission is not clear, it is mainly postnatal and very infrequently transplacental. Importantly, ~60% of mothers whose infants are diagnosed as having RRP report having past or current genital warts. There is no evidence that cesarean delivery decreases the risk of maternal-neonatal transmission of an HPV infection. The presence of multiple lesions in the birth canal is, however, a relative indication for a cesarean section, and it is recommended for cases in which the warts block the birth canal or when vaginal delivery would result in excessive bleeding [17, 24].

16.6 Genital Warts and Neoplastic Risk

HPV types 16, 18, 31, 33, and 35 are also occasionally found in anogenital warts (usually as coinfections with HPV 6 or 11), and they can be associated with foci of high-grade squamous intraepithelial lesions (HSIL), particularly in individuals with HIV infection. Women with STDs, including genital warts, have a higher risk of developing cervical cancer, and so screening for cervical cancer is strongly recommended in this population (cytological screening or HPV testing), but there is no indication for routine screening colposcopy in patients with genital warts [25]. Patients with perianal warts, those who are HIV positive, and those with a history of receptive anal intercourse, are at increased risk for anal HGSIL [26], and anal cytological screening and/or high-resolution anoscopy are indicated for these patients [17].

16.7 Histology

Condyloma acuminatum appears as disruption of the epidermis with hyperkeratosis, coarse keratohyalin granules, and koilocytes in a prominent granular layer (Fig. 16.8).

The epidermis or mucosa of flat condylomata demonstrates acanthosis. Viral multiplication is confined to the nucleus. Koilocytosis (from Greek "koilos" meaning "empty") describes a combination of perinuclear clearing (halo) with a pyknotic or shrunken nucleus, and it is a characteristic feature of productive papillomavirus infection.

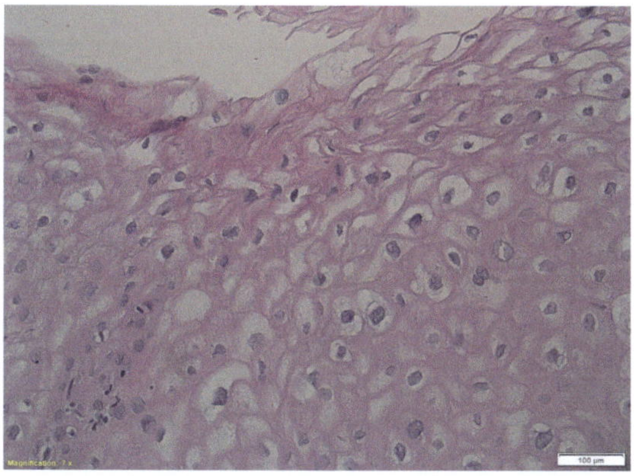

Fig. 16.8 A histologic section of a condyloma, depicting koilocytosis: perinuclear clearing (halo) and a pyknotic or shrunken (raisinoid) nucleus

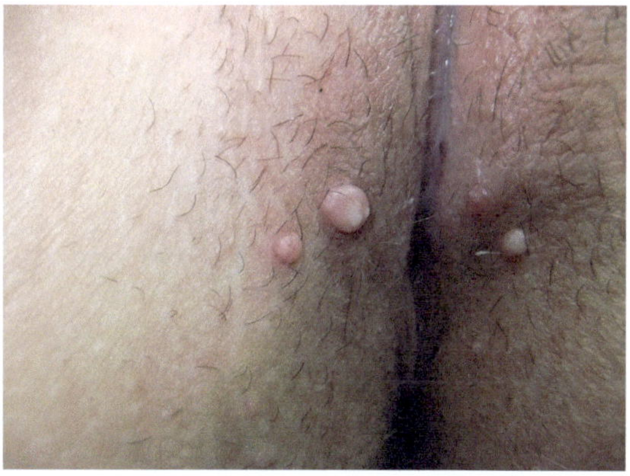

Fig. 16.9 Molluscum contagiosum: small smooth lesion with a dimple or pit in the center. A "look-alike" condyloma acuminata

16.8 Differential Diagnosis

16.8.1 Molluscum Contagiosum

Molluscum contagiosum is an infection caused by a poxvirus (molluscum contagiosum virus). The lesions, known as mollusca, are small, raised, and usually white, pink, or flesh colored, with a dimple or pit in the center (Fig. 16.9). They often have a pearly appearance and are usually smooth. Histopathological examination depicts typical characteristics of intracytoplasmic bodies [27].

16.8.2 Lichen Simplex Chronicus

Lichen simplex chronicus (squamous cell hyperplasia) (see Chap. 26) is a morphologic alteration of the vulvar skin. LSC is characterized by a pink-red coloration with overlying gray-white keratin. Biopsy is mandatory for definitive diagnosis [28].

16.8.3 High-Grade Squamous Intraepithelial Lesion (HGSIL) of the Vulva (Vulvar HGSIL, VIN Usual Type)

HGSIL of the vulva presents as white or erythematous macules or papules, which can coalesce to create verrucous plaques. Around 10% of these lesions are pigmented. Over one-half of affected individuals have multifocal lesions in the vulva.

16.8.4 Differentiated Type VIN (DVIN)

DVIN tends to be unicentric at presentation and produces less bulky lesions compared to vulvar HGSIL. Clinically, the lesions may appear as focal gray-white discolorations with a rough surface, vaguely defined thick white plaques, or elevated nodules [29].

16.9 Treatment

The general treatment strategy is to eliminate as many of the visible lesions as possible until the host immune system can control viral replication. The warts may recur after treatment because of activation of a latent virus present in the healthy skin adjacent to the lesion. There are several treatments that focus on the external lesions, including medication, surgical excision, or destruction by freezing, diathermy, or CO_2 laser vaporization (Fig. 16.10) and Interferon injections (Fig. 16.11).

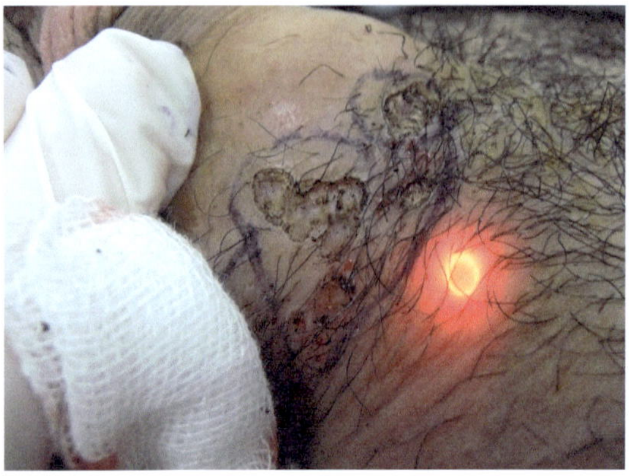

Fig. 16.10 CO_2 laser evaporation treatment, causing superficial skin damage, leaving the basal membrane intact

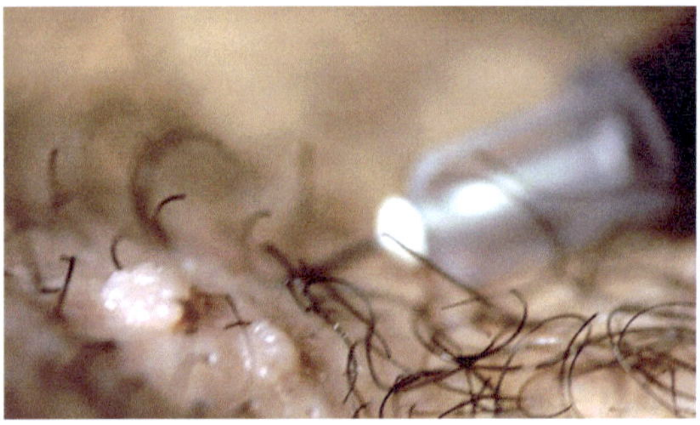

Fig. 16.11 Intralesional interferon injection into a genital condyloma. Courtesy of Professor Jacob Bornstein

16.10 Medical Self-Applied Treatments: Podophyllin (Antiviral)

The commercial preparation Condylox 0.5% contains the active ingredient of podophyllin, an antimitotic product which works by interfering with cell reproduction and by promoting local tissue necrosis. There are reports of wide tissue necrosis when used on nonkeratinized epithelium, and its application is therefore restricted to external keratinized epithelium. The dose is twice daily for 3 days, with a break of 4 days between treatment cycles, up to a maximum of 1 month of treatment. The efficiency ranges between 45% and 77%; the side effects include local inflammation, and the recurrence rates range between 4% and 38% of the patients. Condylox 0.5% must not be used during pregnancy (Fig. 16.12) [30].

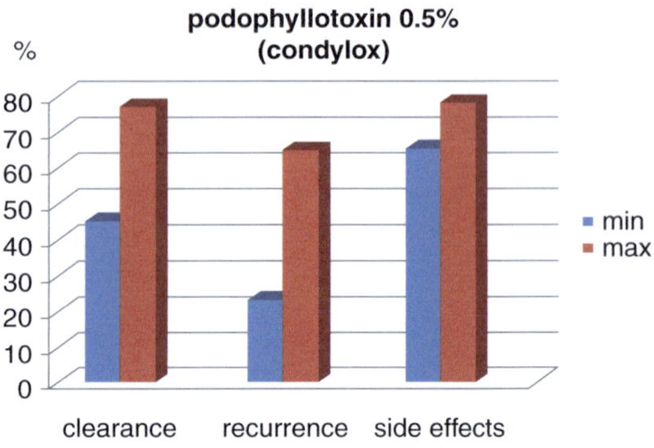

Fig. 16.12 Podophyllotoxin treatment

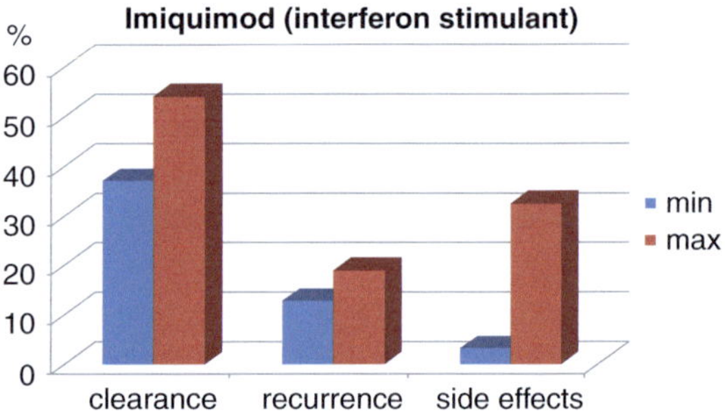

Fig. 16.13 Imiquimod treatment

16.11 Imiquimod (Interferon Stimulant)

This ointment therapy is specific for HPV infections. It induces cytokines and increases the immune response. The dosage is 3 times weekly for up to 16 weeks, and it is recommended to wash the affected area from 6 to 10 h after application. Side effects may include redness and local ulceration that sometimes lead to discontinuation of therapy. Several studies have observed efficiency between 37% and 54% after 16 weeks, with the reported recurrence being between 13% and 19%. It is recommended that the use of imiquimod be avoided during pregnancy (category C) (Fig. 16.13) [31].

16.12 Veregen (Sinecatechins 10% Ointment)

Polyphenon E is an extract originated from tea trees. It is anti-infective. It was approved by the FDA for treating external venereal warts in men and women over the age of 18 years. Early studies observed excellent efficiency: two phase III studies which included 1004 patients showed the disappearance of warts in 55% of cases treated with Veregen ointment 10% 3 times daily for 16 weeks, with relatively low recurrence (approximately 6%) and mild side effects (Fig. 16.14). One meta-analysis published in 2011 concluded that this treatment is effective and safe. It should be noted that it has been tested only on keratinized epithelium and therefore is not indicated for application on mucous membranes [32, 33]. A summary of the outcome of the self-applied methods is brought in Fig. 16.15.

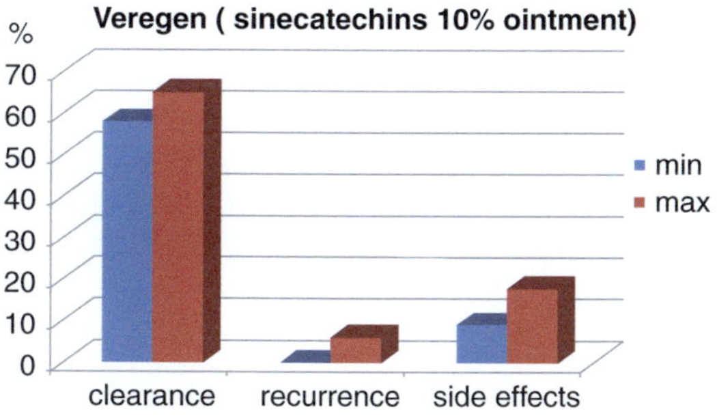

Fig. 16.14 Sinecatechin treatment

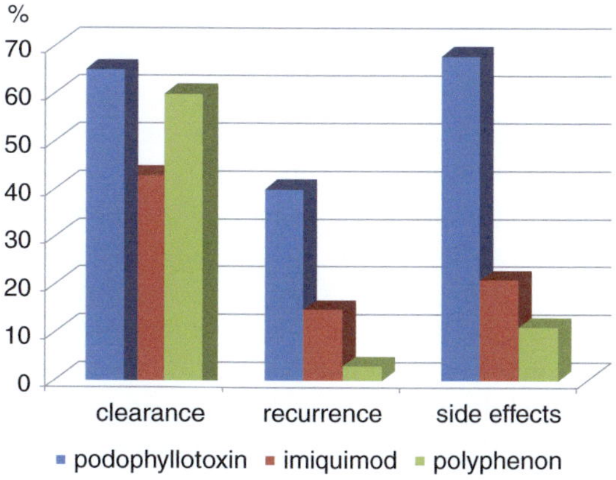

Fig. 16.15 Summary of self-applied medical treatments

16.13 Medical Treatment Applied by Healthcare Provider

16.13.1 Interferon Injections

Several types of interferon were in use in the past for treatment of condylomata. They were administered intralesionally (Fig. 16.11) or systemically. Both approaches included prolonged schedules and caused severe side effects, such as flu-like symptoms and increase in liver enzymes, and therefore are not in general use today.

16.13.2 Local Trichloroacetic Acid (Corrosive Agent)

Treatment by trichloroacetic acid is recommended for external use only and is considered safe in pregnancy. The solution is applied on the lesion with a cotton tip, three times weekly, up to a maximum of 1 month. Inflammation is a common side effect, and it is sometimes not possible to control the depth of the acid activity. The reported effectiveness ranges between 63% and 70%, and there is a relatively high percentage of recurrence (Fig. 16.16) [34].

Medical treatment should not be used on non-keratinized mucosa or during pregnancy, with the exception of trichloroacetic acid.

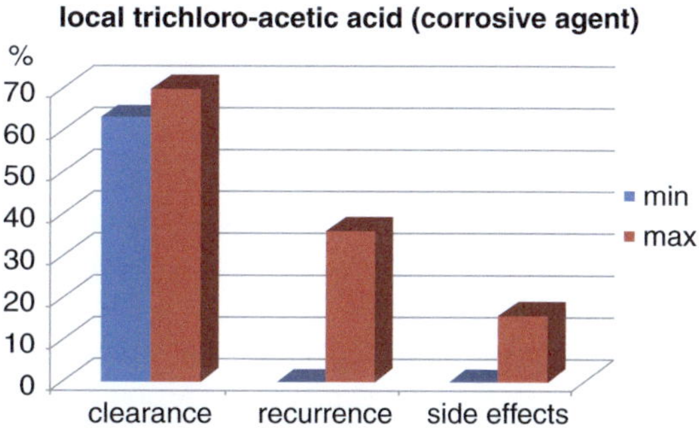

Fig. 16.16 Trichloroacetic acid treatment

16.14 Surgical Treatment

16.14.1 Surgical Excision

Surgery requires either local or general anesthesia. The lesions can be removed by a curette, scalpel, electric loop excision, or electrocautery, with a reported recurrence of approximately 30% within 1 year after removal.

16.14.2 Cryotherapy

The use of liquid nitrogen with a cryoprobe does not require anesthesia and is safe for nonkeratinized areas as well. The cryoprobe is applied directly to the lesions. A gel interface medium often is used between the probe and the skin surface. The freezing time is adjusted according to variables such as skin thickness, vascularity, tissue type, and lesion characteristics. The margin size depends primarily on the thickness of the lesion. Margins for most benign lesions can extend as little as 1–2 mm beyond the visible pathologic border. The reported efficiency ranges between 79% and 71%, and recurrence ranges between 38% and 73%. The main side effect is local inflammation, and the therapy can be repeated after 2 weeks have elapsed [35, 36].

16.14.3 CO_2 Laser Evaporation

In most cases, CO_2 laser vaporization is given as second-line therapy after the failure of initial therapy. It is the preferred method for very widespread lesions. The laser beam makes it possible to accurately control the depth and width of the evaporation and prevent unnecessary damage to healthy tissue while limiting the scarring (Fig. 16.10). However, the equipment is expensive, and the procedure requires a skilled operator. The reported recurrence rate is between 60% and 77% of the patients.

The advantage of laser treatment is that it is possible to control the depth of the lesion so that the damage will be superficial, thus preventing scarring of the skin during the healing process.

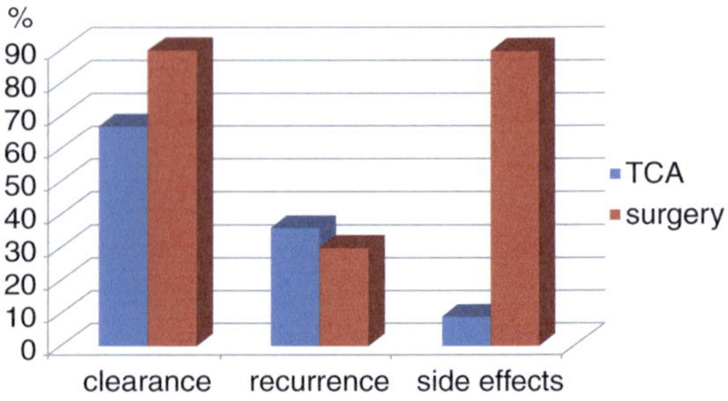

Fig. 16.17 Summary of treatment applied by the medical staff

These treatments are directed solely against warts and have no effect whatsoever on the virus itself, thus the relatively high percentage of recurrence, i.e., ~30%, which is even higher in immunosuppressive states [37, 38].

Figure 16.17 provides a summary of the outcomes of treatments applied by the medical staff.

16.14.4 Primary Prevention

It is now possible to prevent infection by the virus that causes the disease. The HPV vaccines (quadrivalent and nona valent Gardasil) protect against HPV 6 and 11, which are responsible for 90% of all genital warts [39].

16.14.4.1 Prospective Studies

The efficacy of the quadrivalent vaccine in the prevention of genital warts was first validated in prospective controlled trials (FUTURE I and II trials) in more than 17,000 women who were followed for ~4 years. The vaccines prevented up to 100% of genital warts caused by HPV 6 and 11 when provided to young (16–26 years of age) unexposed women (42–44). These studies also proved efficacy in the reduction of condyloma recurrence (i.e., 35% fewer recurrences) and demonstrated that they may provide protection against new exposures [40]. The same efficacy was shown in unexposed women 25–45 years of age [41]. In addition, good efficacy in men was reported in prospective studies, which reported a 90% reduction of external warts caused by HPV 6 and 11 [42].

16.14.4.2 The Real-Life Effect Following Vaccination

The impact of HPV vaccination in real-life settings has become increasingly evident over the last decade, especially among girls vaccinated before HPV exposure in countries with high vaccine uptake. Maximal reductions of genital warts have reached ~90%. Closely tracked declines in the prevalence and incidence of genital warts with decreases in HPV 6 and 11 infections in countries with high vaccine uptake (e.g., Australia and Denmark) recorded considerable reductions in the frequency of genital warts, particularly in the youngest age groups at the time of vaccination. Yearly decreases of ~50% were observed in several studies, and a reduction of up to 92.6% was observed 4 years after the implementation of a vaccination program for Australian women <21 years of age. Furthermore, reductions were observed in unvaccinated young Australian men, consistent with herd protection. In countries with low-to-moderate uptake of the vaccine at the time of the study (including France, the United States, Canada, Sweden, Belgium, Germany, and New Zealand), the reduction in genital warts ranged from 5.5% to 72.1% [43]. The new 9-valent vaccine (Gardasil 9) against HPV 6/11/16/18/31/33/45/52/58 showed similar efficacy for condylomas, closely resembling that of the quadrivalent vaccine [44].

Genital Warts: Condyloma, Breaking the Myths

- One of the long-held beliefs is that intercourse using a condom is safe, but the virus may be transmitted by contact of uncovered skin in the genital area, making the protection for HPV infection partial at best.
- Although many patients have been warned that their condyloma may be a source of malignancy, the HPV types that cause genital warts do not cause malignant changes.
- Classical genital warts can be diagnosed by clinical inspection, and biopsy or HPV-DNA analysis is rarely indicated. The indications for biopsy are treatment failure to standard therapy, atypical warts, ulcerated pigmented lesions, and in immunocompromised patients.
- Genital warts are not trivial; on the quality-adjusted life-year scale, the utility weight of genital warts (0.91) is between uncomplicated type II diabetes and well-controlled asthma or CIN 1 lesions
- Some clinicians recommend that women with genital warts undergo cervical colposcopy. Indeed, women with STDs, including genital warts, have a higher risk of developing cervical cancer, and so screening for cervical cancer is strongly recommended in the form of cytological screening or HPV testing. However, there is no evidence that routine screening colposcopy is indicated for patients with genital warts

References

1. Oriel JD. Natural history of genital warts. 1971. Sex Transm Infect. 2000;76(Suppl 1):S21.
2. Tay SK. Genital oncogenic human papillomavirus infection: a short review on the mode of transmission. Ann Acad Med Singap. 1995;24(4):598–601.
3. Pao CC, Tsai PL, Chang YL, Hsieh TT, Jin JY. Possible non-sexual transmission of genital human papillomavirus infections in young women. Eur J Clin Microbiol Infect Dis. 1993;12(3):221–2.
4. Sonnex C, Strauss S, Gray JJ. Detection of human papillomavirus DNA on the fingers of patients with genital warts. Sex Transm Infect. 1999;75(5):317–9.
5. CDRWkl (Online). 2001;11(35). http://www.hpa.org.uk/cdr/archives/2001/cdr3501.
6. Koutsky L. Epidemiology of genital human papillomavirus infection. Am J Med. 1997;102:3–8.
7. World Health Organization. WHO Office of Information. Sexually transmitted infections increasing—250 million new infections annually. WHO Feature. 1990;152:1–6.
8. Shavit O, Raz R, Stein S, Chodick G, Schejter E, Cohen R, Shalev V. Evaluating the epidemiology and morbidity burden associated with human papillomavirus in Israel: accounting for CIN1 and genital warts in

addition to CIN 2/3 and cervical cancer. Appl Health Econ Health Policy. 2012;10(2):87–97.
9. Insinga RP, Dasbach EF, Myers ER. The health and economic burden of genital warts in a set of private health plans in the United States. Clin Infect Dis. 2003;36(11):1397–403.
10. Koutsky LA, Galloway DA, Holmes KK. Epidemiology of genital human papillomavirus infection. Epidemiol Rev. 1988;10:122–63.
11. Handsfield HH. Clinical presentation and natural course of anogenital warts. Am J Med. 1997;102(5A):16–20.
12. Kjaer SK, Tran TN, Sparen P, Tryggvadottir L, Munk C, Dasbach E, Liaw KL, Nygård J, Nygård M. The burden of genital warts: a study of nearly 70,000 women from the general female population in the 4 Nordic countries. J Infect Dis. 2007;196(10):1447–54.
13. Hansen BT, Kjaer SK, Munk C, Tryggvadottir L, Sparén P, Hagerup-Jenssen M, Liaw KL, Nygård M. Early smoking initiation, sexual behavior and reproductive health – a large population-based study of Nordic women. Prev Med. 2010;51(1): 68–72.
14. Schiffman M, Castle PE. Human papillomavirus: epidemiology and public health. Arch Pathol Lab Med. 2003;127:930–4.
15. Longworth MS, Laimins LA. Pathogenesis of human papillomaviruses in differentiating epithelia. Microbiol Mol Biol Rev. 2004;68(2):362–72.
16. Chiasson MA, Ellerbrock TV, Bush TJ, Sun XW, Wright TC Jr. Increasedprevalence of vulvovaginal condyloma and vulvar intraepithelial neoplasia inwomen infected with the human immunodeficiency virus. Obstet Gynecol. 1997;89(5 Pt 1):690–4.
17. Workowski KA, Berman S, Centers for Disease Control and Prevention (CDC). Sexually transmitted diseases treatment guidelines, 2010. MMWR Recomm Rep. 2010;59(RR-12):1–110.
18. Cook LS, Koutsky LA, Holmes KK. Clinical presentation of genital warts amon circumcised and uncircumcised heterosexual men attending an urSTD clinic. Genitourin Med. 1993;69:262–4.
19. Sonnex C, Schofield JH, Kocjan G, et al. Anal human papillomavirus infection in heterosexuals with genital warts: prevalence and relation with sexual behaviour. Br Med J. 1991;303:1243.
20. Lacey CJ, Woodhall SC, Wikstrom A, Ross J. 2012 European guideline for the management of anogenital warts. J Eur Acad Dermatol Venereol. 2013;27(3):e263–70.
21. Armstrong N, Foley G, Wilson J, Finan P, Sebag-Montefiore D. Successful treatment of a large Buschke-Lowenstein tumour with chemo-radiotherapy. Int J STD AIDS. 2009;20(10):732–4.
22. Drolet M, Brisson M, Maunsell E, Franco EL, Coutlée F, Ferenczy A, Ratnam S, Fisher W, Mansi JA. The impact of anogenital warts on health-related quality oflife: a 6-month prospective study. Sex Transm Dis. 2011;38(10):949–56.
23. Meisels A. Cytologic diagnosis of human papillomavirus. Influence of age and pregnancy stage. Acta Cytol. 1992;36(4):480–2.
24. Silverberg MJ, Thorsen P, Lindeberg H, Grant LA, Shah KV. Condyloma inpregnancy is strongly predictive of juvenile-onset recurrent respiratory papillomatosis. Obstet Gynecol. 2003;101(4):645–52.
25. Workowski KA. Centers for disease control and prevention sexually transmitted diseases treatment guidelines. Clin Infect Dis. 2015;61(Suppl 8):S759–62.
26. Blomberg M, Friis S, Munk C, Bautz A, Kjaer SK. Genital warts and risk of cancer: a Danish study of nearly 50,000 patients with genital warts. J Infect Dis. 2012;205(10):1544–53.
27. Tyring SK. Molluscum contagiosum: the importance of early diagnosis and treatment. Am J Obstet Gynecol. 2003;189(3 Suppl):S12–6.
28. Ambros RA, Malfetano JH, Carlson JA, Mihm MC Jr. Non-neoplastic epithelial alterations of the vulva: recognition assessment and comparisons of terminologies used among the various specialties. Mod Pathol. 1997;10(5):401–8.
29. Hoang LN, Park KJ, Soslow RA, Murali R. Squamous precursor lesions of the vulva: current classification and diagnostic challenges. Pathology. 2016;48(4):291–302.
30. Lacey CJ, Goodall RL, Tennvall GR, Maw R, Kinghorn GR, Fisk PG, Barton S, Byren I, Perstop Pharma Genital Warts Clinical Trial Group. Randomised controlled trial and economic evaluation of podophyllotoxin solution, podophyllotoxin cream, and podophyllin in the treatment of genital warts. Sex Transm Infect. 2003;79(4):270–5.
31. Haidopoulos D, Diakomanolis E, Rodolakis A, Vlachos G, Elsheikh A, Michalas S. Safety and efficacy of locally applied imiquimod cream 5% for the treatment of condylomata acuminata of the vulva. Arch Gynecol Obstet. 2004;270(4):240–3.
32. Tatti S, Stockfleth E, Beutner KR, Tawfik H, Elsasser U, Weyrauch P, Mescheder A. Polyphenon E: a new treatment for external anogenital warts. Br J Dermatol. 2010;162(1):176–84.
33. Tzellos TG, Sardeli C, Lallas A, Papazisis G, Chourdakis M, Kouvelas D. Efficacy, safety and tolerability of green tea catechins in the treatment ofexternal anogenital warts: a systematic review and meta-analysis. J Eur Acad Dermatol Venereol. 2011;25(3):345–53.
34. Ting PT, Dytoc MT. Therapy of external anogenital warts and molluscum contagiosum: a literature review. Dermatol Ther. 2004;17:68–101.
35. Andrews MD. Cryosurgery for common skin conditions. Am Fam Physician. 2004;69(10):2365–72.
36. Abdullah AN, Walzman M, Wade A. Treatment of external genital warts comparing cryotherapy (liquid nitrogen) and trichloracetic acid. Sex Transm Dis. 1993;20:344–5.
37. Yanofsky VR, Patel RV, Goldenberg G. Genital warts: a comprehensive review. J Clin Aesthet Dermatol. 2012;5(6):25–36.

38. Mayeaux EJ Jr, Dunton C. Modern management of external genital warts. J Low Genit Tract Dis. 2008;12(3):185–92. Review.
39. Donovan B, Franklin N, Guy R, et al. Quadrivalent human papillomavirus vaccination and trends in genital warts in Australia: analysis of national sentinel surveillance data. Lancet Infect Dis. 2011;11:39.
40. Joura EA, Garland SM, Paavonen J, Ferris DG, Perez G, Ault KA, Huh WK, Sings HL, James MK, Haupt RM, Future I and II Study Group. Effect of the human papillomavirus (HPV) quadrivalent vaccine in a subgroup of women with cervical and vulvar disease: retrospective pooled analysis of trial data. BMJ. 2012;344:e1401.
41. Luna J, Plata M, Gonzalez M, Correa A, Maldonado I, Nossa C, Radley D, Vuocolo S, Haupt RM, Saah A. Long-term follow-up observation of the safety, immunogenicity, and effectiveness of Gardasil™ in adult women. PLoS One. 2013;8(12):e83431.
42. Giuliano A, et al. Presented at: 25th International Papillomavirus Conference. May 2009. Abstract 0-01.07.
43. Garland SM, Kjaer SK, Muñoz N, Block SL, Brown DR, DiNubile MJ, Lindsay BR, Kuter BJ, Perez G, Dominiak-Felden G, Saah AJ, Drury R, Das R, Velicer C. Impact and effectiveness of the quadrivalent human papillomavirus vaccine: a systematic review of 10 years of real-world experience. Clin Infect Dis. 2016;63(4):519–27.
44. Joura EA, Giuliano AR, Iversen OE, Bouchard C, Mao C, Mehlsen J, Moreira ED Jr, Ngan Y, Petersen LK, Lazcano-Ponce E, Pitisuttithum P, Restrepo JA, Stuart G, Woelber L, Yang YC, Cuzick J, Garland SM, Huh W, Kjaer SK, Bautista OM, Chan IS, Chen J, Gesser R, Moeller E, Ritter M, Vuocolo S, Luxembourg A, Broad Spectrum HPV Vaccine Study. A 9-valent HPV vaccine against infection and intraepithelial neoplasia in women. N Engl J Med. 2015;372(8):711–23.

Part III

Vulvar Lesions: Skin-Colored Plaques

Lichen Simplex Chronicus

17

Despoina Mortaki and Alexander Mortakis

17.1 Definition and Epidemiology

Lichen simplex chronicus (LSC) is an acquired severely itching chronic dermatosis characterized by a nonscarring process of epidermal thickening that develops as a result of repeated rubbing and scratching (the end stage of the itch-scratch-itch cycle). Histologically there is acanthosis with a prominent superficial dermal inflammatory cell infiltrate [1]. Cases previously described with the terms squamous cell hyperplasia, neurodermatitis, and hyperplastic dystrophy are included now under the term lichen simplex chronicus [2, 3].

LSC papules and plaques of thickened lichenified skin can be found on the vulva and the perianal area, but LSC is a common cutaneous disorder occurring also on the pubis, neck, ankles, scalp, and extensor forearms [4].

Vulvar LSC occurs mostly in mid-to-late adulthood, with highest prevalence in persons aged 30–50 years. It is a common disease, although exact incidence and prevalence figures have not been determined. Exact prevalence is unknown, but it is estimated to occur in approximately 0.5–1% of the western European and American populations [5].

D. Mortaki
University Hospital "A. Syggros" for Skin and Venereal Diseases, Athens, Greece

A. Mortakis (✉)
"IASO" Maternity Hospital, Athens, Greece
e-mail: info@mortakis.gr

17.2 Causes and Pathogenesis

Any disorder that causes itch can lead to the development of LSC. The intense, chronic itching leads the patient to repetitively rub and scratch the affected area. When a patient repetitively scratches or rubs a pruritic area of skin over time, lichenification will develop. Lichen simplex chronicus is the end stage of an itch- scratch-itch cycle.

Some skin types are more prone to lichenification, such as skin that tends toward eczematous conditions (i.e., atopic dermatitis, atopic diathesis). There is an altered skin barrier. Up to 75% of patients with LSC have a personal or family history of allergic rhinitis, asthma, or atopic dermatitis. Other studies demonstrate an incidence of between 20% and >90% [5–7]. The itch-scratch cycle, with habitual scratching, is a major component of atopic dermatitis. Disruption of the epidermal barrier, as a result of scratching, allows stimulation of type C non-myelinated nerve endings that convey itch and pain to the CNS, as well as providing the initial driving stimulus for LSC [8].

LSC can be a primary dermatosis (the process arising de novo from normal skin), or secondary, presenting as a reaction to another vulvar disease (superimposed on an underlying disorder such as lichen sclerosus, psoriasis, etc.).

In primary LSC, the skin is normal at the outset. Irritation from any number of originating causes, yeast infection, reaction to a moisturizer, too-tight clothing, over-washing, panty liners,

J. Bornstein (ed.), *Vulvar Disease*, https://doi.org/10.1007/978-3-319-61621-6_17

sweat, urine, etc., starts the process off. Scratching seems mandatory and pleasurable to patients and may occur in their sleep. If scratching causes extensive excoriation, the woman replaces it with rubbing, which also causes lichenification, and a vicious cycle is set up (the itch-scratch-itch cycle) that must be interrupted to allow healing to take place. The patient experiences itching, worse with stress, and persistent habitual scratching results in lichenification and excoriations.

In cases considered as primary LSC, one or multiple patches or plaques arise de novo on normal-appearing skin in the absence of a primary pruritic cutaneous disorder. In these cases the major pruritic triggers are environmental and/or psychological [1, 8]. Primary LSC is the more common condition tending to appear in patients with an atopic diathesis. It may be a consequence of exposure to an irritating or inflammatory agent. The cause of the initiating "itch" that leads to lichen simplex chronicus includes irritation or allergies from chemicals (laundry detergent, fabric softeners, menstrual pads, spermicides, latex condoms, occlusive underwear fabrics with synthetic fibers, tight clothing, over-cleaning with soaps) or infections—most commonly yeast. Intense, chronic itching results in repetitive rubbing and scratching. Usually the inciting agent will remain undetermined. It may be also related to stress, anxiety, depression, and obsessive-compulsive disorder [5, 7, 8].

Secondary LSC may be due to an underlying dermatosis (psoriasis, lichen sclerosus, contact dermatitis), a chronic infection (candidiasis, dermatophytosis), a metabolic cause like diabetes, or even a precancerous lesion (vulvar intraepithelial neoplasia). Some systemic conditions such as renal failure, obstructive biliary disease (primary biliary cirrhosis and primary cholangitis), Hodgkin's lymphoma, hyper- or hypothyroidism, and polycythemia can cause pruritus and thus lead to secondary LSC [9–11].

Stress, heat, sweating, and friction usually increase the itch leading to scratching. Rubbing and scratching relieve the discomfort but damage the protective cutaneous barrier and contributes to thicken the epidermis and perpetuate the lesions.

Scratching seems mandatory and pleasurable to patients and may occur in their sleep. If scratching causes extensive excoriation, the woman replaces it with rubbing, which also causes lichenification, and a vicious cycle is set up (the itch-scratch-itch cycle) that must be interrupted to allow healing to take place. The patient experiences itching, worse with stress, and persistent habitual scratching (the itch-scratch-itch vicious cycle) results in lichenification and excoriations. Generally, emotional tensions, such as in patients with anxiety, depression, or obsessive-compulsive disorder, may play a key role in inducing a pruritic sensation, leading to scratching that can become self-perpetuating [12].

17.3 Diagnostic Approach

17.3.1 Patient History

Characteristic history and physical examination findings are usually sufficient for the diagnosis of LSC. A biopsy is required when the diagnosis is uncertain.

A careful history and thorough vulvar and vaginal examination are paramount to securing the correct diagnosis. Questions should specifically elicit whether the condition is acute or chronic, exposure to common irritants, hygiene practices, sexually transmitted infection exposure risk, current contraceptive method, and previous therapies attempted.

Pruritus is the usual presenting symptom. It may have been present for weeks or months. Patients commonly report that they cannot stop scratching and that it feels pleasurable to scratch. The "itch-scratch" cycle is the most defining characteristic of LSC. Itching is usually well localized on the labial skin and, in most cases, is severe, intractable, worse at night, and exacerbated by heat, sweating, and clothing.

A careful history to evaluate any use of topical medications (antifungals, lotions, soaps, perfumes, lubricants), history of atopy, regular hygienic practices (use of panty liners, baby wipes, douches, shaving, waxing, and laser hair removal), and clothing (noncotton underwear, occlusive undergarments) is essential for identifying triggers.

In many patients the pruritus began during a time of stress, anxiety, or when there is a history of prior psychiatric disorder such as anxiety, depression, obsessive-compulsive disorder, or dissociative experiences. These factors are frequently underrecognized, and they should be inquired about, and addressed if found, in all patients with LSC. In the majority of the cases, an atopic diathesis is defined as a personal or immediate family history of atopic dermatitis, allergic rhinitis, or asthma [7, 12–14].

17.3.2 Physical Examination

LSC most often affects the hair-bearing portion of the labia majora, but involvement of the labia minora, mons pubis, upper inner thighs, and the perianal area is not uncommon.

In early LSC, generalized erythema may be present before lichenification takes place. Inflammation is always present in LSC. In light-skinned women, this will be apparent because of visible redness (Fig. 17.1). In darker-skinned individuals, the natural pigmentation will mask the intensity of the redness and shift the color to a darker, red-brown color.

Later the skin is thickened, erythematous, pale, or pigmented, with accentuated markings secondary to rubbing. Lichenification results from chronic rubbing and scratching of the skin and is characterized by an exaggeration of normal skin markings, forming a crisscross mosaic pattern (Figs. 17.2 and 17.3).

Linear excoriations witness for the scratching. The papules and plaques are bright red initially but develop a dusky, brown-red color as time passes, and at a later stage they may whiten. The margins of the lesions are indistinct. Because the vulva is moist, crusts and scales commonly seen with dermatitis elsewhere on the body may not be seen on the vulva. The final hallmark sign of LSC is lichenification: thickening of the skin with the distinctive pattern of normal skin "hatch markings"

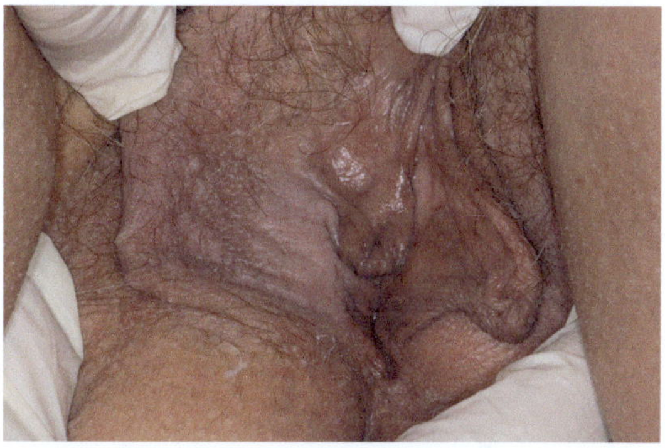

Fig. 17.2 LSC lesions of the right labium. White discoloration of the hydrated hyperkeratotic skin of the wet vulvar area

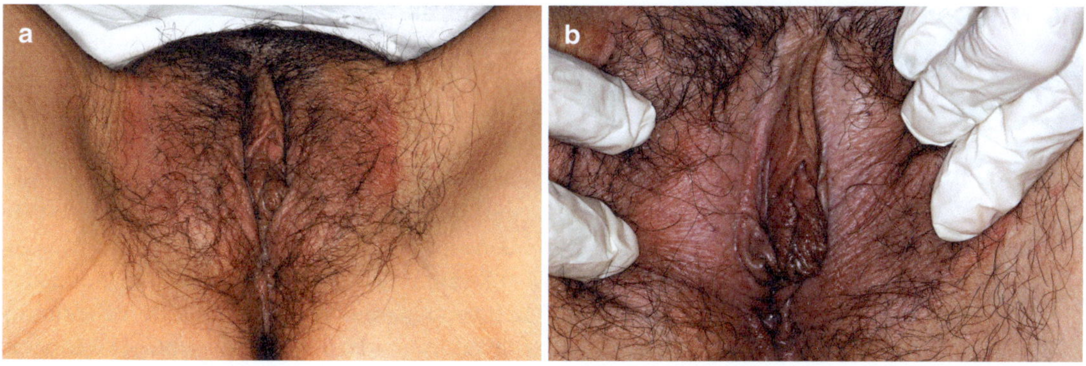

Fig. 17.1 (**a**) Generalized erythema (inflammation) on the vulva of a 38yo atopic patient with chronic candidiasis. Note the lichenification at the lower part of the vulva. (**b**) Same patient: white lesions on the inner aspects of the labia majora, with marked lichenification and linear excoriations. The margins of the lesions are indistinct. Generalized erythema (inflammation) at the periphery

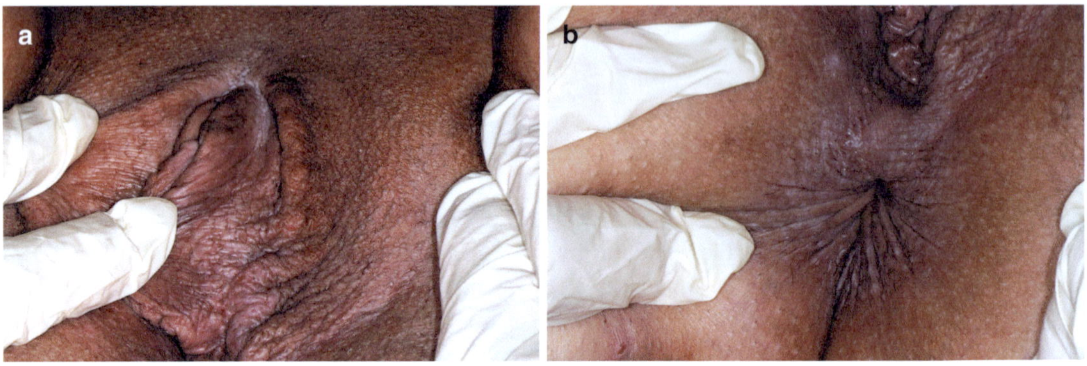

Fig. 17.3 Marked lichenification and hypopigmentation with LSC. (**a**) Vulvar lesions and (**b**) anal lesions on the same patient

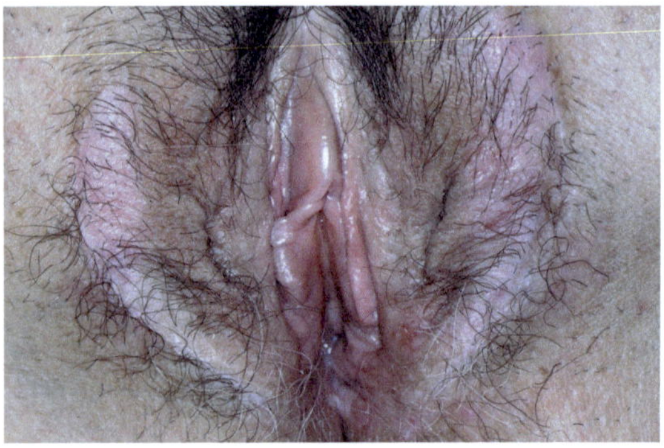

Fig. 17.4 The final hallmark sign of LSC. Thickening of the skin and excoriations because of scratching. The hair is becoming sparse and broken

being exaggerated and deepened when compared with adjacent, non-affected skin. In addition, because of scratching, hair may be absent or broken (Fig. 17.4).

17.3.3 Pathology

Diagnosis is clinical. Biopsy can also make the diagnosis and can rule out other conditions. Histologically, hyperkeratosis, irregular acanthosis (thickening of the epidermis), spongiosis, a prominent granular layer, and lengthened rete ridges are seen with LSC. Parakeratosis and a chronic dermal inflammatory infiltrate can also be seen on histopathologic analysis. There is lamellar thickening of the papillary dermis and sometimes perineural fibrosis. In secondary LSC, the specific features of the triggering dermatosis may be observed [1, 2].

17.3.4 Establishment of Diagnosis

The diagnosis of LSC is usually established on a clinical basis due to the highly characteristic findings described above. When a diagnosis of LSC is established, it is necessary to determine whether the process is primary or secondary (superimposed on an underlying disorder). Lichen simplex chronicus may occur because of itching associated with another skin disease such as lichen sclerosus or may develop as de novo itching. Often when the patient is first seen, the best policy is to break the itch-scratch cycle and re-examine her. If underlying abnormalities remain, the process is presumably secondary, and the underlying disorder must be identified. This can be done by biopsy, by potassium hydroxide smear, or by culture. The underlying disorders most often encountered include candidiasis, lichen sclerosus, tinea cruris, psoriasis, contact dermatitis, warts, and vulvar intraepithelial neoplasia [2, 5].

A careful vulvar skin examination and speculum examination of the vagina are essential to rule out vaginitis. Microscopy with pH testing of any discharge is useful in diagnosing candidiasis, trichomoniasis, or bacterial vaginosis. Given the low sensitivity of wet mounts for all types of candida, a fungal culture is helpful to eliminate candidiasis as a contributing factor in all patients with a negative wet mount [15–17].

17.3.5 Differential Diagnosis

Differential diagnosis includes the causes of secondary lichenification listed earlier (lichen sclerosus, psoriasis, etc.), and these should be ruled out, since they can all present with this almost identical pattern.

Biopsy can be helpful, at times, in differentiating between LSC and lichen sclerosus, which may also cause itching and hypopigmentation. However, LSC will not cause loss of the normal vulvar anatomy as will lichen sclerosus.

Psoriasis can occur in the vulvar area and contribute to the appearance of LSC. Candida must always be ruled out when women report these symptoms because it is often a precipitating factor. Extramammary Paget disease may appear eczematous, like LSC.

17.4 Therapy

The main goals of therapy are:

1. To identify and treat any underlying dermatological or systemic condition (if any) that could be driving the condition in secondary LSC
2. To remove any triggering and exacerbating factors
3. To stop the itch-scratch-itch vicious cycle through reduction of inflammation and controlling the nocturnal pruritus
4. To repair the barrier function of the skin and educate the patient

Although there is no standardized treatment for LSC and management of the condition is very much tailored to the individual patient, the mainstay of treatment usually involves the package of a topical corticosteroid, emollients, and lifestyle modification; a sedating agent for nocturnal pruritus; and the addition of an antipruritic for breakthrough pruritus as required.

17.4.1 Underlying Dermatological or Systemic Conditions

When an underlying disorder can be identified, it should be treated. Concomitant infections can be managed with oral antibiotics and/or fluconazole.

The clinician must identify and treat any underlying infections (*Candida* infections, dermatophytosis, *Streptococcus* A infection), underlying vulvar dermatoses (lichen sclerosus, lichen planus), psoriasis, vulvar intraepithelial neoplasia, Paget's disease, and metabolic causes of itching (diabetes, iron deficiency anemia). It is not uncommon to have psoriasis, contact dermatitis, and LSC in the same patient [2, 9, 16].

Patients with neurologic or psychiatric triggers for LSC should be referred to the appropriate specialists (neurologist, psychiatrist).

Identification of triggering and exacerbating factors:

Environmental triggering and exacerbating factors such as dry or excessively moist skin, chronic friction from tight or rough clothing, and harsh skincare products should be eliminated in all patients.

In most cases no underlying disorder can be found at the initial visit, and it is necessary to treat first the itch-scratch-itch cycle.

17.4.2 Reduction of Inflammation

The presence of inflammation is detrimental because it leads to spongiosis and resultant barrier layer dysfunction.

Topical application of mid to high potency corticosteroids is used to decrease the underlying inflammation. A good policy seems to be starting with fluocinonide 0.05% or triamcinolone acetonide 0.1% ointment and if necessary moving up to the superpotent category of clobetasol propionate 0.05% ointment. Topical steroids should be applied in small amounts twice daily for 2–3 weeks. Close follow-up in the office in a relatively short interval (3 weeks) is helpful to monitor response and determine when tapering of the steroid can begin. In general, ointments are preferred over creams, as they are less irritating and better absorbed and serve additionally as an emollient leaving a protective barrier on the skin's surface [5, 18, 19].

The patients are advised to soak the affected areas in a lukewarm bath before applying the topical corticosteroid followed by a gentle emollient, such as white petrolatum. If skin is very raw, the topical steroids will burn. Start with plain Vaseline, nighttime sedation for 2–3 days, oral antibiotics, and anti-yeast medication (if needed), and then tell her to start using the topical steroids.

If there is little or no improvement using topical steroids for 3 weeks, it is worth considering a short-term course (2 weeks) of systemic steroids (either prednisone or prednisolone). Another alternative is intramuscular injection of triamcinolone (1 mg/kg (up to 80 mg total). Repeat of the injection in 1 month is seldom necessary [5].

Tapering steroid therapy, be it with oral or topical therapy, is essential because long-term steroid therapy can be fraught with negative effects like local tissue thinning and fracturing, blunted immune response, and potential systemic effects. A repeat physical examination shortly after the taper is completed is important to assess tissue response, symptom improvement, and reinforce patient education [18, 19].

A limited place in the treatment of LSC has topical calcineurin inhibitors (tacrolimus ointment and pimecrolimus 1% cream). Their use might be warranted in the event of complete failure of potent topical steroids [5, 20, 21].

17.4.3 Breaking the Itch-Scratch Cycle

Oral antipruritics are often used, such as hydroxyzine or doxepin at night, being mindful of the side effects of sedation of both medications and the medication interactions of doxepin with some psychotropic medications, as doxepin is both an antihistamine and a tricyclic antidepressant.

Amitriptyline can also be used at times for sedation (25 mg po qhs; can be increased to 50 mg po qhs) in patients with severe itch-scratch cycle (caution in the elderly population because of its side effects—arrhythmia, urinary retention, and exacerbation of narrow-angle glaucoma). It puts the patient in a deeper sleep cycle than the other sedation agents listed above. Amitriptyline should not be combined with the other sedation agents above (exacerbation of the anticholinergic side effects). The physician must check for other drug interactions. Due to the side effects of the amitriptyline and doxepin, new-generation antidepressants (citalopram, fluoxetine, or sertraline) have been used successfully [5].

17.4.4 Restoration of the Epidermal Barrier Layer and Educating the Patient

Prompt repair of the epidermal barrier is attempted through the application of emollients and topical corticosteroids, but medication without behavioral modification will not lead to sustained clinical improvement. Counseling the patient about the itch-scratch cycle is of paramount importance. Maintenance of an intact epidermal barrier, especially in the presence of underlying atopic dermatitis, with frequent application of a bland, non-perfumed cream or ointment emollient is extremely important. The most efficacious time to apply an emollient is immediately after showering while the skin is still moist.

Non-pharmacological encouragement to stop scratching, in conjunction with other therapies, is extremely important to help break the itch-scratch cycle characteristic of LSC. Techniques include reinforcing the importance of resisting the urge to scratch, clenching of the fists for 30 s followed by pinching of the pruritic site in lieu of scratching, and applying crushed ice to areas of pruritus [11, 12].

If topical corticosteroid ointments are prescribed, they should be applied directly to the involved skin, most effective when applied immediately after bathing, and a mirror should be used to show the patient the correct area to treat. If an emollient is desired, white petrolatum is recommended because of its lack of allergenicity and irritancy. White petrolatum can be applied several times during the day when a patient feels itch or irritation or applied a few minutes after corticosteroid application. Sitz baths, cold compresses, and showering using a handheld shower head may be soothing. The most efficacious time to apply an emollient is immediately after showering while the skin is still moist. Emollients should be used at least twice a day and more frequently if the patient is able.

Education about appropriate hygiene should be provided. Eliminating common allergens, irritants, or exacerbating behaviors is an essential first step. Patients should be advised to avoid tight-fitting clothes, pantyhose, and synthetic materials and try to sleep without underwear to avoid nighttime occlusion. The use of white cotton underwear and avoiding tight clothing is recommended. The vulva should be cleansed only with warm water, gently with hands; all soaps, detergents, washcloths, and sponges should be eliminated. The vulva should be patted dry to avoid extra friction. The patient should not shave the vulva, as this can cause irritation and epithelial compromise [10, 15].

17.5 Prognosis

As suggested by its name, LSC is often chronic and relapsing and if untreated can go on indefinitely (Fig. 17.5).

Lichen simplex chronicus frequently persists as an itch-scratch cycle, even when environmental and other triggers are removed and the underlying disease is treated.

Vulvar LSC recurs due to sensitive skin in the vulvar area, so it will need repeated management. Even after the clearance of lesions, the condition can recur during a period of psychological stress or in the case of secondary LSC. Some patients may require intermittent therapy for months or years.

Once the acute lesion has been brought under control, patients should be advised that, in the

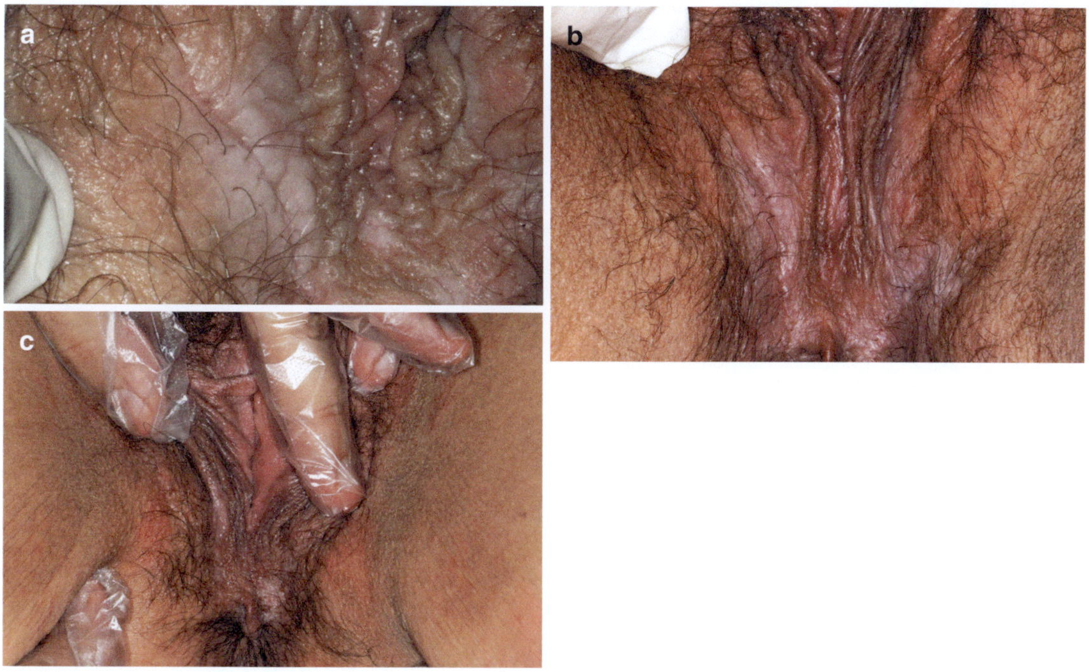

Fig. 17.5 (**a**) Vulvar LSC with white thick lichenified skin lesions. (**b**) Same patient 1 year later with recurrence of the lesions occupying this time a larger area of the vulva and the perineum. (**c**) The same patient after 3 months topical treatment with ointments (clobetasol and tacrolimus)

event of recurrence, they should contact their physician and resume treatment. Lesions may clear completely. Pruritus may resolve, but some pigmentary changes remain after successful treatment. Relapse is more likely in periods of psychic stress or if previously affected skin is stressed by extremes of heat or humidity or by skin irritants or allergens. In patients who do not comply with the treatment regimen and scratching cessation, lesions will not improve.

Vulvar LSC lesions cause little direct morbidity; however, occasionally patients report decreased or interrupted sleep, which affects motor and mental functioning.

Key Points

- Vulvar lichen simplex chronicus is a common dermatosis characterized by skin lichenification following excessive scratching. It is the end stage of an itch-scratch-itch cycle.
- Lichen simplex chronicus (LSC) can be a primary dermatosis (the process arising de novo from normal skin), or secondary, presenting as a reaction to another vulvar disease, like lichen sclerosus, psoriasis, contact dermatitis, etc.
- Paroxysmal pruritus is the usual presenting symptom. The "itch-scratch" cycle is the most defining characteristic of LSC. The final hallmark sign of LSC is lichenification. The skin is thickened, erythematous, pale, or pigmented, with accentuated markings with normal skin (hatch markings).
- Diagnosis of LSC is usually established on a clinical basis. Sometimes biopsy will be necessary to exclude underlying disease.
- The main goals of therapy are to identify and treat any underlying dermatological or systemic condition (if any) that could be driving in secondary LSC, to remove any triggering and exacerbating factors, to stop the itch-scratch-itch vicious cycle (through reduction of inflammation and controlling the nocturnal pruritus), and finally to repair the barrier function of the skin and educate the patient.
- Even after the clearance of lesions, the condition can relapse. Some patients will need repeated management.

Vulvar Lichen Simplex Chronicus: Breaking the Myths

- VLSC has no specific etiology. Any disorder that causes itch can lead to the development of vulvar lichen simplex chronicus
- Although traditional texts emphasize the significance of establishing diagnosis before applying treatment, and despite that vulvar lichen sclerosus and lichen simplex chronicus are two opposing vulvar dermatoses, treatment of these dermatoses is similar: applying potent topical corticosteroids for many weeks. In resistant cases, intralesional corticosteroid injection or calcineurin inhibitors help to break the itch-scratch cycle that often perpetuates this condition

References

1. Lynch PJ. Lichen simplex chronicus (atopic/neurodermatitis) of the anogenital region. Dermatol Ther. 2004;17:8–19.
2. Wilkinson E, Stone K. Atlas of vulvar diseases. Philadelphia: Lippincott Williams and Wilkins; 2008. p. 74–8.
3. Bornstein J, et al. The 2015 International Society for the Study of Vulvovaginal Disease (ISSVD) terminology of vulvar squamous intraepithelial lesions. J Lower Genit Tract Dis. 2016;20(1):11–4.
4. Lebwohl MG, et al. Treatment of skin disease: comprehensive therapeutic strategies. 2nd ed. Philadelphia: Mosby/Elsevier; 2006.
5. Lynch PJ. Vulvar pruritus and lichen simplex chronicus. In: Black M, editor. Obstetric and gynecologic dermatology. Philadelphia: Mosby Elsevier; 2008. p. 157–66.
6. Virgili A, et al. Evaluation of contact sensitization in vulvar lichen simplex chronicus. A proposal for a battery of selected allergens. J Reprod Med. 2003;48:33–6.
7. Crone AM, et al. Aetiological factors in vulvar dermatitis. J Eur Acad Dermatol Venereol. 2000;14:181–6.
8. Liao YH, et al. Increased risk of lichen simplex chronicus in people with anxiety disorder: a nationwide population-based retrospective cohort study. Br J Dermatol. 2014;170:890–4.
9. Schlosser BJ. Contact dermatitis of the vulva. Dermatol Clin. 2010;28(4):697–706.

10. Burrows LJ, et al. The vulvar dermatoses. J Sex Med. 2008;5:276–83.
11. Lotti T, et al. Prurigo nodularis and lichen simplex chronicus. Dermatol Ther. 2008;21:42–6.
12. Rosenbaum MS, Ayllon T. The behavioral treatment of neurodermatitis through habit-reversal. Behav Res Ther. 1981;19:313–8.
13. Moyal-Barracco M, Wendling J. Vulvar dermatoses. Best practice and research. Clin Obstet Gynecol. 2014;28:946–58.
14. Connor CJ, Eppsteiner EE. Vulvar contact dermatitis. Proc Obstet Gynecol. 2014;4(2):1–14.
15. Guerrero A, Venkatesan A. Inflammatory vulvar dermatoses. Clin Obstet Gynecol. 2015;58(3):464–75.
16. ACOG Practice Bulletin. Clinical management guidelines for obstetrician-gynecologists, number 72, May 2006. Vaginitis. Obstet Gynecol. 2006;107:1195–206.
17. Anderson MR, et al. Evaluation of vaginal complaints. JAMA. 2004;291:1368–79.
18. Rodriguez M, Leclair C. Benign vulvar dermatoses. Obstet Gynecol Surv. 2012;67(1):55–63.
19. Datz B, Yawalkar S. A double-blind, multicenter trial of 0.05% halobetasol propionate ointment and 0.05% clobetasol 17-propionate ointment in the treatment of patients with chronic, localized atopic dermatitis or lichen simplex chronicus. J Am Acad Dermatol. 1991;25:1157–60.
20. Aschoff R, Wozel G. Topical tacrolimus for the treatment of lichen simplex chronicus. J Dermatolog Treat. 2007;18:115–7.
21. Goldstein AT, et al. Pimecrolimus cream 1% for treatment of vulvar lichen simplex chronicus: an open-label, preliminary trial. Gynecol Obstet Investig. 2007;64:180–6.

Part IV

Vulvar Lesions: Red Lesions—Eczematous and Lichenified Diseases

Allergic Contact Dermatitis

18

Tanja Bohl

18.1 Introduction

Allergic contact dermatitis (ACD) is an inflammatory dermatosis where the tissue damage is the result of a Type IV, T cell-mediated delayed hypersensitivity reaction [1–9]. It is less common than irritant contact dermatitis (ICD) that is responsible for 80% of all contact dermatitis of the vulva. Vulvar contact dermatitis is common and of which 20% is due to ACD.

Once acquired, the sensitization persists for life. It is not amenable to desensitization as with antibody-mediated allergies (Type I, IgE acute hypersensitivity). Ultimately identification of the allergen by patch testing and complete avoidance is required to prevent recurrences.

18.2 Pathogenesis

ACD involves the presentation of antigens applied to the surface of the skin; dendritic cells (Langerhans cells, LC) within the epidermis process these antigens producing a distinct protein. The LC migrate to the regional lymph nodes where they present this to T cells resulting in their activation into Th1cells. The Th1 cells migrate back to the area of allergen application and initiate an inflammatory cascade resulting in the dermatitis seen clinically. This occurs specifically in the areas of antigen application.

The activated Th1 cells are antigen specific and long lived. Future antigen exposure will result in dermatitis in the site of new and previously exposed areas if they differ.

18.2.1 Allergenicity

Allergenicity is the ability to produce an allergic reaction. Not all potential allergens are equal in this respect.

18.2.2 Number of LC In the Exposed Tissue

The number of LC in the vulvar skin is similar to other body sites with respect to the hair and non-hair-bearing tissues.

18.2.3 Tissue Integrity

The vulva is a unique area of anatomy comprising hair- and non-hair-bearing skin, mucous membranes, and multiple creases that can become reservoirs of perspiration, natural secretions, exfoliated epidermal cells, urine, and feces.

These creases are warm and also undergo friction due to skin touching skin and tight clothing.

T. Bohl (✉)
Jean Hailes for Women's Health,
Clayton, VIC, Australia

J. Bornstein (ed.), *Vulvar Disease*, https://doi.org/10.1007/978-3-319-61621-6_18

These factors can increase the absorption of allergens and susceptibility to irritants.

Atopy and a preexisting vulvar dermatosis are associated with a higher rate of positive results to patch testing.

18.3 Etiology

Anogenital ACD is usually due to topical allergens applied directly to the area, secondary exposure of allergens that are finger borne (e.g., acrylates in nail varnish), and rarely oral allergen exposure.

Both ICD and ACD can complicate dermatoses. This should be considered in all patients with a vulvar dermatosis that becomes recalcitrant to therapy or flares after a period of control.

Vulvar skin is exposed to varying potential irritants and allergens through childhood, puberty, menstruation, sexual activity, reproduction, and ultimately menopause. Most sensitizers are fragrances, preservatives, or medicaments found in sanitary products, intimate products, cosmetics, and self-administered and prescribed topical products. Table 18.1 lists some of the allergens/allergen groups found on patch testing in cases of vulvar ACD to illustrate their diversity and occurrence in sometimes seemingly innocuous items.

Table 18.1 Allergens in vulvar ACD

Fragrances	
Eugenol in moist toilet paper	
Balsam of Peru	
Preservatives	
Methylchloroisothiazolinone (also has antibacterial and antifungal properties) in moist toilet paper	
Phenoxyethanol, formaldehyde releasers, parabens	
Ointment bases/emulsifiers	
Lanolin, a cetylstearyl alcohol (in medicaments, sorbolene cream)	
Topical medications	
Antibiotics	Neomycin
Antimycotics	Clotrimazole
Antivirals	Acyclovir
Corticosteroids	Hydrocortisone, triamcinolone
Anesthetics	Benzocaine
Rubber chemicals	
Condoms and sex toys	
Fabric dyes (in underpants)	
Nail varnishes	
Tosylamide-formaldehyde resin, acrylates	
"Natural" therapies	
Calendula, arnica, propolis	

18.4 Clinical Features

ACD can present as both an acute (Figs. 18.1 and 18.2) and chronic (Figs. 18.3 and 18.4) pruritic

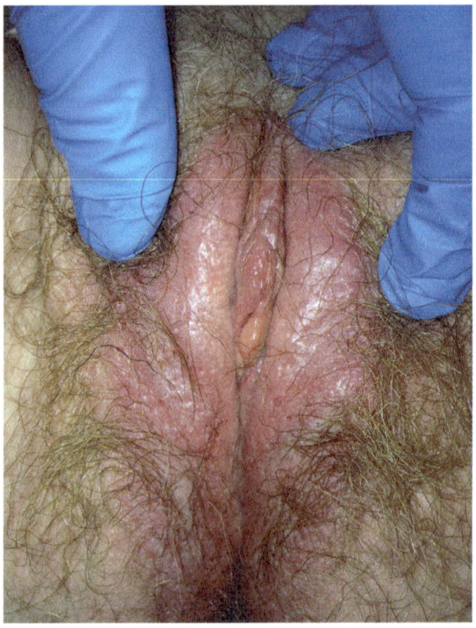

Fig. 18.1 Acute allergic contact dermatitis to benzocaine

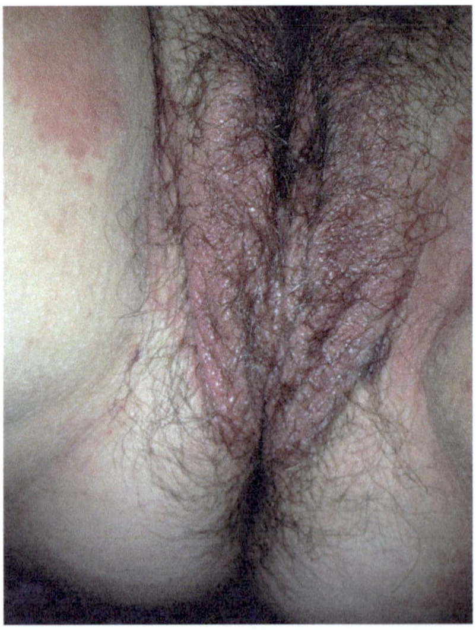

Fig. 18.2 Acute allergic contact dermatitis to benzocaine spreading to the thighs

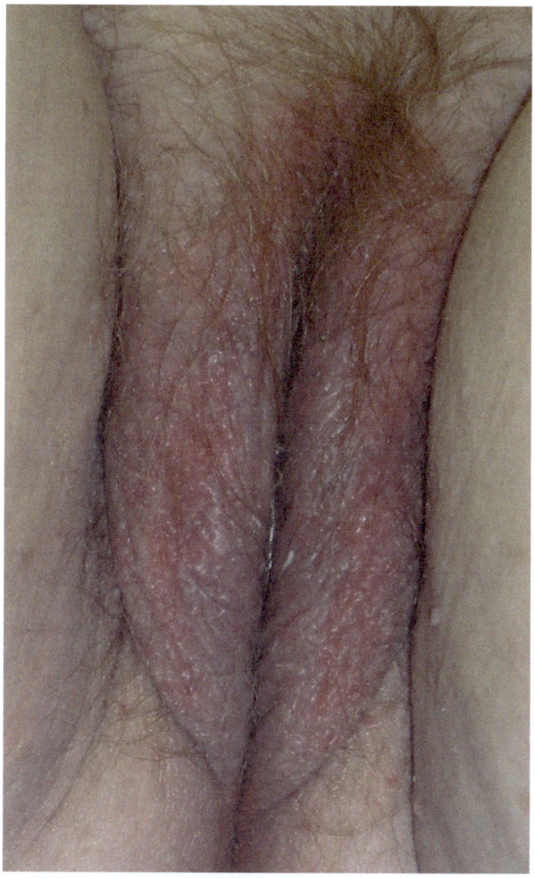

Fig. 18.3 Chronic allergic contact dermatitis

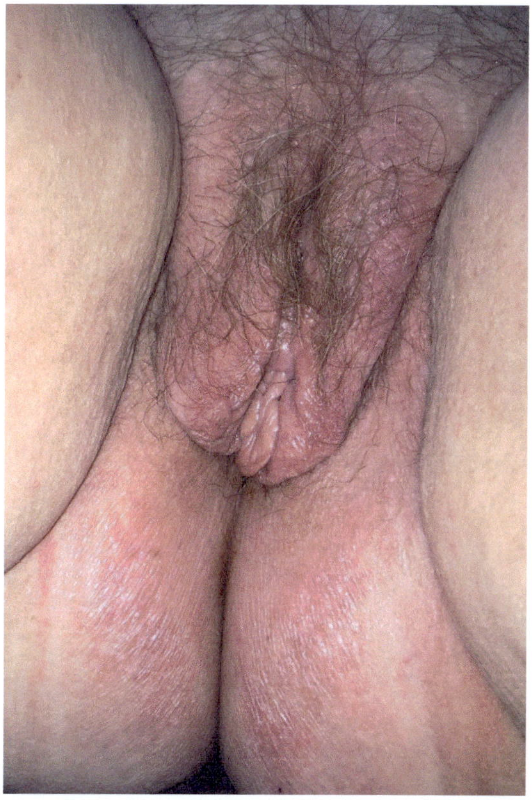

Fig. 18.4 Chronic allergic contact dermatitis spreading to buttocks

dermatoses in contrast to ICD which is usually a cause of burning and stinging sensations and possibly pain.

While the acute lesions may help differentiate ACD from ICD, once the dermatitis becomes chronic, it may be difficult to differentiate the two. A contactant can act as both an irritant and allergen.

Pruritus in a patient with ACD may be due to the ACD or an underlying dermatosis. The presence of an underlying dermatosis will modify the clinical appearance. Scratching damages the epidermal barrier resulting in increased skin vulnerability to both irritants and allergens.

18.5 Diagnosis and Treatment

The most important step in the management of ACD is suspecting it may be present. A possible history of previous reactions to topical medications including emollients should have elicited. Unexplained vulvar eczema and vulvar eczema that doesn't respond as expected to therapy or that worsens with continued appropriate therapy are situations in which the presence of ACD should be considered.

18.5.1 Histopathology

A biopsy is of variable value in establishing the diagnosis but can exclude other pathology. The histopathology will show parakeratosis, spongiosis, and irregular hyperkeratosis of the epidermis. The inflammatory infiltrate is perivascular and lymphocytic. These are all features seen in AD. Eosinophils predominate more than in AD or ICD, but this may not be conclusive.

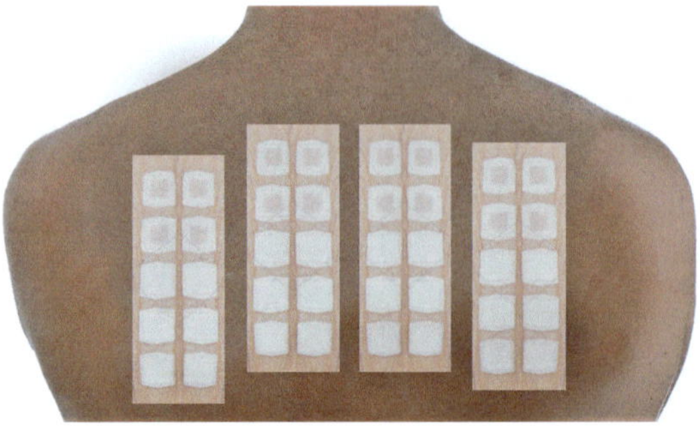

Fig. 18.5 Patch testing application. The strips are taped on the back. Each strip contains several patches. Every patch is coated with a substance (possible allergen) that might cause a skin reaction in sensitive people. Courtesy of Professor Jacob Bornstein

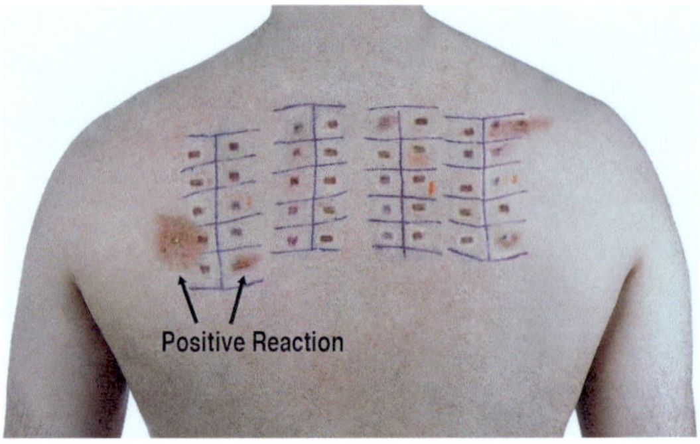

Fig. 18.6 Patch testing after 48 h: The strips are removed. Erythema signifies allergy to a specific allergen. Courtesy of Professor Jacob Bornstein

18.5.2 Patch Testing

Patch testing is required to establish the diagnosis. This should include testing against standard (European) battery which does include some rubber chemicals, fragrance, formaldehyde, clothing dyes, and preservatives but should be supplemented by testing against other recognized potential allergens including the patient's own products.

Standardized concentrations of potential allergens are applied, under occlusion, to the back (Fig. 18.5). These are left for 48 h, removed, and the skin examined for evidence of an eczematous reaction under one or more allergens. The skin is examined another 48 h later for possible late positive reactions. Experience is required to adequately perform the testing and evaluate the results (Fig. 18.6). Sometimes additional testing is required to establish the clinical relevance of a positive patch test result.

Repeat open application testing (ROAT) may be used in this situation. The patient is instructed to apply the suspect product to the volar aspect of their forearm twice a day for 1–2 weeks or until dermatitis develops. Standardized collections of allergens are available to dermatologists and allergists, and patch testing clinics exist in many institutions. Referral for such investigation should be considered if ACD is suspected.

Removing sources of potential allergens should be done with the use of bland emollients instead of soap. It also hydrates the skin. Infections should be excluded or treated if present. If a corticosteroid allergy is suspected changing to a non-hydrocortisone-related, mid- to high-potency corticosteroid such as betamethasone dipropionate 0.05% ointment, with nightly applications for 2 weeks should produce improvement. Mometasone preparations can be irritant in the anogenital area. Clobetasol preparations are also suitable.

Topical pimecrolimus 1.0% and tacrolimus 0.1% are effective in ACD. They may be introduced as steroid sparing alternative treatment once control is achieved and the likelihood of irritation is reduced.

Allergic contact dermatitis to topical corticosteroids does occur and is more common than once thought. Hydrocortisone and similar corticosteroids are usually responsible.

18.6 Prognosis

Avoidance of the causative allergen is the only effective, long-term solution. Allergens may be present in multiple products and may be added to products in the future without warning. Both clinician and patient must remain alert to this possibility and revisit this diagnosis, and patch testing should a recurrence occur.

Allergic Contact Dermatitis: Breaking the Myths

- Allergic contact dermatitis (ACD) and irritant contact dermatitis (ICD) are not the same! In ACD, the lesion develops because of a Type IV, T cell-mediated delayed hypersensitivity reaction
- It is not easy to cure ACD! In fact, the sensitization persists for life. It is not amenable to desensitization as with antibody-mediated allergies.

References

1. Farage M, Maibach H. Lifetime changes in the vulva and vagina. Arch Gynecol Obstet. 2006;273(4):195–202.
2. Farage MA. Vulvar susceptibility to contact irritants and allergens: a review. Arch Gynecol Obstet. 2005;272(2):167–72.
3. Farage MA, Maibach HI. Morphology and physiological changes of genital skin and mucosa. Curr Probl Dermatol. 2011;40:9–19. https://doi.org/10.1159/000321042.
4. Bauer A, Oehme S, Geier J. Contact sensitization in the anal and genital area. Curr Probl Dermatol. 2011;40:133–41. https://doi.org/10.1159/000321065.
5. Brasch J, Becker D, Aberer W, Bircher A, et al. S1-Guidelines of the German Contact Allergy Group (DKG) of the German Dermatology Society (DDG), the Information Network of Dermatological Clinics (IVDK), the German Society for Allergology and Clinical Immunology (DGAKI), the Working Group for Occupational and Environmental Dermatology (ABD) of the DDG, the Medical Association of German Allergologists (AeDA), the Professional Association of German Dermatologists (BVDD) and the DDG. Allergo J Int. 2014;23(4):126–38.
6. Foote CA, Brady SP, Brady KL, Clark NS, Mercurio MG. Vulvar dermatitis from allergy to moist flushable wipes. J Low Genit Tract Dis. 2014;18(1):E16–8. https://doi.org/10.1097/LGT.0b013e31828e499f.
7. O'Gorman SM, Torgerson RR. Allergic contact dermatitis of the vulva. Dermatitis. 2013;24(2):64–72.
8. Vermaat H, Smienk F, Rustemeyer T, Bruynzeel DP, Kirtschig G. Anogenital allergic contact dermatitis, the role of spices and flavour allergy. Contact Dermatitis. 2008;59(4):233–7. https://doi.org/10.1111/j.1600-0536.2008.01417.x.
9. Corazza M, Virgili A, Toni G, Minghetti S, Tiengo S, Borghi A. Level of use and safety of botanical products for itching vulvar dermatoses. Are patch tests useful? Contact Dermatitis. 2016;74(5):289–94. https://doi.org/10.1111/cod.12559.

Irritant Contact Dermatitis 19

Tanja Bohl

19.1 Introduction

Irritant contact dermatitis (ICD) is the more common of the two types of contact dermatitis in all age groups. The second, less frequent, is allergic contact dermatitis (ACD).

19.2 Pathogenesis and Etiology

ICD is the result of skin injury by prolonged pressure and irritation (Fig. 19.1), chemical (Figs. 19.2 and 19.3) or physical agents resulting in inflammation, and a reactive response to produce healing. It occurs and is limited to areas of skin injury and does not involve a delayed immune response. The injury to the skin produces damage faster than the skin can repair itself [1–4].

Vulvar anatomy is conducive to the development of ICD. There are many creases in which perspiration, natural secretions, exfoliated epidermal cells, and feces and urine can collect and irritate the skin. The temperature and humidity in these creases are also increased, stimulating perspiration and reducing epidermal barrier function.

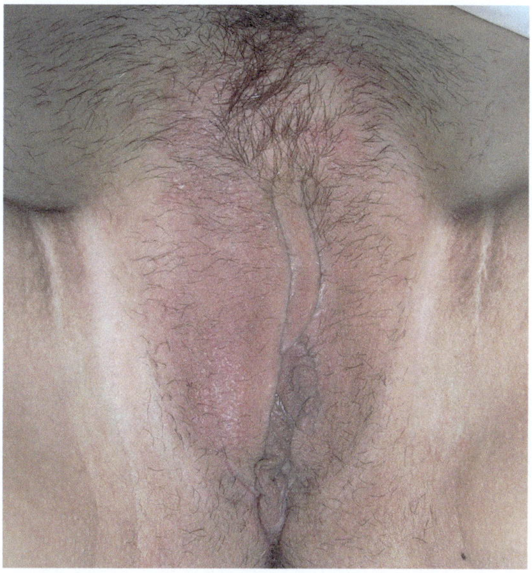

Fig. 19.1 Red plaque of irritant contact dermatitis resulting from wearing tight synthetic underwear

ICD reduces the integrity of the epidermis increasing the irritancy of both the initiating and additional irritants. The epidermal barrier function is reduced in ability to prevent transepidermal water loss (TEWL) and infection.

There are many causes of vulvar ICD that occur more commonly at different times throughout life as part of the "normal" maturation of a female. Some exposures can also produce an allergic response as discussed in the chapter on allergic contact dermatitis.

T. Bohl (✉)
Jean Hailes for Women's Health,
Clayton, VIC, Australia

J. Bornstein (ed.), *Vulvar Disease*, https://doi.org/10.1007/978-3-319-61621-6_19

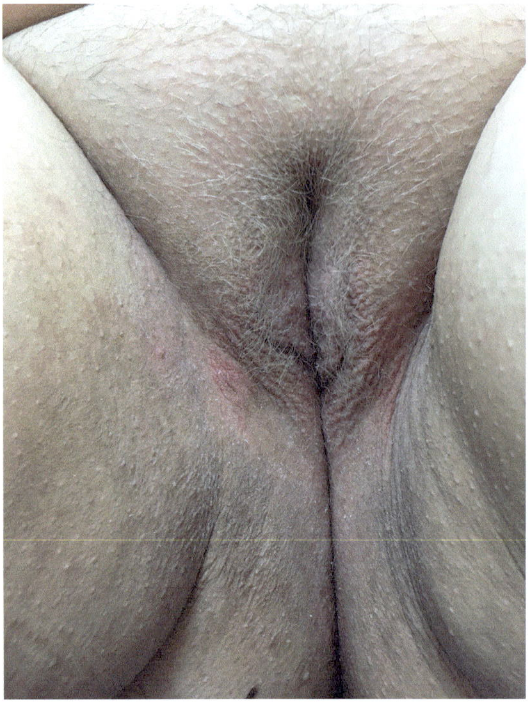

Fig. 19.2 Chronic ICD due to overcleaning the vulva with alkaline soap

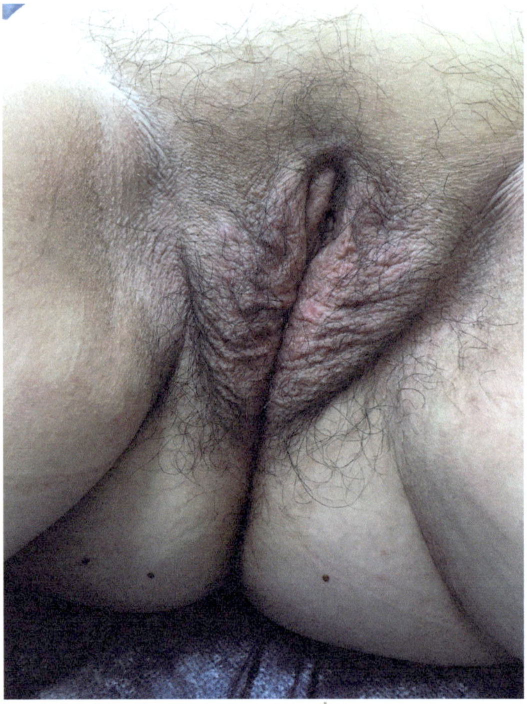

Fig. 19.3 Acute ICD due to chloroxylenol, in healing stages

Friction from skin rubbing on the skin in obesity and with lack of mobility can cause an inflammatory intertrigo. Similarly, rubbing from snug-fitting gym clothes in conjunction with exercise can produce vulvar ICD.

The severity of ICD is determined by the type, strength, and amount of irritant, frequency and duration of exposure in addition to endogenous factors such as atopy, and the presence of a preexisting vulvar dermatosis.

During the reproductive years, a woman is more likely to be exposed to infective agents such as human papilloma virus (HPV) and may require the application of caustic therapeutic agents to her vulva.

19.2.1 Clinical Features

Vulvar ICD is usually the result of multiple exposures to irritants causing cumulative changes such as dryness with fine scale, erythema, altered skin color, and texture (Table 19.1). Distinction from ACD is more difficult in this situation and may coexist.

Early lesions of ICD are the most typical and can usually be distinguished from those of ACD (Table 19.2). They are confined to the area of contact and produce burning and stinging sensations rather than pruritus.

19.3 Diagnosis

As with all vulvar rashes, a careful history is essential. The patient's age, reproductive status, hygiene routine, grooming habits, and use of any products on her vulva should be documented. Any history to suggest an atopic diathesis should also be noted along with a sexual history including any past evidence of HPV-related disease.

19.3.1 Histopathology

This is not likely to be of value in acute vulvar ICD where the history is most likely to yield diagnostic results. It is useful in excluding an underlying dermatosis.

Table 19.1 Potential irritant exposure throughout life

Potential irritant exposure that is "normal"	Stage of life Prepubertal	 Reproductive life	 Post-menopause
Urine	Yes	No	Yes
Feces	Yes	No	Yes
Napkins: infant, sanitary, panty liners, continence aids	Nappies	Panty liners	Panty liners, continence aids
Excessive cleansing, wiping	Yes	Yes	Yes
Cleansers and wipes	Yes	Yes	Yes
Scented products (soap/detergents/fabric softeners/ deodorant sprays)	Yes	Yes	Yes
Vaginal secretions, menstrual fluid	Yes	Yes	Yes (reduced)
Tight clothing	No	Yes	Possibly
Grooming: shaving/plucking/waxing	No	Yes	Possibly
Sexual activity; intercourse: mechanical, semen, lubricant, condoms	No	Yes	Yes

Table 19.2 Clinical features of allergic and irritant contact dermatitis

Clinical features	ACD	ICD
Symptoms	Pruritus most common Increases with multiple exposure May occur at distant sites	Burning/stinging/sensation Pain May develop over time with mild irritant and repeat exposure
Onset after exposure	Delayed; 1–2 days but may seem less with repeated exposure	Rapid, within minutes, possibly hours of contact
Clinical appearance		
(a) Acute		
Margins	Generally diffuse	Well demarcated and reflect area of contact
Lesions	Erythema, edema, vesiculation Erosions; primary, ruptured vesicles on mucous membranes; secondary, due to scratching Scale	Erythema, erosions (not uniform in shape), ulcers, tissue destruction
(b) Chronic		
Lesions	Dry, mild erythema, fine scaling, lichenification	
Course	Waxes and wanes once established even with no further exposure	Individual lesions heal as expected due to cause of trauma New lesions only with repeat exposure

In chronic ICD the histological changes are likely to be very similar to those of ACD: parakeratosis, spongiosis, irregular epidermal hyperplasia, and a perivascular inflammatory infiltrate that is predominantly lymphocytic. Eosinophils are less prevalent than in ACD.

Histological features of epidermal damage are necrotic keratinocytes and intraepidermal neutrophils. It is not possible to determine the cause of irritation from the histology.

If ICD and ACD are thought to be present, patch testing should be considered. This is not useful in ICD, and the application of some irritants may cause undesired damage in areas of testing with repeat open application testing (ROAT).

19.4 Treatment

ICD should improve once the cause of irritation is identified and removed. There are situations in which this cannot be achieved. In the presence of obesity, for example, the presence of deep skin folds usually remains an ongoing problem. Even if substantial weight loss is achieved, skin folds persist and may become deeper, and the problem can become worse.

In this situation, a careful care plan needs to be developed. This should include avoidance of irritants such as soaps or scented products, wearing fitting but not tight cotton underclothes, and regular application of barrier emollients that are essential.

Mild potency topical corticosteroids, such as hydrocortisone 1% ointment, two to three times daily may be of benefit intermittently. If vulvar ICD persists or recurs, reassessment to identify additional irritants, possible infection, the development of ACD, or possibly the development of an additional dermatosis must be undertaken.

19.5 Prognosis

The long-term outlook is generally good but is dependent on ongoing vigilance with careful attention to irritant avoidance, regular use of barrier products, and reassessment if any there is any recurrence of vulvar irritation.

Irritant Contact Dermatitis: Breaking a Myth

- Contact dermatitis is not one condition: there is irritant contact dermatitis (ICD) and allergic contact dermatitis (ACD), and they may present as acute or chronic.

References

1. Gutshall D, Zhou S, Wang B, Farage MA, Hochwalt AE. Assessing the dermal compatibility of a new female incontinence product line. Cutan Ocul Toxicol. 2016;35(4):287–95. https://doi.org/10.3109/15569527.2015.1109519. Epub 2015 Nov 30.
2. Farage M, Stadler A. Cumulative irritation patch test of sanitary pads on sensitive skin. J Cosmet Dermatol. 2005;4(3):179–83.
3. Summers PR, Hunn J. Unique dermatologic aspects of the postmenopausal vulva. Clin Obstet Gynecol. 2007;50(3):745–51.
4. Farage M, Warren R, Wang-Weigand S. The vulva is relatively insensitive to menses-induced irritation. Cutan Ocul Toxicol. 2005;24(4):243–6.

20 Atopic Dermatitis

Tanja Bohl

20.1 Introduction and Terminology

Atopic dermatitis and eczema are often used interchangeably. Other terms used include endogenous eczema and flexural eczema. Atopic dermatitis (AD) is the term that will be used in this article. AD is favoured because it indicates the inflammation of the skin and the presence of atopy in the affected individual.

AD is a common, pruritic, chronic inflammatory dermatosis characterized clinically by relapsing episodes of flares of intensely pruritic, inflammatory skin lesions. Overall incidence in the USA is 17% and varies with 10–20% of children and 2–5% of adults affected in western countries particularly those of European and Asian ethnicity.

The onset is primarily in childhood, and although AD may improve after childhood, dry, easily irritated, sensitive skin persists.

Vulvar AD may occur alone or in the presence of AD elsewhere and is associated with significant impairment of quality of life in either.

20.1.1 Atopic March

Atopic march refers to the progression of AD from a cutaneous disorder alone, to a systemic one.

It begins with AD and a dysfunctional epidermal barrier function. This affects allergen presentation to the cutaneous and systemic immune systems, resulting in systemic effects that include increased IgE-mediated, Type 1 hypersensitivity, allergic reactions. The increased incidence of food allergy in individuals with AD is an example of this.

20.1.2 Atopic Diathesis

Individuals with AD have an increased incidence of extrinsic asthma, allergic rhinitis and allergic conjunctivitis. This is referred to as an atopic diathesis or atopic phenotype. The presence of an atopic diathesis is an important diagnostic criterion for AD.

Common associations seen in this population include ichthyosis vulgaris, keratosis pilaris, *Staphylococcus* colonization, and infection and eczema herpeticum.

T. Bohl (✉)
Jean Hailes for Women's Health, Clayton, VIC, Australia

J. Bornstein (ed.), *Vulvar Disease*, https://doi.org/10.1007/978-3-319-61621-6_20

20.2 Pathogenesis

The aetiology and pathogenesis of AD is multifactorial and incompletely understood [1–18]. It involves a complex interaction of genetic and environmental factors. The mechanisms involved in this interaction are subsequently the focus of research into AD pathogenesis.

AD is predominantly mediated by T-helper cells with T-helper 2 (Th2) primarily in acute AD and T-helper 1 (Th-1) in chronic AD.

A dysfunctional epidermal barrier function is integral to the development of AD and is present in most if not all atopic individuals. Genetic, inflammatory, immunologic and environmental factors affect epidermal barrier function in AD.

20.2.1 Genetics

A genetic component to the aetiology of AD is supported by the familial clustering of the atopic phenotype. Twin studies also support a genetic component. Identical and fraternal twins have a seven- and threefold increase of AD, respectively.

There is no single genetic trait that explains all pathogenetic events in AD. Genome-wide studies have attempted to identify genes related to epidermal barrier function and immune response findings in AD. More than 30 at risk loci have been found to date.

20.2.2 Immunology

AD is predominantly a cytokine-mediated condition. The cytokines involved are the result of different events and in turn have a variety of effects that provide explanations for some of the clinically observed findings in AD-affected individuals.

Th2 inflammation promoters in AD include bacterial colonization and keratinocyte-derived interleukins induced by mechanical injury such as scratching. These interleukins include thymic stromal lymphopoietin (TSLP), IL-25, IL-33, IL-6 and IL-4. IL-4 is also produced by Th2 cells driving the inflammation.

Th2 cytokines have varied roles; IL-4 and IL-5 produce elevated IgE levels and eosinophilia, and IL-4 and IL-13 downregulate skin innate immunity and decreasing filaggrin expression by keratinocytes. This source of IL-4 helps promote further Th2 inflammation.

IL-10 has multiple effects on immune regulation, and IL-31 promotes pruritus and helps trigger cell-mediated immunity against pathogens.

20.2.3 Skin Barrier Defects in AD

Filaggrin (FLG) is the epidermal structural protein that has been investigated the most to date in conjunction with AD. It is integral to epidermal barrier integrity and involved in maintenance of skin hydration. Only 15% of AD-affected individuals carry an FGL mutation. An Asian race-specific mutation has been identified.

The gene that encodes for FGL is located on chromosome 1q21 along with other barrier genes collectively known as the epidermal differentiation complex (EDC) loricrin and involucrin.

Multiple non-functional mutations of the FGL gene have been identified and are associated with more severe AD and conditions seen more commonly in atopy such as ichthyosis vulgaris and keratosis pilaris. FGL mutations are also related to the increased incidence of irritant contact dermatitis and allergic contact dermatitis, recurrent staphylococcal infections and eczema herpeticum.

Epidermal barrier function is also affected by cytokines released after the activation of Th2 cells resulting in reduced filaggrin expression by keratinocytes.

20.2.4 The Microbiome

The skin microbiome inhabits the superficial stratum corneum and is in direct contact with the environment. It is affected by environmental factors such as clothing, hygiene, skin cleansers, other skin care products and topical medicaments as well as endogenous factors such as age and gender.

A healthy microbiome includes *Staphylococcus* epidermidis (SE) which has *Staphylococcus aureus* (SA) inhibiting properties. Disturbances in the skin microbiome are an

Table 20.1 *Staphylococcus aureus* (SA) and AD

Evidence that *Staphylococcus aureus* may cause atopic dermatitis
• Penetrates epidermis in presence of expression of IL-4, IL-13 and IL-22
• SA colonization occurs in 90% of AD lesions
• SA aureus can induce AD flares via Th1 and Th2 pathways
• *Staphylococci* exoproteins and superantigens induce inflammation and impair epidermal barrier function
• Skin barrier function impairment by stimulating production of keratinocyte endogenous serine protease which in turn reduces FGL and other structural proteins
• AD is a risk factor for colonization of the mucous membranes with methicillin-resistant *Staphylococcus aureus* (MRSA)
• Nasal mucosa MRSA colonization acts as reservoir for repeated infections in AD
• MRSA prevalence in AD lesional skin reported 13–24%

independent risk factor for AD. *Staphylococcus aureus*, including methicillin-resistant *Staphylococcus aureus* (MRSA), is the most common bacteria seen in AD and is involved in the pathogenesis of infection, inflammation and epidermal barrier damage (Table 20.1).

20.2.5 Histopathology

A biopsy is useful in confirming a dermatitis and excluding other dermatoses such as psoriasis. The histological features include scale crusts in the stratum corneum, spongiosis and microvesicle formation within the epidermis. The inflammatory infiltrate is mostly perivascular and comprised of lymphocytes and less so eosinophils. Exocytosis into the epidermis is often seen. However, these features are not exclusive to AD.

20.3 Clinical Features and Diagnosis

There is no single diagnostic feature or investigation that establishes a diagnosis of AD. The lack of a singular diagnostic criterion reflects the complex pathophysiology and unknown aetiology of AD.

Table 20.2 Criteria for the diagnosis of atopic dermatitis

Major characteristics
• Pruritus
• Typical morphology and distribution (i.e. flexural lichenification and linearity in adults, facial and extensor involvement in infants and young children)
• Chronic or chronically relapsing dermatitis
• Personal or family history of atopy (e.g. asthma, allergic rhinoconjunctivitis, atopic dermatitis)
Minor characteristics
• Xerosis (dry skin)
• Ichthyosis, palmar hyperlinearity, keratosis pilaris
• Hand dermatitis, foot dermatitis
• Cheilitis
• Nipple eczema
• Susceptibility to cutaneous infection (e.g. with SA, herpes simplex virus [HSV], other viruses, warts, molluscum, dermatophytes)
• Erythroderma
• Perifollicular accentuation
• Pityriasis alba
• Early age of onset
• Impaired cell-mediated immunity
• Recurrent conjunctivitis
• Orbital darkening
• Infraorbital fold (e.g. Dennie pleat, Morgan fold)
• Anterior neck folds
• Keratoconus
• Anterior subcapsular cataracts
• Sensitivity to emotional factors
• Food intolerance
• Pruritus with sweating
• Intolerance of wool
• White dermographism
• Immediate type I skin test response
• Elevated total serum immunoglobulin E (IgE)
• Peripheral blood eosinophilia

By the American Academy of Allergy, Asthma, and Immunology

Appropriate cases must have at least three major characteristics and at least three minor characteristics

The Hanifin and Rajka Criteria and the 'United Kingdom Working Party Criteria' are used predominantly clinical trials although several other criteria have been developed. The American Academy of Allergy, Asthma, and Immunology criteria are useful for the clinician and reflect the main criteria used globally, clinically (Table 20.2).

The lesions may be acute, subacute or chronic and a mixture of these lesions may be present in any individual (Table 20.3).

Table 20.3 Clinical features of eczema

Acute	Subacute	Chronic
Papules	Erythema	Skin thickening
Vesicles	Scaling	Increased skin markings
Erosions		Prurigo nodules aka Besnier's prurigo in AD
Serous exudate—crusts		

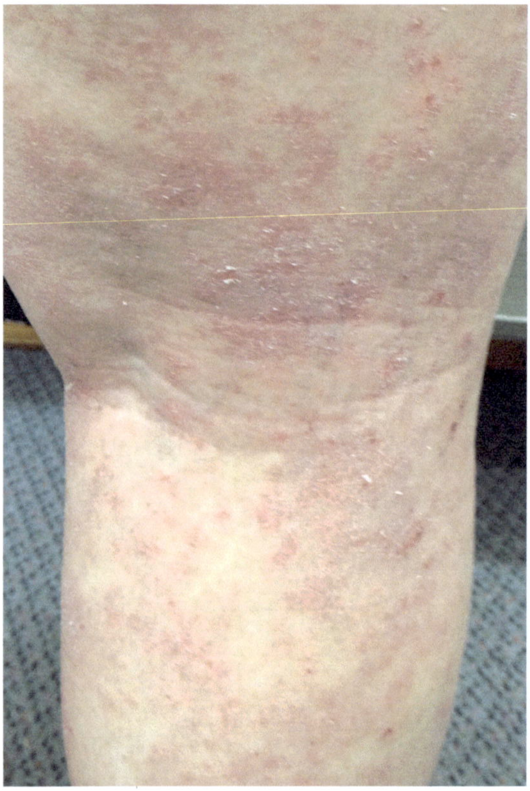

Fig. 20.1 Atopic dermatitis in the popliteal fossa

The 'typical' distribution changes from infancy to adulthood. Some of these changes can be partially explained by altered activities and environmental factors. Extensor surface involvement occurs in the crawling infant is an example of this. Prior to this, the cheeks and scalp are most typical of infantile AD, although it is often generalized.

AD in older children becomes more flexural: neck, wrists, ankles and antecubital and popliteal fossae (Fig. 20.1). Adult AD may be confined to

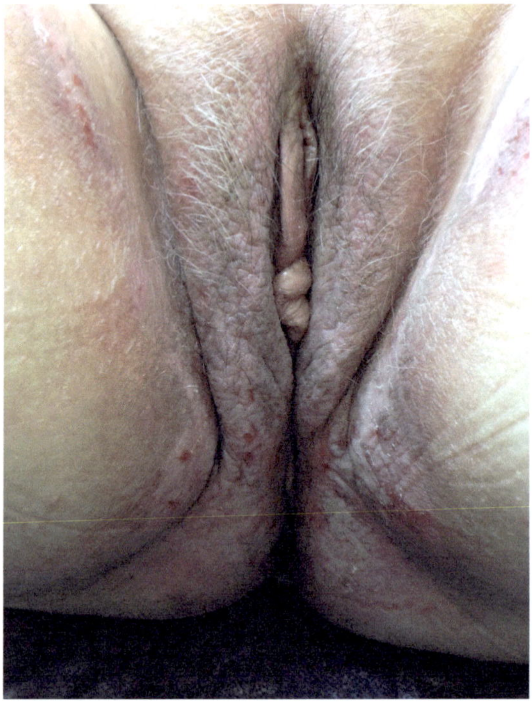

Fig. 20.2 Atopic dermatitis with lichenification and scarring

hand and foot eczema with hyperlinear palms and soles. Severe, generalized AD may persist beyond infancy.

During adolescence there are many changes that can impact of the involvement of the vulva: increased hair growth, change in size and potentially colour of labia, change in odour, physiologic, discharge and menstruation (Fig. 20.2).

It is clinically useful to consider the vulva as an area of creases undergoing skin friction, perspiration, sebaceous secretions, retained vaginal and vulvar secretions, potential irritation and contamination with urine, faeces and the regular presence of menstrual fluid. The dominance of these factors varies over the lifetime.

20.4 Treatment

The principles of management of vulvar AD are the same in all vulvar dermatoses. They include a thorough history and clinical examination to identify and remove any trigger factors, identify and treat any infections and apply bland, non-fragranced, emollients/moisturizers frequently (two to three times a day) and as liberally as tolerable. These should also be used as a soap substitute.

Emollients may be ointments, creams or lotions depending on the amount of water they contain. The aim in AD is to help prevent transepidermal water loss (TEWL), hydrate the skin to reduce pruritus and improve barrier function.

Liquid paraffin 50% in white soft paraffin (emulsifying ointment) is often used; however, the consistency may not be suitable for all vulvar AD patients as it is quite occlusive.

These actions will improve AD substantially and help determine if an irritant or allergic contact dermatitis may be present. Control of pruritus is essential for patient relief and to reduce trauma due to scratching which also is a trigger.

An examination of all the products applied to the skin at any site not just the vulva may be very instructive. Patients should be encouraged to bring these to either their initial or a subsequent consultation.

Initially mild to moderate corticosteroid preparations such as clobetasol butyrate 0.05% ointment applied nightly for up to 2 weeks are often sufficient to establish control. It should be used in conjunction with an emollient and can be used twice daily if required. Potent and ultrapotent corticosteroid preparations can be used for short periods to establish control.

Maintenance therapy should be tailored to the individual. Weaker corticosteroid preparations such as hydrocortisone 1% can be introduced and used daily, or less frequent applications of the initial preparation may be used. Nonsteroidal preparations such as pimecrolimus 1% or tacrolimus 0.01% are less useful on the vulva as they often irritate.

Failure to respond should initiate a reassessment of the vulvar dermatitis to exclude another pathology, intervening infection or the possible development of irritant or contact dermatitis.

20.5 Course and Ongoing Prognosis

AD is chronic, and relapses are frequent. Vulvar involvement follows a similar course. There are multiple potential triggers that occur normally throughout life that can be responsible for the relapses. AD pathogenesis is complex, multifactorial and incompletely understood. The most important factor for clinicians to remember in vulvar AD management is that epidermal barrier function is impaired. Management that does not include attention to this is incomplete.

Atopic Dermatitis: Breaking the Myths

- Specific diagnosis is not always required—the principles of management of vulvar atopic dermatitis are the same in all vulvar dermatoses.

References

1. Hanifin JM, Rajka G. Diagnostic features of atopic dermatitis. Acta Derm Venereol Suppl (Stockh). 1980;92:44–7.
2. Williams HC, Burney PG, Pembroke AC, Hay RJ. The U.K. working Party's diagnostic criteria for atopic dermatitis. III. Independent hospital validation. Br J Dermatol. 1994;131(3):406–16.
3. Samochocki Z, Dejewska J. A comparison of criteria for diagnosis of atopic dermatitis in children. World J Pediatr. 2012;8(4):355–8. https://doi.org/10.1007/s12519-012-0381-1. Epub 2012 Nov 15.
4. Vakharia PP, Chopra R, Silverberg JI. Systematic review of diagnostic criteria used in atopic dermatitis randomized controlled trials. Am J Clin Dermatol. 2017;19(1):15–22. https://doi.org/10.1007/s40257-017-0299-4.
5. Silverberg JI, Thyssen JP, Paller AS, Drucker AM, et al. What's in a name? Atopic dermatitis or atopic eczema, but not eczema alone. Allergy. 2017;72(12):2026–30. https://doi.org/10.1111/all.13225.
6. Malik K, Heitmiller KD, Czarnowicki T. An update on the pathophysiology of atopic dermatitis. Dermatol Clin. 2017;35(3):317–26. https://doi.org/10.1016/j.det.2017.02.006.
7. Weidinger S, Novak N. Atopic dermatitis. Lancet. 2016;387(10023):1109–22. https://doi.org/10.1016/

S0140-6736(15)00149-X. Epub 2015 Sep 13. (Review).
8. Nutten S. Atopic dermatitis: global epidemiology and risk factors. Ann Nutr Metab. 2015;66(suppl 1):8–16.
9. Rerknimitr P, Otsuka A, Nakashima C, Kabashima K. The etiopathogenesis of atopic dermatitis: barrier disruption, immunological derangement, and pruritus. Inflamm Regen. 2017;37:14. Published online 2017 Jun 5. https://doi.org/10.1186/s41232-017-0044-7.
10. Farage MA, Warren R. Emollients on the genital area. Curr Probl Dermatol. 2011;40:101–6. https://doi.org/10.1159/000321059. Epub 2011 Feb 10.
11. Silverberg NB. Typical and atypical clinical appearance of atopic dermatitis. Clin Dermatol. 2017;35(4):354–9. https://doi.org/10.1016/j.clindermatol.2017.03.007. Epub 2017 Mar 24. (Review).
12. Han H, Roan F, Ziegler SF. The atopic march: current insights into skin barrier dysfunction and epithelial cell-derived cytokines. Immunol Rev. 2017;278(1):116–30. https://doi.org/10.1111/imr.12546. (Review).
13. Brunner PM, Silverberg JI, Guttman-Yassky E, Paller AS, Kabashima K, Amagai M, Luger TA, Deleuran M, Werfel T, Eyerich K, Stingl G. Increasing comorbidities suggest that atopic dermatitis is a systemic disorder. J Investig Dermatol. 2017;137:18–25. (Review).
14. Hänel KH, Cornelissen C, Lüscher B, Baron JM. Cytokines and the skin barrier. Int J Mol Sci. 2013;14:6720–45. https://doi.org/10.3390/ijms14046720. (Review).
15. Brandt EB, Sivaprasad U. Th2 cytokines and atopic dermatitis. J Clin Cell Immunol. 2011;2(3):110. https://doi.org/10.4172/2155-9899.1000110. (Review).
16. Bantz SK, Zhu Z, Tao Zheng T. The atopic march: progression from atopic dermatitis to allergic rhinitis and asthma. J Clin Cell Immunol. 2014;5(2):202. https://doi.org/10.4172/2155-9899.1000202. (Review).
17. Bitschar K, Wolz C, Krismer B, Peschel A, Schittek B. Keratinocytes as sensors and central players in the immune defense against Staphylococcus aureus in the skin. J Dermatol Sci. 2017;87(3):215–20pii: S0923-1811(17)30707-7. https://doi.org/10.1016/j.jdermsci.2017.06.003.
18. Dybboe R, Bandier J, Skov L, Engstrand L, Johansen JD. The role of the skin microbiome in atopic dermatitis: a systematic review. Br J Dermatol. 2017;177(5):1272–8. https://doi.org/10.1111/bjd.15390.

Eczematous Changes Superimposed on Other Vulvar Disorders

21

Tanja Bohl

21.1 Introduction

Eczematous changes may be superimposed on other dermatoses at the time of presentation (Fig. 21.1) and complicate the evaluation of the vulvar dermatosis. The superimposed eczematous changes make definitive diagnosis difficult if not impossible.

Eczematous changes may also develop in a patient throughout the course of the management of her vulvar dermatosis. In this scenario the change in symptoms and appearance should alert the clinician to the possibility of the development of an allergic contact dermatitis (ACD) or irritant contact dermatitis (ICD) (Table 21.1).

21.2 Pathogenesis and Etiology

Expression of an underlying atopic diathesis can also lead to eczematous changes and can be precipitated by environmental changes and endogenous changes in general health that result in impairment of epidermal function on the vulva or generally.

These changes can only occur in the presence of an intact epidermis and therefore not present with erosive, bullous, or ulcerative dermatoses. General health conditions that produce or exacerbate xerosis such as hypothyroidism and iron deficiency may also precipitate the development of eczematous changes.

Any chronic dermatosis can be affected, but the most likely are psoriasis, lichen sclerosus, and usual cutaneous lichen planus (LP) [rather than erosive] than less common vulvar dermatoses such as Darier's disease and Hailey-Hailey disease.

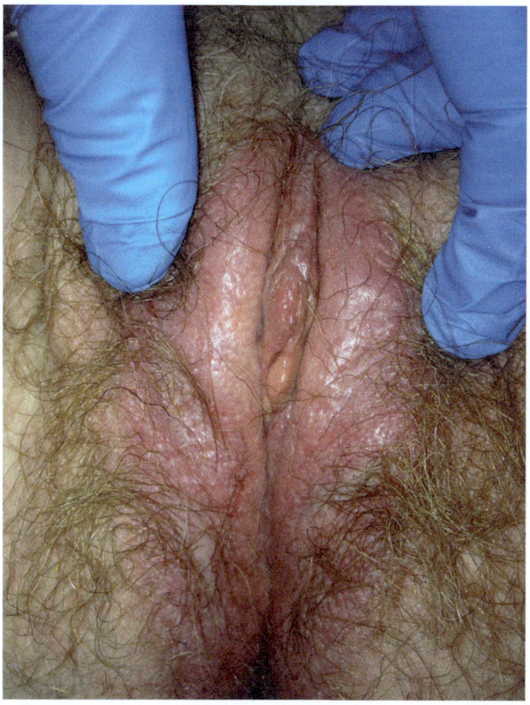

Fig. 21.1 Vulvar eczema developing on existent dermatitis

T. Bohl (✉)
Jean Hailes for Women's Health, Clayton, VIC, Australia

J. Bornstein (ed.), *Vulvar Disease*, https://doi.org/10.1007/978-3-319-61621-6_21

Table 21.1 Causes of eczematous changes

Causes and background conditions that may lead to exematous changes
• Irritant contact dermatitis
• Allergic contact dermatitis
• Underlying atopic diathesis
• Supervening infections
– *Candidiasis*
– Bacterial; streptococcal, *Staphylococcus*
• Environmental
Changes in humidity
• General health factors
– Hypothyroidism
– Iron deficiency
– Medications (cholesterol lowering medications)

Chronic candidiasis can result in eczematous changes.

21.3 Histopathology

The characteristic histology of the underlying dermatosis may be obscured by the eczematous changes. Acute changes include spongiosis with microvesicle formation in the epidermis, and scale crusts due to scratching may also be present. A predominantly perivascular inflammatory infiltrate that may be patchy and predominantly lymphocytic may also be seen. Eosinophils are more likely with superimposed ACD.

There may be clues to the cause of eczematous changes such as pseudo-hyphae among the hyperkeratosis.

21.4 Clinical Features

Acute eczematous changes comprise dryness, fine scale, erythema, edema, vesiculation, excoriations, and possibly serous exudate and crusts. Chronic changes in more established eczematization changes are increased dryness and possibly altered skin color and texture.

The underlying dermatosis will be evident to various degrees. In psoriasis the edge of lesions may be more clearly demarcated with smaller lesions around the periphery. In lichen sclerosus any architectural changes will persist and will establish changes in skin color. Hyperkeratosis is often quite marked.

Patient history and examination of other sites may reveal presence of an atopic diathesis or typical lesions of the underlying dermatosis aiding diagnosis. Pruritus may develop for the first time or be exacerbated at the development of these changes.

21.5 Treatment

Establishing the underlying diagnosis and the reason for supervening eczematous changes is the primary goal. A careful history and examination is essential. The history of development of clinical findings will provide important clues as to the possibility of supervening ACD or ICD and the underlying dermatosis.

Specimens for microbiologic examination looking for the presence of bacterial or *Candida* infection should be taken. A biopsy should be seriously considered, but this could be delayed until the results of the microbiologic investigations are known.

Initially stopping all topical therapy to cease applying potential irritants and allergens and advising the patient on bland emollients for soothing and hydration and as a soap substitute should be initiated. Hopefully the underlying dermatosis will be more evident on review although a biopsy is still indicated.

Unless contraindicated mid-potency topical corticosteroid such as clobetasol butyrate 0.1% will aid in improving the eczematous changes. Additional treatment targeting the underlying dermatosis can be commenced once the diagnosis is established.

21.6 Prognosis

The prognosis will be determined by the underlying dermatosis and the etiology of the eczematous changes. The underlying dermatosis will require specific treatment. In the presence of an ACD, avoidance of the responsible allergen and careful avoidance should see these changes controlled and prevented. ICD can be controlled by careful attention to skin care.

Eczematous Changes Superimposed on Other Vulvar Dermatoses: Breaking the Myths

- A change in symptoms and appearance of a dermatosis is not always due to worsening or improvement of it. Rather consider the possibility of the development of an allergic contact dermatitis (ACD) or irritant contact dermatitis (ICD).

22 Lichenification Superimposed on an Underlying Preceding Pruritic Disease

Tanja Bohl

22.1 Introduction

Clinically, lichenification is thickening of the skin with exaggeration of the skin markings and the development of an altered leathery texture with induration.

Lichenification should not be confused with the term 'lichen' in dermatoses such as lichen sclerosus and lichen planus. The latter refers to the pattern of the inflammatory infiltrate in these dermatoses. 'Lichenoid' infiltrates are located at the dermo-epidermal junction.

22.2 Pathogenesis

Lichenification occurs in pruritic dermatoses of the vulva and other body sites. Overall atopy and atopic dermatitis (AD) is probably the most common.

Skin responds to chronic repetitive trauma such as scratching by thickening, becoming 'lichenified'. In AD the environmental and endogenous factors involved in pathogenesis of pruritus contribute to the development of lichenification.

22.3 Etiology

Lichenification is seen in conjunction with lichen simplex chronicus, lichen sclerosus, atopic dermatitis (AD) and allergic contact dermatitis (ACD). It is often flexural in AD.

Pruritic vulvar dermatoses in which lichenification commonly occurs are lichen simplex, atopic dermatitis (AD), lichen sclerosus and allergic contact dermatitis (ACD).

Not all areas of skin on the body have the same capacity to develop lichenification.

22.4 Clinical Features

Clinically lichenification encompasses a mixture of changes (Table 22.1). They are most marked on the labia majora and perineum (Figs. 22.1, 22.2 and 22.3). The skin texture is altered and appears coarse with exaggerated skin markings. Skin colour can be either increased or decreased in complexion and these changes overly the indurated areas. They can be well demarcated. Broken hairs, excoriations and erosions are evidence of scratching.

Heat, humidity and perspiration aggravate the pruritus associated with lichenification.

T. Bohl (✉)
Jean Hailes for Women's Health,
Clayton, VIC, Australia

J. Bornstein (ed.), *Vulvar Disease*, https://doi.org/10.1007/978-3-319-61621-6_22

Table 22.1 Clinical appearance of vulvar lichenification

Characteristics
• Altered texture
• Exaggerated/increased skin markings (coarseness) of skin
• On glabrous (hair bearing) skin; labia majora more prominently, perineum, natal cleft, inguinal creases, mons pubis
• Broken hairs
• Excoriation marks
• Erosions (due to scratching)
• Variably elevated and indurated
• Altered colour: increased or reduced

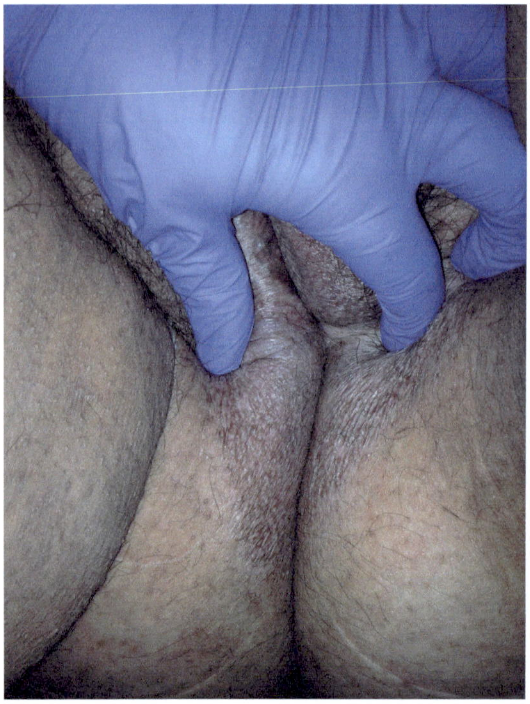

Fig. 22.1 Lichenification on LS focus HSIL arrow

22.5 Diagnosis

As with all patients with a vulvar dermatosis, a clinical examination of the entire vulva and other body sites is essential. A thorough history including the identification of trigger, aggravating and ameliorating factors will suggest the most likely diagnosis as well as provide useful suggestions for management.

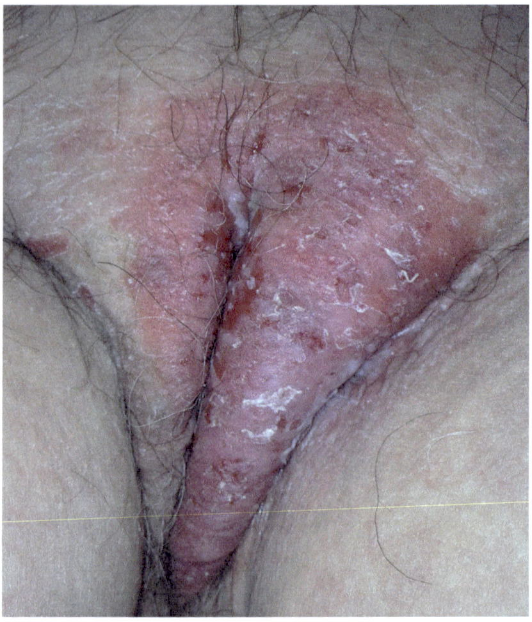

Fig. 22.2 Lichenification and excoriations on pruritic eczema due to Paget's disease

22.5.1 Histopathology

A skin biopsy will help establish the diagnosis of an underlying dermatosis such as lichen sclerosus (LS) and exclude vulvar intraepithelial neoplasia (VIN) associated with LS and Paget's disease.

The histopathological features of lichenification are hyperkeratosis, acanthosis and elongation of the rete ridges with vertical alignment of collagen bundles and blood vessels indicative of long-term scratching. Similar changes are also seen in psoriasis. Scale and crusts are often present and may contain bacterial and fungal elements.

22.5.2 Other Investigations

Additional investigation with microbiological testing to exclude infection should be considered if excoriations and crusting are present. Other investigations such as patch testing may be indicated to exclude ACD.

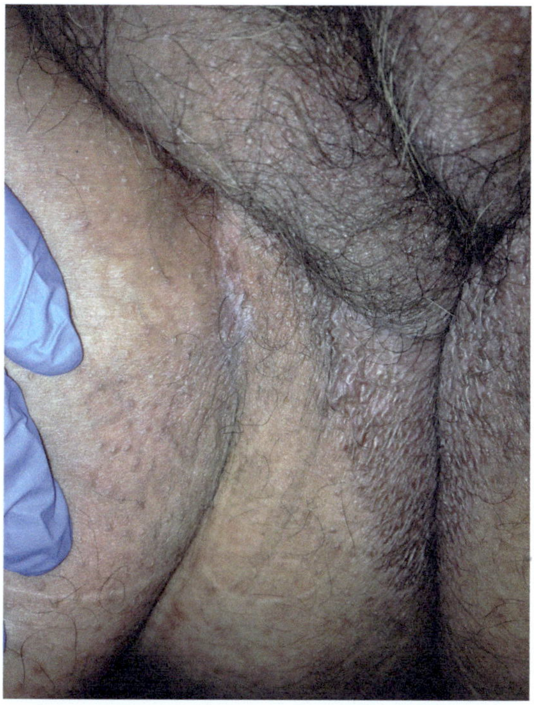

Fig. 22.3 Lichenification on intertrigo in an obese patient

22.6 Treatment

The principles of treatment are the same as for AD: identification and removal of trigger factors, identification and treatment of infection and repair of the epidermal barrier with emollients.

Specific therapy will depend on the underlying dermatoses and is usually a potent or superpotent topical steroid preparation. Attention to the itch-scratch cycle is integral to successful management of lichenification and may require oral medication such a sedating antihistamine, antidepressant or anxiolytic.

22.7 Prognosis

Once lichenification is present, it is unlikely that the changes will be reversed completely. It is a chronic condition that will require maintenance therapy. This should include ongoing attention to avoiding potential triggers and aggravating factors in addition to the underlying dermatosis. Recurrences should each be evaluated in the same manner as initially. Repeat biopsies may be required in the future in women with LS and superimposed lichenification to exclude the potential development of VIN.

Lichenification Superimposed on an Underlying Preceding Pruritic Disease: Breaking the Myths

- 'Lichenification' is not the same as 'lichen' in dermatoses such as lichen sclerosus and lichen planus: Lichenification is thickening of the skin with exaggeration of the skin markings and the development of an altered leathery texture with induration. 'Lichen' refers to the inflammatory infiltrate at the dermo-epidermal junction.

Part V

Vulvar Lesions: Red Lesions—Patches and Plaques

Approach to Diagnosis of Vulvovaginitis

23

Orna Reichman and Shiri Weinberg-Hendel

23.1 Introduction

Vaginal discharge, pruritus, malodor, and dyspareunia are the main reasons for visiting a primary gynecologic clinic [1]. Unfortunately, such symptoms are nonspecific and caused by various etiologies such as hormonal deficiency, several infections, idiopathic inflammation, and contact dermatitis to numerous substances. It is essential to understand that symptoms alone do not provide a sufficient basis for diagnosis [2]. However, by combining medical history with a thorough genital examination, measurements of vaginal pH, and wet mount (microscopy of vaginal secretion), most causes of vaginal discomfort can be diagnosed [2, 3]. Infectious causes that cannot be identified by the microscope can be diagnosed by cultures or molecular biology assays, such as polymerase chain reaction (PCR) [4]. This chapter presents a clinical approach for diagnosing vaginitis by combining point of care tests: pH test, potassium hydroxide (KOH), and wet mount.

23.1.1 Vaginal Epithelium

The vaginal wall is a dynamic stratified squamous epithelium which undergoes maturation in response to estrogen. It is composed of three cell types, all originating from the basal layer. Estrogen induces proliferation of the basal cell layer to form parabasal cells that further undergo cyto-differentiation to form the intermediate cells which are enriched with glycogen. The intermediate cells further differentiate to squamous cells that contain keratin that protects the tissue from the potential damage of friction. The three cell types differentiate in their functional activity and morphology. As the cell differentiates, the cytoplasm-nuclei ratio grows, a phenomenon that helps diagnosing the status of maturation by a microscope, to those women where estrogen is present to these without estrogen (Figs. 23.1 and 23.2) [5]. Lack of estrogen, as seen in premenarchal girls and postmenopausal women, results in an atrophic vaginal epithelium composed by a thin, 3–5-layer stratified epithelia, characterized predominantly by parabasal cells and lacking the intermediate cells and squamous layer. The distribution of the three-cell type (i.e., parabasal, intermediate, and squamous) reflects estrogen levels and could assist in estimating the level of estrogen in the vagina. Meisels developed a scoring system known as the vaginal maturation index (VMI) in which 100 exfoliated vaginal cells are characterized and scored according to their maturation; parabasal cells are scored 0.1, intermediate cells are scored 0.5, and squamous cells receive a score of 1. A score below 50 indicates lack of estrogen and vaginal atrophy where above 65 reflects a well-estrogenized vagina [6].

O. Reichman (✉) · S. Weinberg-Hendel
Shaare Zedek Medical Center, Hebrew University, Jerusalem, Israel

J. Bornstein (ed.), *Vulvar Disease*, https://doi.org/10.1007/978-3-319-61621-6_23

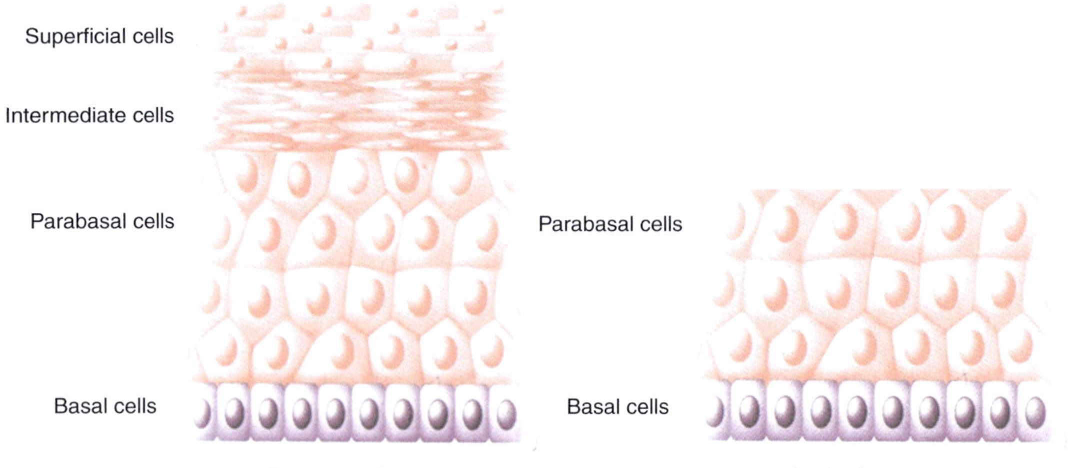

Fig. 23.1 Vaginal multilayer squamous epithelium as a function of estrogen levels. Courtesy of Dr. Orna Reichman

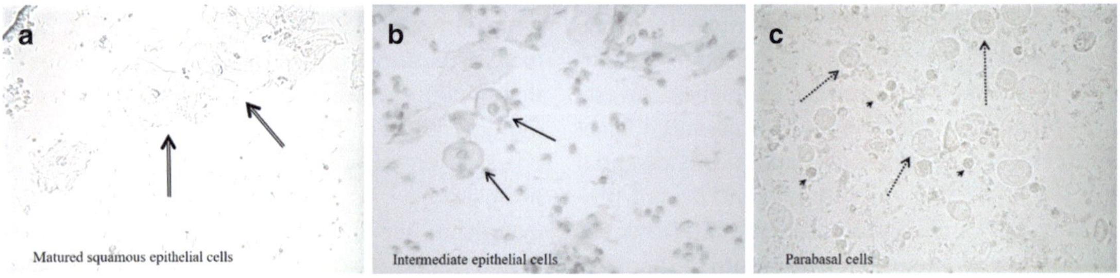

Fig. 23.2 The three morph-type cells of vaginal wall, wet mount ×200. Wet mount samples of three different patients. Each sample presents one of the three morph-type cells of vaginal wall: (**a**) matured squamous epithelial cells (double-lined arrows) located in the upper layers of a healthy vagina when adequate levels of estrogen are present, (**b**) intermediate epithelial cells (black arrows) that store the glycogen required for lactobacillus growth, and (**c**) parabasal cells that are the precursors of the intermediate and squamous cells. These cells are in excess in conditions where the upper layers of vaginal walls are absent such as inflammation, infections, and atrophy (parabasal cells, dashed arrow; inflammatory cells, head arrow). Courtesy of Dr. Orna Reichman

23.1.2 Vaginal Microbiota

Vaginal microbiota is in a delicate equilibrium with hormones. Normal, healthy vaginal flora consists predominantly of hydrogen peroxide-producing *Lactobacilli* and facultative gram-positive rods that ferment pyruvate to lactic acid and induce an acidic environment of pH 4.0 ± 0.5. The acidic environment inhibits growth of anaerobic bacteria that when present cause a troublesome fishy malodorous discharge, a condition known as bacterial vaginosis (BV), which may be associated with obstetrical and gynecological complications [7, 8].

Adequate levels of estrogen facilitate the differentiation of intermediate cells resulting in sufficient levels of glycogen which is the precursor of pyruvate that enables the growth of the hydrogen peroxide-producing *Lactobacilli*. Deficiency of estrogen will reverse the process, resulting in decreased titers of *Lactobacilli* with a shift to an abnormal mixed anaerobic flora [5].

23.2 Wet Mount

23.2.1 Applying a Sample for the Microscope (Wet Mount)

To evaluate vaginal complaints, one needs to sample vaginal discharge. The preference is to perform a full vaginal examination using a speculum, but in rare cases when there is the need to avoid a speculum examination, a sample is obtained easily by applying a cotton-tipped applicator on the mid-lateral vaginal wall without inserting the speculum. The sample is smeared on two separate microscope glasses. On one glass a drop of 0.9% NaCl is applied and on the other a drop of 10% potassium hydroxide (KOH). The latter has the potential to cause lysis of epithelial cells and enables clear visualization of hyphae when present. The samples are covered by microscope cover slides and visualized initially by magnifying the image ×100 followed by ×200 up to ×400 (Figs. 23.3 and 23.4).

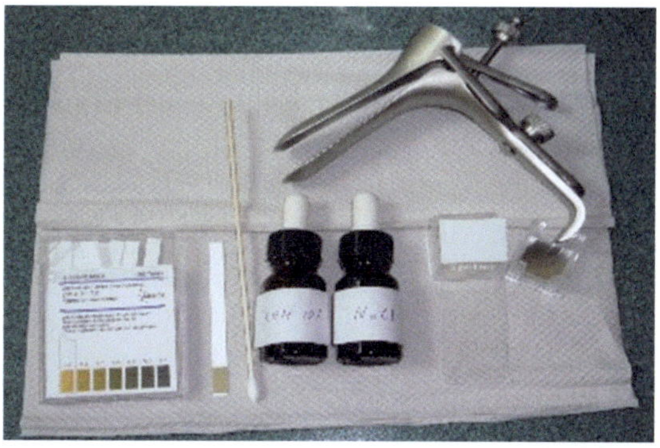

Fig. 23.3 The equipment needed for evaluating vaginal discharge. Courtesy of Dr. Orna Reichman

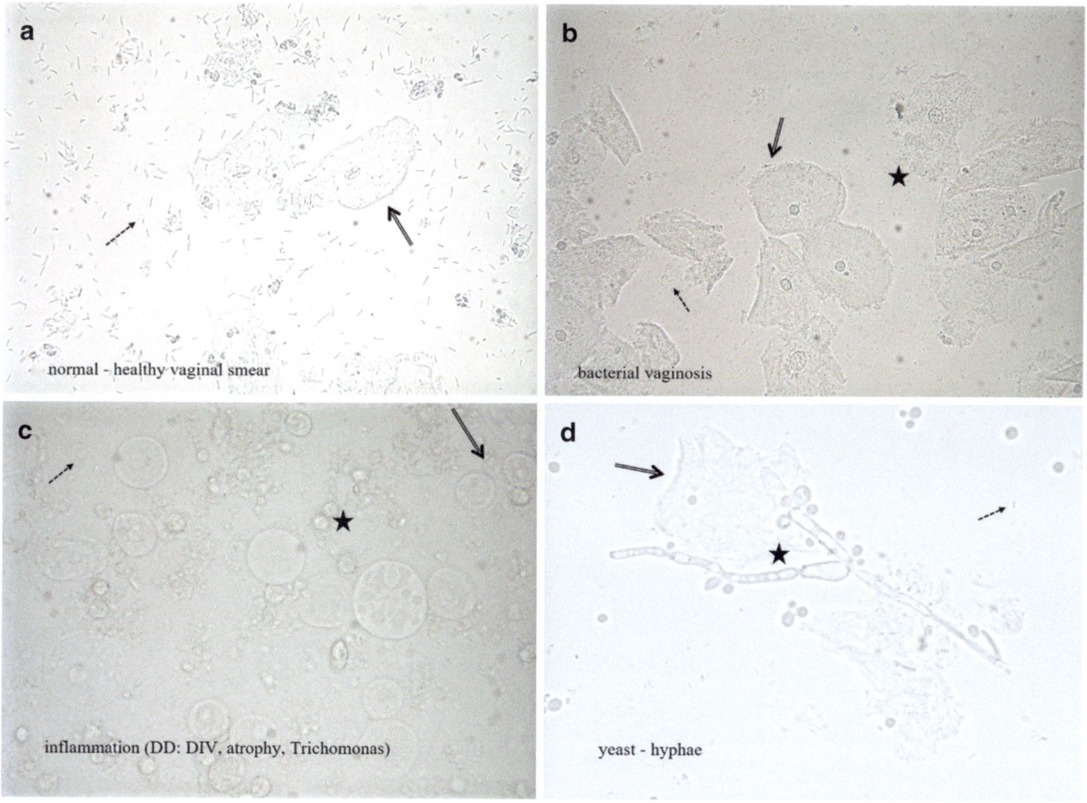

Fig. 23.4 Wet mount of four common vaginal conditions. In all four slides, the double-lined arrow points on the epithelial cells and the dashed arrow on the microbiota, and the asterisk is located next to the hallmark phenomenon of the condition. (**a**) Normal healthy vaginal smear—matured squamous epithelial cells and rod-shaped lactobacilli, (**b**) bacterial vaginosis (BV). Notice that the epithelial cells are matured squamous cells, no inflammation, and the flora is characterized by mixed cocci. The hallmark of BV is the clue cells—a phenomenon unique to this condition, the microbes adhere to the squamous epithelia and cover its borders. (**c**) Purulent vaginitis. Notice the immature parabasal cells and the excess of inflammatory cells. The differential diagnosis (DD) includes desquamative inflammatory vaginitis (DIV) which is an idiopathic inflammation syndrome of the vagina, trichomonas vaginalis, and atrophic vaginitis. Molecular biology assays and response to treatment could narrow down the DD. (**d**) Yeast infection—the presence of hyphae is the hallmark of the pathogenicity of yeast infection. It is important to notice that there are no inflammatory cells and that the epithelial cells are matured squamous cells. Courtesy of Dr. Orna Reichman

23.2.2 Vaginal pH

Vaginal pH reflects the hormonal and bacterial status of the vagina and is an excellent screening tool for evaluating vaginal health. Normal vaginal pH ≤4.5 indicates (1) adequate levels of estrogen, a multilayer epithelium with at least presence of intermediate cells that store the glycogen, and (2) healthy microbiota with predominant hydrogen peroxide-producing *Lactobacilli*. Noteworthy, pH ≤4.5 with a normal wet mount could suggest that the discharge is nonpathogenic and a diagnosis of normal leukorrhea is possible. In such a case, the patient needs reassurance. If discomfort is still present, the cause is probably of non-vaginal origin, such as vulvodynia, vulvitis, cervicitis, etc. If cervicitis is present, it is mandatory to send a PCR test to rule out sexually transmitted disease (STD) as chlamydia, gonorrhea, and trichomonas. However, in most cases, the results are negative, and cervicitis is concluded as non-gonococcal/non-chlamydia cervicitis. Vaginal pH is usually normal in presence of chlamydia. Normal pH in principle rules out trichomonas, bacterial vaginosis, desquamative inflammatory vaginitis, and atrophic vaginitis. A normal pH ≤4.5 narrows the differential diagnosis to yeast infection and contact dermatitis. See Figs. 23.5 and 23.6.

Approach to Diagnosis of Vulvovaginitis: Breaking the Myths

- Vaginal discharge, pruritus, malodor, and dyspareunia are nonspecific symptoms and may be caused by various etiologies.
- The acidic environment of the vagina (pH 4.0 ± 0.5) is essential for prevention of bacterial vaginosis (BV), which is associated with a troublesome fishy malodorous discharge.

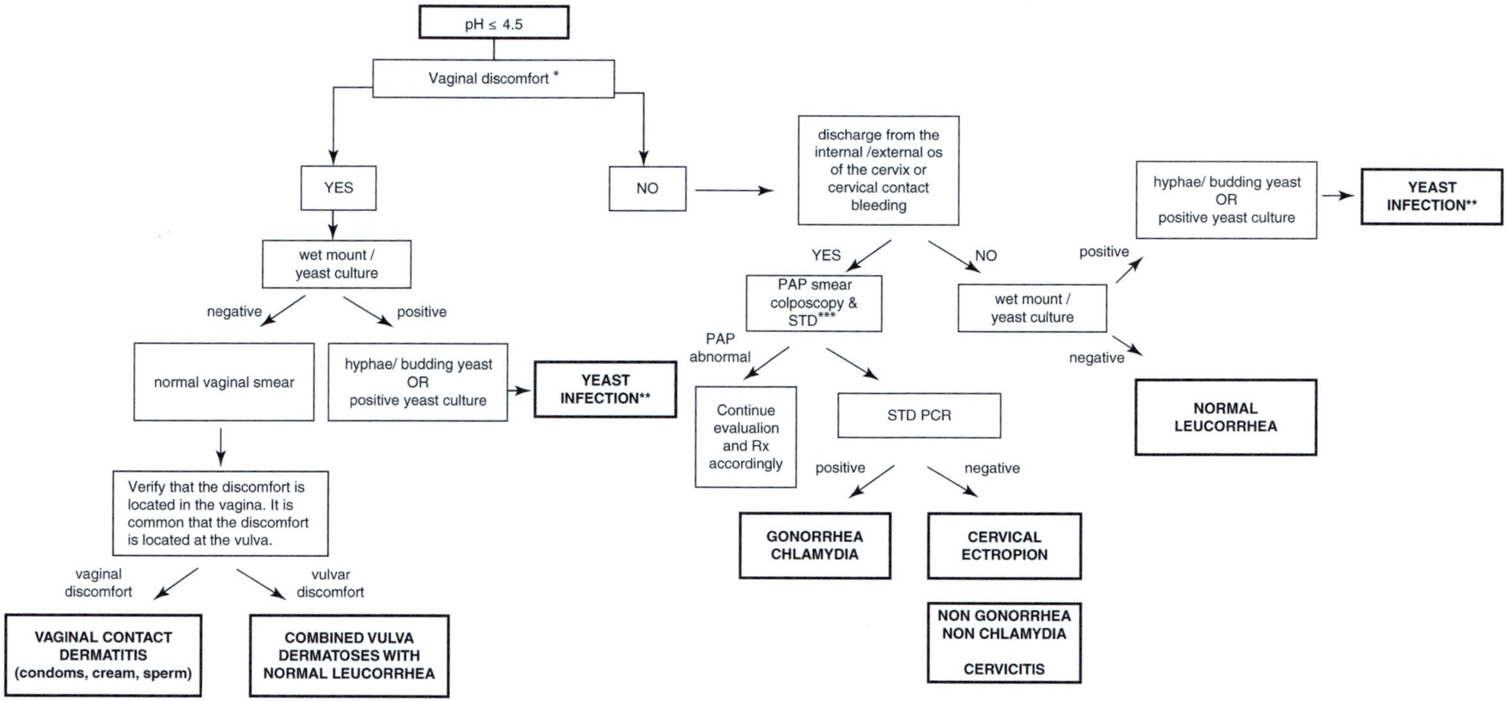

Fig. 23.5 Evaluation of vaginal discharge, combining symptoms, wet mount, and normal pH. * Vaginal discomfort including at least one of the following: itch, pain, dyspareunia, and purulent discharge. ***Yeast infection has a wide clinical presentation*; *symptoms can include discharge only or a combination of discharge itch and dyspareunia*; *some women are asymptomatic*. *PAP* Papanicolaou test, *ASC-US* atypical squamous cells of undetermined significance, *ASC-H* atypical squamous cells cannot exclude, *HGSIL* high-grade squamous intraepithelial lesion, *LGSIL* low-grade squamous intraepithelial lesion, *AGC* atypical glandular cells not otherwise specified. *** STD sexual transmitted disease. Courtesy of Dr. Orna Reichman

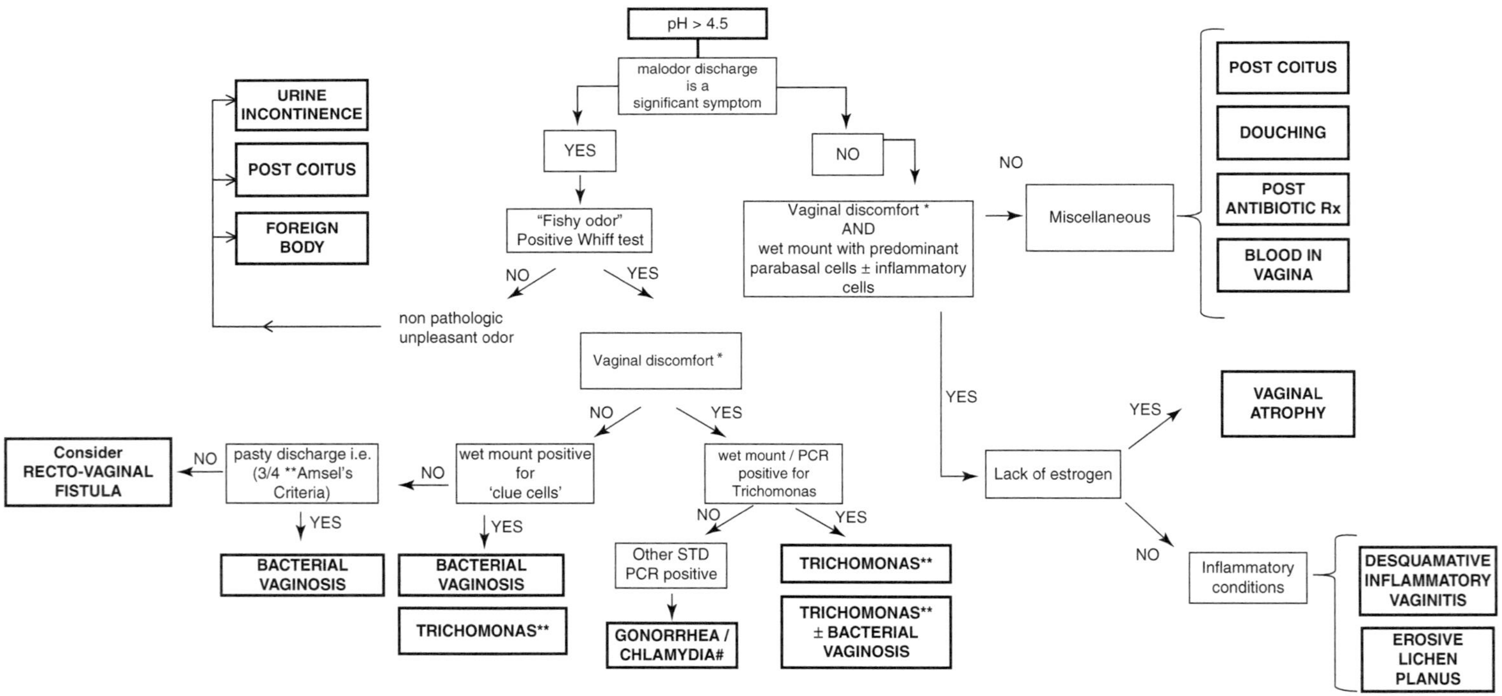

Fig. 23.6 Evaluation of vaginal discharge, combining symptoms, wet mount, and abnormal pH. * Vaginal discomfort including at least one of the following: itch, pain, dyspareunia, and purulent discharge. ** *Trichomonas vaginalis* has a wide clinical presentation; some patients present with acute vaginitis and complain of dyspareunia malodorous, purulent discharge, and itch; the others (up to 50%) are asymptomatic. If clinically indicated a PCR for trichomonas has to be performed. PCR, polymerase chain reaction. *** Amsel's criteria,[18] at least three of the following: (1) pasty discharge, (2) positive "whiff test" a drop of KOH to vaginal discharge will worsen malodor, (3) positive "clue cells" on wet mount, and (4) elevated pH. Courtesy of Dr. Orna Reichman

References

1. Kent HL. Epidemiology of vaginitis. Am J Obstet Gynecol. 1991;165(4 pt 2):1168–76.
2. Anderson MR, Klink K, Cohrssen A. Evaluation of vaginal complaints. JAMA. 2004;291(11): 1368–79.
3. Kottmel A, Petersen EE. Vaginal wet mount. J Sex Med. 2013;10(11):2616–9.
4. Bennett JE, Dolin R, Blaser MJ. Mandell, Douglas, and Bennett's principles and practice of infectious diseases. 8th ed. London: Churchil Livingston; 2015.
5. Buchanan DL, Kurita T, Taylor JA, Lubahn DB, Cunha GR, Cooke PS. Role of stromal and epithelial estrogen receptors in vaginal epithelial proliferation, stratification and cornification. Endocrinology. 1998;139:4345–52.
6. Meisels A. The maturation value. Acta Cytol. 1967;11(4):249.
7. Allsworth JE, Peipert JF. Prevalence of bacterial vaginosis: 2001–2004 National Health and Nutrition Examination Survey data. Obstet Gynecol. 2007;109:114–20.
8. Sobel JD. What's new in bacterial vaginosis and trichomoniasis? Infect Dis Clin N Am. 2005;19:387–406.

Candidiasis, Bacterial Vaginosis, Trichomoniasis and Other Vaginal Conditions Affecting the Vulva

24

Pedro Vieira-Baptista and Jacob Bornstein

24.1 Introduction

The term "vulvovaginitis" encompasses a broad and heterogeneous number of conditions, which, contrarily to what the suffix "-itis" implies, are not necessarily infectious (e.g. cytolytic vaginosis [CyV]) or inflammatory (e.g. bacterial vaginosis [BV]).

The clinical or symptomatic approach to the management of vulvovaginitis is very limited; a significant number of women will not fit the "traditional" diagnosis of candidiasis, BV, or trichomoniasis. A proper approach, encompassing other neglected diagnoses, will reduce the number of women without a diagnosis (reported to be as high as 30%), and lead to more adequate treatments.

These entities, despite not life-threatening, can seriously contribute to impair the quality of life of affected women at all levels, and leave deep and long lasting psychosexual sequelae.

Candidiasis: Breaking the Myths

- A significant number of women will not fit the "traditional" diagnosis of candidiasis, BV, or trichomoniasis
- *Candida albicans* infection does not consist only of vaginal discharge. In fact, its mycelium can penetrate the vaginal mucosa, up to 10 layers of cells deep.
- Despite the long list of risk factors and associations with vulvovaginal candidiasis (VVC), most of the times a precipitating factor cannot be identified.
- Itch is the most notorious symptom of VVC—but most women with itching do not have a VVC.
- Identification of *Candida* in cultures, per se, cannot be assumed as a diagnosis of VVC, as it does not distinguish colonization from infection.

24.2 Vulvovaginal Candidiasis (or Candidosis)

It is debatable whether the symptomatic presence of fungi from the genera *Candida* in the vagina should be referred to as vulvovaginal "candidiasis" or "candidosis" (VVC), since inflammation is not always present, and "-osis" is the suffix usually used for fungal infections.

P. Vieira-Baptista (✉)
Lower Genital Tract Unit, Gynaecolgy and Obstetrics Department, Centro Hospitalar de São João, Porto, Portugal

J. Bornstein
Department of Obstetrics and Gynecology Galilee Medical Center, Bar-Ilan University Faculty of Medicine, Nahariya, Israel

J. Bornstein (ed.), *Vulvar Disease*, https://doi.org/10.1007/978-3-319-61621-6_24

24.2.1 Aetiology and Pathophysiology

Approximately 90% of the cases of VVC are caused by *C. albicans*. The next most common agent is *C. glabrata*; much less frequently (<1–2% of the total), *C. krusei*, *C. tropicalis*, *C. dubliniensis* and *C. parapsilosis*, among others, can also be involved [1]. The non-albicans *Candida* (NAC) species are more commonly encountered in cases of recurrent VVC (in up to 20%), and in diabetic or immunocompromised women.

Co-infection is uncommon (<10% of cases) and usually the involved species are *C. albicans* and *C. glabrata* [1].

Candida is commonly found in the form of blastospores in the mucous layer, as a commensal. Infection starts with adherence to vaginal epithelial cells, mediated by mannoproteins. For the species that form mycelium (*C. albicans*), it is a fundamental step in eliciting an immune response and in causing host cell damage. The mycelium, in a phenomenon mediated, among others, by candidalysin, penetrates the vaginal mucosa, up to 10 layers of cells deep [2].

The first line of defence, innate immunity, includes phagocytosis by neutrophils and macrophages, activation of the complement cascade, direct cellular killing, and promotion of opsonization via complement receptors. This process is mediated by the binding of mannose-binding lectin (MBL) to *Candida* and explains why women with mutations of the MBL gene, especially at the codon 54, are more prone to recurrent VVC [3].

Acquired immunity against *Candida* is mostly mediated by IgA secretion, as well as a Th2 type cytokine profile response. However, an impaired Th1 response has been associated with increased risk of recurrent VVC [4].

A normal lactobacillary flora is protective against VVC due to: (1) competition for nutrients, (2) competition for adhesion sites, (3) production of biosurfactants that decrease the adherence of *Candida*, (4) production of H_2O_2, (5) production of toxic peptides and fatty acids, (6) downregulation of genes responsible for the biofilm production, and (7) inhibition of filamentation [5]. Interestingly however, most cases of VVC occur in women with normal flora [2] (Fig. 24.1).

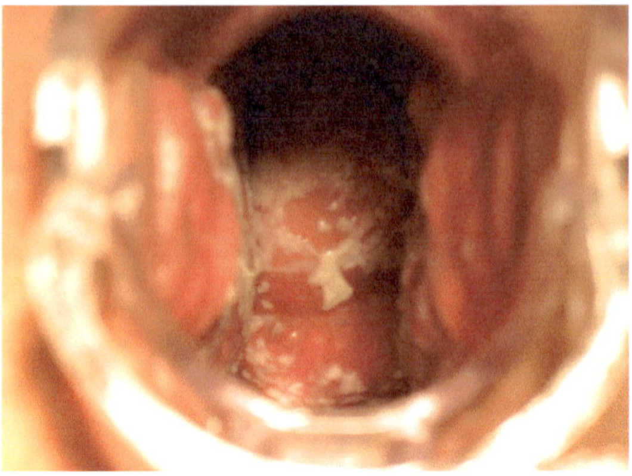

Fig. 24.1 Typical curdy white discharge of VVC (cultures were positive for *C. krusei*)

24.2.2 Prevalence and Epidemiology

VVC is not a reportable disease, thus all prevalence data are based on studies performed in different settings, often not representative of the population, and looking for different outcomes [1].

It is considered the second most frequent cause of "vulvovaginitis" symptoms, after BV. *Candida* can be responsible for the symptoms of vulvovaginitis in up to 30% of cases [6]. However, the perception of its prevalence, from patients' and health care providers' point of view, is higher; most cases are treated with over-the-counter medication, without proper confirmation.

Vaginal *Candida* colonization is found in at least 10–20% of healthy, reproductive age, asymptomatic women [7]. It is higher in pregnant women (20–40%), especially in the third trimester, due to the high levels of estrogens, and in immunocompromised women [8]. The cumulative incidence of colonization over 1 year is as high as 70% [9].

Up to 75% of women will experience at least one episode during their life time [1]. Half of these will suffer at least one additional episode and 5–10% will have recurrent VVC (Table 24.1) [1, 6, 10].

There is no data suggesting an increase in the incidence of VVC over the years [2].

24.2.3 Classification

The majority of episodes of VVC (90%) are considered uncomplicated. When the episodes are recurrent, associated with severe symptoms, caused by NAC species, or occur in diabetic or immunocompromised patients, it is classified as complicated [10] (Table 24.1).

According to most societies' guidelines, recurrent VVC is defined as four or more symptomatic episodes in 1 year. Most do not refer the need for a laboratorial confirmation (wet mount, culture, Gram staining) of every episode. We support that confirmation is necessary, in order to exclude alternative diagnosis (cytolytic vaginosis, allergic vaginitis) or NAC species.

24.2.4 Risk Factors and Associations

Despite the long list of risk factors and associations with VVC (Table 24.2), most of the times a precipitating factor cannot be identified [11].

The presence of *Candida* is highly related to oestrogen levels, and, accordingly it is much less common in prepubertal and postmenopausal women, and, contrarily, more common in pregnant women.

The role of oestrogens is complex: (1) promotes *Candida* proliferation and virulence, (2) induces immunological tolerance, and (3) promotes the production of glycogen by the vaginal epithelium cells. Progesterone, on one side, promotes *Candida* proliferation, but on the other has been shown also to inhibit its ability of forming biofilms and mycelium [12, 13].

The role of oral contraceptives in VVC is controversial. Modern low dose pills seem to pose a low risk, if any. Progestin-only pills and subdermal progestin implants seem to be associated with a lower risk of colonization, probably due to the relative state of hypoestrogenism they induce [14].

Copper intrauterine devices (IUDs) and, more recently, also levonorgestrel-releasing intrauterine systems (LVG-IUS) were associated with an increased risk of colonization by *Candida* [14, 15]. The formation of biofilms in the IUDs/LVG-IUS, to which *Candida* can adhere and act as a reservoir, is a possible explanation. However, this phenomenon does not seem to occur with the vaginal ring [16].

Glycogen, which is increased in cases of high levels of oestrogens, of steroids use, and in diabetic women, is the main growth substrate for Candida [12].

In women colonized with *Candida*, the use of antibiotics and the consequent destruction of the vaginal lactobacilli is a well-established risk factor [6] (Table 24.2).

Factors that can decrease the inflammatory response are associated with VVC. These can be genetic (MBL gene polymorphisms, diabetes) or acquired (HIV, drugs, low zinc levels).

Behavioural and environmental factors are the most complex ones to understand and with the most disparate results across studies. Higher temperatures and increased moisture, whether derived from the climate or local conditions (obesity, non-breathable clothes, etc.) seem to be related to increased rates of VVC. Some authors consider panty liners a risk factor for VVC, but systematic reviews do not support it [17].

Table 24.1 Classification of VVC

Uncomplicated	All 4 criteria must be met: • Sporadic or infrequent • Mild-to-moderate symptoms • Caused by *Candida albicans* • Non immunocompromised woman
Complicated	Any of these criteria present: • Recurrent VVC • Severe (extensive vulvar erythema, oedema, excoriations and fissures) • Non-albicans species involved • Women with diabetes, pregnancy, immunocompromising conditions (e.g. HIV infection), debilitation, or immunosuppressive therapy (e.g. corticosteroids)
Recurrent	• Four or more symptomatic episodes within 1 year • Each episode must have laboratorial confirmation (not recommended by all societies)

Table 24.2 Risk factors associated with VVC

Hormonal factors	Consequences/mechanisms of action
• Increased oestrogen levels (e.g. pregnancy) • Menopausal hormonal replacement therapy • Oral contraceptives (?)	• ↑ Adherence of *Candida* to vaginal cells • ↑ Mycelium formation • ↓ Vaginal immunological response • ↑ Levels of vaginal glycogen • Direct stimulation of *Candida* proliferation
Metabolic factors	
• Obesity • Diabetes *mellitus*	• ↑ Adherence of *Candida* do vaginal cells • ↑ Levels of vaginal glycogen • ↓ Vaginal immunological response
• Low zinc levels	• ↓ Cellular immunity
Host factors	
• Immunosuppression (e.g. HIV) • Debilitating illnesses • Stress	• ↓ Immunological defences
• Genetic polymorphisms (MBL gene, IL4 gene, NALP3, dectin-1 gene, CARD9, STAT1, STAT3)	• ↓ Immunological defences
• ABO-Lewis nonsecretor blood type	• ↓ Inhibition of adherence lectins • ↓ IgA levels • Carbohydrates metabolism abnormalities
• Atopy/allergy history	• Excessive reaction to *Candida* antigens
• Black race	• Genetic factors?
Drugs	
• Antibiotics (topical and systemic) *(mostly beta-lactamics, macrolides, and tetracyclines)*	• Elimination of protective vaginal flora (lactobacilli)
• Steroids • Immunosuppressors • Chemotherapy	• ↓ Immunological defences
Behavioural factors	
• Hot and humid climates • Tight and synthetic clothes • Patny-liners (?) • Obesity	• ↑ Moisture and temperature
• Bad hygienic habits • Vaginal douching • Swimming pools rich in chloride	• ↑ Spore load (from the intestinal reservoir) • ↑ Vaginal pH • Destruction of lactobacilli
• Dietary factors (rapid sugars)	• ↑ Glycogen
• Sexual habits (frequent sexual intercourse, recipient oral sex) (*Controversial: early sexual debut, new or multiple partners, intercourse during menses)*	• ↑ Spore load • Alteration of the flora by semen • Exposure to cytokines, antigens, prostaglandins, and antibodies from semen • Transmission from the oral mucosa (?)
• Copper IUDs/ LNG-IUS	• Formation of biofilms, that increase adherence and act as reservoirs • Changes in the vaginal flora

VVC is not considered STI, but it is sexually related. Sexual intercourse and the deposition of semen in the vagina changes the pH, the interleukin and prostaglandin milieu, exposes the vagina to IgE and antibodies from the male partner, which can be responsible for the development of symptoms of VVC.

24.2.5 Signs and Symptoms

The reservoir of *Candida*, during an active episode of VVC is the vagina, which is devoid of itch receptors, thus the symptoms manifest only in the vulva. It is not known, if itch is caused by the infection itself or secondary to the contact with the vaginal discharge. In severe cases, manifestations of VVC such as redness and oedema may extend up to the perianal area and the intercrural folds (Fig. 24.2). Satellite vulvar lesions can be present.

Itch is the most notorious symptom of VVC—but it must be kept in mind that most women with itching do not have a VVC [18]. Especially in cases of hypoestrogenism, in the absence of immunodepression, VVC is not likely to be the cause of itching.

Other symptoms can include entry dyspareunia, soreness, and irritation. The presence of NAC is usually asymptomatic; if not, it usually causes burning, rather than itching, and the symptoms tend to be milder.

Women can describe a more abundant, curdy, white and thick (cheese-like) or watery discharge, without an offensive smell (Fig. 24.1). It can also be absent, especially in chronic VVC.

Fissures and excoriations can cause vulvar pain and terminal or post-micturition dysuria—derived from the contact of urine with the lesions, rather than from urethral involvement. Oedema can be present, more exuberantly in the *labia minora,* and vulvar redness is seen in up to 40% of cases [2]. The vagina and cervix may be covered with a white, cheesy discharge (Fig. 24.2), but usually do not look inflamed and there is no cervicitis, but minor bleeding can be noticed if removal of the discharge plaque from the vaginal wall is attempted [2].

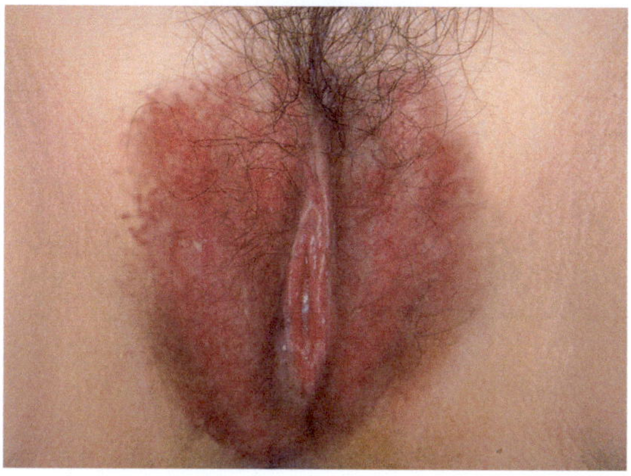

Fig. 24.2 Vulvovaginal candidiasis (VVC), with vulvar erythema in the interlabial sulci Courtesy of Professor Jacob Bornstein

The severity of symptoms can fluctuate along the menstrual cycle, worsening in the week prior to menses and improving during it. It can be explained by the vaginal epithelial cell proliferation and cytolysis, mediated by oestrogens and progesterone, respectively, which ultimately leads to increased levels of glycogen in the vagina. The raising of the pH mediated by the presence of blood and endometrial debris in the vagina leads to a decrease in the symptoms.

24.2.6 Complications

VVC, especially the complicated form, is a major cause of mental suffering, depression, low self-esteem, with impact on sexual and affective relations.

A large majority of newborns who are colonized with *C. albicans* during a vaginal delivery will develop oral candidiasis or napkin dermatitis during their first year of life. This can be diminished by treating colonized mothers during the 3rd trimester [2].

Petricevic et al. have found slight increases in preterm labour and risk of low birth weight rates, especially if colonization is present during the 2nd trimester of pregnancy [19].

Candida chorioamnionitis has been reported, but it is a very rare event and usually related to procedures such as in vitro fertilization, *cérclage*, or amniocentesis [20].

In one study, the presence of *Candida* was significantly associated with an increased risk of seroconversion in HIV negative women, with a seropositive male partner [21].

VVC has been associated with vulvodynia in several studies but most of the reported episodes are based on recall and not laboratory confirmed, thus making it unreliable. Nevertheless, long-term treatment with fluconazole is not an effective treatment of vulvodynia. *Candida* can, however, be the initial aggression to the vestibular mucosa and it has been shown that in vulvodynia patients the inflammatory response to it can be heightened [22].

24.2.7 Diagnosis

Clinical history and a vulvovaginal examination are fundamental parts of the diagnosis, but not sufficient. Self-diagnosis of VVC is wrong in up to 90% of cases and should not be encouraged [6, 23]. "Phone diagnosis" is also an unreliable approach.

The diagnosis is supported by wet mount microscopy (WMM), ideally using phase contrast microscopy [2] and, in some cases, by culture.

24.2.7.1 Microscopy

The most important tool in the diagnosis of VVC is microscopy, which should be performed systematically in women with suspected vulvovaginitis. Not only it allows the diagnosis of VVC, as it is the only way to identify the presence of mixed infections. WMM is cheaper than Gram staining and allows an immediate diagnosis.

There is evidence that collecting the sample from the anterior vaginal wall increases the likelihood of identifying *Candida* [24].

Candida in WMM can present as mycelium and/or blastospores. Mycelium includes both hyphae (filaments that compose the body of the fungus) and pseudohyphae (filaments composed of elongated budding cells that failed to detach) and their presence is highly suggestive of infection, rather than mere colonization (Fig. 24.3). However, some species, like *C. glabrata*, are unable to form mycelium. The blastospores of *C. glabrata* tend to cluster and to have the shape of a bowling pin or a "snowman" (Fig. 24.4). In the presence of clustering blastospores, in the absence of mycelium, NAC should be considered (Fig. 24.5) [4].

Care must be taken not to confuse sperms heads with blastospores. The former tend to be asymmetrical (larger where the tail was attached) and are bicolor (Fig. 24.6) [4].

Some authors recommend the addition of a drop of KOH to the slide, which dissolves the epithelial cells and leukocytes, but not the fungal structures, increasing the sensitivity of WMM to up to 85% [6, 24]. Other measures to try to improve the identification of these structures can include the staining with methylene blue [4].

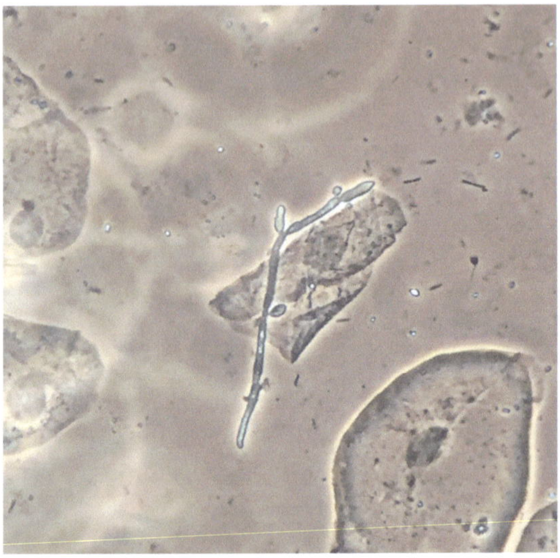

Fig. 24.3 *C. albicans* (pseudohyphae) in wet mount (phase contrast 400×). The background flora is normal, despite some scarcity of lactobacilli. (phase contrast, 400×)

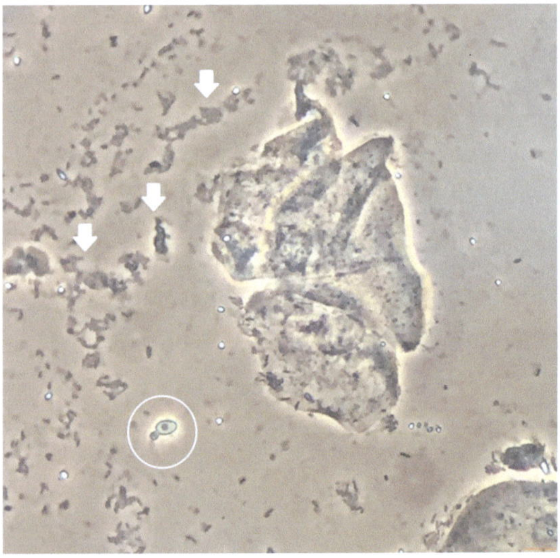

Fig. 24.4 "Snowman" typical of *C. glabrata* (inside the white circle). Anaerobic type background flora (white arrows). (phase contrast, 400×)

The Pap test is specific for the presence of *Candida*, but has a sensitivity of only 25%, making it useless as diagnostic tool. This comes as no surprise, since it is a cervical rather than a vaginal sample [6].

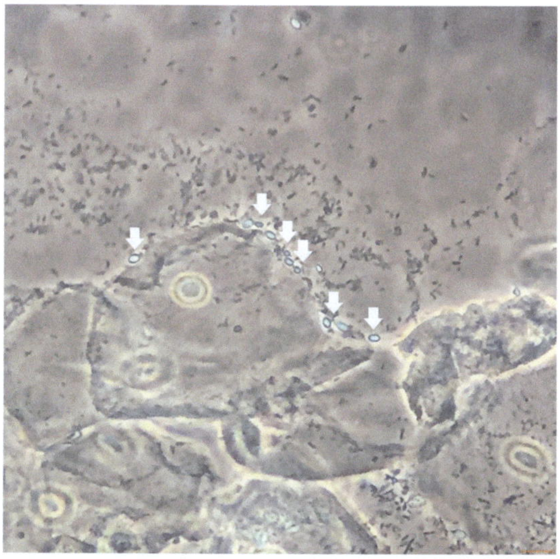

Fig. 24.5 Clustering of blastospores, typical of NAC (white arrows). (phase contrast, 400×)

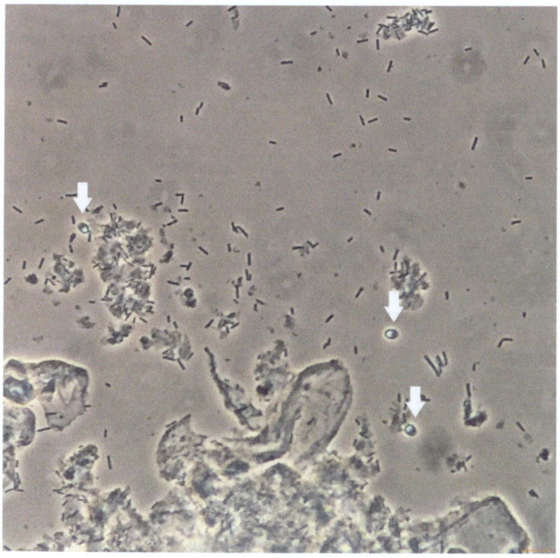

Fig. 24.6 Sperm heads, which can be mistaken by blastospores (white arrows). Notice that these are bicolor and asymmetrical. (phase contrast, 400×)

24.2.7.2 Cultures

Cultures are not needed routinely. Exceptions are recurrent episodes, microscopy negative or uncertain, or no response to treatment [2, 6]. Sensitivity tests are hardly ever needed, except for difficult NAC cases. *C. albicans* strains resistant to fluconazole are uncommon and very rarely pose a clinical problem.

Identification of *Candida* in cultures, per se, cannot be assumed as a diagnosis of VVC, as it does not distinguish colonization from infection.

The swabs can be transported in common transport means (Stuart or Amies)—or even without it, at room temperature, and should be cultivated within 6 h [4]. There seems to be no advantage between the available culture means (Sabouraud agar, Nickerson medium, or Microstix-Candida medium) for *Candida* [6].

24.2.7.3 pH

Candida is more often found with normal pH and is likely to be more symptomatic under those conditions. However, it may co-occur with BV or aerobic vaginitis (AV) (Fig. 24.4), which are typically associated with elevated pH. An elevated pH cannot rule out VVC, and at the same time, typical clinical presentation with a normal pH does not necessarily confirm the diagnosis [4].

However, the pH can guide the next steps in the management of the patient with symptoms suggestive of VVC: If microscopy is positive for *Candida* and the pH is increased, a mixed infection must be considered; if microscopy is negative and pH is normal, cultures are recommended [6].

24.2.7.4 Molecular Tests

The Affirm VPIII is a commercially available test, based on DNA probes, that detects *Candida*, *T. vaginalis*, and *G. vaginalis* in vaginal samples, returning the result in 45 min. The sensitivity and specificity for *Candida*, in comparison with the gold standard (culture) were 82.76% and 98.80%, respectively [25, 26].

The use of nucleic acid amplification tests (NAAT) techniques increases the detection rate of *Candida* in 12.5% [27] and can be an option in those cases of high grade of suspicion, in which wet mount and cultures are negative. In recurrent cases, when microscopy is positive but cultures are negative, molecular techniques lead to the diagnosis of three times more cases [28, 29].

More recently, the BD MAX system, a real time PCR test for the detection of the presence of DNA from lactobacilli, bacteria associated with BV, *T. vaginalis*, and *Candida* (*C. albicans, C. tropicalis, C. parapsilosis, C. dubliniensis, C. glabrata,* and *C. krusei*) was developed. Sensitivity for the different species of *Candida* ranged from 75–91% and specificity was higher than 90%. It showed to perform similarly in self-collected samples [30].

These tests allow for faster results, are less operator dependent, and can improve the diagnostic performance, but pose the risk of overdiagnosis (not distinguishing colonization from infection), not recognizing the full picture (mixed infections), and are still expensive.

24.2.8 Treatment

24.2.8.1 General Principles

Since the symptoms are mostly vulvar, women must be warned that topical medication must be applied inside the vagina, rather than (just) in the vulva. External, vulvar application can lead to transitory relief of symptoms, but not to cure.

Topical antifungals can be oil based and, consequently weaken condoms [10].

Oral azoles can interfere with oral anticoagulants (increasing its levels) and anticonvulsants, such as phenytoin.

There is no indication to treat sexual partners, unless they have symptoms themselves (balanitis); in the latter case, topical antifungals can be used. Redness, in some cases, may be associated with an allergic reaction to *Candida* antigens, rather than infection.

Persistence of symptoms can be the result of a contact dermatitis, resulting from the repeated and long lasting treatments, or from secondary lichen simplex *chronicus*. In some cases, allergy to propylene glycol, a common excipient in vaginal medications can develop.

24.2.8.2 Asymptomatic *Candida*

There is no reason to treat asymptomatic *Candida* in non-pregnant women, independently of being an incidental finding in a Pap test or other laboratorial exam, or being suspected during a clinical examination.

24.2.8.3 Uncomplicated VVC

These cases should be treated with short courses (1–7 days) of vaginal imidazoles (clotrimazole, miconazole, butoconazole, etc.) or single doses of oral triazoles (fluconazole or, alternatively, itraconazole), which have similar efficacy (>80%) and adverse effects profiles [10] (Table 24.3). The choice for oral or topical routes is according to patients' preferences. In some cases, women find a faster relief by using vaginal formulations, as it temporarily increases the pH.

There is no evidence that itraconazole is more effective than fluconazole [31, 32]. Topical polyenes, such as nystatin, have lower cure rates than topical imidazoles [33]. The limited data concerning the use of terbinafine, an allylamine antifungal suggests that it is efficacious if used topically, but not if orally [34, 35]. Data about ciclopirox olamine is also limited, but the few trials in which it was used showed it to be safe and effective.

24.2.8.4 Complicated VVC

Severe cases of VVC should be treated with more prolonged courses of topical antifungals or, if fluconazole is chosen, a second dose after 72 h is recommended (Table 24.3).

Topical, low potency corticosteroids (hydrocortisone) for a couple of days can be helpful in very symptomatic patients.

Cases of recurrent VVC are a truly clinical challenge. Reasonable attempts to control or correct risk factors should be tried: reducing sugar intake, stopping hormonal contraceptives or removing IUDs/LVG-IUSs, correcting excessive washing, stopping the use of tight or synthetic clothes, etc. Each measure should be sequentially tried and, if not efficacious, suspended—otherwise, these changes will just add suffering to someone who already has an impaired quality of life due to a chronic disease [4, 6].

In case of failure of these measures, self-treatment of the episodes or, preferably, suppressive treatment must be considered. The most commonly recommended treatment was proposed by Sobel [36] and consists of taking 150 mg of oral fluconazole weekly, for 6 months, after an induction in the first week (three times 150 mg in the first week). Donders proposed an alternative

Table 24.3 Treatment of VVC

Uncomplicated	Topical (vaginal)	Clotrimazole 1% cream 5 g *id* for 7–14 days Clotrimazole 2% cream 5 g *id* for 3 days Clotrimazole 100 mg suppository, *id* for 7 days Clotrimazole 200 mg suppository, *id* for 3 days Clotrimazole 500 mg suppository, single application Miconazole 2% cream 5 g *id* for 7 days Miconazole 4% cream 5 g *id* for 3 days Miconazole 100 mg suppository, *id* for 7 days Miconazole 200 mg suppository, *id* for 3 days Miconazole 1200 mg suppository, single application Tioconazole 6.5% ointment 5 g single application Tioconazole 300 mg suppository, single application Butoconazole 2% cream (bioadhesive), 5 g in a single application Terconazole 0.4% cream 5 g *id* for 7 days Terconazole 0.8% cream 5 g *id* for 3 days Terconazole 80 mg suppository, *id* 3 days Econazole 150 mg tablets, *id* for 3 days Nystatin 100.000 units suppositories *id* for 14 days Ciclopirox olamine 1% cream 6 days
	Oral	Fluconazole 150 mg, single dose Itraconazole 200 mg *id*, 3 days Itraconazole 200 mg 2 *id*, one day Ketoconazole 200 mg 2 *id*, 5 days (hepatic toxicity)
Pregnancy	Only topical azoles during 7 days	
Breastfeeding	Azoles excreted in milk; avoid during breastfeeding	
Severe VVC	Topical	Prolong treatment for 7–14 days
	Oral	Fluconazole 150 mg day 1 and day 4
Recurrent VVC	Fluconazole suppression for 12 months (ReCiDiF)	Phase 1–200 mg *po* days 1, 4 and 7 Phase 2–200 mg *po* once a week for 2 months Phase 3–200 mg *po* once every other week for 4 weeks Phase 4–200 mg *po* once a month for 6 months Transition from one phase to the other implies: Symptoms free, wet mount/culture negative
	Fluconazole suppression for 6 months (Sobel)	150 mg *po* once a week (100, 150 or 200 mg on day 1, 4 and 7, prior to suppressive therapy)
	Depot medroxyprogesterone acetate	Intramuscular 150 mg every 12 weeks
Non-albicans VVC	Boric acid 600 mg vaginal capsules	Vaginally *id* for 2 weeks Must be compounded by pharmacists Toxic if per mouth Maintenance regimen?
	Gentian violet	Useful in some cases Good antipruritic effect Messy
	High dose fluconazole	800 mg *id* for 2–3 weeks
	Other options may include: • Flucytosine • Posaconazole • Voriconazole • Amphotericin B • Caspofungin • Micafungin	

regimen, after the ReCiDiF trial, lasting 1 year and consisting of progressively increased intervals between fluconazole intake (see scheme in Table 24.3) [28]. In the later, while using the same total dosage of fluconazole and being comparable in terms of efficacy at 6 months, 77% of women were disease free at 12 months, comparing to only 42.9% in the Sobel's scheme [28, 36].

Episodes during suppressive therapy can be managed with topical antifungals; in occasional cases, antihistamines can be helpful.

Dennerstein reported good results in controlling the symptoms by using depo-medroxyprogesterone, probably by inducing a hypoestrogenic state [37]. In our hands, it has been an excellent option when other options fail.

It can be advisable that these patients have swabs with them, for self-collection and confirmation of the episodes.

In difficult cases, consider exclusion of HIV and diabetes.

In women with history of frequent or recurrent VVC after antibiotic intake, beta-lactamics, macrolides, and tetracyclines should be avoided. For urinary tract infections, alternative options include fosfomicine or norfloxacine. Additionally, prophylactic antifungals can be prescribed, to be taken at the beginning and halfway through the course of antibiotics [4].

The most common of the NACs, *C. glabrata*, is not sensible to the usual antifungals. One of the best alternatives is boric acid. Patients must be warned of its toxicity if ingested (gastrointestinal, mental disorders, seizures, anaemia, etc.).

C. krusei is intrinsically resistant to oral triazoles, however, it responds well to topical imidazoles, nystatin, boric acid, and ciclopirox olamine [2].

24.2.8.5 Candida in Pregnancy

Oral triazoles should not be used during pregnancy, as it has been related to spontaneous abortion and to a slight increase in the risk of Fallot's tetralogy.

As discussed previously, *Candida* can be associated with negative obstetrical outcomes and for that reason some authors recommend treatment of asymptomatic women. This recommendation, however, is not universal and more data is needed to support it.

24.2.9 Future Perspectives

Despite the role played by lactobacilli in the prevention of symptomatic VVC, its administration either as treatment or adjuvant of antifungal treatment, has not shown to be useful in acute or recurrent episodes [38]. This line of investigation, however, can prove to have some role in the future, especially if strains that naturally dominate the vagina of healthy women are used.

In the future, vaccines may be the answer to treat recurrent VVC.

24.2.10 *Saccharomyces cerevisiae*

The yeast *S. cerevisiae* can colonize the vagina of healthy women, and very rarely, become symptomatic. Its incidence, however, seems to be rising and, apparently it is not always associated with professional exposure (brewery or bakery) or with consumption of it as a food additive or probiotic [39, 40].

Symptoms are undistinguishable from those of VVC. It is, however, less susceptible to antifungals and is associated with high rates of recurrence. The diagnosis is confirmed by culture, but can be suspected when larger than usual blastospores are seen on WMM [4] (Fig. 24.7). Treatment options can include nystatin, amphotericin B, flucytosine, and boric acid.

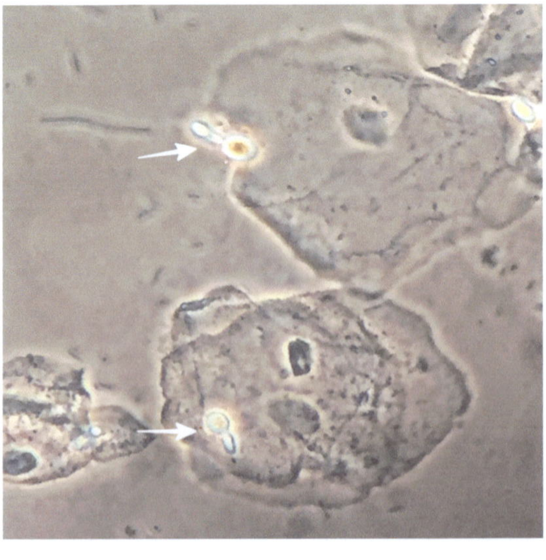

Fig. 24.7 Larger than usual budding blastospores (white arrows). Culture confirmed *S. cerevisiae*

24.3 Trichomoniasis

Trichomoniasis: Breaking the Myths

- Trichomoniasis is not rare—it is the most common non-viral STI and prevalence seems to be rising.
- The classical image of the "strawberry cervix" is seen in less than 5% of the cases with *T. vaginalis*
- Maternal *Trichomonas vaginalis* infection is not only a nuisance. It is a risk factor for low birth weight, premature rupture of membrane, preterm labour, and even intellectual disability. One study related *T. vaginalis* with neonatal death.

24.3.1 Aetiology and Pathophysiology

Trichomoniasis is caused by the extracellular protozoan *Trichomonas vaginalis,* which was first described in 1836, but forgotten in the medical literature for a century.

T. vaginalis is of piriform, round or amoeboid shape, with a distinctive elongated nucleus, four anterior flagella, and a large posterior axostyle to which an undulant membrane is attached. It is motile, with fast and erratic movements.

The amitochondriate and anaerobic parasite is capable of phagocyting bacteria (including lactobacilli), epithelial cells, and erythrocytes (from where it gets iron and cholesterol), but can itself be phagocyted by macrophages [41].

Its only natural hosts are humans, colonizing almost exclusively the genitourinary tract of both men and women. Infection sites in women include the vagina, endocervix, urethra, and paraurethral glands. Very rarely it can be found in the respiratory tract.

In adults, transmission is almost exclusively by sexual route; direct vaginal or urethral inoculation is needed. There are some reports of possible transmission by sharing the bath water, per fomites, or by genital manipulation by another infected person. The parasite can survive outside of the human body for periods of around 3 h, if protected from desiccation [42].

T. vaginalis can be infected by double strand RNA viruses, which, as discussed ahead, can have severe implications in its virulence [43].

24.3.2 Prevalence and Epidemiology

Trichomoniasis is the most common non-viral STI and prevalence seems to be rising [44, 45]. Existing projections are likely to be an underestimation of the true prevalence and burden of the infection, as it is not a reportable disease. This leaves extensive gaps in the understanding of the dynamics of the infection and the true extent of its complications.

Different diagnostic techniques and baseline characteristics of the populations studied preclude comparisons between series. For instance, the very high prevalences found in STI clinics are unlikely to reflect the true picture for the general population [7].

According to World Health Organization, in 2008, in the age range 15–49 years, trichomoniasis led the list of curable STIs, with 276.4 million of new cases in that year: more than the sum of those of *Chlamydia trachomatis*, *Neisseria gonorrhoea* and syphilis. The estimated number of *T. vaginalis* infections at any moment was estimated at 187 million (Table 24.4).

The prevalence is much higher in females (5.6–22.0%) than in males (0.6–2.2%) (Table 24.4). Incidence, however, is similar in both sexes, ranging between 45.6 and 180.60/00 (promil) [45], meaning that the rate of transmis-

Table 24.4 Prevalence and incidence of *T. vaginalis* in 2008, according to the WHO. Adapted from Rowley et al. [45]

	Incidence (‰)		Prevalence (%)	
WHO region	Female	Male	Female	Male
African	146.0	164.8	20.2	2.0
Americas	177.7	180.6	22.0	2.2
South East-Asia	40.3	50.1	5.6	0.6
European	51.7	48.4	5.8	0.6
Eastern Mediterranean	64.0	66.1	8.0	0.8
Western Pacific	45.6	47.0	5.7	0.6

sion and acquisition is similar, but males spontaneous eliminate the infection much faster. It usually takes about 10–21 days in males, while in women it can persist for months or even years [46]. However, in men it too can become chronic or reinfection can occur. The zinc rich milieu of prostatic secretions can account for these differences; chronic infection in men is more likely in those with lower concentrations of zinc in the prostatic secretions [47].

Transmission is more effective from males to female than the other way round (*T. vaginalis* is positive in 66–100% of the female partners of infected men vs. 30–80% of the male partners of infected women [48]).

The incubation period is believed to range between 4 and 28 days [49].

Contrary to other STIs, the prevalence of *T. vaginalis*, at least in some settings, peaks in women after 40 years of age. Possible explanations include: (1) long-standing infection in reservoirs, such as the periurethral and subepithelial glands, (2) increasing resistance to metronidazole, (3) increased pH, due to the falling oestrogen levels, (4) sexual risk factors, and (5) screening artefact. The theory of sexual risk factors is supported by the fact that this peak was also described in men, and in women it only occurred in those who were also positive for high-risk human papillomavirus (HPV) [50].

24.3.3 Risk Factors and Associations

Despite geographical variations, racial, social, sexual, and behavioural factors for trichomoniasis have been identified, disentanglement of the various factors in order to distinguish true risk factors from mere associations is a nearly impossible task.

In the United States, the prevalence of trichomoniasis in women of black race was four times higher than in the general population and, more striking, ten times higher than white non-Hispanic women.

In the same study, positive correlations were found with lower educational level, poverty, greater number of sexual partners, increasing age, and vaginal douching [51]. Other reported factors include early sexual debut, new or multiple sexual partners, having other STIs, incarceration, commercial sex, being an immigrant, intravenous drug use, cigarette smoking, and not using condoms [51, 52].

Sexual factors, per se, cannot account for the full explanation of the different prevalences found in different countries: for instance, European countries with rates of *Chlamydia* similar to those found in the United States have lower rates of TV [41].

One interesting association is that of *T. vaginalis* with BV, which is found in 60–80% of cases. The mechanism is not fully understood: on one side, *T. vaginalis* benefits from the increased pH and anaerobic environment associated with BV, and, on the other side, *T. vaginalis* may disturb the vaginal microbiome and shift it to the anaerobic side [7].

24.3.4 Signs and Symptoms

It is estimated that up to 80–85% of infected women and 77% of men are asymptomatic [41, 45, 48]. Many of the asymptomatic women eventually become symptomatic—sometimes in a very exuberant, highly symptomatic way. Given the long periods during which the infection can be asymptomatic, it is almost impossible to ascertain when infection was acquired.

When symptomatic, women can refer a yellow or green discharge, frequently with a foul smell. Urinary symptoms can be present (frequency, dysuria), as well as lower abdominal pain, dyspareunia, vulvar irritation, itching, and burning. Dysuria, unlikely in women with VVC is not only terminal or post-micturition, as there can be a real urethritis or cystitis (urethral involvement occurs in 90% of cases) [53]. Symptoms tend to worsen during menses, probably due to the increase in the number of parasites, associated with the phagocytosis of erythrocytes.

Some women may suffer from postcoital bleeding, as a consequence of the presence of erosions in the vaginal wall.

On physical examination, this discharge is frothy, more or less abundant and fluid (Fig. 24.8). Erosions, cervical friability, and vaginal enantema

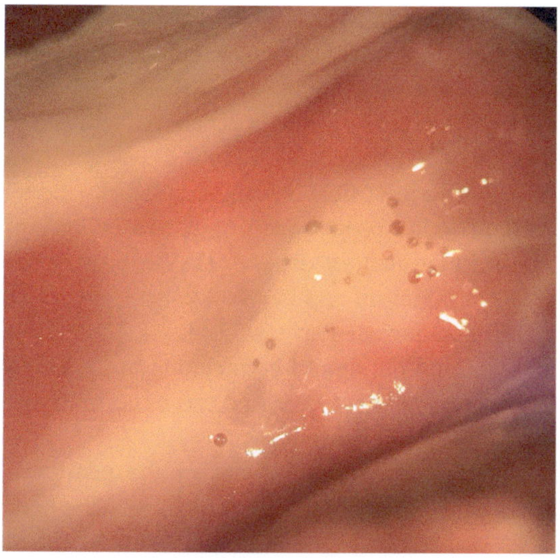

Fig. 24.8 Frothy vaginal discharge in a woman with *Trichomonas vaginalis* and bacterial vaginosis

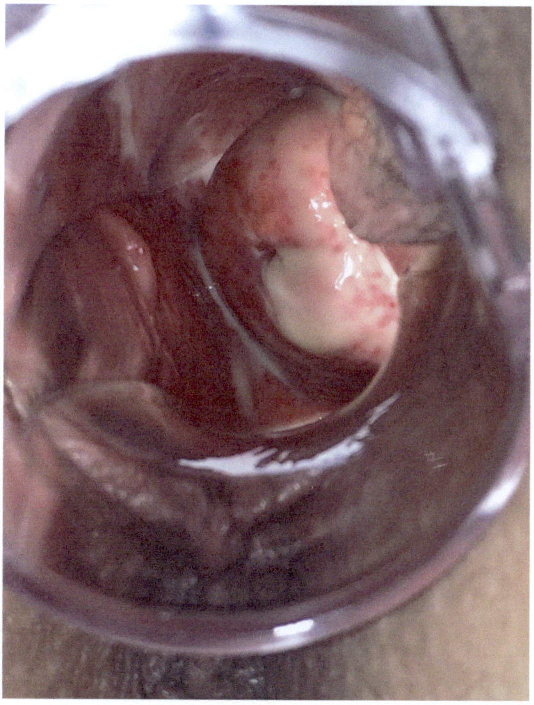

Fig. 24.9 Strawberry cervix, typical of a Trichomonas infection

can be noticed in the vaginal walls and the cervix. The classical image of the "strawberry cervix" is uncommon (<5%) (Fig. 24.9); after the application of Lugol's solution it may gain the typical appearance of "Leopard skin" (Fig. 24.10).

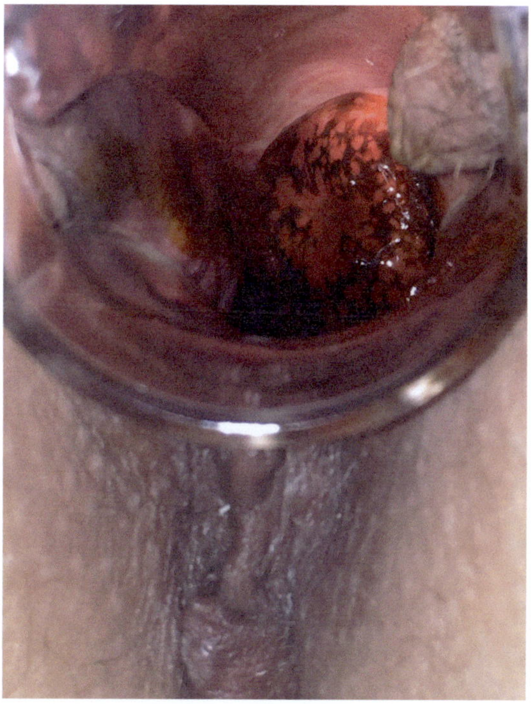

Fig. 24.10 Strawberry cervix after the application of iodine ("leopard skin")

Very rarely, *T. vaginalis* can be associated with the enigmatic condition of emphysematous vaginitis, in which air bubbles form in the vaginal walls, sometimes with crepitus during intercourse or speculum examination [54].

A normal gynaecological examination is not sufficient to exclude the presence of *T. vaginalis*.

24.3.5 Complications

For a long time, *T. vaginalis* was considered a nuisance STI. However, nowadays, it is acknowledged as being associated with severe complications, and considered a public health issue [41].

Maternal *T. vaginalis* infection is a risk factor for low birth weight (RR, 1.51; [95% confidence interval 1.32–1.73, $p < 0.001$]), premature rupture of membranes (RR, 1.41; [95% confidence interval, 1.10–1.82, $p = 0.007$]), preterm labour (RR 1.4 [95% confidence interval, 1.15–1.75; $p = 0.001$]) [55], and even intellectual disability [41]. One study related *T. vaginalis* with neonatal death (1.6% vs. 0.8%, $p = 0.005$) [56].

T. vaginalis infected with *M. hominis*, besides being more cytopathogenic, induce an increased production of IL1β, IL6, IL8, and tumour necrosis factor (TNF) 1α—a similar profile to that associated with preterm labour [57].

Newborns from infected mothers can have a self-limiting vaginitis or pneumonia, but sometimes treatment is required. The symptoms of vaginitis usually disappear as the levels of oestrogens wane.

T. vaginalis is a well-recognized risk factor for the transmission and acquisition of other STIs, namely HIV [58]. *T. vaginalis* increases the risk of acquisition and transmission by several ways: (1) by attracting inflammatory cells to the vagina, (2) by causing breaches in the integrity of the vagina and cervix (facilitating the access of HIV to the bloodstream), (3) by increasing IL-8, which increases HIV1 replication, and (4) by changing the vaginal flora towards BV [41].

Proper management of HIV patients should include regular screening of trichomoniasis (and BV), as it can be asymptomatic and still increase the HIV load in the vagina, as thus promote the transmission. Reducing *T. vaginalis* rates can be an effective, cost-effective measure to reduce HIV transmission, especially in populations such as in sub-Saharan Africa (Table 24.4), where it is believed to increase the risk of infection 2.1–2.8 times; this impact can be extensive to vertical transmission [59].

It has also been linked to increased risk of pelvic inflammatory disease, HSV2, persistence of HPV infection and cervical cancer, and false positive abnormal Pap tests [43, 44, 60]. Some authors claim it should be included in the carcinogenic agents list (increased risk of cervical and prostate cancer) [43].

T. vaginalis infections out of the genitourinary tract are very rare, but a few cases have been described, including a central nervous infection in a premature neonate, leading to death [61].

24.3.6 Diagnosis

Given the burden of complications associated with *T. vaginalis*, low threshold for testing and sensitive tests should be used (Table 24.5).

Table 24.5 Available tests for the diagnosis of *T. vaginalis*

Type of test		Sensitivity	Specificity	Notes
Wet mount microscopy		36–82%	100%	• Results in a few minutes • Easy and cheap • Low sensitivity • Exam must be performed immediately • Not useful in men
Pap test		56–76%%	>95%	• Not recommended for screening • Liquid based cytology performs better than classical cytology • Controversial if further testing is needed before treatment
Culture	Modified diamond medium InPouch (biomed diagnostics, White City, Oregon)	75–96%	>95%%	• Not easily available • Results in up to 7 days for diamond medium • Vaginal secretions preferred • In InPouch, most positive results occur within 3 days, but 17% only after that • InPouch has increased sensitivity over traditional culture mediums (?) • Useful if resistance tests are to be performed

Table 24.5 (continued)

Type of test		Sensitivity	Specificity	Notes
Immunochromatographic assays	OSOM (Sekisui, Framingham, MA)	82–95%	>95%	• Results in 10–15 min • Does not allow to test for other STIs • False positives possible • Self-testing possible (decreased sensitivity) [62]
DNA probes	Affirm VPIII (BD, Sparks, MD)	46.3–63%	>95%	• Results in <1 h • Concomitant test for *C. albicans*, *G. vaginalis* and *T. vaginalis* • Useful in settings where STIs are not prevalent • FDA approved
NAATs	AmpliVue (Quidel, San Diego, CA)	>90%	>95%	• Results in 45 min • Good agreement with PCR • False positives possible? FDA approved
	Solana (Quidel, San Diego, CA)	89.7%	>95%	• Results in >45 min • FDA approved
	Aptima *T. vaginalis* (Hologic, San Diego, CA)	>95%	>95%	• Results in <8 h • Possible cotest of CT/NG • FDA approved
	In-house real time PCR	76–98%	>95%	• Better performance if vaginal swabs are used
	XPert *T. vaginalis* (Cepheid, Sunnyvale, CA)	95% agreement with in-house PCR	100% agreement with in-house-PCR	• Results in 60 min • FDA approved
	BD ProbeTec Q^x (BD, Sparks, Maryland)	>95%	>99%	• Results in <8 h • FDA approved
	BD MAX system (BD, Sparks, Maryland)	>90%	>99%	Results in 3 h

However, that is not the reality most of the times [63]. When comparing studies, it is important to keep in mind if the gold standard used was wet mount/cultures or the much more sensitive NAATs, as these can detect even non-viable protozoans and low loads of microorganisms.

Wet mount microscopy can allow the immediate diagnosis, besides being a cheap and easy technique. However, it relies on documenting motile protozoans (https://www.youtube.com/watch?v=pTL-_Q4S1Og). The observation should be performed immediately after collection of the sample; heating slightly the slide can increase the motility of the parasite. Immotile parasites are difficult to identify, as they have approximately the same size as a leucocyte. Inflammation is not always present (Fig. 24.11), but when present it can be very exuberant. Wet mount microscopy has a rather low sensitivity (36–82%) [64–67], even if using phase contrast and with experienced examiner. The sensitivity may be even lower in asymptomatic women, thus it cannot be recommended as a screening test. However, it can be used in a "cascade" model for symptomatic women: If it is diagnostic for *T. vaginalis*, treatment can be provided immediately; if negative, further laboratory testing must be carried out. Nevertheless, it is an excellent tool to check for the commonly associated presence of BV (Fig. 24.12).

Determination of pH is not a diagnostic tool, but it can work as a triage test; in symptomatic

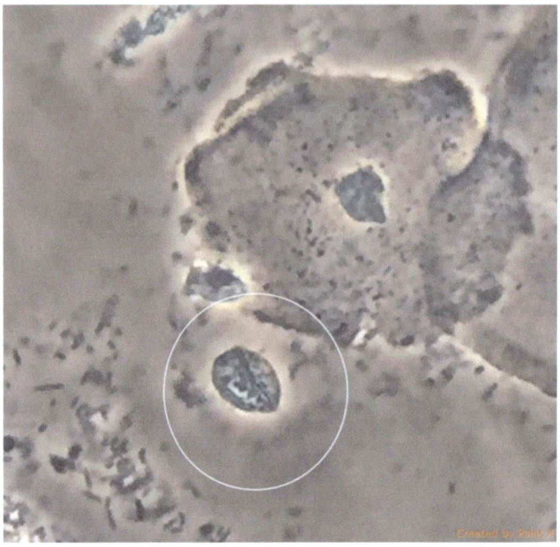

Fig. 24.11 *Trichomonas vaginalis* (inside white circle) (phase contrast, 400×)

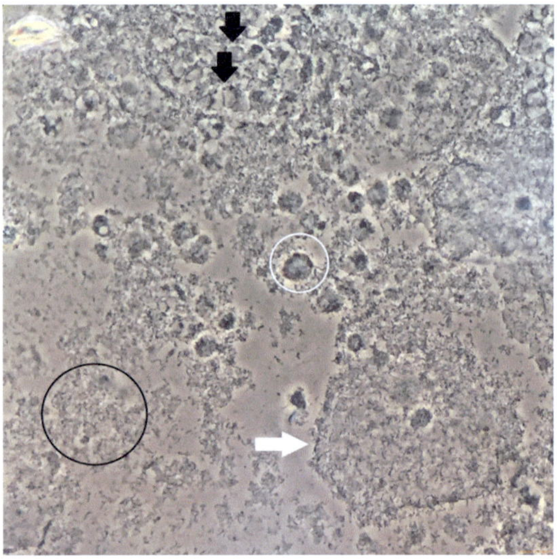

Fig. 24.12 *Trichomonas vaginalis* (white circle) and bacterial vaginosis (granular flora—black circle; clue cell—white arrow). Notice the presence of inflammation (black arrows), which is not a feature of BV (phase contrast, 400×)

trichomoniasis values are higher than 4.5 (frequently even higher than 5) [42]. The sensitivity of pH for the diagnosis of trichomoniasis is very high, but the predictive positive value is very low.

The Whiff test is frequently positive, as the coexistence *T. vaginalis* and BV is very high (60–80%). However, a negative test does not exclude the diagnosis.

The Pap test should not be performed with the objective of diagnosing trichomoniasis. It is controversial if the finding of *T. vaginalis* in a Pap test should be confirmed prior to treatment: Some defend that no further testing is needed if liquid based cytology was used (as specificity is high), while others only accept it in settings where the disease is very prevalent (>10%) [64], and others recommend systematic confirmation [10]. If the diagnosis was made in a conventional Pap test, confirmation should always be performed prior to treatment. In one study from 1972, comparing Pap test to cultures for the diagnosis of trichomoniasis, it was concluded that the former yielded high rates of false negative and false positive results, making it highly unreliable. It was assumed that the source of mistake was the rounded forms that the protozoan can assume, and that are difficult to distinguish from leukocytes [68].

Optimal tests for *T. vaginalis* in terms of sensitivity are NAATs, which can detect 3–5 times more infections than WMM [10]. These tests, however, are expensive and do not produce an immediate result—which is of utmost importance in STI clinics.

Vaginal and endocervical specimens (swabs or liquid based cytology mediums) are the best sampling options. With the use of urine samples, sensitivity drops slightly [66].

In the future, versatile platforms such as the XPert *T. vaginalis* (Cepheid, Sunnyvale, CA) [69] can gain terrain in this field: The results are rapid (60 min) and the cartridge system allows the performance of different analysis using the same platform.

Point of care tests such as OSOM (Sekisui, Framingham, MA) or Affirm VPIII (BD, Sparks, MD) may represent an intermediate option, with a good performance, but cheaper than NAAT tests and allowing faster results, without the need for complex laboratory facilities.

24.3.7 Treatment

Treatment must be considered in all cases, as even if asymptomatic; *T. vaginalis* must not be seen as a commensal. The objectives of treating all cases are: the elimination of symptoms, stopping transmission, and reducing HIV risk.

As male partners of infected women have a high rate of infection [48], simultaneous treatment of those partners without need for confirmatory testing is mandatory.

The standard recommended treatment is a single dose of 2 g of metronidazole or tinidazole. Sexual abstinence for 1 week is recommended.

Patients must be advised to avoid alcohol consumption, as a disulfiram effect is possible for up to 24 h after taking metronidazole and 72 h after tinidazole; however, this risk may be overemphasized in the literature [70]. The most common secondary effects of nitroimidazoles are gastrointestinal symptoms (nausea, vomiting, metallic taste), headache, and dizziness). These are dose dependent and, for that reason, multi-dose schemes, are better tolerated. On the other hand, the compliance is higher for single dose schemes [71].

The success rate of cure with oral metronidazole is high (>90%). Resistance, defined as a failure to eradicate the infection after two consecutive courses of treatment, is a raising problem, estimated to be of up to 5% [71]. For tinidazole it is lower (1%) [10]. Possible factors involved in resistance include: inactivation of metronidazole by vaginal bacteria, inadequate local concentration, and low zinc concentration [47]. It must be kept in mind, however, that many apparent failures of treatment are due to reinfection and non-compliance.

Zinc sulphate douches have been tried in small series, with good efficacy; however, it has been reported that it can cause cervical ulcerations [47] (Table 24.6).

Table 24.6 Treatment options for trichomoniasis

First choice	Metronidazole	• 2 g *per os*, single dose
	Tinidazole	• 2 g *per os*, single dose • Longer half-life • More expensive • Better intestinal tolerance
Alternative regimen	Metronidazole	• 500 mg 2 *id* for 7 days (similar cure rates to single dose schemes) • Better tolerance
	Metronidazole 750 mg/miconazole 200 mg	• Vaginal application 2 *id* for 7 days • Only if oral schemes not tolerated • Very limited data on efficacy (one study)
In case of allergy to nitroimidazoles	Desensitization	
Pregnancy	Metronidazole	• 2 g *per os*, single dose (avoid higher doses in pregnancy) • Consider multiple dose scheme if single dose not tolerated [71] • Treat all symptomatic cases • If asymptomatic, consider treatment only in the first trimester or after 37 weeks of gestation
	(Tinidazole)	• Avoid in the first trimester • Use in the second or third trimester only if no better options available
Breastfeeding women	Metronidazole	• 2 g *per os*, single dose (discard milk for 12–24 h) • 500 mg 2 *id per os* 7 days • 400 mg 3 *id per os* 7 days
	(Tinidazole)	• Avoid • 2 g *per os*, single dose (discard milk for 72 h)
HIV patients	Metronidazole	• 500 mg 2 id for 7 days

(continued)

Table 24.6 (continued)

Alternative treatments in resistant cases (always consider non-compliance or reinfection)	Metronidazole	• 800 mg 3 id for 5–7 days • 2 g *id* for 5–7 days ± intravaginal tinidazole
	Tinidazole	• 2 g *id per os* for 5–7 days • 2–3 g *id per os* for 14 days (same for partners)
	Options needing further studies: • Zinc sulphate 1% (± oral tinidazole) douches • Pessaries (paromomycin/furazolidone/6% non-oxynol-9) • Boric acid (vaginal) • Disulfiram • Nithiamide • Albendazole + nitroimidazole • Coenzyme B12 + nitroimidazole	

The rate of clinical cure can be improved by using sensitivity tests and tailoring the treatment according to it (higher doses of metronidazole or changing to tinidazole).

Topical metronidazole is not recommended for treatment, as it is associated with very low rates of cure (<50%), probably due to the fact that only insufficient concentrations are achieved in the urethra and periurethral glands, which can act as reservoirs of the parasite. However, higher doses of vaginal metronidazole (750 mg), combined with miconazole can lead to cure rates comparable to oral metronidazole [72].

It is still uncertain which is the impact of the coexistence of BV and *T. vaginalis* on the results of treatment, despite that both situations usually respond to nitroimidazole therapy [7].

Treatment during pregnancy, in one study increased the risk of preterm delivery three times (RR 3.0; 95% confidence interval, 1.5–5.9) but this is still controversial and not confirmed in other studies [73, 74]. One of the theories sustains that the exposition of *T. vaginalis* infected with *M. hominis* to antibiotics leads to a massive release of the latter. These, once released, can infect the membranes and the amniotic fluid, thus initiating a preterm labour [73]. Treatment, however, reduces the risk of transmission to the newborn and decreases the risk of HIV infection. One reasonable option is treating all cases in the first trimester (to reduce HIV risk), the symptomatic cases at any time, and the asymptomatic ones after 37 weeks of gestational age (to reduce the risk of transmission, without increasing that of preterm labour) [53].

Women who test positive for *T. vaginalis* during pregnancy should be counselled to consistently use condoms, besides the adequate treatment of all sexual partners.

A test of cure can be performed 2–3 weeks after the treatment; prior to that, NAATs can be positive due to the presence of non-viable organisms. In pregnant women, given that *T. vaginalis* is a risk factor for HIV, the CDC recommends retesting after 3 months. In HIV women, retesting is also recommended [10].

24.4 Dysbiosis

Vaginal Lactobacilli: Breaking the Myths

- Bacterial vaginosis is not the only cause for absent lactobacilli in non-hypoestrogenic women. Aerobic vaginitis is another cause, which is much less recognized
- Despite the important role of Lactobacilli in vaginal health, they are absent in nearly one third of asymptomatic women

Vaginal dysbiosis refers to the conditions in which there is a flora disturbance or imbalance, characterized by a severe depletion or even absence of lactobacilli [75]. Traditionally, it has been assumed that BV is "the" cause for absent lactobacilli in non-hypoestrogenic women. However, clinical practice, especially with the use of WMM, has shown that it is not necessarily true. An increased pH (a marker of lactobacilli depletion and, thus, dysbiosis) is found not only in BV, but also in conditions in which aerobic, rather than anaerobic, bacteria predominate. Besides the overgrowth of aerobic bacteria, these women usually also have atrophy and inflammation (which are not part of BV) [76]. This entity was named aerobic vaginitis (AV) by Donders et al. in 2002 [77].

The non-recognition of AV may have led to serious drawbacks in clinical investigation, namely in the areas of preterm labour, sexually transmitted infections, and cervical dysplasia [78].

The concept of the essential role of the dominance of lactobacilli in the vaginal flora during reproductive age has been challenged, as it has been shown that it does not happen in nearly one third of asymptomatic women [79]. This is the rule in other species of mammals, in which lactobacilli represent only 1% of the vaginal microbiota, while one similar to that associated with BV dominates (*Gardnerella*, *Mobiluncus*, *Sneathia*, and *Prevotella*). Bacteriocins are not of exclusive production by lactobacilli; other bacteria such as *Streptococcus*, *Prevotella*, and *Corynebacterium* may fulfil that function [80].

24.4.1 Bacterial Vaginosis

Some authors have suggested that the condition should be named anaerobic vaginosis, rather than bacterial, as it overemphasizes a mere bacterial aetiology [81].

Bacterial Vaginosis (BV): Breaking the Myths

- BV may go unnoticed—it is asymptomatic in 50–85% of the cases
- BV is a sexually associated condition but not an STI, as no disease has been identified in the male partners, the condition cannot be attributed to a single microorganism, and treatment of the partner does not prevent recurrences in women.

24.4.1.1 Aetiology and Pathophysiology

BV is a polymicrobial syndrome, characterized by the absence of lactobacilli and overgrowth of a variable mixture of predominantly anaerobic and facultative bacteria, which in low loads are part of the normal vaginal flora. These can include *G. vaginalis, Atopobium vaginalis, Mobiluncus, Prevotella, Megasphaera, Leptotrichia, Sneathia, Bifidobacterium, Dialister, Peptostreptococcus, Fusobacterium, Clostridium,* non-cultivable "BV-associated bacteria" (BVAB) 1–3, and *M. hominis*, among others, in loads 100–1000 times higher than the normal. Identifiable modifications in the microbiota precede the development of BV by weeks or months [82].

Given that these bacteria are sensitive to lactic acid and hydrogen peroxide, the initial step for the development of BV is likely to be the reduction or disappearance of lactobacilli. Several endogenous and exogenous factors, including phages and some *Mollicutes*, can be responsible for this [81, 83].

According to the model proposed by Nasioudis et al., it all starts with a transitory state of diminished lactobacillary dominance. During this stage, if the disturbing factor is enough to prevent the recovery of the lactobacilli or gives advantage to other bacteria in the competition for glycogen, a biofilm starts to be produced. The biofilm further deprives lactobacilli from having access to manganese, inhibiting their recovery, and allows the eviction of the already depressed innate immune system defences (low levels of H_2O_2 and lactic acid) [58, 84]. Additionally, the production of sialidase leads to the degradation of IgA, impairing the acquired immune system response. The immunological response is typically absent or scarce [58, 84].

24.4.1.2 Prevalence and Epidemiology

BV is the most common cause of symptomatic vulvovaginal discharge in childbearing age women, accounting for nearly half of the cases. It is rarely encountered in children and becomes less common during menopause. Prevalence is lower during pregnancy [85].

As BV is asymptomatic in 50–85% of the cases, when comparing epidemiological data, it must be checked whether it refers to microbiological or clinical (symptomatic) disease and how the diagnosis was established.

Global prevalence (symptomatic and asymptomatic) varies widely according to the population studied (12–55%), being consistently higher in black women (50–55%) [86, 87]. BV is much rarer in non-sexually experienced women, especially in those without any kind of sexual contact [88], but is very high (20–50%) in women with female partners [89].

24.4.1.3 Risk Factors and Associations

BV is a sexually associated condition (Table 24.7). It cannot be considered an STI, as no disease has been identified in the male partners, the condition cannot be attributed to a single microorganism, and treatment of the partner does not prevent recurrences in women. However, there is a growing evidence that BVAB can be exchanged during intercourse, and it has been isolated from the penis, seminal fluid, and even urine of male partners of women with BV. The bladder may act as a reservoir for recurrences [90]. Circumcision can decrease the load of BVAB and, consequently the risk of BV in partners [91].

Table 24.7 Risk factors and associations for BV

Demographic factors	• Lower educational level • Poverty • Black race • Childbearing age
Sexual factors	• New partner(s) • Multiple partner(s) • Higher number of lifetime sexual partners • Having female partner(s) • Receptive oral sex • Anal sex • Higher frequency of intercourse • Early sexual debut • Unprotected sex • Sharing sex toys
Behavioural factor	• Smoking • Vaginal douching • IUD • Not using oral contraceptives • Having an STI (HIV, HSV2, *C. trachomatis*, *M. genitalium*) • Uncircumcised partner • Antibiotic use • Stress • Dietary factors (increased fat, low calcium, folate, and vitamin A)

While women usually do not consider it an STI themselves, they can link sexual activity to the development or recurrence of symptoms [92].

Phages can be the "missing link" between BV and its association with sexual activity: hypothetically, a partner may transmit it, leading to the depletion of lactobacilli [81]. Interestingly, phages are promoted by smoking, which is also a risk factor for BV, by direct toxicity to lactobacilli, and by inducing hormonal changes [93].

While *L. crispatus* is associated with a lower risk for BV, *L. iners* can be identified during dysbiosis. It is uncertain whether it predisposes to dysbiosis or is part of the recovery process [82, 94]. Interestingly, female couples share lactobacilli strains [95].

Progesterone seems to play a protective role, as the rates of BV are lower and the cure rates higher during pregnancy, and less cases are detected during the luteal phase [96].

24.4.1.4 Signs and Symptoms

More than half of the women with BV type flora are asymptomatic. If not, symptoms tend to be mild, fluctuating and sometimes with a longstanding duration (weeks or months).

The most common symptom is an offensive fishy smell, which typically worsens with menses and sexual intercourse, as the release of volatile amines (putrescine and cadaverine) is increased in elevated pH. Sometimes women tend to wash more frequently or to use perfumed products, which paradoxically further worsen the smell.

The discharge associated with BV is yellow or grey, homogeneous, thin, and adherent to the vaginal walls (Fig. 24.13a). Mild burning or dysuria are sometimes described, but are not typical features of BV.

The vulvar and vaginal exam, apart from the presence of discharge, are usually unremarkable (Fig. 24.13b).

BV can be considered recurrent if a woman has 3 or more episodes during 1 year.

24.4.1.5 Complications

The risk of complications is independent of whether or not a woman is symptomatic.

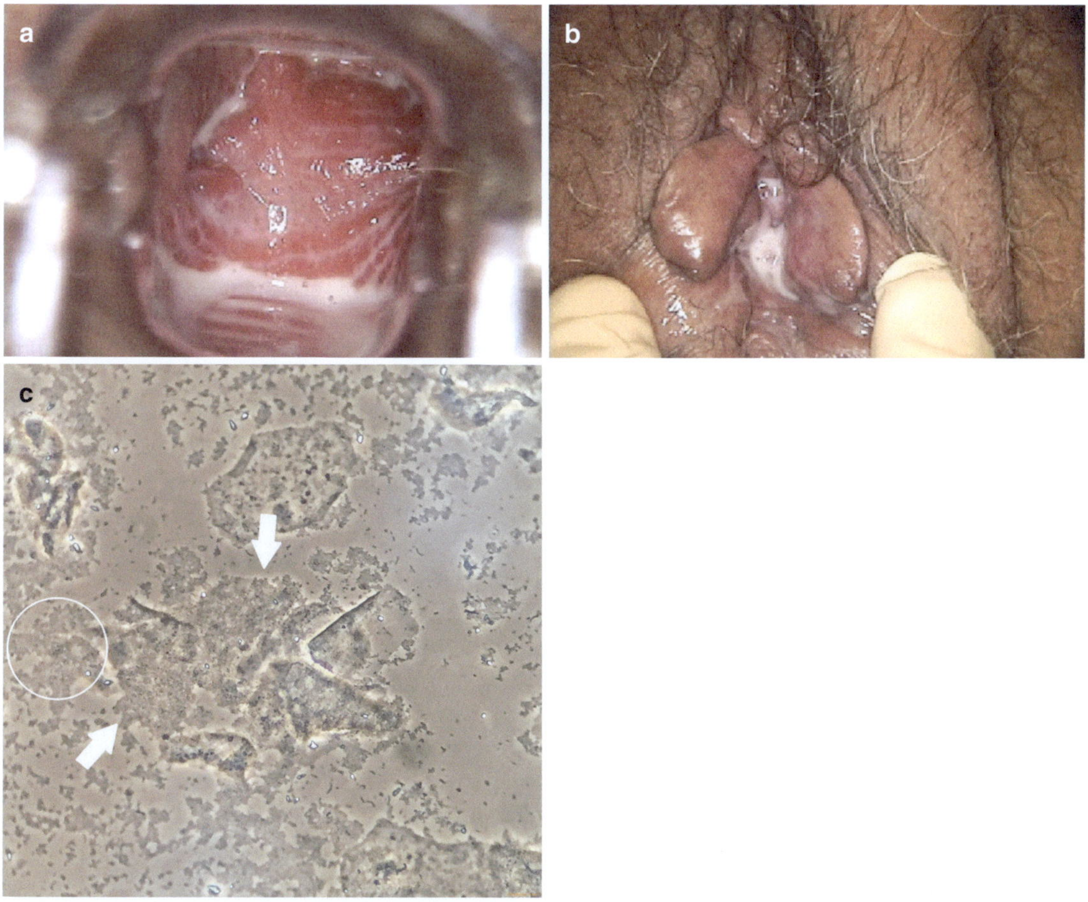

Fig. 24.13 (**a**) Homogenous vaginal discharge in a woman with bacterial vaginosis. (**b**) At the vulva, the homogenous vaginal discharge can be easily detected in women with bacterial vaginosis. (**c**) Bacterial vaginosis with all typical features: no lactobacilli, granular floor (white circle) and clue cells (white arrows) (phase contrast, 400×)

Most studies failed to distinguish BV from AV, as the diagnosis was frequently based on an increased pH and/or absence of lactobacilli. This can explain different results between studies and why, for instance, treatment failed to reduce the risk of preterm labour in women with the diagnosis of BV. The listed complications most likely represent those of abnormal vaginal flora or dysbiosis, rather than just of BV.

BV was first associated with adverse pregnancy outcomes in 1984, namely with preterm labour. Following that, other obstetrical and neonatal complications were added to the list: spontaneous abortion, low birth weight and increased neonatal morbidity [97].

Pelvic inflammatory disease, post-hysterectomy cuff infection and post C-section endometritis are also more common in women with BV. Interestingly, there are theories sustaining that one of the roles of vaginal lactobacilli may be the reduction of the infectious risks related to pregnancy and delivery [80].

The risk of acquiring an STI, including *C. trachomatis, N. gonorrhoea*, HSV2 and HIV infection, is double in women with BV [98]. *U. urealyticum*, *U. parvum* and *M. hominis*, but not *M. genitalium*, are frequently found associated with BV [99].

Additionally, it increases the risk of transmission of HIV to male partners [100]. Several studies link BV to HPV persistence, cervical dysplasia and cancer.

More recently, there is increasing data relating BV with infertility and lower success rates of assisted reproduction techniques [101].

24.4.1.6 Diagnosis

BV should not be screened in asymptomatic women; it can be considered, but without enough evidence to recommend it, in pregnant women, prior to pelvic surgery or uterine cavity instrumentation, or in those with STIs, especially HIV.

Clinical Diagnosis

Clinical criteria allow the diagnosis of BV in settings of limited resources or expertise. To fulfil the Amsel criteria [102], 3 out of the following 4 must be fulfilled:

1. Homogeneous grey or white discharge coating the vaginal walls (Fig. 24.13a, b);
2. Vaginal pH increased (>4.5);
3. Fishy smell (before or after 10% KOH addition—Whiff test);
4. Clue cells on wet mount (cells with a heavy coating of bacteria, leading to blurring of the peripheral borders; must be present in >20% of cells) (Fig. 24.13c).

The sensitivity and specificity of the Amsel criteria is around 80 and 90%, respectively. The first three criteria are also frequently positive in women with trichomoniasis. The combination of only pH and Whiff test may perform better than the traditional criteria [103]. However, odour is too subjective to base a diagnosis on; in the future, it may be overcome by the use of "electronic noses" [104].

In our opinion, in settings where a microscope is available, it should be used for the proper diagnosis of BV by WMM, rather than just for the mere evaluation of the presence of clue cells.

pH

The pH based point of care tests available for self-testing have a sensitivity and specificity of 73% and 67%, respectively [105].

The VI-SENSE is a pH test, based on a strip placed in a panty liner; clinical trials showed good performance for BV or trichomoniasis, but not allowing distinction between both conditions [106].

Microscopy

In WMM, BV is characterized by absent lactobacilli, granular flora or abundant motile small, curved, rod shaped bacteria (*Mobiluncus*), absence of inflammation, and presence of clue cells (Fig. 24.13c).

WMM has several advantages relatively to Gram staining based Nugent score: (1) it is cheaper, (2) allows the diagnosis during the appointment, (3) requires less expertise, (4) allows the distinction of full-blown from partial BV (in which in the same slide areas of granular flora can coexist with areas with lactobacilli, and frequently clue cells represent <20% of the total number of epithelial cells) and the overcome of the problem of "intermediate scores" from Nugent score, and (5) the evaluation of the bacteria may be more accurate, since there is no fixation and washing of the slides.

The Nugent score, an improvement from the Spiegel score, was described in 1991 [107], and is considered the gold standard for the diagnosis of BV. It is based on the proportion of bacterial morphotypes, using Gram staining:

- Lactobacilli (large Gram-positive rods)—0 to 4 points (higher scores if less abundant);
- *G. vaginalis* and bacteroides (small Gram variable rods)—0 to 4 points (higher scores if more abundant;
- *Mobiluncus*-like morphotypes (curved Gram negative rods)—0 to 2 points (higher scores if more abundant);
- (Gram-positive cocci are not considered in this scoring system).

The diagnosis of BV is established if the final score is equal or higher than seven. If it is equal or lower than three, it is considered normal. A score between 4 and 6 is the troublesome "intermediate score". It does not correspond to partial BV; part of the cases classified in this grey area, which usually do not respond to metronidazole treatment, may represent AV. For this reason, Donders proposed that "undetermined flora" would be a more accurate description [108].

The Hay and Ison criteria [109], also based on Gram staining may allow a more complete and realistic evaluation of the vaginal flora:

- Grade 0—epithelial cells with no bacteria seen;
- Grade I—lactobacillus morphotypes only (normal flora);
- Grade II—reduced lactobacillus morphotypes with mixed bacterial morphotypes (intermediate flora);
- Grade III—mixed bacterial morphotypes with few or absent lactobacillus morphotypes (BV);
- Grade IV—epithelial cells covered with Gram-positive cocci only (AV type flora).

Cultures

G. vaginalis can be cultivated from the large majority of women with BV, but also from more than half of the women without it [110]. This translates into a high sensitivity, but a low positive predictive value and thus should not be used.

Pap Test

The Pap test is not intended for the diagnosis of vaginitis. The sensitivity for BV is low, and likely to be even lower when using liquid based cytology, due to centrifugation and filtering of the sample.

Enzymatic Tests

The OSOM BVBlue is a point of care test, based on the chromogenic determination of the presence of sialidase, which is produced by bacteria commonly involved in BV (*Gardnerella, Prevotella* and *Bacteroides*). The results are available within 10 min. The sensitivity of the test is variable (38–100%), while the specificity is systematically high (>90%) [111]. In AV, sialidase is also increased and it may explain part of the differences in sensitivity across studies.

Tests to evaluate the activity of proline aminopeptidase have also been designed, giving the results in 10 min. Sensitivity and specificity are higher than 90% [112]. It has also been evaluated in combination with pH and amines determination (FemExam).

Molecular Tests

The use of DNA tests in BV is very complex, as it is polymicrobial and most of the involved agents commonly colonize the vagina of healthy women in low loads. These techniques are usually highly sensitive, but with low predictive positive values. In the future, combinations of evaluation of the proportion of selected anaerobic bacteria and lactobacilli may increase the specificity of this methodology [113].

Nevertheless, the Affirm VPIII, which tests not only BV, but also *T. vaginalis* and *Candida*, has been shown to be a good alternative in settings where a microscope is not available [25, 26].

24.4.1.7 Treatment

BV can heal spontaneously [53]. Treatment aims at resolving the symptoms associated with BV; there is no indication to treat asymptomatic women. It can, however, be considered in high-risk populations for STIs, as it can reduce the risk of acquiring HIV, *T. vaginalis*, *C. trachomatis, N. gonorrhoea* and HSV2, and before pelvic surgery.

Therapeutic options for BV include oral and topical antibiotics (metronidazole, tinidazole and clindamycin), and antiseptics (dequalinium chloride) (Table 24.8). The rates of cure are high for all drugs and routes (around 80%), but relapses are common [10, 114].

The vaginal levels achieved with topical medication can be 30 times higher than those achieved with oral medication. This translates into cure rates equal or slightly higher than those achieved with the oral route, with the advantage of having less adverse effects. Combinations of oral and vaginal treatment can increase the cure rates [115].

Despite the perceived increased resistance to metronidazole and clindamycin, it does not seem yet to be a major clinical issue [85, 116]. Some *Gardnerella* strains have been shown to be intrinsically resistant to metronidazole [117]. Several of the bacteria involved in BV cannot be cultivated, thus making it impossible to test its susceptibility profiles.

The cure rates achieved with the antiseptic dequalinium chloride are non-inferior to those of clindamycin [116]. It has the advantages of being less toxic for lactobacilli, and not increasing the risk of VVC, contrarily to antibiotics [118].

Table 24.8 Treatment of BV

First line	Metronidazole tablets	500 mg *per os* 2 *id* 7 days
	Metronidazole gel 0.75%	5 g *id* intravaginally 5 days
	Clindamycin cream 2%	5 g *id* intravaginally 7 days
	Dequalinium chloride	10 mg tablets *id* intravaginally 6 days
Second line	Tinidazole	2 g *id* 2 days
	Tinidazole	1 g *id* 5 days
	Clindamycin	300 mg *per os* 2 *id* 7 days
	Clindamycin	100 mg vaginal ovules *id* for 3 days
Alternatives	Secnidazole	2 g *per os*, single dose
	Polyhexamethylene biguanide hydrochloride	1–2 *id* for 7 days
	Chlorhexidine	Vaginal douche once a day
	Rifaximin	25–100 mg *id* intravaginally
Recurrent BV	Metronidazole 0.75% gel	2 times/week for 4–6 months
	Triple phase regimen: Oral nitroimidazole, vaginal boric acid, and vaginal metronidazole	• Oral nitroimidazole for 7 days • Vaginal boric acid for 3 weeks • Vaginal metronidazole gel twice a week for 16 weeks
	Metronidazole 2 g + fluconazole 150 mg	Once a month
	Ascorbic acid	250 mg vaginal tablets *id* 6 days/month for 6 months

Additionally, it is not expected that bacteria develop resistance to it and can have some effect in other causes of "vaginitis" other than BV, thus making it at least partially useful for mixed infections, including AV, VVC and trichomoniasis [116]. However, long-term studies concerning recurrences are still lacking.

Women must be warned about the possible interaction between alcohol and nitroimidazoles. Clindamycin is associated with pseudomembranous colitis, and topical formulations may weaken latex condoms.

The use of H_2O_2 irrigations has resulted in contradictory results, but it seems to be less effective than metronidazole, and associated with a risk of development of severe lesions in the vaginal mucosa, due to its caustic effects [119].

The use of acidifying agents, though tempting, has not proven to be efficacious. Only the use of ascorbic acid has some clinical support [120].

There is no evidence that the use of probiotics in acute episodes, isolated or concomitantly with antibiotics improves the rate of success [121].

Pregnancy

Treatment of BV during pregnancy with metronidazole failed to decrease the risk of preterm labour and, in some studies, even lead to an increase. On the contrary, in most series in which clindamycin was used showed a decrease in the rate of preterm labour [122–124]. Difference in terms of outcomes may be related to the antibiotics spectrum: clindamycin covers Gram-positive bacteria, frequently involved in AV. New studies with a more accurate classification of the vaginal flora may settle the question in the near future.

While treatment of symptomatic women during pregnancy is recommended, the available data does not allow the recommendation of screening and treating asymptomatic cases.

All first line schemes recommended for non-pregnant women can safely be used during all trimesters of pregnancy. There was some concern about the use of clindamycin during the second half of pregnancy, but it has been shown that there is no reason for that [10, 53, 125].

Recurrent BV

Antibiotic treatment is usually effective, but relapses are common, estimated at 50–70% at 6–12 months [126]. There is contradictory data associating *A. vaginae* and specific strains of *G. vaginalis* with failure of treatment and recurrences [85, 127, 128]. Bacterial strains that produce more sialidase have a higher potential of developing a biofilm and adhering to epithelial cells [129].

Higher loads of bacteria also seem to correlate with an increased risk of recurrence [130].

Recurrent episodes can be managed by using a different antibiotic/antiseptic from the previous episode, for a longer duration. The use of repeated options in the subsequent episodes is an acceptable approach [131].

Some patients will opt for a suppressive treatment. The use of metronidazole 0.75% gel twice a week for 4–6 months is one of the most commonly used regimens, with an efficacy of 70%. However, the rate of relapse severely increases once it is stopped and VVC is not uncommon during treatment (43.1%) [132]. A regimen in which 2 g of oral metronidazole and 150 mg of oral fluconazole monthly was used, in HIV1 women showed to be effective, and the risk of VVC was lower than in the placebo arm [133].

There is no advantage in the treatment of male partners, however this recommendation is not based on good quality studies [10, 134]. If the phages theory proves to be correct, the male treatment will not be effective indeed.

Using oral contraceptives continuously for 3 months is a strategy that can be tried; it may work both by reducing the levels of oestrogens and by eliminating the exposure to blood [85].

A triple sequential scheme, including oral metronidazole or tinidazole, vaginal boric acid, and vaginal metronidazole, has shown a cure rate of 65% at 28 weeks, but it has a failure rate of 50% at 36 weeks [135].

Recurrences/treatment failures seem to be associated with inability to eradicate the biofilm. Boric acid is one of the agents capable of destroying it; other options may include tobramycin, DNases, octenidine, and retrocyclin, among others [98].

The concept of using probiotics to restore the vaginal health is intuitive and appealing, however the studies have not supported its use. It does not seem to affect the cure rate, but may increase the time to recurrence in 50% [136, 137]. Failure to improve the vaginal flora with probiotics may be due to the use of inadequate species (the ones commercially available usually are not dominant ones in healthy women) and/or inability to colonize the vagina.

There is no data supporting the use of acidifiers of the vagina for the purpose of avoiding recurrences [138].

Future options may include oral or vaginal lactoferrin, which can act by immunomodulation, disruption of the cell membranes, and by binding to iron and thus making it unavailable for bacteria (without affecting lactobacilli, which rely on manganese for their metabolism) [126].

24.4.2 Aerobic Vaginitis, Desquamative Inflammatory Vaginitis, GBS Vaginitis

Aerobic Vaginitis: Breaking the Myth

- Group B streptococcus (GBS) infection and desquamative inflammatory vaginitis (DIV) are not separate entities. They are a part of aerobic vaginitis (AV).

In 2002, Donders et al. named a condition characterized by lack of lactobacilli, presence of aerobic (enteric) bacteria, and atrophy as aerobic vaginitis, thus stressing the main differences between this entity and its anaerobic, non-inflammatory, counterpart: BV [77]. Its most severe forms of presentation correspond to the desquamative inflammatory vaginitis (DIV), described by Gardner in 1968 [139] (probably the same as Scheffey's "exudative vaginitis" [140]). While DIV is an extreme form of the disease, AV shows the full spectrum of the disease [141].

Group B streptococcus (GBS) vaginitis is also included in the spectrum of AV. GBS is today considered one of the agents commonly found in women with AV.

Even though it is more and more recognized as a nosologic entity, unfortunately it still is not the rule. Failure to recognize it may be a missed opportunity to help women with otherwise "untreatable" or "unspecific" vaginitis, and to diminish the associated gynaecological and obstetrical risks associated with it.

As we consider these entities as subtypes of AV, AV will be used to discuss it as a whole.

24.4.2.1 Aetiology

The aetiology of AV remains unknown. Although the isolation of bacteria other than lactobacilli is one of the features of AV, it cannot be assumed straightforward that AV is an infection—its presence may be secondary to the abnormal local conditions. The most commonly isolated bacteria are *Streptococcus* spp., *S. aureus*, coagulase negative staphylococci, *E. coli* and *E. faecalis* [142].

The lack of lactobacilli, namely the H_2O_2 producing strains which are capable of reducing the levels of IL-1β [143] can, partially, explain the inflammatory response found in AV.

Host immunity factors can also be involved, as not only the levels of IL-1β are increased (higher than in women with BV), but also those of IL-6 and -8 (while in BV they are within normal range) [144, 145]. Sialidase, which leads to diminished local immunity by ultimately causing IgA proteolysis, is increased in both AV and BV [144].

The presence of intermediate or even parabasal cells suggests a role for hypoestrogenism. However, it must be a local phenomenon, given that it can be seen in women without further evidence of low oestrogens, and systemic treatment is ineffective.

Other theories include that AV/DIV might be localized forms of lichen planus, or that it is a consequence of low levels of vitamin D [142].

24.4.2.2 Prevalence and Epidemiology

Data concerning the epidemiology of AV is still scarce, however we are starting to see the broad picture. Comparing data on prevalence is not easy, as studies considered different grades of AV, some looked only into symptomatic women, and others considered only pregnant women.

In Europe, the prevalence rate of moderate or severe AV (msAV) seems to range between 7.4 and 12.0%, while it seems to be less common in South America (2.0–2.9%), and more common in Africa (11.0–25.8%) [142]. The prevalence is systematically lower in pregnant women (4.0–8.0%) [57], and in one study it has been shown to be very high in a cohort of 123 HIV positive women (26.8% with msAV and 20.4% with light forms) [146].

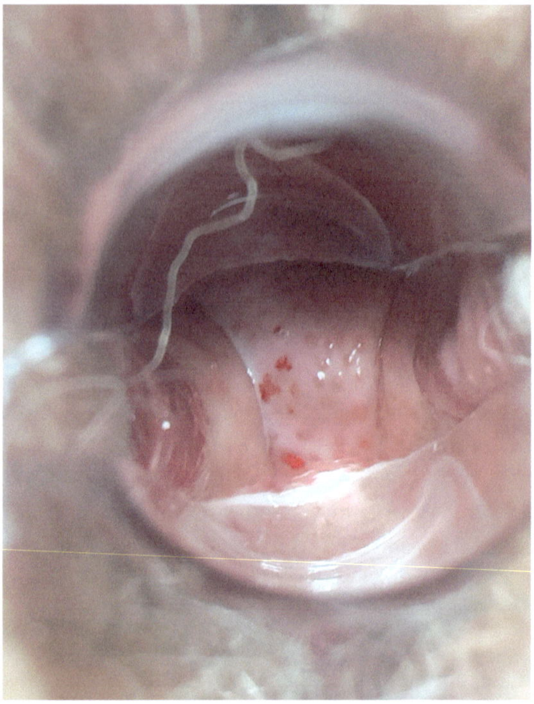

Fig. 24.14 Erosions of the vaginal walls in a patient with severe aerobic vaginosis

It can be found in women of all ages (not studied in children), but there seems to exist a peak in the peri-menopausal period.

24.4.2.3 Risk Factors and Associations

Up to the moment, the studies concerning risk factors and associations with AV are very limited. One Chinese study associated AV with being unmarried, using an IUD, long-term use of antibiotics, and vaginal douching; on the contrary, higher education and systematic use of condoms were protective [147]. The latter was not confirmed in a European study [78].

24.4.2.4 Signs and Symptoms

AV can range from asymptomatic to highly symptomatic. Symptoms can include yellowish or yellow-green vaginal purulent discharge (in 20% with a rotten smell—different from the fishy one typical of BV), dyspareunia, burning and stinging. The vagina and the vestibule can be reddish and with erosions (Fig. 24.14) [57, 77]. Symptoms can be present for months with variable intensity [142].

24.4.2.5 Complications

The number of studies linking AV with severe gynaecological and obstetrical complications has been growing the last years [142].

Among gynaecological complications, there are studies relating it to an increased risk of having an abnormal Pap test and of acquiring STIs. The presence of inflammation and erosions, the lack of lactobacilli, and the associated increased levels of sialidase can easily explain the increased risk for STIs; diagnosing and treating AV can be highly relevant in populations at elevated risk, namely in Africa [87, 118].

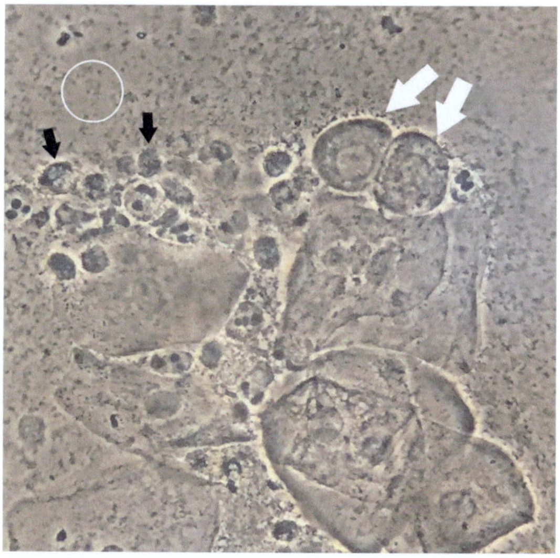

Fig. 24.15 Severe aerobic vaginosis/desquamative inflammatory vaginitis: absent lactobacilli, basal/parabasal cells (white arrows), cocci (white circle), and inflammation (black arrows) (phase contrast 400×)

In terms of obstetrics, it can be the explanation for the contradictory results found when relating flora changes to preterm labour. It has also been linked to premature rupture of membranes, chorioamnionitis and even neonatal sepsis.

The interleukin profile associated with these complications, as well as that associated with cervical intraepithelial neoplasia and cervical cancer are near perfect matches with that of AV [78, 142, 148].

24.4.2.6 Diagnosis

The diagnosis of AV is made with the aid of a microscope, ideally with phase contrast (Fig. 24.15). A composite score must be calculated, including: (1) relative quantity of lactobacilli; (2) presence of inflammation; (3) relative quantity of toxic leucocytes (active, swollen leucocytes); (4) presence of other bacteria and (5) proportion of parabasal cells (Table 24.9). WMM is a better tool than Gram staining, as the former allows a more precise evaluation of the lactobacillary grades.

Cultures are not useful, as it is not informative of the relative proportion of lactobacilli and other bacteria and colonization is common [113].

The pH is usually increased, in a more pronounced way than in BV [149].

Rumyantseva et al. have shown that molecular diagnosis, using real time PCR is feasible and, in the future, can be an option in settings where health care professionals are not trained to perform microscopy [113]. Enzymatic test has already been developed, but validation is still needed [150].

Table 24.9 AV score

Score	Lactobacillary grade	Inflammation (leucocytes)	Toxic leucocytes	Presence of other bacteria	Proportion of parabasal cells
0	I or IIa	≤10 per HPF	Absent	Unremarkable or cytolysis	<1%
1	IIb	>10 per HPFand ≤10 per cell	≤50%	Small coliform bacilli	1–10%
2	III	>10 per cell	>50%	Cocci or chains of cocci	>10%

Score <3—no AV; score 3 to 4—light AV; score 5 to 6—moderate AV; score >6—severe AV. Lactobacillary grades: I—only numerous pleomorphic lactobacilli; IIa—dominance of lactobacilli, but other bacteria present; IIb—dominance of other bacteria, but still some lactobacilli present; III—lactobacilli absent or severely depressed and dominance of other bacteria. Use 400× magnification. *HPF* high power field. Adapted from Donders et al. [145]

Table 24.10 Treatment of Aerobic Vaginosis. Donders et al. [142]

Antiseptics	Dequalinium chloride	*id* for 6 days
	Iodopovidone	(Transient effect, low impact on lactobacilli, washing effect?)
	Chlorhexidine	
Topical antibiotics	Clindamycin cream 2%	*id* for 2 weeks
	Rifaximin 25–100 mg	*id* for 6 days
Systemic antibiotics	Moxifloxacin 400 mg	*id* for 6 days (repeat if absence of microscopic cure)
Topical steroids	Hydrocortisone cream 10%	3–5 times/week (vaginal) advisable to concomitantly use antifungals?
Topical oestrogens	Estriol Estradiol	According to usual schemes
Probiotics	*L. acidophilus* + estriol 30 μg	*id* for 6–12 days
Other	Nifuratel 500 mg	*id* 10 days (topical or oral)

24.4.2.7 Treatment

Treatment of AV is not yet standardized and further studies are needed in this specific field. The treatment is guided by the microscopy findings: It must be attempted to correct the atrophy (topical oestrogens), the inflammation (topical steroids) and the presence of bacteria (antiseptics, topical and antibiotic antiseptics). In one study, probiotics have shown to increase the time to recurrence [136] (Table 24.10).

If antibiotics are chosen, preference should be given to topical formulations, to those active against Gram negative bacilli and Gram-positive cocci, and as innocuous as possible to lactobacilli. The use of the antiseptic dequalinium chloride was less associated with *Candida* at the end of the treatment, when compared to antibiotics [118].

24.5 Cytolytic Vaginosis, Lactobacillosis and "Leptothrix"

Cytolytic Vaginosis: Breaking the Myths

- Lactobacilli are not always protective—Increase in lactobacilli may cause cytolytic vaginosis, a special form of sometimes symptomatic vaginal discharge
- Cytolytic vaginosis symptoms closely mimic those of vulvovaginal candidiasis

The dominance of the vaginal milieu by lactobacilli species and the consequent low pH is unique to the human species. Its main goal seems to be the protection against sexually transmitted infections (STIs) and, ultimately, the consequences of it in the offspring. In evolutionary terms, it may have happened as a consequence of the continuous ovarian cycle (and, consequently, an increased risk of exposure to STIs, when compared to other species) or due to the high consumption of starch, which occurred after the agricultural revolution [80, 151]. Other authors have highlighted the need for a protective environment during delivery, as due to the disproportion between the head and the pelvis, the likelihood of vaginal wall lacerations is higher than in other species. However, this unique situation can turn against the host [80].

Higher levels of oestrogens, as seen just before ovulation, are directly linked to the lactobacilli abundance, lower vaginal pH, thickening of the vaginal epithelium, and increased production of glycogen [80].

For still unknown reasons, sometimes the lactobacilli can be a cause of cytolysis (cytolytic vaginosis [CV]), can be increased in number (lactobacillosis), or longer than normal (previously denominated "leptothrix"). These are controversial entities, and it is still unknown whether or not they are part of the same spectrum. Some authors consider lactobacillosis and "leptothrix" as one single entity.

These are not infectious causes of "vaginitis", but are important differential diagnosis of VVC, which are commonly found in women with suspected "resistant" or recurrent candidiasis.

24.5.1 Cytolytic Vaginosis

24.5.1.1 Aetiology

It has not been fully understood what leads to the overgrowth of lactobacilli in some women or why does it lead to the destruction of the intermediate cells of the vaginal epithelium. It is highly likely that hormones play a role in the development of CV, as it is more common—or more symptomatic, during the luteal phase, pregnancy or perimenopause [152].

The cytolysis may be the consequence of the very low pH, due to the increased degradation of glycogen by the large number of lactobacilli.

Lactobacilli, except for *L. iners,* produce both L- and D-lactic acid (*L. iners* produces only the L-isomer); vaginal cells produce only the L-isomer. An imbalance in the local ratio between the two isomers, in favour of the L-isomer, can be involved in the development of VC, by altering the expression of the extracellular matrix metalloproteinase inducer [153].

Most women with symptomatic CV were previously treated with repeated courses of antifungals, which lead some authors to try to establish an association. However, this association is more likely to be due to the fact that they were previously misdiagnosed as *Candida* and thus treated as so.

24.5.1.2 Prevalence and Epidemiology

The prevalence of CV in asymptomatic women ranges between 1 and 7%, peaking during the reproductive years [152]. Despite the now acknowledged racial differences in terms of vaginal microbiome composition, it is not known if it has any impact in the prevalence of CV.

24.5.1.3 Risk Factors and Associations

One study suggested that less sexually active women were more likely to have CV, but it can be biased, as the comparison group was with sexual workers [154]. It has been suggested, also in one isolated study, that women with CV are less likely to have an abnormal Pap test, but we could not confirm it [155].

24.5.1.4 Signs and Symptoms

VC mimics the symptoms of VVC; almost all patients were previously treated with antifungals, either for a suspected diagnosis performed by a physician or by self-diagnosis.

The clinical history most of the times is enough to raise a high level of suspicion for CV.

The most striking symptom is burning, rather than pruritus. The typical discharge is white, sometimes lumpy and abundant (Fig. 24.16); some women will describe that it smells like vinegar. Dysuria and dyspareunia may also be among the list of symptoms. Symptoms tend be cyclic, aggravating in the luteal phase, peaking just before the menses. There is usually a great relief associated with menstruation or withdrawal bleeding. It is common that women report a transitory relief with the use of topical antifungals, but not oral formulations, probably due to a buffering effect.

The vulvar exam may be unremarkable, or some degree of erythema and/or oedema can be present. Fissures are an uncommon feature.

24.5.1.5 Complications

The very few studies about CV usually did not address the issue of complications. In one single study, we found that CV is much more prevalent

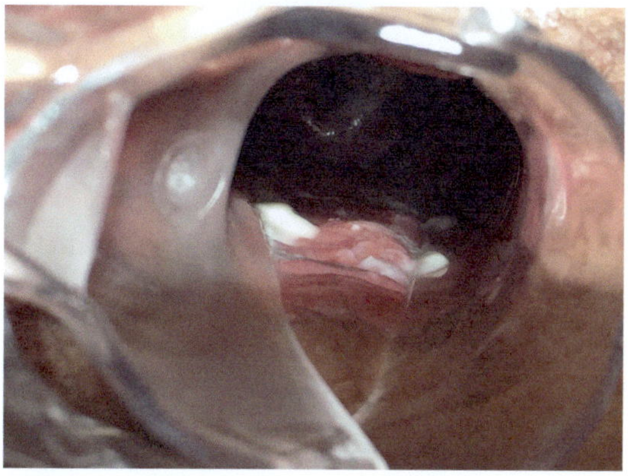

Fig. 24.16 Abundant, lumpy discharge in a woman with cytolytic vaginosis

in women with localized provoked vulvodynia, when compared to healthy controls (16.5% vs. 4.1%, $p = 0.000$) [156]. However, women with vulvodynia tend to have less frequent intercourse and, as referred before, CV has been found to be more common in less sexually active women [154]. On the other side, there is a biological plausibility that the chronic exposure of the vestibule to a very low pH, excessive amounts of H_2O_2, or the association to a specific lactobacillus species can be involved in the development of some cases of vulvodynia. Ventolini et al. associated *L. gasseri* with vulvodynia, which can lead to the speculation that this can be a common link between the two entities [157].

24.5.1.6 Diagnosis

The diagnosis is made using the microscope (Table 24.12). It is characterized by the presence of an abundant number of lactobacilli, bare nuclei and cellular debris (in extreme cases, no intact cells are seen in the slide). Inflammation, clue cells, bacteria other than lactobacilli, and *T. vaginalis* are typically absent (Fig. 24.17). Although, per definition, the diagnosis implies the exclusion of the presence of *Candida*, given the typically low pH (<4.0–4.2) the coexistence of both is not rare.

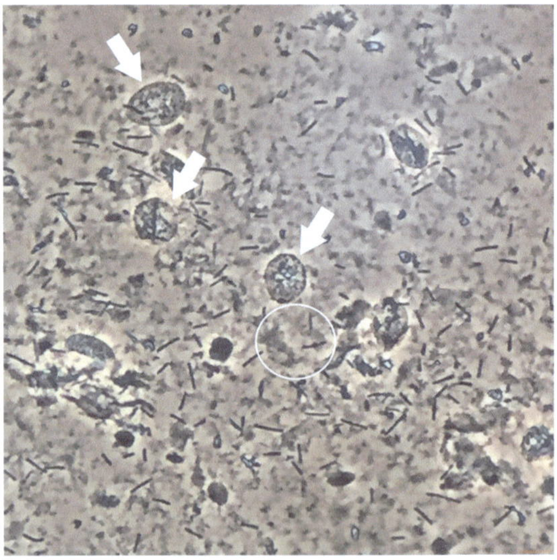

Fig. 24.17 Cytolytic vaginosis. Bare nuclei (white arrows), cellular debris (white arrows) and abundant lactobacilli

Cultures for fungi can be used to exclude the presence of *Candida*.

24.5.1.7 Treatment

The treatment consists of increasing the pH of the vagina (buffer effect), which will diminish the load of lactobacilli in the vagina and ameliorate the symptoms.

Vaginal irrigations with sodium bicarbonate are highly effective in controlling the symptoms. While some authors recommend sitz baths, in our experience irrigations are much more effective (Table 24.11). In recurrent cases, if a pattern is identified, treatment should be started 24–48 h prior to the anticipated moment of onset [159].

24.5.2 Lactobacillosis

This entity is characterized by the overgrowth of lactobacilli, without cellular lysis (Fig. 24.18). When symptomatic, it is very similar to CV. There is no epidemiological data in the literature concerning lactobacillosis.

The diagnosis is established by a normal or reduced pH, cultures negative for *Candida*, and, most important, by an increased number of lactobacilli in microscopy, without other types of

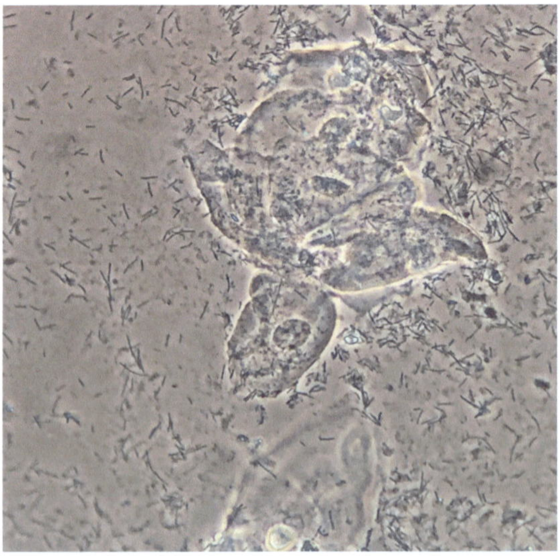

Fig. 24.18 Lactobacillosis (phase contrast 400×)

bacteria, cytolysis, inflammation, clue cells, or *T. vaginalis* (Table 24.12).

It is believed that it is self-limited, thus expectant management is an option. In cases in which treatment is needed, it is similar to that of CV (Table 24.11).

24.5.3 "Leptothrix"

Leptothrix is a controversial entity; even those who acknowledge its existence do not agree in how it should be designated (alternative names include "fusiform lactobacilli") [160]. It is characterized

Table 24.11 Treatment of CV, lactobacillosis and leptothrix

Cytolytic vaginosis	Sodium bicarbonate	30–40 mg should be diluted in 1 L of warm water and vaginal irrigations performed daily for 2 weeks Maintenance, if needed, should be kept as the minimum required to control the symptoms
Lactobacillosis		
Leptothrix	Amoxicillin + clavulanate 500/125	First choice 3 *id* for 7 days
	Doxycycline 100 mg [158]	If allergic to penicillin 2 *id* for 10 days
	Nifuratel 200 mg	Alternative needing further tests 3 *id* for 7 days

Table 24.12 Wet mount characterization and differential diagnosis of vulvovaginitis

	Presence of parabasal/ basal cells	Lactobacilli	Inflammation	Other	Notes
Candidiasis or candidosis	–	Normal	Can be present	Hyphae, pseudohyphae, spores	Inflammation, if present, usually without toxic leucocytes *C. glabrata* presents only as blastospores Presence of pseudohyphae is highly suggestive of infection rather than colonization Blastospores of *C. parapsilosis* and *S. cerevisiae* are larger than those of *C. glabrata*
Trichomoniasis	–/+	Frequently decreased	+ (frequently exuberant and with toxic leukocytes)	Motile protozoarians can be seen (10–20 by 2–14 μm)	Frequently associated with BV. If slide kept warm and microscopy performed immediately after collection, the likelihood of seeing motile TV is higher
Bacterial vaginosis	–	Decreased/ absent	–	Clue cells	If inflammation is present, exclude other causes for it
Aerobic vaginitis	+	Decreased/ absent	+	Toxic leucocytes can be present	–
Cytolytic vaginosis	–	Increased	–	Bare nuclei and cellular debris	–
Lactobacillosis	–	Increased and long	–	–	–
Leptothrix	–	Long	–	–	Lactobacilli longer than in lactobacillosis Can coexist with normal lactobacilli, BV, or even TV

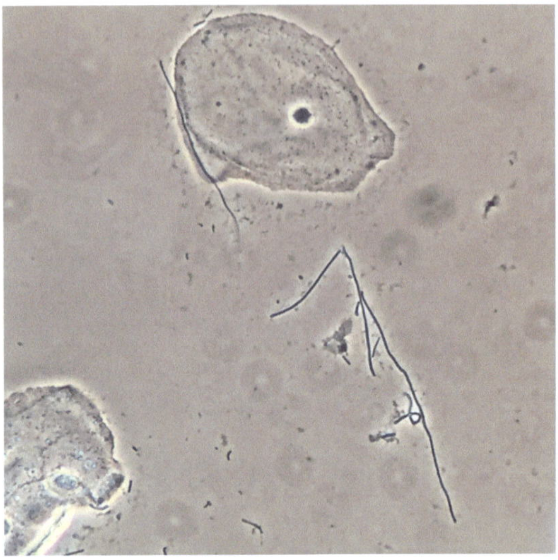

Fig. 24.19 Leptothrix (phase contrast 400×)

by the presence of long, filamentous lactobacilli, sometimes with segmentation and/or sporulation (Fig. 24.19). Its size can be 8–15 times that of a normal lactobacillus [161]. It can totally dominate the flora or be associated with normal lactobacilli, lactobacillosis [158], or even BV type flora and *T. vaginalis*. In a Swedish study, its prevalence in a cohort of women without BV was 8%. These authors identified these bacteria as *L. gasseri* [160].

There is some speculation that these lactobacilli may be the consequence of the previous use of antibiotics or antifungals.

Horowitz et al. described women with cyclical symptoms of vulvar discomfort and vaginal discharge during the luteal phase, associated with the presence of long and serpiginous lactobacilli.

The diagnosis is easily made by microscopy, by the presence of the typical long bacteria, that should not be confused with *Candida* or *Actinomyces* (Table 24.12).

Treatment with oral antibiotics has proven to be highly effective, both in the control and symptoms and in the elimination of the bacteria [158]. The first choice is amoxicillin + clavulanate; in women allergic to penicillin, doxycycline is an alternative [158]. Nifuratel has also been tested, but with much higher rates of relapse [162] (Table 24.11).

In contrast to other authors' experience, we have seen recurrences, even after successful treatment.

24.6 Other Conditions to Consider in the Differential Diagnosis of Vaginal Discharge

Several other conditions can present in similar ways to vulvovaginitis and must be considered in the differential diagnosis.

Vaginal Atrophy: Breaking the Myth

"Vaginal atrophy" and "atrophic vaginitis" may be associated with vaginal discharge. These terms have recently been renamed: "genitourinary syndrome of menopause". However, no minimum number of criteria was defined, the list of signs and symptoms is not specific, and some of the mainstays for its creation are highly debatable.

Postmenopausal vaginal atrophy can present in two ways: (1) without discharge (on microscopy there is paucity of epithelial cells and no inflammation) and (2) with purulent discharge (abundance of deep layer cells and inflammation—"atrophic vaginitis"). In 2014, the North American Menopause Society and the International Society for the Study of Women's Sexual Health proposed that "vaginal atrophy" and "atrophic vaginitis" should be replaced by "genitourinary syndrome of menopause". However, we disagree with this concept, as it cannot be considered a syndrome (which, by definition, is a particular abnormality or condition), no minimum number of criteria was defined, the list of signs and symptoms is not specific, and some of the mainstays for its creation are highly debatable (like "atrophy" having a negative connotation or "vagina" not being a well accepted term) [163].

Vaginal involvement of erosive lichen planus can manifest itself also with by a purulent discharge, sometimes with more or less extensive formation of synechia.

Other causes to be considered include allergic and contact vaginitis, as well as cervical ectopy [53] (Table 24.13).

Table 24.13 Clinical characteristics and potential risks of different causes of vulvovaginitis

	pH	Whiff test	Variation of symptoms during ovarian cycle	Symptoms	Signs	Risks
Candidiasis	Normal (but can occur at any pH; most likely to be symptomatic at low pH)	–	Worsening during the luteal phase and improving with menses	Pruritus, terminal/ post-micturition dysuria, dyspareunia. If burning is the main symptom consider *C.* non-*albicans* or alternative diagnosis	Erythema and enantema, fissures, oedema, white, curdy discharge, without foul smell	• Limited data relating it to bad obstetrical outcomes • Increased risk of HIV
Trichomoniasis	Increased (≥5)	+ (frequently)	Worsening of symptoms during menses	Can be asymptomatic Dysuria, burning, itching, irritation, discharge	Erythema, enantema, erosions, fissures, strawberry cervix, yellow or green purulent discharge (sometimes with bubbles), discharge can have a rotten smell	• Adverse obstetrical outcomes • STIs (HIV)
Bacterial vaginosis	Increased (>4.5)	+	Worsening of symptoms during menses	Fishy smell, mild burning	Grey or yellow, thin, adherent discharge	• Adverse obstetrical and neonatal outcomes • STIs • Cervical dysplasia/ cancer
Aerobic vaginitis	Increased (usually more than in BV: >5)	–	Worsening of symptoms during menses?	Rotten wood smell discharge; burning, stinging, dyspareunia	Yellow or green purulent discharge; erosions, enantema	• Adverse obstetrical and neonatal outcomes • STIs • Abnormal pap tests
Cytolytic vaginosis	Lower than normal	–	Worsening during the luteal phase and marked improvement with menses	Burning, abundant discharge	White, curdy, abundant discharge	• Vulvodynia (?)
Lactobacillosis	Lower than normal	–	Worsening during the luteal phase and marked improvement with menses	Burning	Normal/white discharge	• Not reported
Leptothrix	Normal/low (?)	–	?	Asymptomatic most of time times Burning	Normal	• Not reported

References

1. Sobel JD, et al. Vulvovaginal candidiasis: epidemiologic, diagnostic, and therapeutic considerations. Am J Obstet Gynecol. 1998;178:203–11.
2. Mendling W, et al. Guideline: vulvovaginal candidosis (AWMF 015/072), S2k (excluding chronic mucocutaneous candidosis). Mycoses. 2015;58:1–15.
3. Nedovic B, et al. Mannose-binding lectin codon 54 gene polymorphism and vulvovaginal candidiasis: a systematic review and meta-analysis. Biomed Res Int. 2014;2014:1–7.
4. Donders GGG, Bellen G, Mendling W. Management of recurrent vulvo-vaginal candidosis as a chronic illness. Gynecol Obstet Investig. 2010;70:306–21.
5. Matsubara VH, Wang Y, Bandara HMHN, Mayer MPA, Samaranayake LP. Probiotic lactobacilli inhibit early stages of *Candida albicans* biofilm development by reducing their growth, cell adhesion, and filamentation. Appl Microbiol Biotechnol. 2016;100:6415–26.
6. Sobel JD. Vulvovaginal candidosis. Lancet. 2007;369:1961–71.
7. Sobel JD, Subramanian C, Foxman B, Fairfax M, Gygax SE. Mixed vaginitis-more than coinfection and with therapeutic implications. Curr Infect Dis Rep. 2013;15:104–8.
8. Lindner JG, Plantema FH, Hoogkamp-Korstanje JA. Quantitative studies of the vaginal flora of healthy women and of obstetric and gynaecological patients. J Med Microbiol. 1978;11:233–41.
9. Beigi RH, Meyn LA, Moore DM, Krohn MA, Hillier SL. Vaginal yeast colonization in nonpregnant women: a longitudinal study. Obstet Gynecol. 2004;104:926–30.
10. Workowski KA, Bolan GA, Centers for Disease Control and Prevention. Sexually transmitted diseases treatment guidelines, 2015. MMWR Morb Mortal Wkly Rep. 2015;64:1–137.
11. Ventolini G. Progresses in vaginal microflora physiology and implications for bacterial vaginosis and candidiasis. Women's Health (Lond Engl). 2016;12:283–91.
12. Dennerstein GJ, Ellis DH. Oestrogen, glycogen and vaginal candidiasis. Aust N Z J Obstet Gynaecol. 2001;41:326–8.
13. Alves CT, et al. Effect of progesterone on *Candida albicans* vaginal pathogenicity. Int J Med Microbiol. 2014;304:1011–7.
14. Donders G, et al. Influence of contraceptive choice on vaginal bacterial and fungal microflora. Eur J Clin Microbiol Infect Dis. 2017;36:43–8.
15. Erol O, Simavlı S, Derbent AU, Ayrım A, Kafalı H. The impact of copper-containing and levonorgestrel-releasing intrauterine contraceptives on cervicovaginal cytology and microbiological flora: a prospective study. Eur J Contracept Reprod Health Care. 2014;19:187–93.
16. Lete I, Cuesta MC, Marín JM, Guerra S. Vaginal health in contraceptive vaginal ring users – a review. Eur J Contracept Reprod Health Care. 2013;18:234–41.
17. Farage M, Bramante M, Otaka Y, Sobel J. Do panty liners promote vulvovaginal candidiasis or urinary tract infections? Eur J Obstet Gynecol Reprod Biol. 2007;132:8–19.
18. Anderson MR, Klink K, Cohrssen A. Evaluation of vaginal complaints. JAMA. 2004;291:1368–79.
19. Holzer I, Farr A, Kiss H, Hagmann M, Petricevic L. The colonization with Candida species is more harmful in the second trimester of pregnancy. Arch Gynecol Obstet. 2017;295:891–5.
20. Garcia-Flores J, et al. Candida chorioamnionitis: report of two cases and review of literature. J Obstet Gynaecol. 2016;36:843–4.
21. Hester RA, Kennedy SB. Candida infection as a risk factor for HIV transmission. J Womens Health. 2003;12:487–94.
22. Foster DC, et al. Site-specific mesenchymal control of inflammatory pain to yeast challenge in vulvodynia-afflicted and pain-free women. Pain. 2015;156:386–96.
23. Ferris DG, Dekle C, Litaker MS. Women's use of over-the-counter antifungal medications for gynecologic symptoms. J Fam Pract. 1996;42:595–600.
24. Emmerson J, et al. Sampling for vaginal candidosis: how good is it? Int J STD AIDS. 1994;5:356–8.
25. Cartwright CP, et al. Comparison of nucleic acid amplification assays with BD affirm VPIII for diagnosis of vaginitis in symptomatic women. J Clin Microbiol. 2013;51(11):3694–9. https://doi.org/10.1128/JCM.01537-13.
26. Brown HL, Fuller DD, Jasper LT, Davis TE, Wright JD. Clinical evaluation of affirm VPIII in the detection and identification of *Trichomonas vaginalis*, *Gardnerella vaginalis*, and candida species in vaginitis/vaginosis. Infect Dis Obstet Gynecol. 2004;12:17–21.
27. Weissenbacher T, et al. Relationship between clinical diagnosis of recurrent vulvovaginal candidiasis and detection of candida species by culture and polymerase chain reaction. Arch Gynecol Obstet. 2009;279:125–9.
28. Donders G, et al. Individualized decreasing-dose maintenance fluconazole regimen for recurrent vulvovaginal candidiasis (ReCiDiF trial). Am J Obstet Gynecol. 2008;199:613.e1–9.
29. Donders GGG, et al. Role of molecular biology in diagnosis and characterization of Vulvo-vaginitis in clinical practice. Gynecol Obstet Investig. 2017;82:607–16.
30. Gaydos CA, et al. Clinical validation of a test for the diagnosis of vaginitis. Obstet Gynecol. 2017;130:181–9.
31. Martin Lopez JE. Candidiasis (vulvovaginal). BMJ Clin Evid. 2015. pii: 0815. https://www.ncbi.nlm.nih.gov/pubmed/25775428.

32. Pitsouni E, Iavazzo C, Falagas ME. Itraconazole vs fluconazole for the treatment of uncomplicated acute vaginal and vulvovaginal candidiasis in nonpregnant women: a metaanalysis of randomized controlled trials. Am J Obstet Gynecol. 2008;198(2):153–60. https://doi.org/10.1016/j.ajog.2007.10.786.
33. Consolaro MEL, Albertoni TA, Svidzinski AE, Peralta RM, Svidzinski TIE. Vulvovaginal candidiasis is associated with the production of germ tubes by *Candida albicans*. Mycopathologia. 2005;159:501–7.
34. Mahmoudabadi AZ, Najafyan M, Moghimipour E, Alwanian M, Seifi Z. Lamisil versus clotrimazole in the treatment of vulvovaginal candidiasis. Iran J Microbiol. 2013;5:86–90.
35. Ferahbas A, et al. Terbinafine versus Itraconazole and fluconazole in the treatment of vulvovaginal candidiasis. Am J Ther. 2006;13(4):332–6. https://doi.org/10.1097/00045391-200607000-00010.
36. Sobel JD, et al. Maintenance fluconazole therapy for recurrent vulvovaginal candidiasis. N Engl J Med. 2004;351:876–83.
37. Dennerstein GJ. Depo-Provera in the treatment of recurrent vulvovaginal candidiasis. J Reprod Med. 1986;31:801–3.
38. Vieira-Baptista P, Donders G. Is it possible to prevent recurrent vulvovaginitis? The role of lactobacillus plantarum I1001 (CECT7504). Eur J Clin Microbiol Infect Dis. 2017;36(3):593–4. https://doi.org/10.1007/s10096-016-2861-z.
39. Papaemmanouil V, et al. Prevalence and susceptibility of *Saccharomyces cerevisiae* causing vaginitis in Greek women. Anaerobe. 2011;17:298–9.
40. Nyirjesy P, et al. *Saccharomyces cerevisiae* vaginitis: transmission from yeast used in baking. Obstet Gynecol. 1995;86:326–9.
41. Kissinger P. Epidemiology and treatment of trichomoniasis. Curr Infect Dis Rep. 2015;17:31.
42. Petrin D, Delgaty K, Bhatt R, Garber G. Clinical and microbiological aspects of *Trichomonas vaginalis*. Clin Microbiol Rev. 1998;11:300–17.
43. Fichorova R, Fraga J, Rappelli P, Fiori PL. *Trichomonas vaginalis* infection in symbiosis with Trichomonasvirus and mycoplasma. Res Microbiol. 2017;168(9–10):882–91. https://doi.org/10.1016/j.resmic.2017.03.005.
44. Menezes CB, Amanda Piccoli Frasson AP, Tasca T. Trichomoniasis – are we giving the deserved attention to the most common non-viral sexually transmitted disease worldwide? Microb Cell. 2016;3:404–18.
45. Rowley J, Toskin I, Ndowa F, World Health Organization. Reproductive health and research. Global incidence and prevalence of selected curable sexually transmitted infections, 2008. Geneva: World Health Organization; 2012.
46. Krieger JN. Trichomoniasis in men: old issues and new data. Sex Transm Dis. 1995;22:83–96.
47. Byun JM, et al. Experience of successful treatment of patients with metronidazole-resistant *Trichomonas vaginalis* with zinc sulfate: a case series. Taiwan J Obstet Gynecol. 2015;54:617–20.
48. Sena AC, et al. *Trichomonas vaginalis* infection in male sexual partners: implications for diagnosis, treatment, and prevention. Clin Infect Dis. 2007;44:13–22.
49. Schwebke JR, Burgess D. Trichomoniasis. Clin Microbiol Rev. 2004;17:794–803.
50. Donders GGG, Depuydt C. Increased prevalence of *Trichomonas vaginalis* in mid-aged women is linked to sexual activity and not to hormonal changes. J Low Genit Tract Dis. 2013;17:e31–2.
51. Sutton M, et al. The prevalence of *Trichomonas vaginalis* infection among reproductive-age women in the United States, 2001–2004. Clin Infect Dis. 2007;45:1319–26.
52. Freeman AH, et al. Prevalence and correlates of *Trichomonas vaginalis* among incarcerated persons assessed using a highly sensitive molecular assay. Sex Transm Dis. 2010;37:165–8.
53. Sherrard J, Donders G, White D. European (IUSTI/WHO) guideline on the management of vaginal discharge, 2011. Int J STD AIDS. 2011;22:421–9.
54. Lima-Silva J, Vieira-Baptista P, Cavaco-Gomes J, Maia T, Beires J. Emphysematous vaginitis. J Low Genit Tract Dis. 2015;19:e43–4.
55. Silver BJ, Guy RJ, Kaldor JM, Jamil MS, Rumbold AR. *Trichomonas vaginalis* as a cause of perinatal morbidity: a systematic review and meta-analysis. Sex Transm Dis. 2014;41:369–76.
56. Cotch MF, et al. *Trichomonas vaginalis* associated with low birth weight and preterm delivery. The vaginal Infections and Prematurity Study Group. Sex Transm Dis. 1997;24:353–60.
57. Donders G, Bellen G, Rezeberga D. Aerobic vaginitis in pregnancy. BJOG. 2011;118:1163–70.
58. Fastring DR, et al. Co-occurrence of *Trichomonas vaginalis* and bacterial Vaginosis and vaginal shedding of HIV-1 RNA. Sex Transm Dis. 2014;41:173–9.
59. Mavedzenge SN, et al. Epidemiological synergy of *Trichomonas vaginalis* and HIV in Zimbabwean and south African women. Sex Transm Dis. 2010;37:460–6.
60. Donders GGG, Depuydt CE, Bogers J-P, Vereecken AJ. Association of *Trichomonas vaginalis* and cytological abnormalities of the cervix in low risk women. PLoS One. 2013;8:e86266.
61. Hamilton H, et al. *Trichomonas vaginalis* brain abscess in a neonate. Clin Infect Dis. 2017;66(4):604–7. https://doi.org/10.1093/cid/cix908.
62. Jones HE, Lippman SA, Caiaffa-Filho HH, Young T, van de Wijgert JHHM. Performance of a rapid self-test for detection of *Trichomonas vaginalis* in South Africa and Brazil. J Clin Microbiol. 2013;51:1037–9.
63. Van Der Pol B. Clinical and laboratory testing for *Trichomonas vaginalis* infection. J Clin Microbiol. 2016;54:7–12.
64. Wiese W, Patel SR, Patel SC, Ohl CA, Estrada CA. A meta-analysis of the Papanicolaou smear and

wet mount for the diagnosis of vaginal trichomoniasis. Am J Med. 2000;108:301–8.
65. Nathan B, et al. Microscopy outperformed in a comparison of five methods for detecting *Trichomonas vaginalis* in symptomatic women. Int J STD AIDS. 2015;26:251–6.
66. Nye MB, Schwebke JR, Body BA. Comparison of APTIMA *Trichomonas vaginalis* transcription-mediated amplification to wet mount microscopy, culture, and polymerase chain reaction for diagnosis of trichomoniasis in men and women. Am J Obstet Gynecol. 2009;200:188.e1–7.
67. Gaydos CA, et al. Rapid diagnosis of *Trichomonas vaginalis* by testing vaginal swabs in an isothermal helicase-dependent AmpliVue assay. Sex Transm Dis. 2016;43:369–73.
68. Perl G. Errors in the diagnosis of *trichomonas vaginalis* infections as observed among 1199 patients. Obstet Gynecol. 1972;39:7–9.
69. Badman SG, et al. A preliminary evaluation of a new GeneXpert (Gx) molecular point-of-care test for the detection of *Trichomonas vaginalis*. Sex Transm Infect. 2016;92:350–2.
70. Visapää J-P, Tillonen JS, Kaihovaara PS, Salaspuro MP. Lack of disulfiram-like reaction with metronidazole and ethanol. Ann Pharmacother. 2002;36:971–4.
71. Sobel R, Sobel JD. Metronidazole for the treatment of vaginal infections. Expert Opin Pharmacother. 2015;16:1109–15.
72. Schwebke JR, Lensing SY, Sobel J. Intravaginal metronidazole/miconazole for the treatment of vaginal trichomoniasis. Sex Transm Dis. 2013;40:710–4.
73. Klebanoff MA, et al. Failure of metronidazole to prevent preterm delivery among pregnant women with asymptomatic *Trichomonas vaginalis* infection. N Engl J Med. 2001;345:487–93.
74. Gülmezoglu AM, Azhar M. Interventions for trichomoniasis in pregnancy. Cochrane Database Syst Rev. 2011;11:CD000220. https://doi.org/10.1002/14651858.CD000220.pub2.
75. Crucitti T. Eve's garden: myths, legends and secrets unmasked. Res Microbiol. 2017;168(9–10):773–81. https://doi.org/10.1016/j.resmic.2017.07.004.
76. Donders G, Vieira-Baptista P. Bacterial vaginosis and inflammatory response showed association with severity of cervical neoplasia in HPV-positive women. Diagn Cytopathol. 2016;45(5):472–3.
77. Donders GGG, et al. Definition of a type of abnormal vaginal flora that is distinct from bacterial vaginosis: aerobic vaginitis. BJOG. 2002;109:34–43.
78. Vieira-Baptista P, et al. Bacterial vaginosis, aerobic vaginitis, vaginal inflammation and major pap smear abnormalities. Eur J Clin Microbiol Infect Dis. 2016;35:1–8. https://doi.org/10.1007/s10096-016-2584-1.
79. Ravel J, et al. Vaginal microbiome of reproductive-age women. Proc Natl Acad Sci U S A. 2011;108(Suppl 1):4680–7. https://doi.org/10.1073/pnas.1002611107.
80. Miller EA, Beasley DE, Dunn RR, Archie EA. Lactobacilli dominance and vaginal pH: why is the human vaginal microbiome unique? Front Microbiol. 2016;7:1936.
81. Blackwell AL. Vaginal bacterial phaginosis? Sex Transm Infect. 1999;75:352–3.
82. Marrazzo JM, Thomas KK, Fiedler TL, Ringwood K, Fredricks DN. Risks for acquisition of bacterial vaginosis among women who report sex with women: a cohort study. PLoS One. 2010;5:e11139.
83. Harada K, et al. Vaginal infection with Ureaplasma urealyticum accounts for preterm delivery via induction of inflammatory responses. Microbiol Immunol. 2008;52:297–304.
84. Nasioudis D, Linhares I, Ledger W, Witkin S. Bacterial vaginosis: a critical analysis of current knowledge. BJOG An Int J Obstet Gynaecol. 2017;124:61–9.
85. Hay P. Bacterial vaginosis. F1000Res. 2017;6:1761.
86. Allsworth JE, Peipert JF. Prevalence of bacterial vaginosis. Obstet Gynecol. 2007;109:114–20.
87. Vieira-Baptista P, et al. Genital tract infections in an isolated community: 100 women of the Príncipe Island. Infect Dis Obstet Gynecol. 2017;2017:3058569.
88. Yen S, et al. Bacterial vaginosis in sexually experienced and non-sexually experienced young women entering the military. Obstet Gynecol. 2003;102:927–33.
89. Marrazzo JM, Thomas KK, Agnew K, Ringwood K. Prevalence and risks for bacterial vaginosis in women who have sex with women. Sex Transm Dis. 2010;37:335–9.
90. Gottschick C, et al. The urinary microbiota of men and women and its changes in women during bacterial vaginosis and antibiotic treatment. Microbiome. 2017;5:99.
91. Gray RH, et al. The effects of male circumcision on female partners' genital tract symptoms and vaginal infections in a randomized trial in Rakai, Uganda. Am J Obstet Gynecol. 2009;200(42):e1–7.
92. Bilardi JE, et al. Women view key sexual behaviours as the trigger for the onset and recurrence of bacterial vaginosis. PLoS One. 2017;12:e0173637.
93. Brotman RM, et al. Association between cigarette smoking and the vaginal microbiota: a pilot study. BMC Infect Dis. 2014;14:471.
94. Petrova MI, Reid G, Vaneechoutte M, Lebeer S. Lactobacillus iners: friend or foe? Trends Microbiol. 2017;25:182–91.
95. Marrazzo JM, Antonio M, Agnew K, Hillier SL. Distribution of genital lactobacillus strains shared by female sex partners. J Infect Dis. 2009;199:680–3.
96. Taylor-Robinson D, McCaffrey M, Pitkin J, Lamont RF. Bacterial vaginosis in climacteric and menopausal women. Int J STD AIDS. 2002;13:449–52.
97. Eschenbach DA, Gravett MG, Chen KC, Hoyme UB, Holmes KK. Bacterial vaginosis during pregnancy. An association with prematurity and post-

partum complications. Scand J Urol Nephrol Suppl. 1984;86:213–22.
98. Unemo M, et al. Sexually transmitted infections: challenges ahead. Lancet Infect Dis. 2017;17:e235–79.
99. Donders GGG, Ruban K, Bellen G, Petricevic L. Mycoplasma/Ureaplasma infection in pregnancy: to screen or not to screen. J Perinat Med. 2017;45:505–15.
100. Cohen CR, et al. Bacterial vaginosis associated with increased risk of female-to-male HIV-1 transmission: a prospective cohort analysis among African couples. PLoS Med. 2012;9:e1001251.
101. Babu G, Singaravelu BG, Srikumar R, Reddy SV, Kokan A. Comparative study on the vaginal flora and incidence of asymptomatic vaginosis among healthy women and in women with infertility problems of reproductive age. J Clin Diagn Res. 2017;11:DC18–22.
102. Amsel R, et al. Nonspecific vaginitis. Diagnostic criteria and microbial and epidemiologic associations. Am J Med. 1983;74(1):14–22. https://doi.org/10.1016/0002-9343(83)91137-3.
103. Mittal V, Jain A, Pradeep Y, Pradeep Y. Development of modified diagnostic criteria for bacterial vaginosis at peripheral health centres in developing countries. J Infect Dev Countries. 2012;6:373–7.
104. Hay P, Tummon A, Ogunfile M, Adebiyi A, Adefowora A. Evaluation of a novel diagnostic test for bacterial vaginosis: 'the electronic nose'. Int J STD AIDS. 2003;14:114–8.
105. Huppert JS, et al. Accuracy and trust of self-testing for bacterial vaginosis. J Adolesc Health. 2012;51:400–5.
106. Geva A, Bornstein J, Dan M, Shoham HK, Sobel JD. The VI-SENSE–vaginal discharge self-test to facilitate management of vaginal symptoms. Am J Obstet Gynecol. 2006;195:1351–6.
107. Nugent R, Krohn M, Hillier S. Reliability of diagnosing bacterial vaginosis is improved by a standardized method of gram stain interpretation. J Clin Microbiol. 1991;29:297–301.
108. Donders GGG. Definition and classification of abnormal vaginal flora. Best Pract Res Clin Obstet Gynaecol. 2007;21:355–73.
109. Ison CA, Hay PE. Validation of a simplified grading of gram stained vaginal smears for use in genitourinary medicine clinics. Sex Transm Infect. 2002;78:413–5.
110. Stockdale CK. A positive culture result for gardnerella is not diagnostic of bacterial vaginosis. J Low Genit Tract Dis. 2016;20:281–2.
111. Madhivanan P, et al. Performance of BVBlue rapid test in detecting bacterial vaginosis among women in Mysore, India. Infect Dis Obstet Gynecol. 2014;2014:908313.
112. Calderón E, Rivera R. Evaluation of a fast test to identify the presence of proline aminopeptidase in women with bacterial Vaginosis. Infect Dis Obstet Gynecol. 1997;231:226–31.
113. Rumyantseva T a, Bellen G, Savochkina YA, Guschin a E, Donders GGG. Diagnosis of aerobic vaginitis by quantitative real-time PCR. Arch Gynecol Obstet. 2016;294(1):109–14. https://doi.org/10.1007/s00404-015-4007-4.
114. Oduyebo OO, Anorlu RI, Ogunsola FT. In: Oduyebo OO, editor. Cochrane database of systematic reviews. Hoboken: Wiley; 2009. p. CD006055. https://doi.org/10.1002/14651858.CD006055.pub2.
115. Donders GG, Zodzika J, Rezeberga D. Treatment of bacterial vaginosis: what we have and what we miss. Expert Opin Pharmacother. 2014;15:645–57.
116. Mendling W, Weissenbacher ER, Gerber S, Prasauskas V, Grob P. Use of locally delivered dequalinium chloride in the treatment of vaginal infections: a review. Arch Gynecol Obstet. 2015;293(3):469–84. https://doi.org/10.1007/s00404-015-3914-8.
117. Schuyler JA, et al. Identification of intrinsically metronidazole-resistant clades of Gardnerella vaginalis. Diagn Microbiol Infect Dis. 2016;84:1–3.
118. Donders G, et al. Improvement of abnormal vaginal flora in Ugandan women by self-testing and short use of intravaginal antimicrobials. Eur J Clin Microbiol Infect Dis. 2016;36(4):731–8. https://doi.org/10.1007/s10096-016-2856-9.
119. Chaithongwongwatthana S, Limpongsanurak S, Sitthi-Amorn C. Single hydrogen peroxide vaginal douching versus single-dose oral metronidazole for the treatment of bacterial vaginosis: a randomized controlled trial. J Med Assoc Thail. 2003;86(Suppl 2):S379–84.
120. Krasnopolsky VN, et al. Efficacy of vitamin C vaginal tablets as prophylaxis for recurrent bacterial vaginosis: a randomised, double-blind, placebo-controlled clinical trial. J Clin Med Res. 2013;5:309–15.
121. Tan H, Fu Y, Yang C, Ma J. Effects of metronidazole combined probiotics over metronidazole alone for the treatment of bacterial vaginosis: a meta-analysis of randomized clinical trials. Arch Gynecol Obstet. 2017;295:1331–9.
122. Ugwumadu A, Manyonda I, Reid F, Hay P. Effect of early oral clindamycin on late miscarriage and preterm delivery in asymptomatic women with abnormal vaginal flora and bacterial vaginosis: a randomised controlled trial. Lancet. 2003;361:983–8.
123. Larsson P-G, et al. Late miscarriage and preterm birth after treatment with clindamycin: a randomised consent design study according to Zelen. BJOG. 2006;113:629–37.
124. Lamont RF, Jones BM, Mandal D, Hay PE, Sheehan M. The efficacy of vaginal clindamycin for the treatment of abnormal genital tract flora in pregnancy. Infect Dis Obstet Gynecol. 2003;11:181–9.
125. Yudin MH, Money DM. No. 211-screening and management of bacterial vaginosis in pregnancy. J Obstet Gynaecol Canada. 2017;39:e184–91.

126. Bradshaw CS, Sobel JD. Current treatment of bacterial vaginosis-limitations and need for innovation. J Infect Dis. 2016;214(Suppl 1): S14–20.
127. Verstraelen H, Swidsinski A. The biofilm in bacterial vaginosis: implications for epidemiology, diagnosis and treatment. Curr Opin Infect Dis. 2013;26:86–9.
128. Ferreira CST, et al. Treatment failure of bacterial vaginosis is not associated with higher loads of Atopobium vaginae and Gardnerella vaginalis. J Med Microbiol. 2017;66:1217–24.
129. Alves P, Castro J, Sousa C, Cereija TB, Cerca N. Gardnerella vaginalis outcompetes 29 other bacterial species isolated from patients with bacterial vaginosis, using in an in vitro biofilm formation model. J Infect Dis. 2014;210:593–6.
130. Marrazzo JM, Thomas KK, Fiedler TL, Ringwood K, Fredricks DN. Relationship of specific vaginal bacteria and bacterial vaginosis treatment failure in women who have sex with women. Ann Intern Med. 2008;149:20–8.
131. Bunge KE, Beigi RH, Meyn LA, Hillier SL. The efficacy of retreatment with the same medication for early treatment failure of bacterial vaginosis. Sex Transm Dis. 2009;36:711–3.
132. Sobel JD, et al. Suppressive antibacterial therapy with 0.75% metronidazole vaginal gel to prevent recurrent bacterial vaginosis. Am J Obstet Gynecol. 2006;194:1283–9.
133. McClelland RS, et al. Improvement of vaginal health for Kenyan women at risk for acquisition of human immunodeficiency virus type 1: results of a randomized trial. J Infect Dis. 2008;197:1361–8.
134. Mehta SD. Systematic review of randomized trials of treatment of male sexual partners for improved bacteria vaginosis outcomes in women. Sex Transm Dis. 2012;39:822–30.
135. Reichman O, Akins R, Sobel JD. Boric acid addition to suppressive antimicrobial therapy for recurrent bacterial vaginosis. Sex Transm Dis. 2009;36:732–4.
136. Heczko PB, et al. Supplementation of standard antibiotic therapy with oral probiotics for bacterial vaginosis and aerobic vaginitis: a randomised, double-blind, placebo-controlled trial. BMC Womens Health. 2015;15:115.
137. Xie HY, et al. Probiotics for vulvovaginal candidiasis in non-pregnant women. Cochrane Database Syst Rev. 2017;11:CD010496.
138. Verstraelen H, Verhelst R, Roelens K, Temmerman M. Antiseptics and disinfectants for the treatment of bacterial vaginosis: a systematic review. BMC Infect Dis. 2012;12:148.
139. Gardner HL. Desquamative inflammatory vaginitis: a newly defined entity. Am J Obstet Gynecol. 1968;102:1102–5.
140. Oates JK, Rowen D. Desquamative inflammatory vaginitis. A review. Genitourin Med. 1990;66:275–9.
141. Lima-silva J, Tavares S, Vieira-baptista P, Beires J. Desquamative inflammatory vaginitis. Acta Obstét Ginecol Port. 2016;10:317–25.
142. Donders GG, Bellen G, Grinceviciene S, Ruban K, Vieira-Baptista P. Aerobic vaginitis: no longer a stranger. Res Microbiol. 2017;168(9–10):845–58. https://doi.org/10.1016/j.resmic.2017.04.004.
143. Mitchell C, Fredricks D, Agnew K, Hitti J. Hydrogen peroxide-producing lactobacilli are associated with lower levels of vaginal interleukin-1β, independent of bacterial vaginosis. Sex Transm Dis. 2015;42:358–63.
144. Marconi C, et al. Sialidase activity in aerobic vaginitis is equal to levels during bacterial vaginosis. Eur J Obstet Gynecol Reprod Biol. 2013;167:205–9.
145. Donders GGG, Vereecken A, Bosmans E, Spitz B. Vaginal cytokines in normal pregnancy. Am J Obstet Gynecol. 2003;189:1433–8.
146. Vieira-Baptista P, et al. Wet mount characterization of the vaginal flora of HIV women. In: 2nd ISIDOG meeting; 2017.
147. Geng N, et al. Analysis of the risk factors for aerobic vaginitis: a case-control study. Gynecol Obstet Investig. 2015. https://doi.org/10.1159/000431286.
148. Iwata T, et al. Cytokine profile in cervical mucosa of Japanese patients with cervical intraepithelial neoplasia. Int J Clin Oncol. 2015;20:126–33.
149. Donders GGG, et al. Increased vaginal pH in Ugandan women: what does it indicate? Eur J Clin Microbiol Infect Dis. 2016;35:1297–303.
150. Wang Z-L, et al. Diagnosis and microecological characteristics of aerobic vaginitis in outpatients based on preformed enzymes. Taiwan J Obstet Gynecol. 2016;55:40–4.
151. Witkin SS. Lactic acid alleviates stress: good for female genital tract homeostasis, bad for protection against malignancy. Cell Stress Chaperones. 2017;23(3):297–302. https://doi.org/10.1007/s12192-017-0852-3.
152. Soares R, Vieira-Baptista P, Tavares S. Cytolytic vaginosis: an underdiagnosed pathology that mimics vulvovaginal candidiasis. Acta Obstet Ginecol Port. 2017;11:106–12.
153. Witkin SS, et al. Influence of vaginal bacteria and D- and L-lactic acid isomers on vaginal extracellular matrix metalloproteinase inducer: implications for protection against upper genital tract infections. MBio. 2013;4:e00460–13.
154. Giraldo PC, et al. Influência da freqüência de coitos vaginais e da prática de duchas higiênicas sobre o equilíbrio da microbiota vaginal. Rev Bras Ginecol Obstet. 2005;27:257–62.
155. Vieira-Baptista P, Lima-Silva J, Beires J, Donders G. Cytolytic Vaginosis does not have an impact on human papilloma virus (HPV) infection and cervical dysplasia. Int J Low Genit Tract Dis. 2017;21:S27.

156. Vieira-Baptista P, Lima-Silva J, Xavier J, Beires J, Donders G. Vaginal Flora influences the risk of Vulvodynia. J Low Genit Tract Dis. 2017;21:S26.
157. Ventolini G, Gygax SE, Adelson ME, Cool DR. Vulvodynia and fungal association: a preliminary report. Med Hypotheses. 2013;81:228–30.
158. Horowitz BJ, Mårdh PA, Nagy E, Rank EL. Vaginal lactobacillosis. Am J Obstet Gynecol. 1994;170:857–61.
159. Cibley LJ, Cibley LJ. Cytolytic vaginosis. Am J Obstet Gynecol. 1991;165:1245–9.
160. Platz-Christensen JJ, Påhlson C, Larsson PG. Long, uniform lactobacilli (Döderlein's Bacteria): a new risk factor for postoperative infection after first-trimester abortion. Infect Dis Obstet Gynecol. 1995;3:102–9.
161. Ventolini G. Vaginal leptothrix: from fungi to lactobacillosis. J Genit Syst Disord. 2015;4. https://www.scitechnol.com/vaginal-leptothrix-from-fungi-to-lactobacillosis-oPa9.php?article_id=2738.
162. Cepický P, Malina J, Kuzelová M. Treatment of aerobic vaginitis and clinically uncertain causes of vulvovaginal discomfort. Ceska Gynekol. 2003;68:439–42.
163. Vieira-Baptista P, Marchitelli C, Haefner HK, Donders G, Pérez-López F. Deconstructing the genitourinary syndrome of menopause. Int Urogynecol J. 2017;28:675–9.

25 Psoriasis

Darion Rowan

25.1 Introduction

Psoriasis is a chronic inflammatory condition in which there is rapid proliferation of the epidermis (approximately 4 days compared with the normal 28 days) resulting in localized erythematous scaly plaques of skin [1–3].

It affects about 2–5% of the population and no ethnic group is spared. There is variance in incidence in different populations. Most commonly it develops in the second and third decades of life, but onset can be at any age.

Psoriasis is familial in about 40% of those affected suggesting a genetic predisposition. Its onset may be triggered by infection such as measles and streptococcal throat infection, traumatic injury, some drugs or a stressful life event. However, in many affected individuals, it arises spontaneously.

Inflammatory arthritis is present in approximately 10% of patients (estimates are from 7–42%) with psoriasis. It is also associated with signs of the metabolic syndrome which suggests that psoriasis is a multisystem chronic inflammatory disorder.

D. Rowan (✉)
Omnicare Women's Health, Auckland, New Zealand

25.2 Pathogenesis

In the past it was thought that the pathogenesis was primarily related to changes in the keratinocytes stimulated to excessive proliferation by extravasation of neutrophils into the epidermis from dilated capillaries of the dermal papillae. However, that simplistic view is only a small part in the pathogenesis and the end result of dysregulation of the immune system. It is now thought to be a T-cell-driven disorder, and some consider it to be an autoimmune disorder.

Both innate and adaptive immunity is altered in psoriasis. Interactions between cutaneous dendritic cells, T-cells, keratinocytes, neutrophils and the cytokines released from the immune cells contribute to the initiation and ongoing inflammation. Upregulation of interferon-alpha (IFNα) produced by plasmacytoid dendritic cells which are present in increased numbers in early psoriatic lesions stimulates the activation of myeloid dendritic cells. These cells produce cytokines including interleukin (IL)-23 and IL-12 that attract and activate T-cell differentiation, particularly Th17 and Th1 cells. These activated T-cells produce cytokines that stimulate keratinocytes to proliferate and produce pro-inflammatory antimicrobial peptides (AMPs). Other cytokines including tumour necrosis factor-alpha (TNFα) produced by immune cells and keratinocytes perpetuate the inflammatory process with the result that it becomes chronic. Biologic drugs which target specific cytokines

J. Bornstein (ed.), *Vulvar Disease*, https://doi.org/10.1007/978-3-319-61621-6_25

help to support the current theories of pathogenesis of psoriasis [1].

25.3 Clinical Presentation

There are many types of psoriasis and lesions. The most common is plaque psoriasis, but others include guttate psoriasis, flexural psoriasis, palmoplantar psoriasis, pustular psoriasis, keratoderma, erythrodermic psoriasis and nail disease.

Symptoms of vulval involvement are pruritus, irritation, burning and dyspareunia. In some patients psoriasis of the vulva may be the initial manifestation of the condition.

On the vulva the common areas involved are the pubis and labia majora, but no site is spared. Adjacent flexural areas, the genitocrural folds, natal cleft and perianal skin are also often affected. The lesions are well-demarcated erythematous patches or plaques, small or large (Figs. 25.1 and 25.2). Often involvement is bilateral and symmetrical but unilateral lesions occur (Fig. 25.3). In flexural areas the typical scaling of plaque psoriasis is lacking because of the moist occluded environment (Fig. 25.4). There may be fissuring and secondary infection with yeasts or bacteria.

The majority of patients will have psoriasis at sites other than the anogenital skin. Other flexural areas including retroauricular and submammary folds, limbs flexures and umbilicus demonstrate "inverse psoriasis" so called because

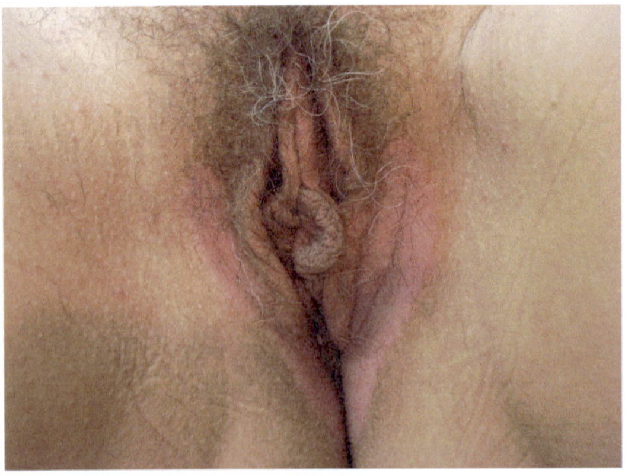

Fig. 25.1 Symmetrical psoriasis of anogenital area with well-defined border and lack of scaling

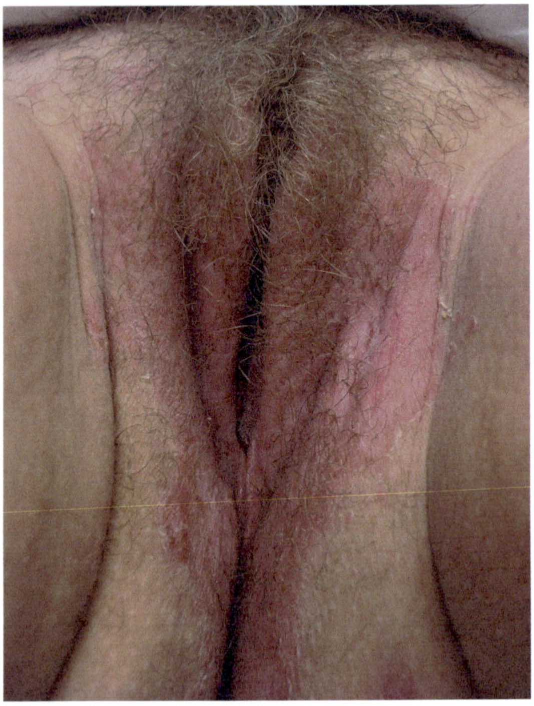

Fig. 25.2 Inflamed symmetrical psoriasis of anogenital area with peripheral scaling. Plaques present in adjacent pubic area

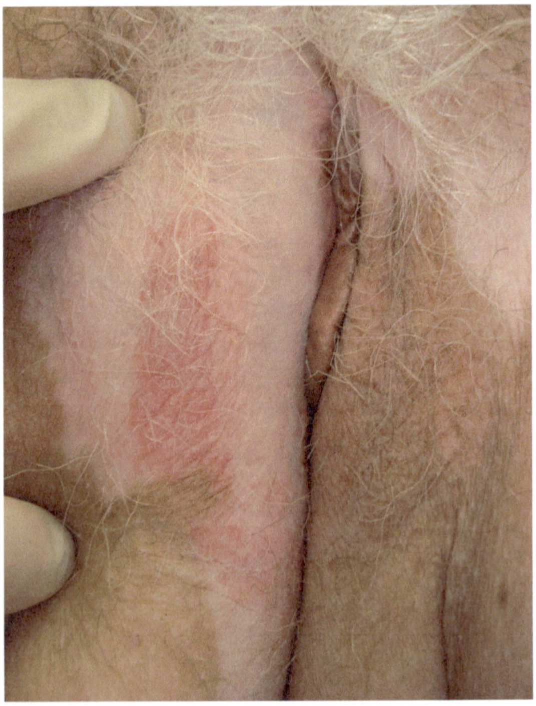

Fig. 25.3 Unilateral psoriatic plaque with adjacent vitiligo

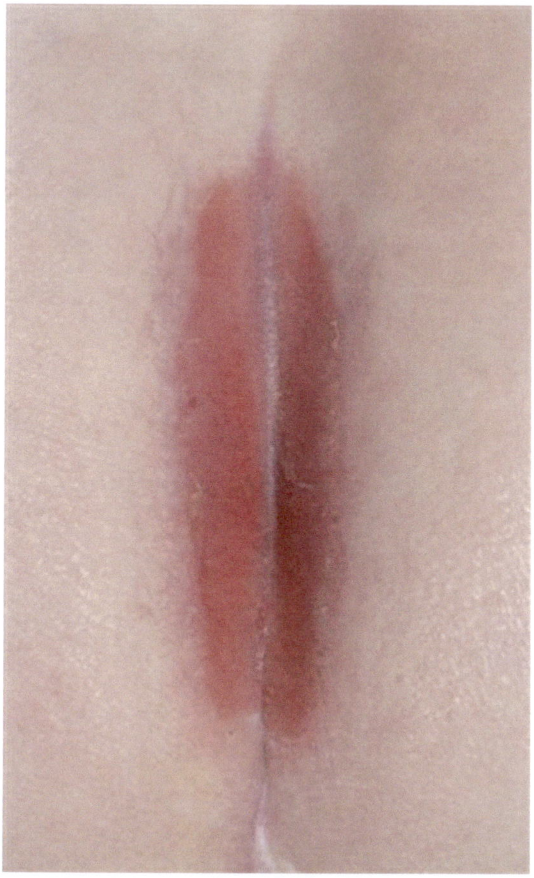

Fig. 25.4 Symmetrical erythematous, non-scaling asymptomatic plague of psoriasis in the natal cleft

of the distribution in body creases rather than over the dorsal aspects of limbs, trunk and scalp which are the most common sites. Fingernails commonly show pitting or other dystrophy such as thickened or yellowish discolouration, rough surface of the nail plate or onycholysis [2].

Vulval lichen sclerosus, an autoimmune condition, may be present. 10–17% of women with lichen sclerosus have psoriasis. Vitiligo, another autoimmune condition, may also be present on adjacent skin (Fig. 25.3).

If the affected areas are very itchy and been excessively scratched, chronic dermatitis (lichen simplex chronicus) develops on the surface. However, the lesions may be asymptomatic and the patient unaware of their presence.

Quality of life in patients with vulval psoriasis is frequently impaired, and this is more severe than if the genitalia are not affected. There is impairment of sexual functioning (sexual intercourse exacerbates vulval psoriasis in some patients) as well as concerns about other symptoms such as pruritus, irritation and soreness together with the abnormal appearance of the skin. This has negative social and psychological effects on patients [3].

25.4 Histopathology

Histopathology of psoriasis in typical cases shows epidermal hyperplasia resulting in elongated rete ridges of similar lengths with prominent capillary loops high in the papillary dermis, where there is overlying thinning of the epidermis, and parakeratosis. Neutrophils enter the epidermis and form neutrophilic abscesses in the subcorneal layer (Munro microabscesses). The stratum corneum is thickened which produces the scaling seen clinically. If the affected area has been rubbed excessively, the histologic appearance will show features of chronic dermatitis (lichen simplex chronicus), and the two can require expert dermatopathologists to distinguish them. However, in a typical case with evidence of psoriasis elsewhere, biopsy will not be required to confirm the diagnosis.

25.5 Differential Diagnosis

The differential diagnosis includes dermatitis of various types including seborrhoeic, atopic, chronic dermatitis, irritant or allergic chronic dermatitis; intertrigo; tinea; vulval candidiasis; squamous intra-epithelial lesion (formerly called vulval intra-epithelial neoplasia); and extramammary Paget's disease.

25.6 Treatment

Because the vulva is in a flexural area, usually clothed, and where moisture can be maintained, treatment with topical corticosteroid cream or ointment is usually effective. A weak tar preparation such as 2% coal tar solution in emulsifying ointment or calcipotriol ointment is an alternative. Intermittent therapy will be required by many patients. However, some have a poor response to topical treatment, and if there is recalcitrant disease, consideration should be given to systemic treatments such as methotrexate, acitretin or cyclosporine. These drugs are usually reserved for patients who have extensive skin surface involvement with psoriasis. Biologic agents can be used in those with a poor response to these second-line drugs and who have widespread disease but are not particularly effective in vulval psoriasis.

Psoriasis: Breaking the Myths

- Psoriasis may affect the vulva—but not the vagina.
- In many women it is triggered by a trauma or infection.
- Psoriasis is not only a skin condition—arthritis and metabolic syndrome are frequent comorbidities.
- T-cell-driven malfunction or autoimmune process leading to excess production of various cytokines and TNF is currently considered to cause psoriasis.
- On the vulva, psoriasis usually involves the pubis and labia majora, but no site is spared.
- The typical scaling is lacking because of the moist occluded vulvar environment.

References

1. Van de Kerkhof P and Nestlé F Psoriasis. In: Bolgnia Dermatology, 3rd ed. Section 3, Psoriasis 8; 2012. p. 135–156.
2. Kapila S, Bradford J, Fischer G. Vulvar psoriasis in adults and children: a clinical audit of 194 cases and review of the literature. J Low Genit Tract Dis. 2012;16:364–71.
3. Ryan C, et al. Genital psoriasis is associated with significant impairment in quality of life and sexual functioning. J Am Acad Dermatol. 2015;72:978–83.

Plasma Cell Vulvitis

26

Darion Rowan

26.1 Introduction

Zoon first described glazed erythema of the glans penis in 1952. A female counterpart was recognized 3 years later. The histology showed a plasma cell-rich dermal infiltrate.

Plasma cell vulvitis is a rare, benign condition of the introitus that most often affects postmenopausal women. It can develop in the presence of lichen sclerosus or other dermatoses of the vulva, and the course can be one of relapses and remissions. The cause is not known, but some consider it is a variant of lichen planus. Spontaneous remission may occur.

26.2 Clinical Presentation

The most common symptom is soreness but burning and pruritus may be experienced. It causes dyspareunia and often leads to apareunia because of severe pain experienced with intercourse. Dysuria, a pinky brown discharge, and bleeding on wiping are other symptoms. Some women are asymptomatic [1–5].

Examination findings are of shiny or glistening erythematous or orange macules with brown or purpuric spots affecting the medial labia minora, posterior fourchette, and periurethral mucosa. These changes are usually multifocal (Figs. 26.1, 26.2, and 26.3). The lateral vulva is less commonly affected, and the anatomy is not altered (unless by concomitant lichen sclerosus or lichen planus).

26.3 Histopathology

On histological examination, there is epidermal atrophy with an underlying dense inflammatory dermal infiltrate. The predominant cells are plasma cells: 50% or more is diagnostic of plasma cell vulvitis; if there are 25–50%, the diagnosis is likely. There are dilated capillaries and hemosiderin deposition which is the cause of the brown

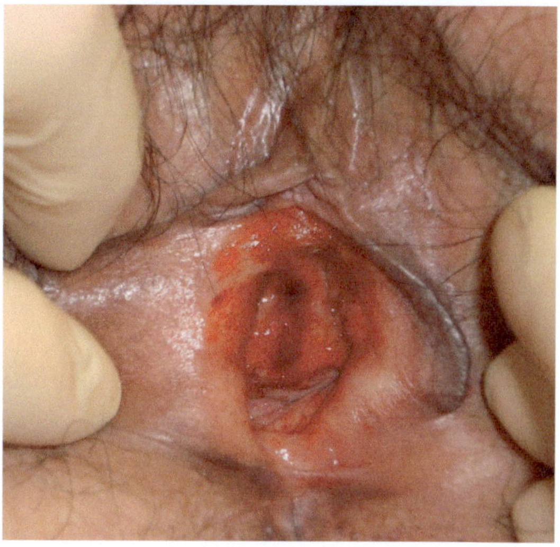

Fig. 26.1 Plasma cell vulvitis with patchy orange-red discoloration of the introitus and periurethral mucosa

D. Rowan (✉)
Omnicare Women's Health, Auckland, New Zealand

J. Bornstein (ed.), *Vulvar Disease*, https://doi.org/10.1007/978-3-319-61621-6_26

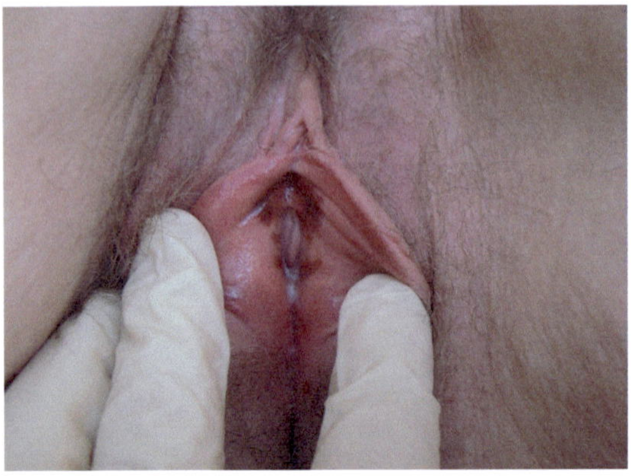

Fig. 26.2 Dark red-brown patches and macules localized to anterior introitus in plasma cell vulvitis

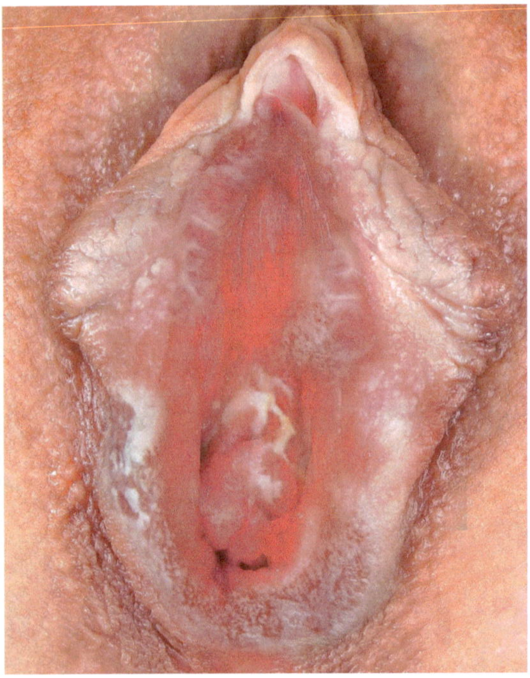

Fig. 26.3 Plasma cell vulvitis. Red patches at the vestibule and inner labia minora. Courtesy of Professor Jacob Bornstein

discoloration. The diagnosis requires confirmatory histopathology.

26.4 Differential Diagnosis

The differential diagnosis includes lichen planus; autoimmune blistering disorders such as bullous pemphigoid, cicatricial pemphigoid, and pemphigus vulgaris; fixed drug eruption; and trauma.

26.5 Treatment

Treatment for plasma cell vulvitis is often not effective. Topical preparations which may be beneficial are corticosteroids, tacrolimus, misoprostol (compounded 0.1% in white soft paraffin), and imiquimod. Intralesional steroids and interferon have been used, as have systemic steroids, antibiotics, methotrexate, and retinoids. Laser ablation and surgical excision have sometimes been used.

Plasma Cell Vulvitis: Breaking the Myths

- When an erythematous lesion is present on the medial vulva and vestibule, do not consider only lichen planus—it may also be plasma cell vulvitis.
- Histopathological examination reveals dense inflammatory dermal infiltrate. When 50% or more of the leucocytes are plasma cells, it is diagnostic of plasma cell vulvitis.
- Although most texts preach for detailed examination and the importance of making a definite diagnosis of any vulvar lesion, treatment of many red, white and ulcerative vulvar lesion is idem: topical steroids, calcineurin inhibitors, systemic steroids, immune suppresants etc.

References

1. Gunter J, Golitz L. Topical misoprostol therapy for plasma cell vulvitis: a case series. J Reprod Med. 2005;9:176–80.
2. Gurumurthy M, Cairns M, Cruickshank M. Case series of Zoon vulvitis. J Low Genit Tract Dis. 2010;14:56–8.
3. Neill SM, Lewis FM. Non-infective cutaneous conditions of the vulva. In: Ridley's the vulva. 3rd ed. London: Wiley-Blackwell; 2009. p. 127–8.
4. Toeima E, Sule M, Warren R, Igali L. Diagnosis and treatment of Zoon's vulvitis. J Obstet Gynaecol. 2011;31:473–5.
5. Virgili A, Levratti A, Marzola A, Corazza M. Retrospective histopathologic reevaluation of 18 cases of plasma cell vulvitis. J Reprod Med. 2005;50:3–7.

Part VI

Vulvar Lesions: Red Lesions—Papules

Folliculitis

27

Amanda Selk and Sara Wood

27.1 Introduction

Folliculitis can be defined by inflammation of the superficial area of the hair follicle and pilosebaceous unit within the epidermis [1]. While any region with hair may be affected, areas with friction and perspiration, such as the inguinal and vulvar area, may be particularly bothersome to women [1–3]. Both noninfectious and infectious causes can produce the signs and symptoms of folliculitis as purulence alone does not necessarily denote an infectious etiology. The physical exam generally reveals a classic erythematous pustule associated with a hair follicle often in clusters although progressive and deeper inflammatory nodules or furuncles may be visualized as well [1, 4]. Integral to the identification of the inciting etiology, a thorough history should be conducted and include investigation of risk factors, such as prior skin infections, immunosuppression, and environmental work and home exposures. Lesions that do not or incompletely resolve may be managed in consultation with dermatologic experts who may utilize more advanced diagnostic and treatment modalities.

Folliculitis often occurs when the hair follicle has been damaged. A common cause of trauma to the hair follicle is hair removal practices such as shaving, waxing, etc. [1]. Clothing that is constricting and rubs the skin can also lead to irritation and subsequent inflammation. If the hair follicles are blocked by sweat, they are also more likely to become irritated and inflamed.

Some risk factors for developing folliculitis include:

- The use of hot tubs, whirlpools, and swimming pools that are inadequately chlorinated.
- Using oily products on the skin that can block follicles.
- Any cut or microabrasion to the skin.
- When "hot tub folliculitis" appears, it is often caused by a *Pseudomonas aeruginosa* infection [4]. It will appear within a few days after bathing in a hot tub, swimming pool, or whirlpool and often occurs in the distribution of a bathing suit or other areas that were submersed in contaminated water. It usually resolves within 10 days with good hygiene and supportive care. Oral antibiotics are rarely required.

27.2 Diagnosis

Folliculitis is an inflammation of the hair follicle. It can occur anywhere on the body but is common in the groin as well as the buttock. It commonly

A. Selk (✉)
Women's College Hospital, Mount Sinai Hospital, University of Toronto, Toronto, ON, Canada

S. Wood
OBGYN Residency Program, Division of Female Pelvic Medicine and Reconstructive Surgery, Department of Obstetrics and Gynecology, Mercy Hospital St. Louis, St. Louis, MO, USA

J. Bornstein (ed.), *Vulvar Disease*, https://doi.org/10.1007/978-3-319-61621-6_27

presents as red or white bumps or pimple-like areas (papules or pustules) in hair-bearing skin (Fig. 27.1). On close examination, a hair can often be seen at the center of the lesion. Patients usually complain of itch or pain in the affected area. When the lesions burst, blood or pus may drain from them.

Diagnosis can be aided by culture with sensitivities and possible cytology of the purulent area to distinguish bacterial, viral, and fungal etiologies [2]. Consideration for sexually transmitted infections, such as herpes or secondary syphilis, should remain within the differential in patients with risk factors for these infections, emphasizing the importance of a careful history [1]. An algorithm to aid in the evaluation of folliculitis lesions is given in Fig. 27.2 [1]. A swab to identify possible methicillin-resistant *Staphylococcus aureus* (MRSA) avoids overlooking this diagnosis and facilitates appropriate treatment. In particular, athletes who undergo direct skin-to-skin contact or share personal items (razors, deodorant, etc.) may have an increased risk for transmission of MRSA [5, 6]. Folliculitis can also be misdiagnosed as insect bites given their pleomorphic appearance; thus, taking note of environmental exposures is key.

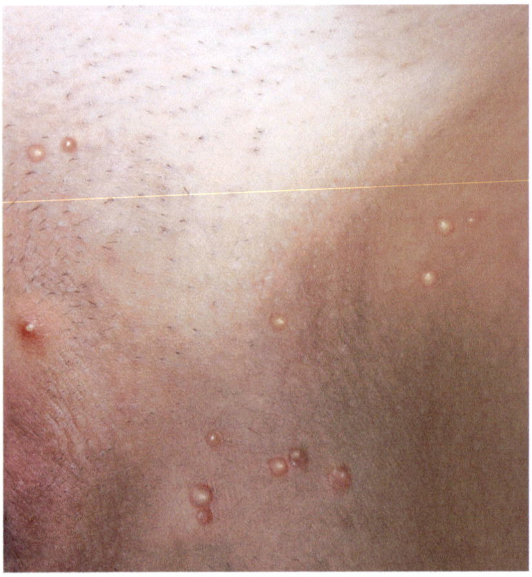

Fig. 27.1 Folliculitis, small pustules that may burst. They are usually located in hair-bearing skin. Sometimes a hair can often be seen at the lesion. Courtesy of Professor Jacob Bornstein

27.3 Treatment

Treatment for folliculitis encompasses both pharmacologic and lifestyle modifications. Counseling on hygiene measures with good handwashing and eradication of predisposing factors, such as cessation of aggressive scratching and avoidance of skin-to-skin contact in affected areas, should be provided to the patient along with vulvar skin care guidelines [5, 7]. Individualizing treatment to the inciting agent if

Fig. 27.2 Algorithm for the clinical evaluation of folliculitis. Reproduced with permission from Luelmo-Aguilar, 2004

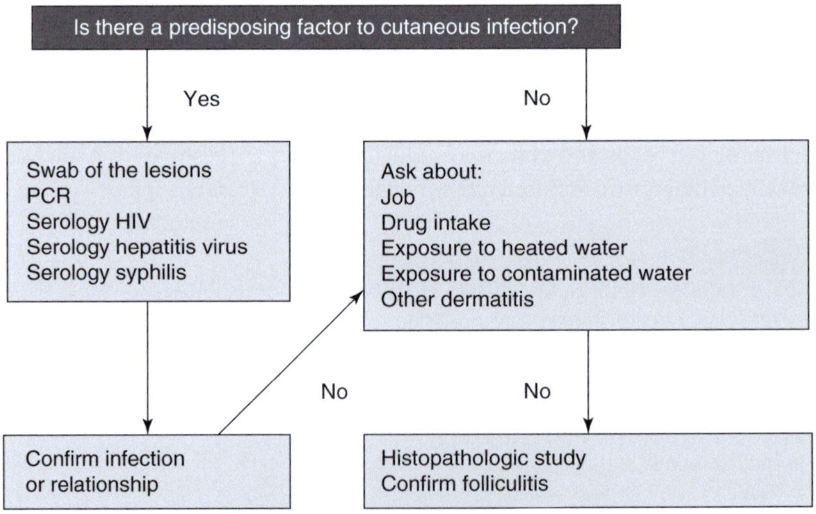

infectious is central to elimination of folliculitis. Options for treatments by pathogen are noted in Table 27.1 [1].

Treatment of bacterial folliculitis due to gram-positive cocci will often include a topical mupirocin or clindamycin ointment. Pseudomonal folliculitis associated with whirlpools can resolve spontaneously within 7–10 days by abstaining from whirlpool use or may require topical dilute acetic acid baths, oral ciprofloxacin, or isotretinoin [1, 4]. In some cases, simple folliculitis progresses to involve the deeper portion of the pilosebaceous unit producing a furuncle, which can coalesce to form a larger boil called a carbuncle [4]. These lesions can be treated with oral antibiotics, and if an abscess is apparent, incision and drainage is appropriate [1, 8].

Prior reviews reveal that significant delays in correct diagnosis and treatment commonly occur for non-bacterial causes of folliculitis [2]. Cytology may help differentiate between various infectious causes in addition to biopsy, which is important for diagnosis of noninfectious causes of folliculitis [1, 2]. Pseudofolliculitis from shaving and wax epilation appears to resemble a foreign body inflammatory reaction caused by the newly cut hair shaft reentering the epidermis and not represent a true folliculitis [1, 9]. However, severe infections post-waxing have been reported in the literature, and patients reporting worsening folliculitis symptoms should undergo prompt examination [10].

Folliculitis: Breaking the Myths

- Unexpected causes of folliculitis are constrictive, skin-irritative underwear or hair removal by shaving or the usage of oily products on the skin that can block follicles.
- Methicillin-resistant *Staphylococcus aureus* (MRSA) may also be involved with folliculitis. It is therefore important to culture for this bacterium and treat appropriately.

Table 27.1 Infectious folliculitis treatment options. Reproduced with permission from Luelmo-Aguilar, 2004

Type of folliculitis	Topical	Systemic
Staphylococcal and streptococcal	Fusidic acid or mupirocin ointment (tid)	Dicloxacillin, flucloxacillin, fusidic acid, azithromycin
Gram-negative bacteria (pseudomonas)[a]	Dilute acetic acid baths	Ciprofloxacin
Dermatophytes	Antifungal shampoo	Griseofulvin, terbinafine, itraconazole
Pityrosporum	Topical azoles, shampoos with sulfur of selenium	
Candidal		Itraconazole
Herpetic		Aciclovir, valaciclovir, antihistamines
Molluscum (poxvirus)	Curettage, cryotherapy, cantharidin, podophyllotoxin, trichloroacetic acid	
Demodicidosis	5% permethrin cream	Itraconazole, ivermectin

tid three times daily

[a]Usually resolves spontaneously

References

1. Luelmo-Aguilar J, Santandreu M. Folliculitis: recognition and management. Am J Clin Dermatol. 2004;5(5):301–10.
2. Durdu M, Ilkit M. First step in the differential diagnosis of folliculitis: cytology. Crit Rev Microbiol. 2013;39(1):9–25.
3. Breen J. Skin and soft tissue infections in immunocompetent patients. Am Fam Physician. 2010;81(7):893–9.
4. Chiller K, Selkin B, Murakawa G. Skin microflora and bacterial infections of the skin. J Investig Dermatol Symp Proc. 2001;6(3):170–4.
5. Cohen P. Community-acquired methicillin-resistant *Staphylococcus aureus* skin infections: a review of epidemiology, clinical features, management, and prevention. Int J Dermatol. 2007;46:1–11.
6. Cohen P. The skin in the gym: a comprehensive review of the cutaneous manifestations of community-acquired methicillin-resistant *Staphylococcus aureus* infection in athletes. Clin Dermatol. 2008;26:16–26.
7. University of Iowa Hospitals and Clinics. "Vulvar Skin Care Guidelines". 2016. Accessed at: https://uihc.org/health-library/vulvar-skin-care-guidelines.
8. Stevens D, Bisno A, Chambers H, et al. Practice guidelines for the diagnosis and management of skin and soft tissue infections: 2014 update by the Infectious Diseases Society of America. Clin Infect Dis. 2014;59(2):e10–52.
9. Perry P, Cook-Bolden F, Rahman Z, et al. Defining pseudofolliculitis barbae in 2001: a review of the literature and current trends. J Am Acad Dermatol. 2002;46:S113–9.
10. Khanna N, Chandramohan K, Khaitan B, et al. Post waxing folliculitis: a clinicopathological evaluation. Int J Dermatol. 2014;53(7):849–54.

28 Angiokeratoma

Amanda Selk and Sandra Ronger Savle

28.1 Introduction

Angiokeratomas are benign skin lesions. They are composed of superficial dilated blood vessels (capillaries) with a hyperkeratotic epidermis overlying the vessels [1]. They usually appear as dome-shaped papules (Fig. 28.1). Most of the time, they are smooth, but sometimes they have a scale on the surface [1].

Angiokeratomas are usually small, measuring between 2 and 5 mm. They can be solitary or multiple lesions can be present. They are usually dark-red, blue, or purple papules [1, 2] (Figs. 28.2 and 28.3). They are soft and easily compressible, and as they age, they darken to brown or black, and they become keratotic and non-compressible. The disseminated angiokeratomas are also called angiokeratoma corporis diffusum (Fabry disease) and are associated with deficiency of galactosidase A. The localized type includes angiokeratoma of the vulva (angiokeratoma of Fordyce), circumscribed angiokeratoma, and angiokeratoma of Mibelli. If there is a clot in the vessel, the lesion can turn black or dark purple.

A. Selk (✉)
Women's College Hospital, Mount Sinai Hospital, University of Toronto, Toronto, ON, Canada

S. Ronger Savle
Department of Dermatology and Gynecology, Lyon 1 University and Centre Hospitalier Lyon Sud, Lyon, France

28.2 Pathophysiology

The etiopathogenesis is related to increased local venous pressure and consequent subepithelial vascular dilatation. The labia majora are embryologically similar to the scrotum, since both derive from the labioscrotal folds. The loss of support of the local vessels, secondary to congenital deficiency of elastic tissue, is one of the associated factors. The role of increased local venous pressure caused by venous malformations, varicocele, or thrombosis, in addition phlebectasia secondary to chronic inflammation, is also postulated. Dilatation would therefore be induced by stasis, retrograde pressure, or venous injury. Therefore, excess weight, increased parity, hemorrhoids, pelvic inflammatory disease,

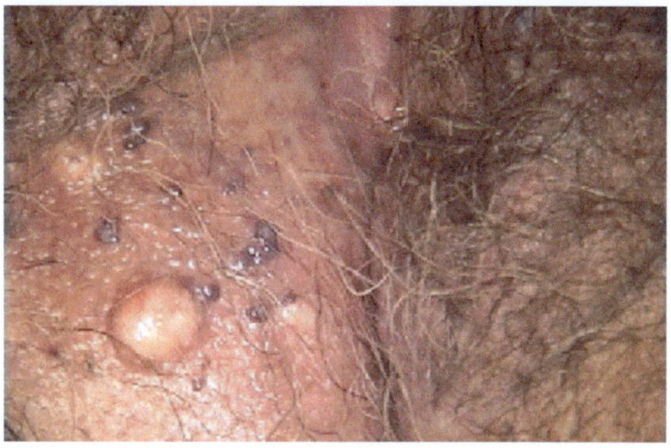

Fig. 28.1 Multiple angiokeratomas cover the vulvar labia majora. They are benign lesions consisting of superficial dilated blood vessels. An epidermal cyst also exists. Courtesy of Professor Jacob Bornstein

J. Bornstein (ed.), *Vulvar Disease*, https://doi.org/10.1007/978-3-319-61621-6_28

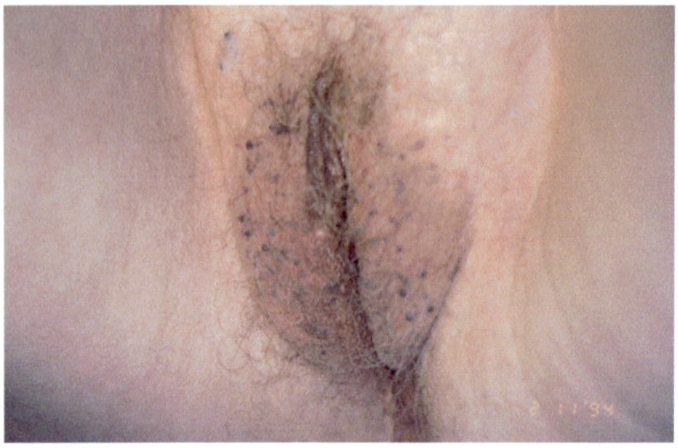

Fig. 28.2 Multiple minute angiokeratomas covering both labia majora. Courtesy of Professor Jacob Bornstein

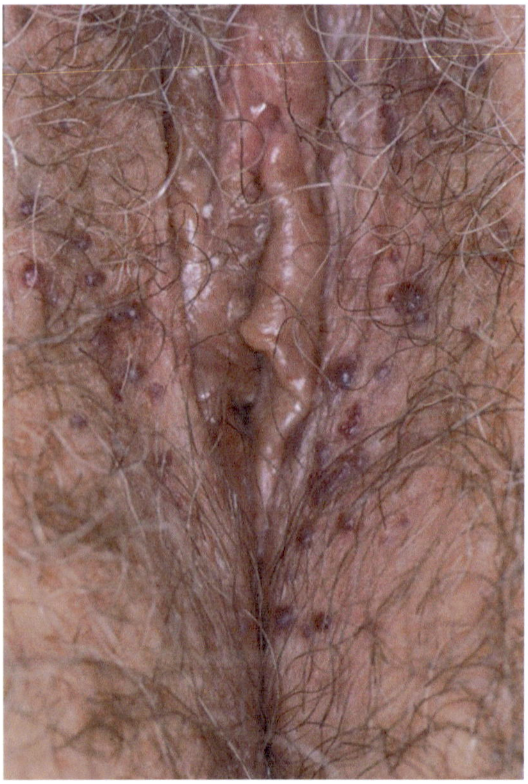

Fig. 28.3 Angiokeratomas of both labia majora. Courtesy of Dr. Sandra Ronger Savle

prior hysterectomy, varicose veins, and vascular varicosity are considered risk factors for the occurrence of angiokeratomas of the vulva.

The presence of black, warty, bleeding lesion can arouse suspicious of a malignant melanoma, which can be rapidly dispelled by dermoscopy or histopathology.

28.3 Clinical Presentation

Angiokeratomas are often asymptomatic but they can bleed if trauma occurs to them. Sometimes they bleed after they have been scratched or squeezed, or they bleed after they get rubbed during sexual activity [1].

They tend to appear in adulthood and often increase in pregnancy. They appear more commonly over the age of 40 [3]. The prevalence tends to increase with age. They are not hereditary. Their etiology is unknown.

Fabry disease is a rare x-linked condition where angiokeratomas are present [4]. This disease should be considered when lesions appear in young people, are multiple, spread quickly, and involve mucosal surfaces or if they are associated with burning, tingling, or pricking sensations or numbness in the extremities present on awaking (acroparesthesia), hypohidrosis (diminished sweating), or heat intolerance [4].

In most cases of angiokeratoma, diagnosis is made through history and physical exam. In the genital area of women, they most commonly appear on the labia majora. A biopsy is required if there is a concern for a possible malignancy. Concerning features are those seen in melanoma such as asymmetry, irregular border, color variation, or diameter greater than 6 mm [2].

28.4 Histopathology

Histopathological examination shows that dilated capillary vessels, often converted into a solitary, sinusoidal vascular channel, are present in the papillary dermis: the overlying epidermis shows a variable degree of hyperkeratosis and acanthosis with elongated rete ridges growing down to surround the dilated vascular channels in the dermis.

28.5 Dermoscopy Features

Dermoscopy is a valuable tool for diagnosis [5]. A study evaluated 32 patients with solitary angiokeratomas, and the dermoscopic findings showed dark lacunae (94%), whitish veil (91%), erythema (69%), peripheral erythema (53%), red lacunae (53%), and hemorrhagic crusts (53%).

It is helpful in improving the diagnostic accuracy of solitary angiokeratomas and allows the observer to differentiate them from other cutaneous tumors such as malignant melanomas and pigmented basal cell carcinomas.

28.6 Treatment

It is important to reassure patients that angiokeratomas are benign and are not contagious or sexually transmitted. Treatment is generally not recommended. Treatment can be done through surgical excision or physical and chemical cauterization. Angiokeratomas can be removed by simple excision with closure if lesions are few. Cryotherapy, electrocautery, and radiofrequency may be applied for multiple lesions. Laser Yag or CO_2 are effective with less scarring [6].

Angiokeratoma: Breaking the Myths

- Although angiokeratomas are benign, dark, finding dilated capillary vessels, and the presence of malignant melanoma should be ruled out by dermoscopy or histopathology.
- When angiokeratomas are disseminated and develop in the young, they may actually represent Fabry disease, an x-linked deficiency of galactosidase A.
- Since the etiopathogenesis may be related to increased local venous pressure and consequent subepithelial vascular dilatation, the risk factors may contain excess weight and past hysterectomy.

References

1. Buljan M, Poduje S, Situm M, Bulat V, Bolanca Z, Tomas D. Multiple angiokeratomas of the vulva: case report and literature review. Acta Dermatovenerol Croat. 2010;18(4):271–5.
2. Cohen PR, Young AW Jr, Tovell HM. Angiokeratoma of the vulva: diagnosis and review of the literature. Obstet Gynecol Surv. 1989;44(5):339–46.
3. Koufakis T, Gabranis I. Fordyce angiokeratoma. Pan Afr Med J. 2014;19:376.
4. Luna PC, Boggio P, Larralde M. Dermatologic aspects of Fabry disease. J Inborn Errors Metab Screen. 2016;1(2016):4.
5. Zaballos P, Daufí C, Puig S, Argenziano G, Moreno-Ramírez D, Cabo H, Marghoob AA, Llambrich A, Zalaudek I, Malvehy J. Dermoscopy of solitary angiokeratomas: a morphological study. Arch Dermatol. 2007;143(3):318–25.
6. Oni G, Mahaffey P. Treatment of angiokeratoma of the vulva with pulsed dye laser therapy. J Cosmet Laser Ther. 2010;12(1):51–2.

Part VII

Vulvar Lesions: Red Lesions—Nodules

Furunculosis

29

Amanda Selk

29.1 Introduction

Furuncles and carbuncles are deep infections of the hair follicles, and thus they only occur in hair-bearing skin. With furuncles, the infection is deeper than in folliculitis, and there is often a small collection of pus (an abscess) in the subcutaneous tissue [1]. The pus collecting causes the furuncle to grow. If multiple inflamed hair follicles coalesce with infected material draining into a single inflammatory mass, they are referred to as a carbuncle [1].

29.2 Clinical Presentation

Furuncles present as painful red nodules. The skin surrounding the nodule is also commonly red. As furuncles grow, they usually become increasingly painful. A white yellow tip develops which eventually bursts and pus drains from the area. This often gives patients relief.

Furuncles are diagnosed based on history and physical examination. They occur most often in areas that are affected by sweat and friction. They can occur in any individual but are more common in those who are immunosuppressed [1].

A. Selk (✉)
Women's College Hospital, Mount Sinai Hospital, University of Toronto, Toronto, ON, Canada

29.3 Pathogenesis

They often occur when bacteria enter damaged skin (such as cuts or bites). The most common bacteria involved is *Staphylococcus aureus* [1]. However, in the vulvar area, multi-organism infections occur more often and can include gram negatives and anaerobes [2]. Infections caused by methicillin-resistant *Staphylococcus aureus* (MRSA) are increasingly common and can be difficult to treat [3, 4].

29.4 Treatment

In general, the treatment of furuncles involves instructing patients to apply warm compresses four times a day to help aid in drainage. Patients should be reminded not to squeeze the lesions. They should wash their hands with soap and water after touching the furuncle to prevent spreading to other areas or people. A furuncle that is large or not resolving may require an incision and drainage [1]. If drained, the contents should be sent for culture and sensitivities to help guide antibiotic treatment [1].

Rare complications include the development of cellulitis or sepsis [1]. In these circumstances, systemic antibiotics in addition to incision and drainage are warranted.

Although recurrences are common, immunosuppression should be considered in those cases. In addition, recurrences can require searching for

J. Bornstein (ed.), *Vulvar Disease*, https://doi.org/10.1007/978-3-319-61621-6_29

reservoirs of *Staphylococcus* in household contacts or other areas of the body (like the nose or vagina) and treating those reservoirs [3, 4].

Furunculosis: Breaking the Myths

- In contrast to folliculitis, furuncles are deep rather than superficial infections of the hair follicle.
- *Staphylococcus aureus* and methicillin-resistant *Staphylococcus aureus* (MRSA) may be the causative agents.
- Multi-organism infections are more common in the vulvar area and can include gram negatives and anaerobes.

References

1. Stulberg DL, Penrod MA, Blatny RA. Common bacterial skin infections. Am Fam Physician. 2002;66(1):119–24.
2. Summanen PH, Talan DA, Strong C, et al. Bacteriology of skin and soft-tissue infections: comparison of infections in intravenous drug users and individuals with no history of intravenous drug use. Clin Infect Dis. 1995;20(Suppl 2):S279–82.
3. Ibler KS, Kromann CB. Recurrent furunculosis - challenges and management: a review. Clin Cosmet Investig Dermatol. 2014;7:59–64.
4. Reichman O, Sobel JD. MRSA infection of buttocks, vulva, and genital tract in women. Curr Infect Dis Rep. 2009;11(6):465–70.

Prurigo Nodularis

30

Amanda Selk

30.1 Introduction

Prurigo nodularis is a condition involving itchy hard nodules on the skin and occurs most commonly in adults. It can affect men and women of any age.

30.2 Clinical Presentation

Often multiple lesions are present (Fig. 30.1). The distribution of lesions is often symmetric, and they commonly first appear on the arms and legs [1].

Patients often have an atopic history [2]. Prurigo nodularis occurs in 5% of patients with human immunodeficiency virus (HIV), especially in those with low CD4 counts [3].

Affected individuals often complain of intense itching.

30.3 Treatment

Treatment is often multimodal and needs to address both the itching and healing of the lesions [1]. The itch-scratch cycle that occurs is often difficult to treat.

Treatment can include topical or intralesional steroids [1]. When steroids fail, lesions may respond to treatment with calcineurin inhibitors or UV phototherapy [1]. There is also randomized controlled trial (RCT) evidence supporting the use of topical calcipotriol ointment [4].

Daily systemic antihistamines are also an important component in treatment. In cases of intractable itching, topical capsaicin has been used [1]. Case series have been published promoting the use of pregabalin or gabapentin to treat

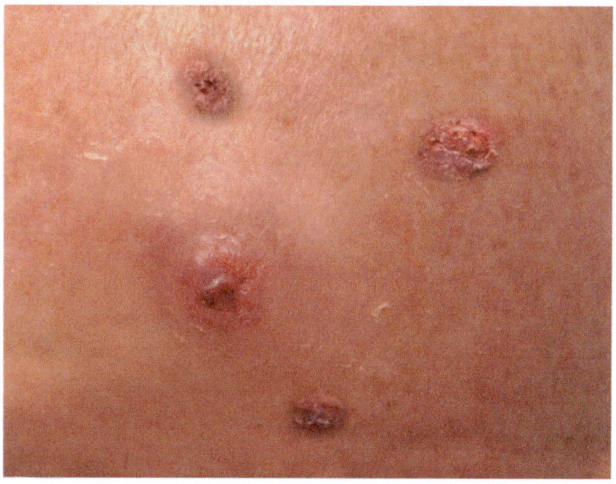

Fig. 30.1 Prurigo nodularis: multiple itchy hard nodules on the skin. They are excoriated as a result of constant pruritus. Courtesy of Professor Jacob Bornstein

A. Selk (✉)
Women's College Hospital, Mount Sinai Hospital, University of Toronto, Toronto, ON, Canada

J. Bornstein (ed.), *Vulvar Disease*, https://doi.org/10.1007/978-3-319-61621-6_30

itch that is unresponsive to other treatments [1]. In very resistant cases, some small series of patients have been treated with thalidomide, cyclosporine, and methotrexate [5–7].

It is very important to stop the itch-scratch cycle which can involve daily antihistamines, keeping nails short, wearing gloves, etc. [1]. The use of sedating antihistamines a few hours before bed can help with nighttime itching. Cooling agents are sometimes used for relief such as those with menthol or camphor or simply the application of cold compresses [8].

In general, prurigo nodularis is a disease that recurs after treatment, and complete resolution of lesions is uncommon [1].

Prurigo Nodularis: Breaking the Myths

- Prurigo nodularis is a rare cause of vulvar pruritus.
- It consists of symmetric distribution of hard nodules on the vulva but also on the arms and legs.
- The pruritus is intractable to many treatments. Among the various therapeutic options that have been described are topical or intralesional steroids, calcineurin inhibitors, UV phototherapy, topical calcipotriol (a vitamin D derivative) ointment, systemic antihistamines, topical capsaicin, oral pregabalin, gabapentin, thalidomide, cyclosporine, or methotrexate. Cooling agents with menthol or camphor or cold compresses have also been used.

References

1. Tsianakas A, Zeidler C, Stander S. Prurigo Nodularis management. Curr Probl Dermatol. 2016;50:94–101.
2. Tanaka M, Aiba S, Matsumura N, Aoyama H, Tagami H. Prurigo nodularis consists of two distinct forms: early-onset atopic and late-onset non-atopic. Dermatology. 1995;190(4):269–76.
3. Zancanaro PC, McGirt LY, Mamelak AJ, Nguyen RH, Martins CR. Cutaneous manifestations of HIV in the era of highly active antiretroviral therapy: an institutional urban clinic experience. J Am Acad Dermatol. 2006;54(4):581–8.
4. Wong SS, Goh CL. Double-blind, right/left comparison of calcipotriol ointment and betamethasone ointment in the treatment of Prurigo nodularis. Arch Dermatol. 2000;136(6):807–8.
5. Lim VM, Maranda EL, Patel V, Simmons BJ, Jimenez JJ. A review of the efficacy of thalidomide and Lenalidomide in the treatment of refractory Prurigo Nodularis. Dermatol Ther (Heidelb). 2016;6(3):397–411.
6. Siepmann D, Luger TA, Stander S. Antipruritic effect of cyclosporine microemulsion in prurigo nodularis: results of a case series. J Dtsch Dermatol Ges. 2008;6(11):941–6.
7. Spring P, Gschwind I, Gilliet M. Prurigo nodularis: retrospective study of 13 cases managed with methotrexate. Clin Exp Dermatol. 2014;39(4):468–73.
8. Burkhart CG, Burkhart HR. Contact irritant dermatitis and anti-pruritic agents: the need to address the itch. J Drugs Dermatol. 2003;2(2):143–6.

31 Urethral Caruncle and Prolapse

Amanda Selk

31.1 Introduction

Urethral caruncles are benign lesions that measure less than 1 cm in size and appear as bright red papules most commonly on the posterior edge of the urethra [1] (Fig. 31.1). A urethral prolapse can be identified by tissue that appears bright red circumferentially in a doughnut shape around the distal urethral meatus.

Urethral caruncles are the most common benign tumor of the female urethra [2].

31.2 Clinical Presentation

The diagnosis of a caruncle or prolapse is based on clinical exam findings of a soft pink or red mass protruding for the urethral meatus often <1 cm in size.

Most commonly, urethral caruncles and urethral prolapse are asymptomatic lesions that are found incidentally on clinical exam [3]. Alternatively, the presentation can involve the patient noticing small amounts of blood on their underwear or the toilet paper when wiping [2, 3]. Some patients complain of irritation when they are voiding or when they are wiping the area. In general, urethral caruncles and prolapse are usually not painful.

A. Selk (✉)
Women's College Hospital, Mount Sinai Hospital, University of Toronto, Toronto, ON, Canada

31.3 Pathogenesis

The etiology of caruncles and prolapse is unknown, but they seem to be related to low estrogen states as they occur predominantly in women who are postmenopausal. They are also seen in school-age prepubertal girls [2]. In the

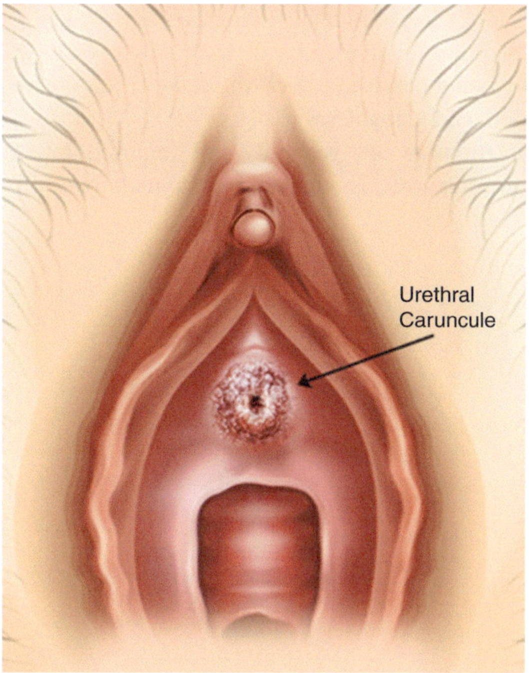

Fig. 31.1 A drawing depicting a urethral caruncle. This is the most common benign tumor of the female urethra. It should be differentiated from urethral prolapse. Courtesy of Professor Jacob Bornstein

J. Bornstein (ed.), *Vulvar Disease*, https://doi.org/10.1007/978-3-319-61621-6_31

pediatric population, most cases are seen in black females [2]. Rare cases have been reported in premenopausal women [4].

Other risk factors for developing urethral prolapse are chronic cough, obesity, and constipation [2, 4].

31.4 Differential Diagnosis

A differential diagnosis for distal urethral lesions also includes urethral diverticulum, leiomyoma, paraurethral gland abscess, and cancer [5, 6].

31.5 Treatment

Treatment is not required if patients are asymptomatic. If treatment is desired, it usually involves topical estrogen to the affected area for several months. The dose is often tapered from daily for a few weeks to maintenance therapy 2–3×/week similarly to the treatment for vaginal atrophy [3]. Surgery has been reported in cases that are symptomatic and fail medical therapy and in rare cases of strangulation and necrosis, acute urinary retention, and malignancy [3, 4].

Biopsies are generally not required unless the diagnosis is uncertain or a malignancy is suspected.

Urethral Caruncle and Prolapse: Breaking the Myths

- Many clinicians do not differentiate between urethral caruncle and prolapse; a urethral caruncle is a benign lesion of the distal urethra. Urethral prolapse occurs when the urethral mucosa is everted circumferentially all the way around the urethral meatus.
- Urethral caruncles are the most common benign tumors of the female urethra.
- Urethral prolapse should be considered in the differential diagnosis of vaginal bleeding due to estrogen deficiency, mainly in the postmenopausal.

References

1. Ozkurkcugil C, Ozkan L, Tarcan T. The effect of asymptomatic urethral caruncle on micturition in women with urinary incontinence. Korean J Urol. 2010;51(4):257–9.
2. Chiba M, Toki A, Sugiyama A, et al. Urethral caruncle in a 9-year-old girl: a case report and review of the literature. J Med Case Rep. 2015;9:71.
3. Kleinjan JH, Vos P. Strangulated urethral prolapse. Urology. 1996;47(4):599–601.
4. Jessop ML, Zaslau S, Al-Omar O. A case of strangulated urethral prolapse in a premenopausal adult female. Case Rep Urol. 2016;2016:1802623.
5. Schneider E, Sims SM, Davis JD. An unusual-appearing suburethral diverticulum resulting from trauma: a case report. J Reprod Med. 2014;59(3–4):174–6.
6. de Lima Junior MM, Sampaio CB, Ticianeli JG, de Lima MM, Granja F. Leiomyoma--a rare benign tumor of the female urethra: a case report. J Med Case Rep. 2014;8:366.

Mammary-Like Gland Adenoma: Hidradenoma Papilliferum

32

Amanda Selk, David Nunns, and Sandra Ronger Savle

32.1 Introduction

Mammary-like gland adenoma (hidradenoma papilliferum) is a rare benign tumor. These tumors were previously thought to arise from apocrine sweat glands but are now thought to be adenomas of mammary-like anogenital glands [1].

32.2 Pathogenesis

The etiology of hidradenoma papilliferum is unknown. In a single institution review, they were found to be the most common vulvar adnexal lesions [2]. Excised vulvar specimens have shown histologic and immunochemical staining similar to that seen in breast tissue [3–5]. Hidradenoma is usually seen between 30 and 49 years.

A. Selk (✉)
Women's College Hospital, Mount Sinai Hospital, University of Toronto, Toronto, ON, Canada

D. Nunns
Department of Gynaecological Oncology, Nottingham University Hospital, Nottingham, UK

S. Ronger Savle
Department of Dermatology and Gynecology, Lyon 1 University and Centre Hospitalier Lyon Sud, Pierre Bénite, Lyon, France

32.3 Clinical Presentation

Hidradenoma papilliferum usually presents as an asymptomatic, slow-growing nodule, in middle-aged women [1]. The lesions are skin colored or red and located on the vulva or perianal area [1]. When lesions appear in the vulva, they often develop in the interlabial sulcus or adjacent on the perineum [1, 6] (Figs. 32.1 and 32.2). The lesions can ulcerate or bleed which can lead them

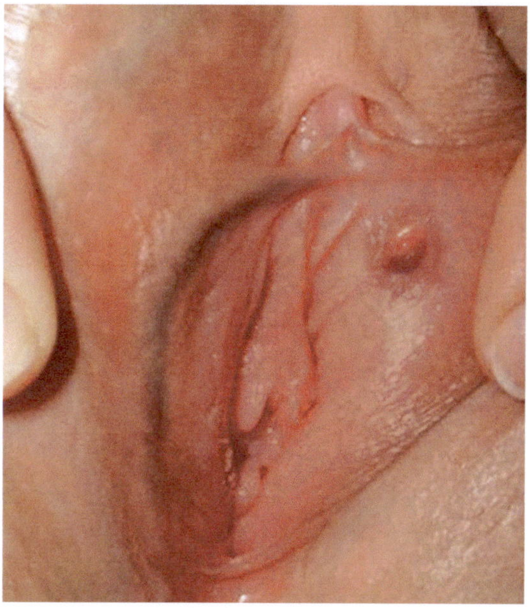

Fig. 32.1 Hidradenoma papilliferum, a skin-colored 3 mm nodule on the left labia minora

J. Bornstein (ed.), *Vulvar Disease*, https://doi.org/10.1007/978-3-319-61621-6_32

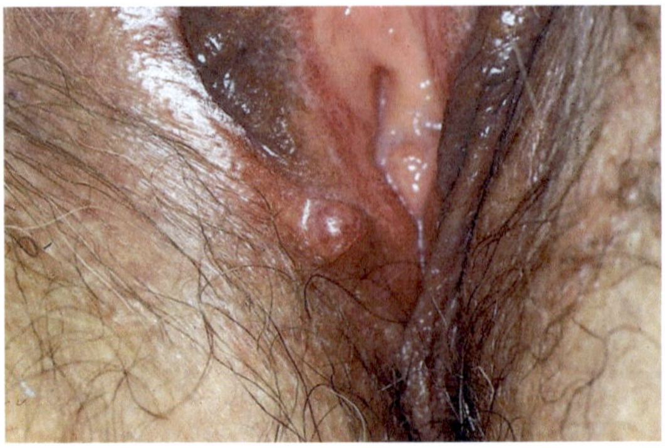

Fig. 32.2 Hidradenoma papilliferum between the right labia minora and labia majora

to be confused with malignancy, and they should be excised or biopsied in this circumstance [7].

32.4 Treatment

Treatment is not required except for cosmetic reasons or if there are concerning signs for malignancy such as ulceration, bleeding, pain, a lesion that is growing, etc. [1, 7, 8].

If treatment is desired, the lesion is excised surgically, and the condition is generally cured and not recurrent.

Hidradenoma Papilliferum: Breaking the Myth

- Hidradenoma papilliferum may have alarming glandular features in histopathological examination. However, it is a benign tumor.

References

1. El-Khoury J, Renald MH, Plantier F, Avril MF, Moyal-Barracco M. Vulvar hidradenoma papilliferum (HP) is located on the sites of mammary-like anogenital glands (MLAGs): analysis of the photographs of 52 tumors. J Am Acad Dermatol. 2016;75(2):380–4.
2. Baker GM, Selim MA, Hoang MP. Vulvar adnexal lesions: a 32-year, single-institution review from Massachusetts General Hospital. Arch Pathol Lab Med. 2013;137(9):1237–46.
3. Konstantinova AM, Kyrpychova L, Belousova IE, et al. Anogenital mammary-like glands: a study of their normal histology with emphasis on glandular depth, presence of columnar epithelial cells, and distribution of elastic fibers. Am J Dermatopathol. 2016;39(9):663–7.
4. Konstantinova AM, Michal M, Kacerovska D, et al. Hidradenoma Papilliferum: a Clinicopathologic study of 264 tumors from 261 patients, with emphasis on mammary-type alterations. Am J Dermatopathol. 2016;38(8):598–607.
5. Konstantinova AM, Stewart CJ, Kyrpychova L, Belousova IE, Michal M, Kazakov DV. An immunohistochemical study of anogenital mammary-like glands. Am J Dermatopathol. 2016;39(8): 599–605.
6. Kurashige Y, Kishida K, Kurashige K, Minemura T, Nagatani T. Hidradenoma papilliferum of the vulva in association with an anogenital mammary-like gland. J Dermatol. 2014;41(5):411–3.
7. Duhan N, Kalra R, Singh S, Rajotia N. Hidradenoma papilliferum of the vulva: case report and review of literature. Arch Gynecol Obstet. 2011;284(4): 1015–7.
8. Scurry J, van der Putte SC, Pyman J, Chetty N, Szabo R. Mammary-like gland adenoma of the vulva: review of 46 cases. Pathology. 2009;41(4):372–8.

Part VIII

Vulvar Lesions: White Lesions—Papules and Nodules, Patches and Plaques

33 White Papules and Nodules: Fordyce Spots, Sebaceous Cyst, Milia, and Hailey–Hailey Disease

Gayle Fischer

33.1 Fordyce Spots

Fordyce spots is the name given to a normal feature of the non-keratinising epithelium of the vestibule and are visible sebaceous glands containing the same lipids found in the sebaceous glands of the skin. They appear as yellow micropapules just below the mucosal surface (Fig. 33.1).

Although found in all individuals, they are more visible in some than others; however, this is part of the normal spectrum. They are also found on the buccal mucosa.

Fordyce spots are benign and normal, but their significance is that patients may become concerned about them, and they can be confused with disease states.

Sebaceous gland hyperplasia can occur on the inner aspects of the labia minora. In this condition patients have numerous, prominent sebaceous glands. These glands contain androgen receptors and may become enlarged and painful, particularly in the premenstrual week. This condition is known as sebaceous adenitis [1] and is often mistaken for genital herpes.

No treatment other than reassurance is required.

Fordyce spots, which are normal, should not be confused with Fox-Fordyce disease.

G. Fischer (✉)
Dermatology, Sydney Medical School Northern, The University of Sydney, Sydney, Australia
e-mail: gayle.fischer@sydney.edu.au

33.2 Sebaceous Cysts

33.2.1 Introduction

These benign lesions are quite common on the vulva and are often multiple, involving the labia majora bilaterally. The age of onset can be any time from adolescence onward, but they are most common in middle age and increase in number with time.

33.2.2 Clinical Presentation

The cysts appear as yellow, ovoid, mobile dermal nodules with a punctum. The size varies from a few millimetres to 20 mm. The content of the cyst

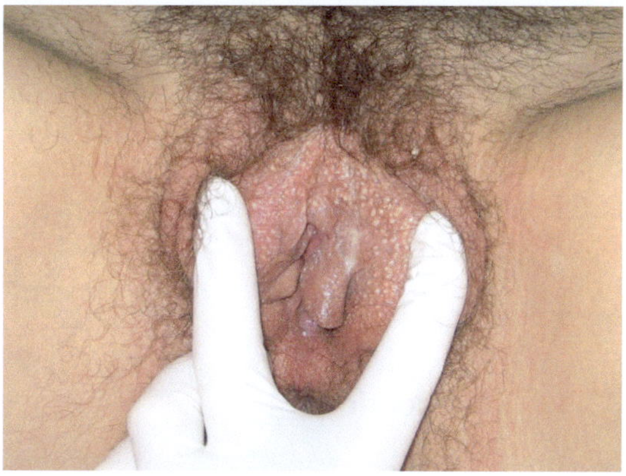

Fig. 33.1 Fordyce spots in this case very prominent yellow micropapules on the inner surface of the labia minora

J. Bornstein (ed.), *Vulvar Disease*, https://doi.org/10.1007/978-3-319-61621-6_33

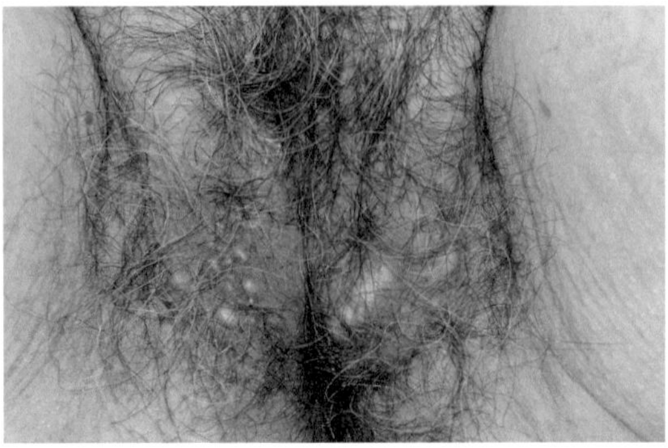

Fig. 33.2 Sebaceous cysts: yellow, nodular lesions found on the labia majora

is lipid material which has an unpleasant odour (Fig. 33.2).

Sebaceous cysts of the vulva are usually a cosmetic problem but may become inflamed and secondarily infected and then rupture. Attempting to squeeze out the contents inexpertly can potentiate this situation.

Patients with sebaceous cysts present for one of two reasons: either they are embarrassed about the appearance or the cyst has become inflamed and painful. If the latter has occurred incision and drainage, relieve the discomfort immediately. If there is secondary cellulitis, this should be treated with antibiotics.

33.2.3 Treatment

Sebaceous cysts of the vulva are very easily excised if the patient wants them removed for cosmetic reasons. A small incision is made over the cyst which can then be extracted with fine forceps. For large lesions some dissection is required, and the resulting cavity may need to be sutured.

33.3 Milia

33.3.1 Introduction

Milia are small subepidermal keratin-filled cysts which may form on any part of the skin surface.

33.3.2 Clinical Presentation

Milia are spherical, white, or yellow in colour and usually only 1–2 mm in diameter [2]. They do not have a punctum, unlike sebaceous cysts. Milia often form in the ruptured duct of glands during the healing process of blistering diseases but may appear in any healed wound.

33.3.3 Differential Diagnosis

On the vulva, milia may be confused with Fordyce spots, small sebaceous cysts, genital warts, and mollusca contagiosa.

33.3.4 Treatment

If treatment is required, the lesion can be pierced with a needle and extruded. Diathermy is also effective.

33.4 Hailey–Hailey Disease

33.4.1 Introduction

This is a rare dominantly inherited disorder. Patients with it have an inherited tendency to fragile skin in certain areas of the body, particularly areas that are prone to friction and maceration, like the genital area.

33.4.2 Clinical Presentation

The appearance on the genital area is of a nonspecific erythematous and eroded eruption involving the labia majora and minora [3] (Fig. 33.3). Superinfection with bacteria and herpes simplex is a recurrent problem in many patients, and overheating is an exacerbating factor as it increases epidermal fragility. Patients may report blistering and erosions after intercourse.

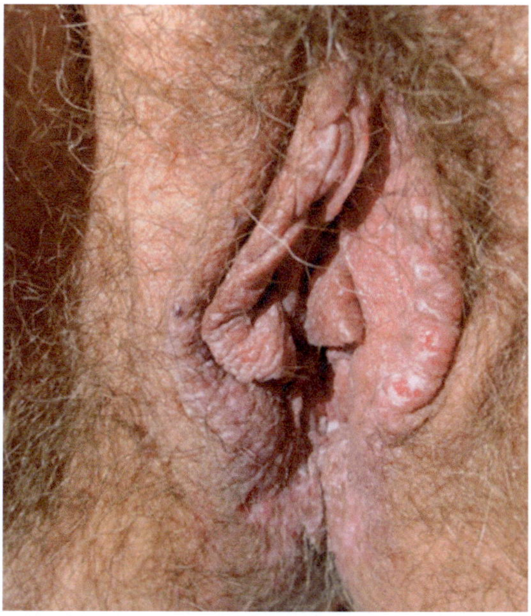

Fig. 33.3 Hailey–Hailey disease showing multiple erosions

33.4.3 Histopathology

Hailey–Hailey disease has a very characteristic histopathology which is diagnostic. The epidermal cells appear disjointed, and this is often described as a "dilapidated brick" wall by the pathologist. Most patients have a positive family history, but as with all genetic conditions, this is not invariable [4].

33.4.4 Treatment

This condition is aggravated by overheating so treatment involves climate control.

Antiviral and antibiotic medications may be needed for superinfection. Some patients improve with systemic retinoids.

Fordyce Spots: Breaking the Myths

- Visible sebaceous glands do need treatment; they are a normal finding.
- Fordyce spots, which are normal, should not be confused with Fox-Fordyce disease.

References

1. Dixit S, Olsson A, Fischer G. A case series of 11 patients with hormone-responsive sebaceous adenitis of the labia minora. Australas J Dermatol. 2014;55(1):80–3.
2. Adotama P, Susa J, Glass DA 2nd. Primary milia localized to the vulva. Dermatol Online J. 2014;20(4):22339.
3. Wieselthier JS, Pincus SH. Hailey–Hailey disease of the vulva. Arch Dermatol. 1993;129(10):1344–5.
4. Hadjicharralambous E, Diamond S, Mehregan D. Papular acantholytic dyskeratosis of vulva in setting of Hailey–Hailey. Int J Dermatol. 2017;56(6):e126–8.

34 White Patches and Plaques: Lichen Sclerosus, Vitiligo, Postinflammatory Hypopigmentation and Lichenified Diseases

Gayle Fischer

34.1 Lichen Sclerosus

34.1.1 Introduction

Lichen sclerosus (LS) is an uncommon skin disease that has a predilection for the genital skin. It is an important condition of the vulva with a reported prevalence between 1 in 300 and 1 in 1000 women and 1 in 900 girls.

34.1.2 Aetiology

The true aetiology of LS remains unknown; however, there is a well-documented association with autoimmune disease, particularly thyroiditis with about 15% of patients having thyroid autoantibodies. Other associated autoimmune conditions include alopecia areata, vitiligo, pernicious anaemia and Addison's disease.

Antibodies to extracellular matrix protein 1 (ECM-1), and basement membrane zone (BMZ) components, have also been found in patients with LS, but the significance of it is unclear as there is no clinical correlation with the presence of these autoantibodies.

Lichen sclerosus has been reported to run in families, and the HLA class II antigen HLA-DQ7 has the strongest association. Whilst these documented HLA associations are of interest, there remains a lack of clinical significance.

Vulvar LS can affect the perianal region, clitoris, internal surface of the labia majora, labia minora and the vaginal introitus. Patients with significant involvement have a figure of eight patterns encircling the vagina and anus. Early and usually before there are significant symptoms, white polygonal papules with central indentation appear which over time coalesce into plaques. The typical plaque of LS develops a smooth, atrophic, porcelain-white, cigarette-paper surface. Oedema, telangiectasia, purpura and fissures may be seen at any time (Fig. 34.1). More severe inflammation leads to blistering with haemorrhagic bullae or erosions. With time, scarring appears with loss of vulval architecture including disappearance of the labia minora and clitoris (Fig. 34.2). The appearance in children is the same as in adults, and atrophy as well as loss of vulvar architecture also occurs in children.

Symptomatically LS has a different presentation in children to adults. The average age of presentation is about 5 years of age and there is often a delay in diagnosis. Although, as in adults, itching and soreness are common, constipation and urinary symptoms are also a form of presentation that may result in children being referred to gastroenterology or urology. As in adults, some children are asymptomatic.

G. Fischer (✉)
Dermatology, Sydney Medical School Northern, The University of Sydney, Sydney, NSW, Australia
e-mail: gayle.fischer@sydney.edu.au

J. Bornstein (ed.), *Vulvar Disease*, https://doi.org/10.1007/978-3-319-61621-6_34

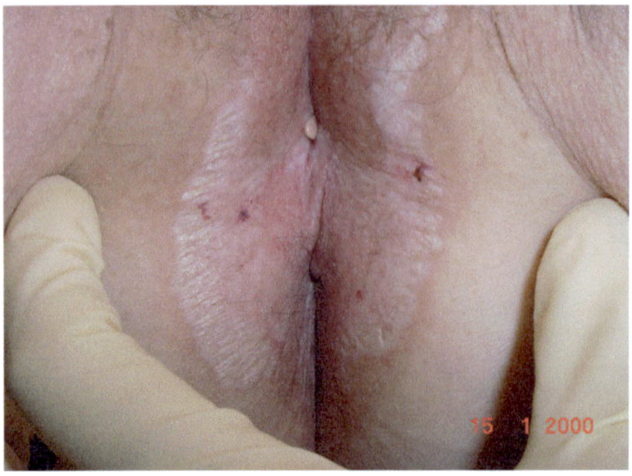

Fig. 34.1 Lichen sclerosus: typical morphology with well demarcated, white wrinkled plaque with telangiectasia

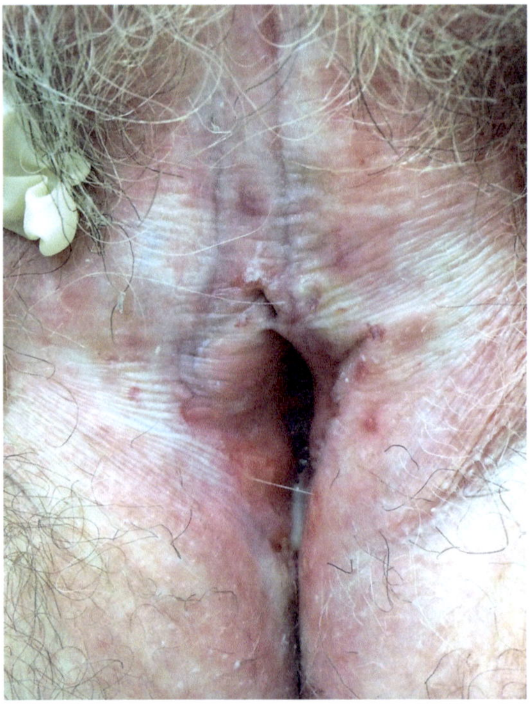

Fig. 34.2 Severe lichen sclerosus with scarring, erosions and loss of vulvar architecture

34.1.3 Clinical Presentation

Lichen sclerosus may be asymptomatic, discovered by chance by the patient or by the physician when she has a pap smear. However, it is usually extremely itchy and, because there is a tendency for the involved skin to split, also painful.

The appearance of a well-defined white plaque with an atrophic wrinkled surface and areas of purpura and erosion is classical. With time and sometimes alarmingly quickly, change in the shape of the vulva occurs in about 50% of affected patients. The labia minora are resorbed and may fuse together anteriorly and posteriorly, and the clitoris is buried beneath scar tissue so that it is not possible to retract the clitoral hood. Although the vagina is not involved, the vestibule is and stenosis of the introitus may occur.

Although LS occurs in all age groups, it is most common in postmenopausal women with only about 5% of cases occurring in children. Once it has occurred, it is very unlikely to regress spontaneously. In the past, it was believed that it could resolve at puberty; however, more recent studies have shed considerable doubt on this [1, 2]. The belief that LS will spontaneously resolve in children can lead to therapeutic nihilism and should never be relied upon. In children, as in adults, there is a high rate of scarring which can occur in the meantime [3]. As detailed below, this condition requires the same treatment in children as it does in adults.

LS also runs a cancer risk and is linked to squamous cell carcinoma of the vulva, with the lifetime risk of untreated or inadequately treated disease being 2–6%. Therefore, in order to prevent complications, patients require lifelong treatment and surveillance.

34.2 Diagnosis

Vulvar LS has a characteristic clinical presentation; however, a skin biopsy from the affected site will give a definitive diagnosis provided the lesion has not been completely suppressed with topical corticosteroid.

The histology of LS is distinctive and uniform across ages and genders. The epidermis is atrophic with hydropic degeneration of basal cells and a homogenous pale zone in the upper dermis. There is a lichenoid infiltrate of mainly mononuclear cells in the dermis.

In children, a clinical diagnosis is sufficient with a biopsy only used as a last resort because there is little to consider in the differential diagnosis and genital biopsy is likely to be traumatic.

34.2.1 Differential Diagnosis

The differentials in adults include lichen simplex chronicus, irritant or allergic dermatitis, lichen planus and neoplasia such as vulvar intraepithelial neoplasia and extra-mammary Paget's disease. Psoriasis may co-exist, causing diagnostic confusion because of superimposed erythema. Superinfection with candida is not seen in prepubertal children; however, bacterial infection with Group A streptococcus may occur causing sudden onset of pain, discharge and erythema.

Sexual abuse can be a consideration in children. The erosions, fissures, hematomas, bleeding and scarring that accompany LS can cause these concerns. There have been numerous case reports of patients with the classic presentation of LS undergoing extensive evaluation for sexual abuse; however, a diagnosis of LS does not either rule out or prove it.

34.3 Associated Malignancy

Many studies have confirmed that LS is associated with vulvar squamous cell malignancy, 'differentiated vulvar intraepithelial neoplasia' and frank squamous cell carcinoma in adults.

The long-term risk of vulvar malignancy for adults is reported to be between 4% and 6% in untreated or under-treated disease. SCC of the vulva has been reported prior to the age of 40 in patients with childhood onset LS. Recent research demonstrates that regular, suppressive treatment with topical corticosteroids markedly reduces the risk of malignancy [4].

Malignant melanoma accounts for 2% of all vulvar cancers and is considered a rare association with LS in the paediatric setting. In fact, only six cases of malignant melanoma of the vulva seen in combination with LS in a prepubescent child have previously been reported in the literature [5]. It is important to bear in mind that melanocytic proliferations associated with LS are very common and harmless. However, if there is any doubt about pigmentary change in a patient with LS, a biopsy should be performed.

34.4 Treatment

The gold standard treatment to induce and maintain remission in LS is topical corticosteroid. It was first demonstrated in 1991 that the potent corticosteroid clobetasol propionate could effectively induce a symptomatic and clinical remission in adults with LS [6]. Subsequently, this was also demonstrated in children [7].

It therefore became an accepted fact that ultrapotent topical corticosteroid was a safe and effective initial treatment in the short term, but there remained questions about subsequent steps in long-term management and whether treatment could modify the course of disease and prevent the complications of scarring and development of squamous cell carcinoma and dVIN.

The majority of patients of all age groups require long-term treatment to maintain remission of LS. Although older literature suggested that childhood onset disease would resolve at puberty, this has now been shown not to be true [7, 8].

For over two decades, virtually all publications on the treatment of LS have focussed on the use of clobetasol propionate; however, a consensus on what is the best regimen for long-term treatment was never developed. Commonly patients were told to use clobetasol daily for up to 3 months and then as needed when they experienced symptoms. Because of the potency of clobetasol, more regular treatment ran the risk of side effects such as irritation, redness and atrophy.

Recent research demonstrates however that there are viable, safer alternatives to clobetasol. In fact, it is only required in the most severe, hyperkeratotic variants. The majority of cases remit using treatment with superpotent rather than ultrapotent steroids such as clobetasol.

Superpotent products on which there have been publications include, for example, betamethasone dipropionate 0.05% or mometasone furoate 0.1% [9, 10]. The time required for the skin to return to normal ranges from approximately 3 to 18 months with a mean of about 6 months [7]. Ongoing preventative treatment with mild to moderate products, titrated to patient response so that the skin remains normal, not only prevents return of symptoms but also markedly reduces the risk of cancer and scarring. It has been shown to have virtually no side effects [9].

The target endpoint of any topical corticosteroid treatment of LS is skin of normal texture, healing of all fissures and ulcers and colour as close to normal as possible. In some cases, postinflammatory hyperpigmentation and hypopigmentation mean that this cannot be achieved completely. However, there should be considerable improvement. Some degree of erythema as a side effect is acceptable unless the patient complains of irritation or burning. In this scenario, the potency of the topical corticosteroid should be reduced. Once a regime is determined that achieves the target, it should not be changed unless this occurs or conversely the disease progresses.

Details of lichen sclerosus treatment regimen are shown in Table 34.1.

Provided patients are treated in this way and kept under regular surveillance, the prognosis of LS is very good, and it is very rare for any patient to be treatment resistant (Figs. 34.3 and 34.4). If LS is left untreated or partially treated so that only symptoms and not signs are suppressed, the risk of scarring is approximately 50% and of cancer approximately 5% [8].

Table 34.1 Flow chart for long-term lichen sclerosus management *TCS* **topical corticosteroid**

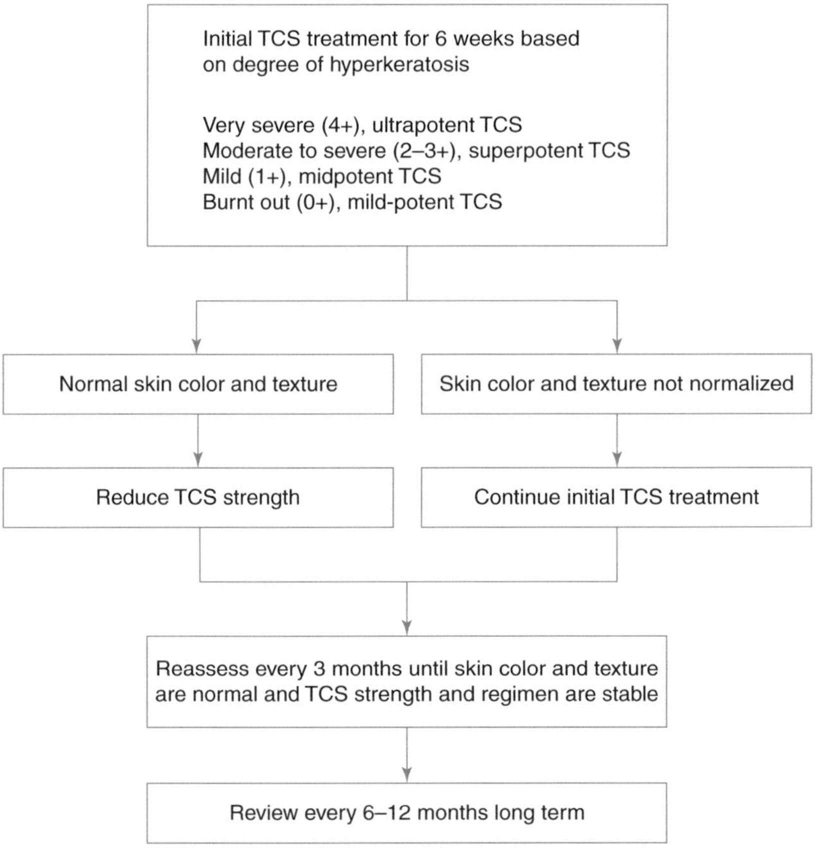

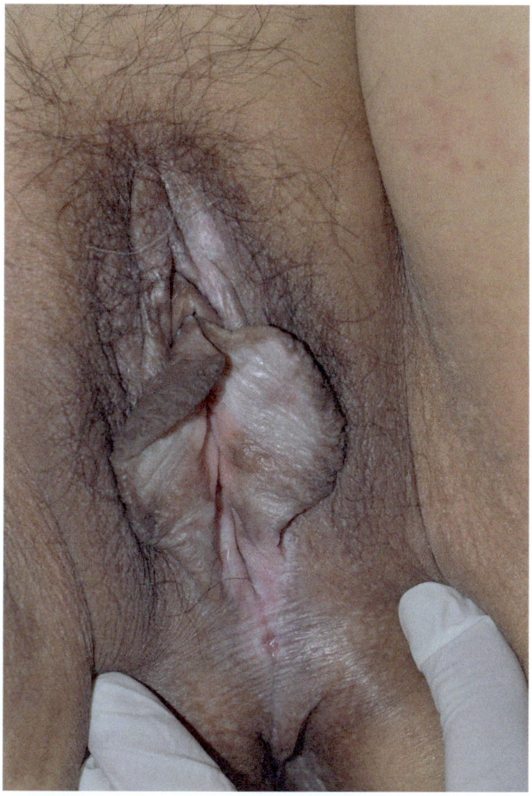

Fig. 34.3 Lichen sclerosus before topical corticosteroid treatment

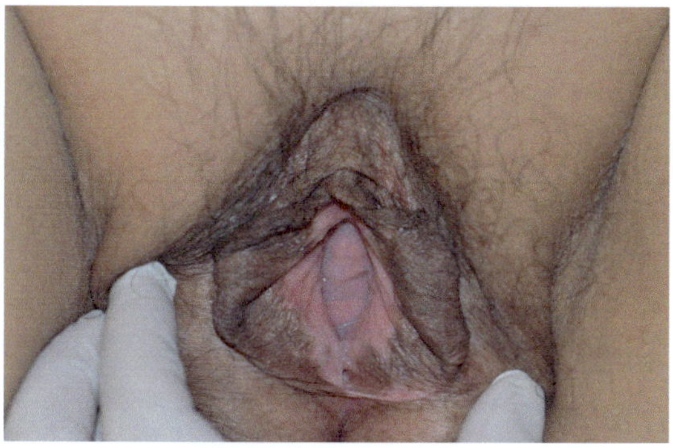

Fig. 34.4 Lichen sclerosus after superpotent induction treatment. The disease is inactive

Approach to Management: Lichen Sclerosus

- Clinical Diagnosis—White plaque with an atrophic wrinkled surface with variable degree of lichenification and areas of purpura and erosion. If untreated, the labia minora may be resorbed and may fuse anteriorly and posteriorly. The clitoris may be buried beneath scar tissue, and it may not be possible to retract the clitoral hood.
- Histopathology—Atrophic epidermis with hydropic degeneration of basal cells and a homogenous pale zone in the upper dermis. Lichenoid infiltrate of mainly mononuclear cells is in the dermis.
- Differential Diagnosis—Lichen simplex chronicus, lichen planus, chronic lichenified dermatitis (endogenous or exogenous) and neoplasia such as vulvar intraepithelial neoplasia and extramammary Paget's disease.
- Treatment—Commence treatment with ultrapotent topical corticosteroid clobetasol propionate if severely lichenified or superpotent topical corticosteroid if moderately or mildly lichenified. When the skin returns to normal (which may take several months), reduce to a moderate topical corticosteroid for maintenance therapy. Long-term follow-up is required.

34.4.1 Other Treatments

Topical immunosuppressives (TIMS), such as tacrolimus and pimecrolimus, have been described as potentially playing a role in the treatment of LS in children and adults [10]. However, the theoretical disadvantage of these topical calcineurin inhibitors is an increased risk of malignant transformation due to local immunosuppression. This is an important consideration given the association of LS and malignancy. Vulvar SCC has been reported in an adult with LS in association with pimecrolimus treatment [11]. TIMS offer no advantage over topical corticosteroids, are much more likely to cause irritation and are more expensive [12].

Historically topical testosterone has been used to treat vulvar LS. However, there is no longer any role for topical testosterone, which is ineffective and may produce androgenisation.

Vulvectomy has no role in the management of LS. However, surgical procedures have been used to divide adherent labial and periclitoral lesions and relieve introital stenosis. This must be followed with intensive topical corticosteroid treatment to prevent recurrence of scarring.

CO_2 laser treatment can occasionally play an adjunctive role in the treatment of hyperkeratotic disease which is commonly slow to respond to treatment. However, topical corticosteroid treatment must be continued afterwards.

There have been claims that platelet-rich plasma ('stem-cell') treatment has the potential to induce a cure of LS. This is not evidence based. Further work is required before this can be recommended.

In postmenopausal women, particularly those who are sexually active, vaginal oestrogen, whilst having no direct treatment effect on LS, is as useful as in any other postmenopausal woman to relieve dryness and prevent dyspareunia.

34.4.2 Follow-Up

When a patient of any age presents with LS, it is important to acknowledge that this patient will need long-term treatment and follow-up. LS is very treatment responsive in most cases, and once the vulvar skin has been returned to normal, patients require ongoing encouragement to continue with preventative treatment.

Ideally every adult patient should have the diagnosis confirmed by vulvar biopsy prior to a commitment to lifelong treatment and follow-up.

There is no single regime that suits every patient nor is there a need to compare regimes. The clinical endpoint of treatment is skin of normal texture with colour as close to normal as possible. Any topical corticosteroid regimen that achieves this is acceptable.

If scarring had already occurred prior to the diagnosis, this will not improve; however, treatment that maintains normal skin will prevent progression in most cases.

During the first year of treatment, a patient will typically require follow-up at 6 weeks, 6 months and 12 months. Once a steady state has been reached and the patient is in a good routine of regular treatment, follow-up should be yearly.

34.5 Vitiligo

34.5.1 Introduction

Vitiligo is a relatively common autoimmune disease, which results in patchy, very well-defined areas of complete loss of pigment on the skin resulting in striking white decolouration.

34.5.2 Clinical Presentation

The surface of the skin retains its normal texture (Fig. 34.5). Vitiligo is asymptomatic and harmless and is predominantly a cosmetic issue.

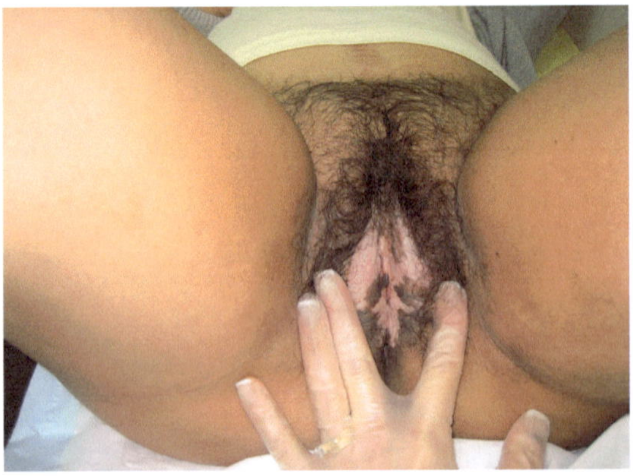

Fig. 34.5 Vitiligo showing typical well-defined macular lesion without textural change

Vitiligo may be confined to the vulva. In this location, cosmesis is less of an issue than on the skin that is normally visible to others, but in some patients, the perception is that it is still a cosmetic problem. On the exposed skin, areas of vitiligo burn easily and thus become prone to skin cancer. This is not an issue in vulvar disease.

Vitiligo can co-exist with LS. When both LS and vitiligo are found together on the vulva, the clinical presentation may be confusing. However, the key to differentiating vulval vitiligo from vulval LS is that there is no textural change. A biopsy will distinguish the two. In vitiligo, all melanocytes have disappeared. Therefore, even if LS has been treated and the classic inflammatory signs have resolved, it will still be histologically different to LS.

A useful diagnostic tool to identify vitiligo is an ultraviolet light (also known as a Wood's light). It may be obtained very inexpensively. Melanin, the pigment in the skin, is what is known as a chromophore or a substance that absorbs light. Because there is no melanin in the skin affected by vitiligo, blue light will be completely reflected, resulting in fluorescence.

34.5.3 Treatment

Vitiligo is difficult to treat, and all treatments are slow to respond, requiring many months to become effective. When vitiligo occurs on the genital area, it is doubtful that it requires treatment and patients are usually happy to be told that their condition is harmless. The treatments available are likely to be irritating, and prolonged use of potent topical corticosteroid on the vulval skin unaffected by LS will result in atrophy and peri-orificial dermatitis. Topical tacrolimus may be a better option.

When vitiligo and LS occur together on the vulva, corticosteroid treatment of the LS can result in re-pigmentation of the vitiligo after prolonged treatment. However, in the absence of LS, potent topical corticosteroids should not be used on vulvar vitiligo.

34.5.4 Postinflammatory Hypopigmentation

Any inflammatory dermatosis can result in loss of pigment from the skin. This is most often seen in and is most obvious in non-Caucasians and Caucasians with darker skin (also known as Fitzpatrick types IV and V; see Table 34.).

34.5.5 Clinical Presentation

When postinflammatory hypopigmentation occurs, the edges of the white areas are not well defined, and there is often some textural change present because of the underlying dermatosis that caused it. The patient gives a history of a previous erythematous dermatosis in the same area, including symptoms of itch. Unlike vitiligo, there is not complete loss of melanin, and therefore, the appearance is of colour attenuation, not loss. This means it looks paler than the surrounding skin rather than white and will not fluoresce when exposed to ultraviolet light.

The dermatoses that occur on the vulva that result in loss of pigment include psoriasis, any form of dermatitis and LS.

When this type of colour loss occurs after LS has been treated, it can cause confusion about when to reduce treatment. When treating LS therefore, the key is to observe very carefully for loss of textural change (thickening, atrophy, wrinkling). In some patients, it may take many months for normal colour to return, and in some, it never returns to normal.

Table 34.2 Fitzpatrick skin type

Skin type	Reaction to ultraviolet light exposure
I Very fair or redheaded	Always burns, cannot tan
II Fair	Usually burns, sometimes tans
III Medium	Sometimes burns, usually tans
IV Olive	Rarely burns, always tans
V Brown	Never burns, always tans
VI Black	Never burns, always tans

34.5.6 Treatment

Postinflammatory hypopigmentation is harmless and does not specifically require treatment. It usually resolves spontaneously once the underlying dermatosis is treated.

34.6 Lichenified Diseases

34.6.1 Introduction

Lichenification is a normal response of the skin to recurrent friction, rubbing and scratching to thicken, with an increase in the width of the epidermis. The most obvious examples of this are callouses on the hands of manual workers and corns on feet in areas of friction with footwear. To a lesser extent, any chronically itchy dermatosis may, with time, become hyperkeratotic so that the surface feels rough and thickened to the touch. This is a process called lichenification and the resultant effect is called lichen simplex chronicus.

34.6.2 Clinical Presentation

Lichenification often produces a surface that is lighter than the surrounding skin, although some forms of lichenification may be darker. It is commoner in patients of Asian descent and in atopic patients; however, not all patients are capable of lichenification.

Lichenification may superimpose on any itchy skin condition including dermatitis, psoriasis and lichen sclerosus. However, lichenification may occur in isolation, presenting as white nodules and plaques. The former has been termed pseudoverrucous papules and nodules and is rare but harmless. More often what has been termed lichen simplex chronicus is long-standing, untreated dermatitis.

The clinical appearance of vulvar lichen simplex is of white, scaly patches and papules usually on the labia majora, minora and perineum. On the perianal skin, it presents as the pale, thickened and rugose skin surrounding the anal verge. Because of the hyperkeratosis that is part of the condition, fissuring is common and painful. Persistent scratching may result in excoriation or even ulceration.

34.6.3 Histopathology

Histologically lichenified skin demonstrates a hypertrophic keratin layer, hyperplasia of the whole epidermis (acanthosis) and in long-standing cases dermal fibrosis.

34.6.4 Treatment

Treatment of most forms of lichenification is of the underlying condition, and this usually requires the use of potent topical corticosteroids for many weeks. In resistant cases, intralesional corticosteroid injection helps to break the itch-scratch cycle that often perpetuates this condition. This should be followed by ongoing prolonged preventative treatment similar to that used to maintain remission in lichen sclerosus.

Lichen Sclerosus: Breaking the Myths

- Although traditional texts emphasise the significance of establishing diagnosis before applying treatment and despite that vulvar lichen sclerosus and lichen simplex chronicus are two opposing vulvar dermatoses, treatment of these dermatoses is similar: applying potent topical corticosteroids for many weeks. In resistant cases, intralesional corticosteroid injection or calcineurin inhibitors help to break the itch-scratch cycle that often perpetuates this condition.
- If LS is left untreated or partially treated so that pruritus prevail, the risk of scarring is approximately 50% and of cancer approximately 5%.

References

1. Smith S, Fischer G. Childhood onset vulvar lichen sclerosus does not resolve at puberty: a prospective case series. Pediatr Dermatol. 2009;26(6):725–9.
2. Powell J, Wojnarowska F. Childhood vulvar lichen sclerosus. The course after puberty. J Reprod Med. 2002;47(9):706–9.
3. Ellis E, Fischer G. Prepubertal-onset vulvar lichen sclerosus: the importance of maintenance therapy in long-term outcomes. Paediatr Dermatol. 2015;32(4):461–7.
4. Lee A, Bradford J, Fischer G. Long-term management of adult vulvar lichen sclerosus: a prospective cohort study of 507 women. JAMA Dermatol. 2015;151(10):1061–7.
5. La Spina M, Meli MC, De Pasquale R, et al. Vulvar melanoma associated with lichen sclerosus in a child: case report and literature review. Pediatr Dermatol. 2016;33(3):e190–4.
6. Dalziel KL, Millard PR, Wojnarowska F. The treatment of vulval lichen sclerosus with a very potent topical steroid (clobetasol propionate .05%) cream. Br J Dermatol. 1991;121(5):461–4.
7. Virgili A, Borghi A, Minghetti S, Corazza M. Mometasone furoate 0.1% ointment in the treatment of vulvar lichen sclerosus: a study of efficacy and safety on a large cohort of patients. J Eur Acad Dermatol Venereol. 2014;28(7):943–8.
8. Garzon MC, Paller AS. Ultrapotent topical corticosteroid treatment of childhood genital lichen sclerosus. Arch Dermatol. 1999;135(5):525–8.
9. Dalziel KL, Wojnarowska F. Long-term control of vulval lichen sclerosus after treatment with a potent topical steroid cream. J Reprod Med. 1993;38(1):25–7.
10. Fischer G, Bradford J. Topical immunosuppressants, genital lichen sclerosus and the risk of squamous cell carcinoma: a case report. J Reprod Med. 2007;52(4):329–31.
11. Broeders J, Ali U, Fischer G. Systematic review and meta-analysis of randomized clinical trials (RCTs) comparing topical calcineurin inhibitors with topical corticosteroids for atopic dermatitis: a 15-year experience. J Am Acad Dermatol. 2016; https://doi.org/10.1016/j.jaad.2016.02.1228.
12. Dixit S, Scurry J, Fischer G. A vesicular variant of pseudoverrucous papules and nodules in the genital area of an incontinent 4-year-old. Australas J Dermatol. 2013;54(4):e92–4.

Part IX

Vulvar Lesions: Dark Colored (Brown, Blue, Gray or Black) Lesions—Patches, Papules and Nodules

35 Dark-Colored (Brown, Blue, Gray, or Black) Lesions: Patches

Sandra Ronger Savle

Pigmented vulvar lesions are estimated to occur in 10–12% of the general population and account for approximately 20% of vulvar disease [1]. Vulvar melanosis is the most frequent lesion among these pigmented disorders.

Pigmented vulvar lesions mainly arise on the labia majora and minora and clitoris, although they can also occur at the perineum or mons pubis.

They include melanocytic and nonmelanocytic proliferations. The differential diagnosis includes benign and malignant melanocytic proliferations, such as nevi and melanoma. Other entities marked by increased pigmentation include melanosis, post-inflammatory and physiological hyperpigmentation, and acanthosis nigricans. Nonmelanocytic proliferations such as basal cell carcinoma, vascular tumors, and seborrheic keratosis can also present as pigmented vulvar lesions (Table 35.1).

Vulvar nevi, melanosis, and melanoma are particularly challenging because of the similarity of their clinical and histopathological presentation. As such, they may be a cause of patient and physician anxiety and can result in unnecessary surgical procedures [2]. Pigmented lesions on mucosa and especially in genitalia are usually alarming. Very frequently, the diagnosis has to be performed by histologic examination. Dermoscopy is a helpful tool for the selection of the best site to perform the biopsy.

Table 35.1 Differential diagnosis and classification of pigmented vulvar lesions

	Melanocytic lesion		Nonmelanocytic lesion
	Melanocytic hyperplasia	Epithelial hyperpigmentation without melanocytic hyperplasia	
Benign lesion	Nevus	Melanosis Post-inflammatory pigmentation Acanthosis nigricans	Angiomas, angiokeratomas Seborrheic keratosis Papillary hidradenoma Mucous cyst, blackheads
Malignant or premalignant lesion	Melanoma		Basal cell carcinoma vHSIL

S. Ronger Savle (✉)
Department of Dermatology and Gynecology, Lyon 1 University and Centre Hospitalier Lyon Sud, Pierre Bénite, Lyon, France

J. Bornstein (ed.), *Vulvar Disease*, https://doi.org/10.1007/978-3-319-61621-6_35

Dark-Colored Lesions: Breaking the Myths

- Once a vulvar pigmented lesion is detected, it causes anxiety for both patient and health-care giver. For the patient, it is especially alarming. For the health-care giver, differential diagnosis is difficult. Vulvar nevi, melanosis, and melanoma are particularly challenging because of the similarity of their clinical and histopathological presentation. These situations may result in needless surgical procedures.

References

1. Hosler GA, Moresi JM, Barrett TL. Naevi with site-related atypia: a review of melanocytic naevi with atypical histopathological features based on anatomic site. J Cutan Pathol. 2008;35:889–98.
2. Venkatesan A. Pigmented lesions of the vulva. Dermatol Clin. 2010;28:795–805.

Melanocytic Nevus

36

Sandra Ronger Savle

36.1 Clinical Presentation

36.1.1 Common Nevus

A common nevus represents only 2.3% of clinically pigmented vulvar lesions [1].

They are more likely noted in young patients, especially in premenopausal women. Common nevi appear at age of 28–33 years, whereas atypical melanocytic nevus of genital type (AMNGT) at the age of 17–26 years.

Common nevi are asymptomatic and discovered incidentally during routine physical examination or self-examination. They present as symmetric macules or papules, ranging in color from pink to dark brown, black, or rarely blue. They are well-defined lesions, usually single, round to oval, and basically monochromatic. They can be acquired [2]. Their diameter is typically less than 1 cm (Figs. 36.1 and 36.2). They are often located on the labia majora, labia minora, and clitoral hood.

Most vulvar nevi are compound or intradermal nevi, but other variants such as congenital, dysplastic, blue, and Spitz nevi have rarely been reported [2].

Nevus can appear on lesions with lichen sclerosus, making the diagnosis difficult [3].

Sometimes a nevus could be asymmetric, with irregular colors. ABCDE criteria can't be applied on mucosal areas like on cutaneous lesions (Fig. 36.3).

36.1.2 Atypical Melanocytic Nevus of Genital Type (AMNGT)

An uncommon but distinctive melanocytic lesion presenting in the genital area of premenopausal women was first reported by Friedman and Ackerman in 1981. To reflect the often-worrying histologic features, which can suggest a diagnosis of melanoma, the term atypical melanocytic nevus of genital type was proposed by Clark et al. in 1998; this is frequently abbreviated to atypical genital nevus (AGN) [4]. AMNGT may be regarded as a melanocytic nevus with site-specific features and atypia similar to atypical acral nevi, flexural nevi, nevi from the breast, or conjunctival nevi.

The precise incidence of AGN is unclear, but it represents approximately 10% of all pigmented lesions and 5% of melanocytic nevi in the genital area [5].

It is most often found in the vulva of premenopausal women, and more than 50% of patients are younger than 20 years. Moreover, a personal or familial history of dysplastic nevi or melanoma may be found at increased rates in patients with AMNGT.

S. Ronger Savle (✉)
Department of Dermatology and Gynecology, Lyon 1 University and Centre Hospitalier Lyon Sud, Pierre Bénite, Lyon, France

J. Bornstein (ed.), *Vulvar Disease*, https://doi.org/10.1007/978-3-319-61621-6_36

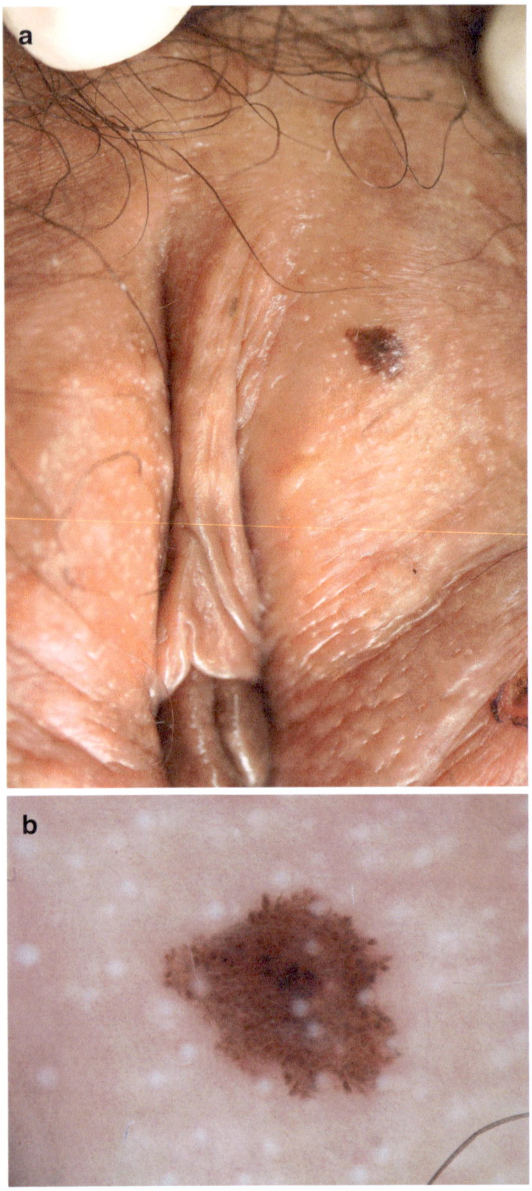

Fig. 36.1 (**a**) Intradermal nevus on the left labia majora. (**b**) The dermoscopy shows a globular pattern

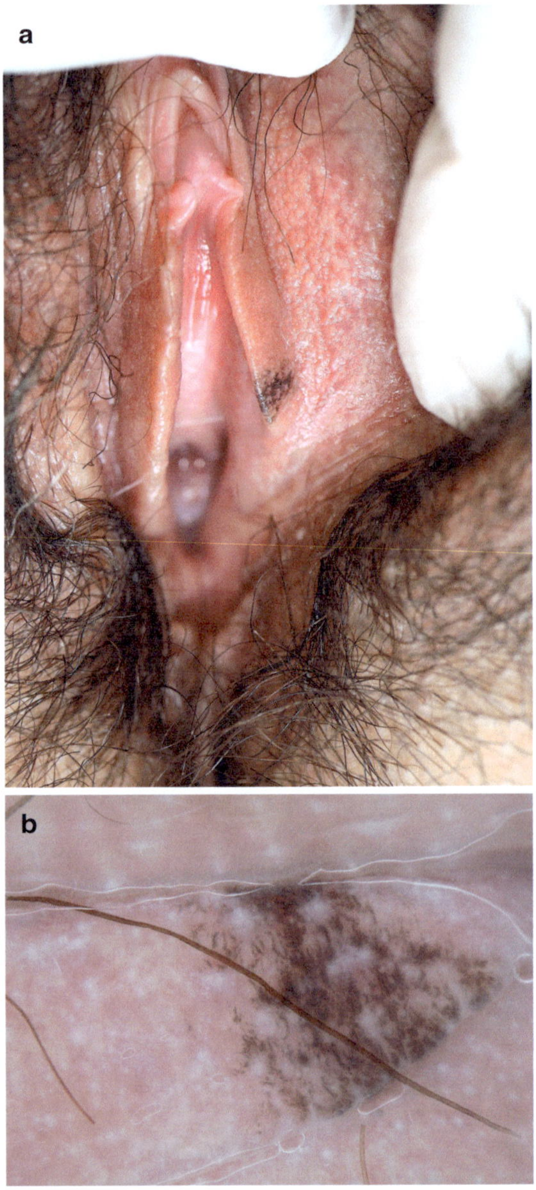

Fig. 36.2 (**a**) Compound nevus on the left labia minora. (**b**) On dermoscopy, we can see a parallel fingerprint pattern

The clinical appearances are often atypical, with hyperpigmentation and increased lesion size of up to 2 cm in diameter (median, 5.9 mm). It may present as a macule or a papule. They are often black, with different colors. The ABCDE criteria can't be applied because they may be positive on melanoma lesions, and on AMNGT, and on a nevus.

They are located mostly on the labia minora.

36.2 Dermoscopy Features

Dermoscopy may be helpful in the diagnosis of vulvar nevi. Globular and homogeneous patterns predominate among common vulvar nevi [6]. Parallel pattern is also seen but less frequently. Vascular pattern is homogeneous, and we can see generally one or two colors.

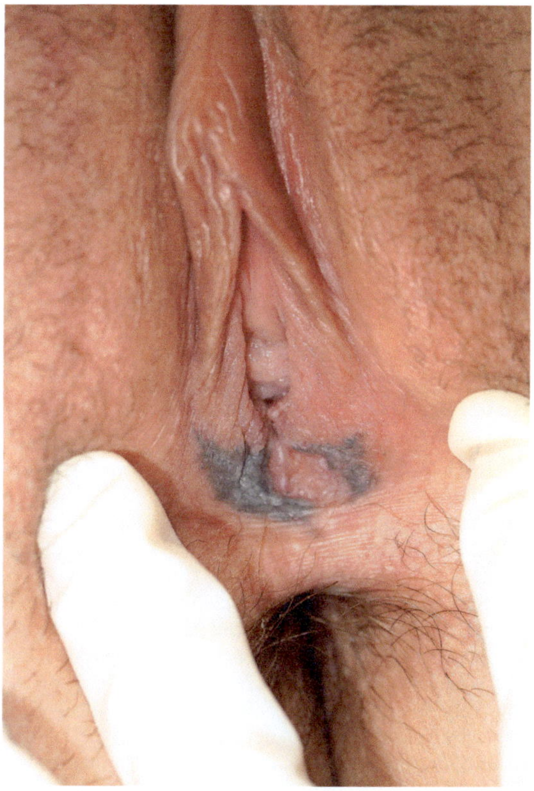

Fig. 36.3 Compound nevus of the fourchette. The ABCDE criteria can't be applied because they are positive on this nevus

36.3 Reflectance Confocal Microscopy

Reflectance confocal microscopy (RCM) is a relatively new noninvasive imaging technique that has shown promise as a diagnostic aid in many dermatologic conditions. It helps to bridge the gap between dermoscopy and histologic analysis, allowing horizontal evaluation of a lesion while producing in vivo images of the epidermis and superficial dermis at a resolution that approximates that of histopathologic specimens.

Reflectance confocal microscopy can play a role in noninvasive diagnosis of vulvar nevi, but only one paper has been published about six cases. Further broader studies are required to validate these observations [7].

36.4 Histopathology

36.4.1 Common Vulvar Nevi

They exhibit regularly sized, evenly distributed nests of melanocytes, which show no cytologic atypia.

Most vulvar nevi are compound or intradermal nevi, but other variants such as congenital, dysplastic, blue, and Spitz nevi have rarely been reported [2].

Vulvar nevi with lichen sclerosus pose an additional challenge as they can demonstrate a lichenoid lymphocytic infiltrate and melanophages with pigment incontinence that may mimic features of melanoma regression [8].

36.4.2 Atypical Melanocytic Nevus of Genital Type (AMNGT)

Most AMNGT are compound melanocytic lesions with well-demarcated and symmetric contours; the tumors appear nodular.

The junctional component is florid and composed of large melanocytic nests of variable size and shape. They are classified by Clark et al. into three patterns: nested pattern, dyshesive nest pattern, and crowded pattern [9]. Melanocytic atypia of the junctional component is present, ranging from mild to severe, but it is uniform rather than random. There is sometimes focal pagetoid spread.

The dermal component is often prominent and mushroom-shaped. Rare mitotic activity may be observed. There are additional findings: broad bands of eosinophilic fibrosis of the superficial dermis, pigment incontinence in areas, and coarse melanin pigmentation of the junctional and superficial dermal melanocytes.

There is no evidence of malignant transformation [9].

Awareness and recognition of this group are important to avoid overdiagnosis as melanoma with subsequent wide excision and possibly sentinel lymph node biopsy.

Table 36.1 Histopathologic differences among vulvar nevi, AMNGT, and melanoma

	Nevus	Atypical genital nevus	Melanoma
Lentiginous growth	Absent	Minor component	Prominent
Pagetoid spread	Absent	+/− focal and central	++ prominent
Ulceration	Absent	Absent	++
Dermal Atypia	Absent	Superficial	Confluent and deep
Dermal mitoses	Absent	Rare, superficial	Abundant and deep
Dermal maturation	Present	Preserved	Absent
Necrosis	Absent	Absent	Prominent

Data from Brenn [9]. Atypical genital nevus

In Table 36.1, we summarize the histopathologic differences between nevus, AMNGT, and melanoma.

36.5 Treatment

Vulvar nevi have benign clinical course. There is conflicting evidence regarding the presence of vulvar nevi as risk markers for vulvar melanomas. AMNGT are also believed to have low malignant potential.

The problem is that clinical examination is not helpful to discriminate nevus or AMNGT from melanoma. Moreover, the ABCDE rule can't be applied on mucosa. Dermoscopy can help, but in case of doubt, it is recommended to perform an exeresis of the lesion. If the patient is against excision, follow-up with photographies and photodermoscopy should be applied once a year.

Melanocytic Nevi: Breaking the Myths

- A common nevus represents only 2.3% of clinically pigmented vulvar lesions.
- Vulvar nevi with lichen sclerosus pose clinical and pathologic challenges as they can demonstrate a lichenoid lymphocytic infiltrate and melanophages with pigment incontinence that may mimic features of melanoma regression.
- Clinical examination is not helpful to discriminate nevus or AMNGT from melanoma. Dermoscopy can help, but in case of doubt, it is recommended to perform an exeresis of the lesion.

References

1. Rock B. Pigmented lesions of the vulva. Dermatol Clin. 1992;10(2):361–70.
2. Christensen WN, Friedman KJ, Wooduff JD, Hood AF. Histologic characteristics of vulvar nevocellular nevi. J Cutan Pathol. 1987;14(2):87–91.
3. Neri I, Dika E, Fanti PA, Misciali C, Patrizi A. Genital melanocytic naevus on lichen sclerosus: an uncommon occurrence and a management proposal. J Eur Acad Dermatol Venereol. 2016;30(5):794–7.
4. Clark WH, Hood AF, Tucker MA, Jampel RM. Atypical melanocytic nevi of genital type with a discussion of reciprocal parenchymal stromal interactions in the biology of neoplasia. Hum Pathol. 1998;29(Suppl 1):S1–S24.
5. Gleason BC, Hirsch MS, Nucci MR. Atypical genital nevi: a clinicopathological analysis of 56 cases. Am J Surg Pathol. 2008;32(1):51–7.
6. Ronger Savle S, Julien V, Duru G, Raudrant D, Dalle S, Thomas L. Features of pigmented vulvar lesions on dermoscopy. Br J Dermatol. 2011;164:54–61.
7. Cinotti E, Couzan C, Perrot JL, Labeille B, Bahadoran P, Puig S, Wantz M, et al. Reflectance confocal microscopy for the diagnosis of vulvar nevi: six cases. J Eur Acad Dermatol Venereol. 2016;30(1):30–5.
8. El Shabrawi-Caelen L, Soyer HP, Schaeppi H, Cerroni L, Schirren CG, Rudolph C. Genital lentigines and melanocytic nevi with superimposed lichen sclerosus: a diagnostic challenge. J Am Acad Dermatol. 2004;50:690–4.
9. Brenn T. Atypical genital nevus. Arch Pathol Lab Med. 2011;135:317–20.

Vulvar Melanosis (Vulvar Lentiginosis)

37

Sandra Ronger Savle

37.1 Clinical Presentation

37.1.1 Vulvar Melanosis

Vulvar melanosis is also called vulvar lentiginosis or vulvar melanotic macules. These lesions represent 68% of pigmented vulvar lesions in women. They are more commonly found among perimenopausal women with a median age of 40–44 years. The labia minora is the most commonly affected site.

When they are present in children or young adults, one should consider that they represent systemic dermatoses:

- In Peutz-Jeghers syndrome, the oral mucosa, perianal area, hands, and feet may be involved. The genetic mutation is STK11. In this syndrome one may find gastrointestinal hamartomatous polyps. An increased risk of breast, ovarian, pancreatic, and gastrointestinal cancer has been reported.
- LEOPARD syndrome or multiple lentigines syndrome is associated with the genetic mutations: PTPN11, RAF1, and BRAF. Pigmentation is located also on the face, neck, and trunk. Electrocardiographic abnormalities, ocular hypertelorism, pulmonary stenosis, abnormal genitalia retardation of growth, and sensorineural deafness may also coexist.
- The Carney complex is a mutation of PRKAR1A. It involves the eyelids, conjunctivae, and oral mucosa. Cardiac myxomas, endocrine tumors, blue nevus, and psammomatous melanotic schwannoma may also coexist.
- The Dowling-Degos disease is associated with reticulated hyperpigmentation, follicular papules, comedo-like lesions, perioral scars, and hypopigmented or erythematous macules. The pigmentation sites are axillae, groin, flexural folds, and neck. A mutation of KRT5 is found.
- Bannayan-Riley-Ruvalcaba is located on the face. It is associated with macrocephaly, intestinal hamartomatous polyposis, lipomas, hemangiomas, intellectual disability, joint hyperextensibility, pectus excavatum, and scoliosis.

Laugier-Hunziker syndrome is an acquired disorder involving 10% of the population, characterized by benign macular hyperpigmentation of the oral and genital mucosa, which is associated with longitudinal melanonychia in 50–60% of cases.

These lesions are benign melanocytic macules characterized by single or often numerous lesions with a tendency to confluence. They can be variegated in color (light brown, dark brown, slate gray, blue, or black) and with a geographic aspect (Fig. 37.1). They are mostly bilateral but

S. Ronger Savle (✉)
Department of Dermatology and Gynecology, Lyon 1 University and Centre Hospitalier Lyon Sud, Pierre Bénite, Lyon, France

J. Bornstein (ed.), *Vulvar Disease*, https://doi.org/10.1007/978-3-319-61621-6_37

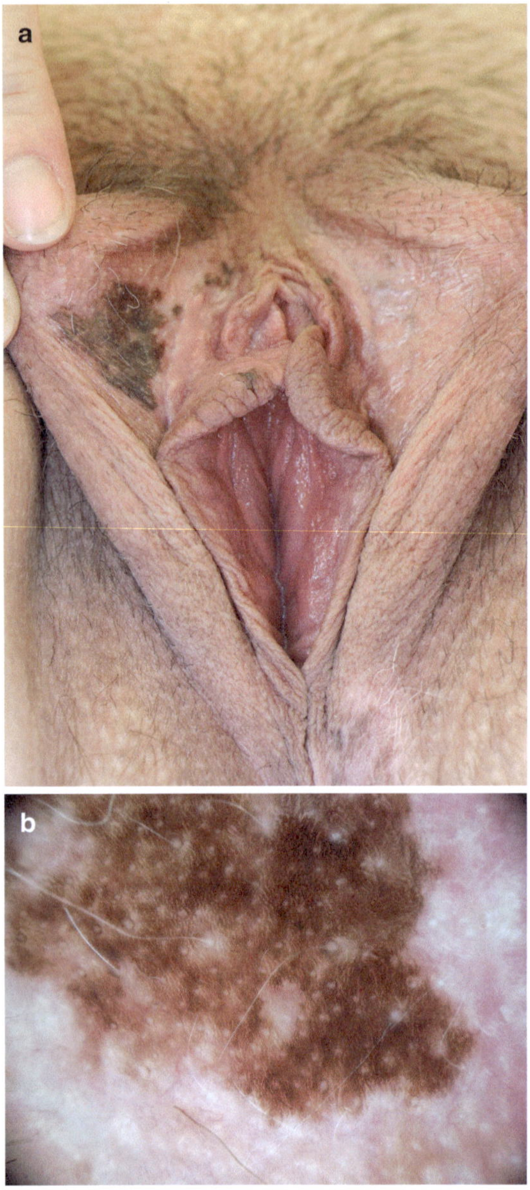

Fig. 37.1 (**a**) Melanosis on the right labia minora. (**b**) Dermoscopy shows a parallel pattern

sometimes unilateral. These lesions arise in adulthood and persist for years without changing in size or shape. They are more frequent in pigmented skin patients (phototypes IV, V, or VI of Fitzpatrick classification); their clinical aspect may resemble a melanoma in situ, being frequently misdiagnosed by non-dermatologists: it shows overlapping features with melanoma at times being characterized by asymmetry, irregular borders, multifocality, variegated pigmentary patterns, and large size [1–3].

The origin of mucosal melanosis is unclear. The excessive pigmentation could be secondary to a chronic stimulus in the area or due to a defect in the normal transport of melanin to suprabasal keratinocytes [4].

37.1.2 Lentigines, Lentigo

They may be sporadic or part of a syndrome.

It is the most common pigmented lesions of the vulva and occurs as homogeneous dark brown macules, measuring less than 5 mm in diameter on the labia minora and around the introitus.

37.2 Dermoscopy Features

It may aid in the diagnosis. The different patterns are ringlike, homogeneous, globular-like, parallel, cobblestone, and reticular-like [5]. There is the presence of aligned brown to slate gray regular globules in a more or less parallel pattern conferring a fingerprint aspect [6].

The vascular pattern is homogeneous, and there are one or two colors (mostly on lentigines).

37.3 Reflectance Confocal Microscopy

It may be used to facilitate the diagnosis of vulvar melanosis. The cells around the papillae appeared more refractive than in vulvar mucosa. We can see ringed pattern characterized by round or polycyclic papillae, with a hyper-reflective basal layer. Sparse bright dendritic cells are in the basal layer [7].

37.4 Histopathology

There is an increase in the amount of melanin in basal cells without hyperplasia of melanocytes or the presence of nevus cells. Other possible features include elongation of the rete ridges, dendritic melanocytes at the dermoepidermal junction, and melanophages in the papillary dermis [8].

When the increase of pigmentation of basal cells is associated with elongation of the rete ridges, the lesion is classified as lentigo simplex.

37.5 Treatment

Vulvar melanosis typically follows a benign clinical course. Whether vulvar melanosis is a risk factor for the development of melanoma remains unknown.

Clinical follow-up with baseline photography/photodermoscopy and sequential imaging is a conservative management approach. Biopsy should be considered if the distinction between melanosis and melanoma cannot be made on clinical or if the lesion changes over the time or new-onset melanosis in advanced age.

Vulvar Melanosis: Breaking the Myths

- These lesions represent 68% of pigmented vulvar lesions in women. They are benign melanocytic macules characterized by single or often numerous lesions with a tendency to confluence.
- When they are present in children or young adults, do not assume that they are solitary lesions. They may represent systemic dermatoses.

References

1. Barnhill RL, Albert LS, Shama SK, Goldenhersh MA, Rhodes AR, Sober AJ. Genital lentiginosis. J Am Acad Dermatol. 1990;22(3):453–60.
2. Rock B. Pigmented lesions of the vulva. Dermatol Clin. 1992;10(2):361–70.
3. Lenane P, Keane CO, Connell BO, Loughlin SO, Powell FC. Genital melanotic macules. J Am Acad Dermatol. 2000;42(4):640–4.
4. Veraldi S, Cavicchini S, Benelli C, Gasparini G. Laugier-Hunziker syndrome: a clinical histopathological and ultrastructural study of 4 cases and review of the literature. J Am Acad Dermatol. 1991;25:632–6.
5. Ferrari A, Zalaudek I, Argenziano G, Buccini P, De Simone P, Silipo V. Dermoscopy of pigmented lesions of the vulva: a retrospective morphological study. Dermatology. 2011;222:157–66.
6. Blum A, et al. Dermoscopy of pigmented lesions of the mucosa and the mucocutaneous junction: results of a multicenter study by the International Dermoscopy Society (IDS). Arch Dermatol. 2011;147(10):1181–7.
7. Debarbieux S, Perrot JL, erfan N, Ronger Savle S, Labeille B, Cinotti E. Reflectance confocal microscopy of mucosal pigmented macules : a review of 56 cases including 10 macular melanoma. Br J Dermatol. 2014;170:1276–84.
8. Heller DS. Pigmented vulvar lesions- a pathology review of lesions that are not melanoma. J Low Genital Tract Dis. 2013;17:320–5.

38 Postinflammatory Hyperpigmentation

Sandra Ronger Savle

38.1 Clinical Presentation

This acquired excess of pigment can be attributed to various preceding disease processes that affect the skin such as infections, allergic reactions, mechanical injuries, reactions to medications, phototoxic eruptions, trauma-like burning, and inflammatory diseases. This frequently follows lichen planus or lichen sclerosus in which the pigmentation may be persistent. It can develop on scars (obstetrical, gynecological).

It is more common in individuals with darker skin (Fitzpatrick skin types III to VI). The classification known as the Fitzpatrick skin type (or phototype) depends on the amount of melanin pigment in the skin. This is determined by constitutional color (white, brown, or black skin) and the result of exposure to ultraviolet radiation (tanning). Type I is pale or white skin that burns easily and tans slowly and poorly: it needs more protection against sun exposure. Type VI is darker skin that burns less and tans more easily. It is also more prone to develop postinflammatory pigmentation after injury (brown marks).

The lesions are macular pigmentation macules, unilateral or bilateral, and with tendency to confluence, on site of inflammatory lesions or on scars. The color of the lesions ranges from light brown to black, with a lighter brown appearance if the pigment is within the epidermis (i.e., epidermal melanosis) and a darker gray to bluish appearance if lesions contain dermal melanin (i.e., dermal melanosis).

Furthermore, lesions of postinflammatory hyperpigmentation can darken with exposure to UV light and various chemicals and medications, such as tetracycline, bleomycin, doxorubicin, 5-fluorouracil, busulfan, arsenicals, silver, gold, antimalarial drugs, hormones, and clofazimine.

38.2 Histopathology

The epidermal inflammatory response results in the release and subsequent oxidation of arachidonic acid to prostaglandins, leukotrienes, and other products. These products of inflammation alter the activity of both immune cells and melanocytes.

Specifically, these inflammatory products stimulate epidermal melanocytes, causing them to increase the synthesis of melanin and subsequently to increase the transfer of pigment to surrounding keratinocytes. Such increased stimulation and transfer of melanin granules result in epidermal hypermelanosis.

On the contrary, dermal melanosis occurs when inflammation disrupts the basal cell layer, causing melanin pigment to be released and subsequently be trapped by macrophages in the

S. Ronger Savle (✉)
Department of Dermatology and Gynecology, Lyon 1 University and Centre Hospitalier Lyon Sud, Pierre Bénite, Lyon, France

J. Bornstein (ed.), *Vulvar Disease*, https://doi.org/10.1007/978-3-319-61621-6_38

papillary dermis, also known as pigmentary incontinence.

38.3 Treatment

Postinflammatory hyperpigmentation tends to fade with time and therapy. Remnants of epidermal hyperpigmentation may persist for indefinite periods, typically 6–12 months, after the initial inflammatory process resolves. Dermal postinflammatory hyperpigmentation may even persist for years.

When it is clear that there have been a preceding inflammatory dermatosis, the diagnosis is easy, but if there is any doubt, or atypical features are present, a biopsy should be performed.

Post Inflammatory Hyperpigmentation: Breaking the Myths

- These lesions are pigmentation macules, unilateral or bilateral, and with tendency to confluence, on site of inflammatory lesions or on scars.
- They become darker with exposure to UV light and various chemicals and medications.
- If the diagnosis is doubtful, or atypical features are present, a biopsy should be performed.

Acanthosis Nigricans

39

Sandra Ronger Savle

39.1 Clinical Presentation

The exact incidence of Acanthosis Nigricans (AN) is unknown. In an unselected population of 1412 children, AN were present in 7.1%.

In children, it is benign and may be hereditary. In 2000, the American Diabetes Association declared that acanthosis nigricans may be a risk factor for the development of diabetes in children.

All forms of this disease, including pseudoacanthosis nigricans, seen in obese patients are now thought to be related to insulin resistance. Related disorders are type 2 diabetes, metabolic syndrome, and polycystic ovarian syndrome. Early recognition of these conditions is essential for prevention of disease progression. Obesity is closely associated with AN, and more than half the adults who weigh more than 200% of their ideal body weight have lesions consistent with AN.

In adults, some cases may be linked with malignancy, usually an adenocarcinoma. The malignant form of AN is far less common, and in one study, only 2 of 12,000 patients with cancer had signs of AN. The most frequent associations were with adenocarcinomas of the gastrointestinal tract (70–90%), particularly gastric cancer (55–61% of malignant AN cases). Approximately, 61.3% of cases are diagnosed simultaneously with the cancer manifestation, while 17.6% of malignant AN cases predate the diagnosis of malignancy.

AN may also appear as an adverse effect of medications that promote hyperinsulinemia such as glucocorticoids, niacin, insulin, oral contraceptives, and protease inhibitors.

The lesions chiefly affect the neck, the mucosa, and the flexural areas in the groin, knees, and elbows. The genital area is a site of predilection, and the vulva is involved in 5–10%. AN may also affect the eyelids, lips, mucosal surfaces, and dorsal hands.

They are dark, at first, velvety, and then warty. We can see papillomatous, brownish-black, and hyperkeratotic plaques. All aspects of the vulva may be involved [1].

While usually asymptomatic, AN is occasionally pruritic.

39.2 Histopathology

Histopathology reveals a thickened stratum corneum with minimal involvement of the dermis except for thickened and elongated dermal projections. Despite the term “acanthosis,” the actual amount of acanthosis or thickening of the stratum spinosum is variable and typically mild. The dark color of AN is likely due to hyperkeratosis rather than a mild increase in melanin

S. Ronger Savle (✉)
Department of Dermatology and Gynecology, Lyon 1 University and Centre Hospitalier Lyon Sud, Pierre Bénite, Lyon, France

J. Bornstein (ed.), *Vulvar Disease*, https://doi.org/10.1007/978-3-319-61621-6_39

pigmentation. There is papillomatosis. A subtle infiltrate composed of lymphocytes, plasma cells, or neutrophils may be present, as well as horn pseudocyst formation. Tissue staining with colloidal iron often shows infiltration of the papillary dermis with glycosaminoglycans such as hyaluronic acid, particularly in patients with gonadal disease such as polycystic ovarian syndrome (PCOS). AN is linked to variety of syndromes. Most are associated with insulin resistance or fibroblast growth factor receptor (FGFR) mutations.

39.3 Treatment

Improvement of the skin lesions is often the patient's primary concern. No randomized, controlled trials exist for any treatment of AN. Multiple case reports suggest that AN improves with treatment of its underlying condition. Treatment of the lesions of AN is for cosmetic reasons only. Correction of hyperinsulinemia often reduces the burden of hyperkeratotic lesions. Likewise, weight reduction in obesity-associated AN may result in resolution of the dermatosis. Cessation of inciting agent in drug-induced AN often results in resolution. Acipimox may be used in place of nicotinic acid to induce AN regression while improving the lipid profile. Topical medications that have been effective in some cases of AN include keratolytics (e.g., topical tretinoin 0.05%, ammonium lactate 12% cream, or a combination of the two) and triple combination depigmenting cream (tretinoin 0.05%, hydroquinone 4%, fluocinolone acetonide 0.01%) nightly with daily sunscreen. Calcipotriol, podophyllin, urea, and salicylic acid also have been reported, with variable results.

Acanthosis Nigricans: Breaking the Myths

- Acanthosis Nigricans may be a risk factor for the development of diabetes in children.
- All forms of this disease seen in obese patients, are related to insulin resistance.
- In adults, some cases may be linked with gastric adenocarcinoma.
- Acanthosis Nigricans improves with treatment of its underlying condition.

Reference

1. Grasinger CC, Wild RA, Parker IJ. Vulvar acanthosis nigricans: a marker for insulin resistance in hirsute women. Fertil Steril. 1993;59(3):583–6.

Seborrheic Keratosis

40

Sandra Ronger Savle

40.1 Clinical Presentation

Seborrheic keratosis, a benign growth lesion, is a very common cutaneous lesion encountered in white races in the fourth and fifth decade. They usually form warty proliferations that appear pasted onto the surface, are usually pigmented, and may have a waxy appearance owing to extruded keratin (Fig. 40.1).

The occurrence of this lesion on the vulva is rare, as an isolated lesion or in association with lesions elsewhere. The classical clinical features, distinct keratotic and follicular plugging and stuck on appearance, disappear because of the friction and maceration typical of this area. The mean age is over 60 years [1].

The differential diagnosis between seborrheic keratosis, malignant melanoma and genital wart is difficult.

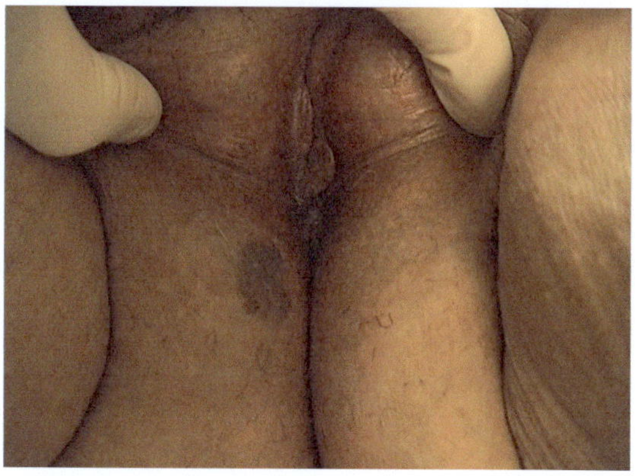

Fig. 40.1 Seborrheic keratosis on the perineum

40.2 Dermoscopy Features

We can see gland openings which created a pseudonetwork. There are multiple milia-like cysts. A cerebriform pattern is noted, like on VHSIL.

40.3 Histopathology

Broad columns of highly pigmented basaloid cells intermingled with horn cysts. They have delicate fibrovascular cores. Melanin pigment is frequently present throughout the proliferation, and the surface is usually hyperkeratotic. Mitoses are absent or rare. When irritated, there may be prominent inflammation and atypia that is characterized by mild nuclear atypia and a more squamoid appearance. But unlike vulvar HSIL, mitotic figures remain confined to the basal layers, and atypical mitoses are absent [2].

S. Ronger Savle (✉)
Department of Dermatology and Gynecology, Lyon 1 University and Centre Hospitalier Lyon Sud, Pierre Bénite, Lyon, France

J. Bornstein (ed.), *Vulvar Disease*, https://doi.org/10.1007/978-3-319-61621-6_40

Sebohrreic Keratosis: Breaking the Myths

- This is a very common cutaneous lesion.
- The classical clinical features disappear because of the friction and maceration typical of the vulva.
- The lesion sometimes look alike vulvar intraepithelial neoplasia. However, here mitotic figures remain confined to the basal layers and atypical mitoses are absent.

References

1. Giogi V, Massi D, salvini C, Mannone F. Pigmented seborrheic keratoses of the vulva clinically mimicking a malignant melanoma: a clinical, dermoscopic-pathologic case study. Clin Dermatol. 2005;30:17–9.
2. Reutter JC, Geisinger KR, Laudadio J. Vulvar seborrheic keratosis: is there a relationship to human papillomavirus? J Low Genit Tract Dis. 2014 Apr;18(2):190–4.

41 Melanoma

Sandra Ronger Savle

41.1 Clinical Presentation

Melanomas are malignant tumors arising from pigment cells: melanocytes. They arise from the neural crest, a transitory embryological structure at the dorsal borders of the neural plate.

Melanoma is the second most common malignancy of the vulva after squamous cell carcinoma, accounting approximately 10% of vulvar malignancies [1].

Vulvar melanoma accounts for approximately 1.4% of all body melanomas [2]. The Surveillance Epidemiology and End Results database of the US National Cancer Institute noted only 644 cases of vulvar melanoma from 1973 to 2003.

The incidence of mucosal melanomas remains stable over the years, in contrast to cutaneous melanoma. It is 0.1 per 100,000 females per year [3]. Its incidence is increasing with age: the median age is 68 years. However, it may be diagnosed at any age with cases reported in girls as young as 10 and women as old as age 99.

Malignant melanoma in children has been reported in lichen sclerosus, but it must be noted that junctional and compound nevi may be mistaken for malignant melanoma when they are superimposed on lichen sclerosus in children and adolescents [4]. There are six cases of melanoma on girls [5].

Family history of melanoma is noted in 15% of cases. Women are generally Caucasian and in the fifth to eighth decades of life. Compared with cutaneous melanoma, it has less marked difference in incidence across racial ethnic groups.

Risk factors for development have not been identified. HPV, HSV, and polyomavirus have no role in the ethiopathogenesis. Unlike most cutaneous melanoma, ultraviolet radiation doses do not appear to play a role in the pathogenesis of vulvar melanoma.

The etiology of vulvar melanoma is complex and multifactorial. From molecular genetic perspective, it more closely resembles acral lentiginous rather than cutaneous melanoma. KIT is the most commonly mutated gene found with sequence variants detected in up to 35% of vulvar melanomas [6]. More rarely, NRAS and BRAF mutations have been described [7].

Melanoma has high levels of chromosomal instability, with many copy number aberrations when comparing with Atypical melanocytic nevi of genital type (AMNGT) [8].

Chronic inflammation such as lichen sclerosus has been linked to vulvar melanoma, but this association is controversial [9].

Melanoma arises mainly in the clitoral area and labia majora, followed by labia minora and periurethral area. Sometimes a multifocal origin is observed.

It may present as macules, papules, or nodules of irregular coloration, asymmetric borders, and diameter larger than 7 mm [10] (Fig. 41.1).

S. Ronger Savle (✉)
Department of Dermatology and Gynecology, Lyon 1 University and Centre Hospitalier Lyon Sud, Lyon, France

J. Bornstein (ed.), *Vulvar Disease*, https://doi.org/10.1007/978-3-319-61621-6_41

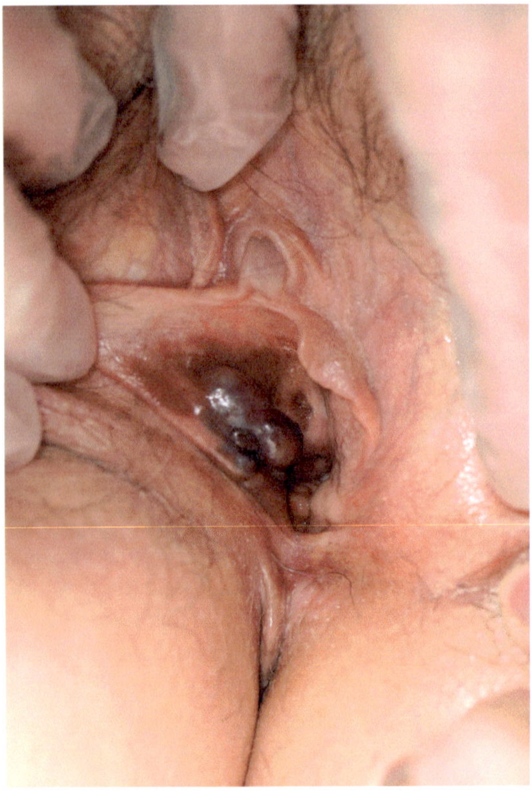

Fig. 41.1 Nodular melanoma. The prognosis is poor but the diagnosis is easy

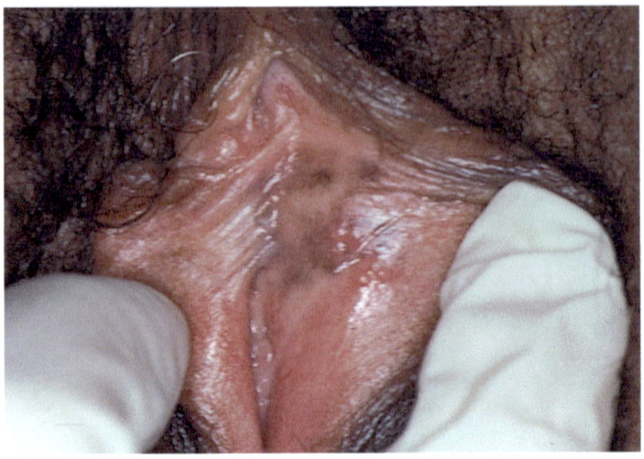

Fig. 41.2 Melanoma in situ of the left labia minora

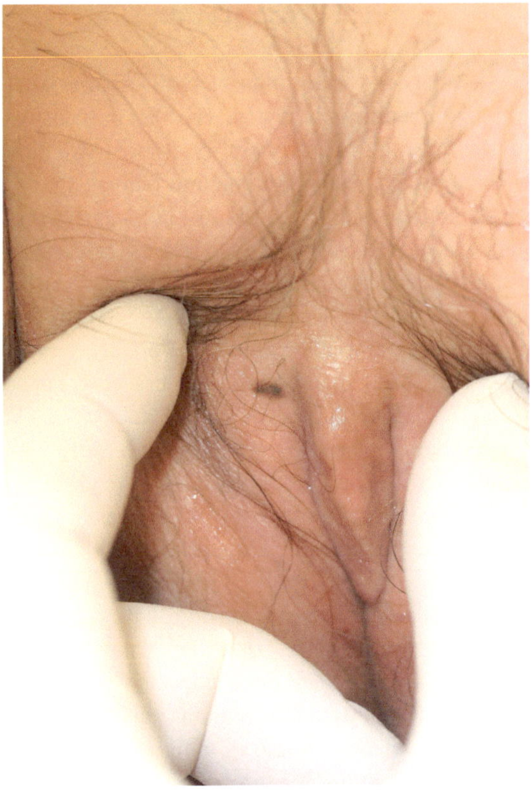

Fig. 41.3 Melanoma Breslow 0.3 mm on the right labia minora. Good prognosis, but difficult diagnosis

Melanosis may be indistinguishable from melanoma in situ clinically (Fig. 41.2). Sometimes melanoma can mimic a nevus and clinical diagnosis is impossible (Fig. 41.3). Achromic melanoma represents 27–39% of vulvar melanomas. In this form, diagnosis is almost impossible and is made late with biopsy. It is thought that about 10% arise in preexisting vulvar nevi.

Non-specific symptoms include bleeding, pruritis, discharge, irritation, lymphadenopathy, pain, or urination discomfort [11].

Metastases are commonly found in the inguinal lymph nodes. Other reported metastatic sites are the vagina, lungs, liver, and brain.

Pelvic MRI and PET scan are important in the initial evaluation of patients with vulvovaginal melanoma because of the high propensity for local, regional, and distant spread.

The scale that is generally confirmed to be the most predictive of the overall survival for vulvar melanoma is the 2009 American Joint Committee on Cancer (AJCC) melanoma staging system, which puts emphasis on the tumor invasion rather than the FIGO classification of gynecological tumors. It considers the tumor size.

A few cases of vulvar melanomas arising in a preexisting vulvar nevus have been recorded in the literature.

41.2 Dermoscopy Features

Dermoscopy helps for early detection of melanoma. Dermoscopic combination of blue, gray, or white color plus structureless zones may be predictive of melanoma. Findings are similar to those in cutaneous melanoma, including a multicomponent pattern, irregular dots and globules, multiples colors, a blue white veil, and atypical vessels. There are more than three colors.

Indeed one of the important uses of dermoscopy in genital locations is to identify atypical areas for biopsy to differentiate melanoma from melanosis.

41.3 Reflectance Confocal Microscopy

Some characteristics include loss of dermic papillae architecture; high density of dendritic cells, pagetoid cells, and melanocytes arranged in sheets and nests; and cytologic atypia with large, pleomorphic shape, bright cytoplasm, and hyporefractive nucleus [12].

41.4 Histopathology

Most of the melanoma lesions are of the mucosal lentiginous subtype. Other types are superficial spreading or nodular subtypes. Atypical melanocytes arranged as confluent nests and sheets, prominent pagetoid spread, and absent dermal maturation are typically seen. Ulceration, cell necrosis, and abundant and reticular dermal mitoses are often present.

Demonstration of melanocytes with thick dendrites, found also in the upper part of the epidermis, is a clue for the diagnosis of genital melanoma in situ [13].

41.5 Treatment

Vulvar melanomas are often diagnosed late and carry a poor prognosis, with a mean 5-year survival ranging from 27% to 60%. They are known to behave more aggressive and have less favorable prognosis compared to other melanoma subtypes. Breslow thickness, ulceration, and lymph node involvement are important prognostic indicators [14].

If melanoma is suspected, a biopsy should include as much as possible of the lesion.

There is limited data on specific treatment of vulvar melanomas, and the majority of treatment decisions are based on extrapolation from data regarding cutaneous melanomas of other sites [15].

Classification of mucosal melanomas is exactly the same as that of cutaneous melanomas, consistent with the recommendations of the American Joint Committee on Cancer (AJCC) 2009 (Table 41.1). Multivariate analysis was performed on nearly 40,000 melanoma patients from multiple treatment centers (the Melanoma Task Force). This resulted in a new guideline in January 2010. Primary tumor thickness continues to be the factor most closely correlated with prognosis. Within each thickness category, the presence of ulceration upgrades the tumor classification (from a to b). Ulceration is associated with poor prognosis, and an ulcerated tumor has equivalent prognosis to a nonulcerated tumor in the next higher (increased depth) category. Based on emerging data, mitotic rate was introduced into analyses as an independent variable and was determined to be an important predictor of outcome, second only to the primary tumor thickness. Accordingly, for the first time in over 40 years, Clark level has been excluded from the staging system. The mitotic rate (in conjunction with ulceration) has

Table 41.1 The American Joint Committee on Cancer (AJCC) melanoma classification: 7th édition, 2009/2010

Table 1. Seventh (2010) TNM staging system for cutaneous melanoma	
Primary tumor (T)	
TX	Primary tumor cannot be assessed (e.g., curettaged or severely regrassed primary)
To	No evidence of primary tumor
Tis	Melanoma in situ
T1	≤1.0 mm a: without ulceration and mitoses <1/mm² b: with ulceration or mitoses ≥ 1/mm²
T2	1.01–2.0 mm a: without ulceration b: with ulceration
T3	2.01–4.0 mm a: without ulceration b: with ulceration
T4	> 4.0 mm a: without ulceration b: with ulceration
Regional lymph nodes (N)	
NX	Patients in whom the regional nodes cannot be assessed (e.g., Previously removed for another reason)
N0	No regional metastases detected
N1	One lymph node a: micrometastases* b: macrometastases.
N2	Two or three lymph nodes a: micrometastases* b: macrometastases. c: in-transit met(s)/satellite(s) without metastatic lym ph nodes
N3	Four or more metastatic lymph nodes, or matted lymph nodes. or in-transit met(s)/satellite(s) with metastatic lymph node(s)
Distant metastasis (M)	
M0	No detectable evidence of distant metastases
M1a	Metastases to skin, subcutaneous, or distant lymph node. normal serum LDH
M1b	Lung metastases, normal LDH
M1c	Metastasis to other visceral metastases with a normal LDH, or any distant metastases and an elevated LDH

Table 2. Seventh TNM staging groupings for cutaneous melanoma			
Stage	**Primary tumor (T)**	**Regional lymph node (N)**	**Distant metastasis (M)**
Clinical staging*			
Stage 0	Tis	NO	MO
Stage IA	T1a	NO	MO
Stage IB	T1b T2a	NO NO	MO MO
Stage IIA	T2b T3a	NO NO	MO MO
Stage IIB	T3b T4a	NO NO	MO MO
Stage IIC	T4b	NO	MO
Stage III	Any T	N1, N2, or N3	MO
Stage IV	Any T	Any N	M1
Pathologic staging*			
Stage 0	Tis	NO	MO
Stage IA	T1a	NO	MO
Stage IB	T1b T2a	NO	MO MO
Stage IIA	T2b T3a	NO	MO MO
Stage IIB	T3b T4a	NO	MO MO
Stage IIC	T4b	NO	MO
Stage IIIA	T1-4a T1-4a T1-4b	N1a N2a N1a	MO
Stage IIIB	T1-4b T1-4b T1-4a T1-4a T1-4a	N1a N2a N1b N2b N2c	MO
Stage IIIC	T1-4b T1-4b T1-4b Any T	N1b N2b N2c N3	MO
Stage IV	Any T	Any N	Any M

replaced Clark level IV as a determinant of T1a vs. T1b disease.

The mainstay of treatment for these tumors is primary surgical resection with the goal of achieving negative margins. Radical surgery does not improve long-term survival time and should be performed only in large tumors.

Management of mucosal melanomas is also the same as for cutaneous melanomas; the excision margins are the same: 0.5 cm for in situ melanoma and 1 cm for T1 and 2 cm after that; however, surgery is adapted to anatomical sites, and we try to preserve essential organs, such as the urethra and clitoris. More radical procedures have not resulted in better locoregional control or survival compared with wide local excision.

The role of sentinel lymph node (SLN): [16] The Multicenter Selective Lymphadenectomy Trial 1 (MSLT 1) noted a disease-free survival advantage; however, no benefit was noted in either overall survival (OS) or melanoma-specific survival for the cohorts as a whole. SLN mapping is recommended by experienced surgeons. Sentinel node biopsy (SLNB) is recommended for T1b, T2, T3, and T4. It is a recommended requirement for inclusion in clinical trials.

Radiotherapy was not proven to improve the overall survival, but it can reduce the local recurrence rate [17]. A study on mucosal melanoma of the head and neck recommended postoperative radiotherapy to optimize local control.

Radiation treatment has customarily been used in the palliative setting for women with advanced and symptomatic disease.

There is lack of consensus as to the benefit of adjuvant therapies for high-risk melanomas (AJCC stage II or III) after surgical excision. There is a suggestion that adjuvant interferon alpha provides an improved recurrent-free survival but not an overall survival benefit.

Traditional cytotoxic therapies have resulted in a very poor improvement in survival (dacarbazine, platinum). Standard chemotherapeutics like dacarbazine show limited activity in the metastatic setting [18].

The treatment of metastatic melanoma dramatically changed over the last years. Two therapeutic revolutions emerged in parallel, *targeted anti-BRAF and anti-MEK therapies*, for patients BRAFV600 mutated, and *immunotherapy* with immune checkpoint blockers using anti-CTLA-4 then anti-PD1 monoclonal antibodies. Ipilimumab (anti-CTLA4), authorized in 2011, was the first drug which showed a benefit of overall survival in patients with metastatic melanoma in spite a low response rate (10–15) and the occurrence of about 25% of serious toxicity. Anti-PD1 appear as a new generation of immune checkpoint blockade with response rates between 30 and 40% of the patients, a proven overall survival benefit as compared with chemotherapy or ipilimumab and less toxicity than ipilimumab. Two molecules, pembrolizumab and nivolumab, were recently approved in monotherapy, for metastatic melanoma. Several questions remain unresolved: the respective indications of anti-PD1 and targeted therapies in first-line therapy in patients with BRAF mutant melanoma, the benefit of combining immunotherapy with radiotherapy or with targeted therapies, the optimal treatment duration, and the benefit of the anti-PD1 in the adjuvant setting. The combination of ipilimumab and nivolumab, recently approved by the FDA but not yet in Europe, shows an improvement of the objective response rates (50–57%) and progression-free survival compared with nivolumab but is associated with a higher incidence of serious adverse events (more than 50%). For immunotherapy, overall survival seems to be low on mucosal melanomas. For targeted therapies, vulvar melanomas have more frequently a cKIT mutation than a BRAF mutation, and the use of a cKIT-targeted therapy (e.g., imatinib) is under investigation, but rarity of mucosal melanomas and the fact that cKIT mutations are present only in a few patients make it difficult to conduct large clinical trials. A current phase II trial from the ECOG group is assessing the use of dasatinib, a multi-tyrosine kinase inhibitor, in melanomas harboring a c kit mutation [19].

41.6 Work-Up of a Pigmented Vulvar Lesion

There are various delays in the detection of melanoma: the first regards the absence of vulvar inspection, since patients and sometimes dermatologists are reluctant to examine.

The second delay concerns the clinical markers: regarding the skin, the ABCDE criteria may be helpful (asymmetry, irregular borders, color, diameter more than 6 mm, and evolutionary changes), but this algorithm does not work for mucous membranes, palms, or plants. In our experience the ABCDE criteria do not work for unique lesions or even multiple lesions. Given that clinical diagnosis is often hard to make, the clinical approach needs to be rationalized by analyzing lesions, which may be in a single or multiple form. Single pigmented lesions include flat or raised lesions and multiple pigmented lesions as well.The third delay concerns diagnostic aids. We saw that the clinical distinction is hard to make between melanoma and nevus, lentigo, post-inflammatory pigmentation, and single melanosis. That is why dermoscopy is important.

On the mucous membranes, dermoscopy may be difficult to perform since the dermatoscope is in contact with the skin, which means that the practitioner is very close to the skin. Therefore, we can use a video dermatoscope to ensure larger distance from the patient, and also DermLite dermatoscope to be able to observe the lesions from a comfortable distance. The instruments must either be covered with a transparent film and/or cleaned with antibacterial agents after use, so as to avoid viral spread.

Three major articles were published on dermoscopy and vulvar pigmented lesions: one from our team, one from Iris Zalaudek's team, and one from the International Dermoscopy Society (IDS). To summarize, to diagnose melanoma, one needs to see more than three colors—especially gray, blue, and white colors like on this example. You can see irregular globules and regression signs, zones without structure. There are irregular vessels like on this photo. When you see a lesion, you have different patterns on dermoscopy: parallel one, annular, homogeneous, globular, and reticular which are benign patterns. The polymorphous one is in favor of melanoma. The last pattern cerebriform is found in VHSIL and seborrheic keratosis. So dermoscopy is very helpful to diagnose vascular lesions and permits an immediate diagnosis and localization of preferred biopsy sites.

Confocal microscopy, which is still in research phase, is a noninvasive microscopy which now has handpieces. It does not require sagittal cutting as for normal histology but horizontal cutting of the different epidermal layers. The images are black and white. In melanosis the confocal microscope reveals dermal papillae have shinier monomorphic cells, with a polycyclic or round architecture; there are some dendritic cells in the basal epidermal layers that are triangular- or star-shaped. In melanoma, there is a loss of dermal papilla architecture; there are typical shiny basal cells. They are round and fusiform in the epidermis.

The fourth issue regards excisional biopsy.

If a lesion is *flat or raised*, a complete excision is recommended. Biopsy will only be acceptable if the lesion is large in size. If excision is delicate, dermoscopy and/or confocal microscopy are to be used as well. However, recommendations may include dispensations, in particular light brown macules less than 4 or 5 mm long (lentigo) and nevi obviously benign like certain tuberous dermal nevi.

For *flat multiple pigmented lesions*, mostly post-inflammatory, for instance, on vulvar lichen sclerosus, if the color of the lesions is uniform and if there are inflammatory lesions, a biopsy is recommended. Several biopsies should be performed, with the help of dermoscopy, if there is no inflammation, if there are several shades of pigmentation, or if there are other types of associated lesions.

On *raised multiple pigmented lesions*, one must suspect HPV or VHSIL. If there is only one type of lesion, a biopsy should be performed from the lesion with the highest point, and if there are different associated lesions, several biopsies will be performed.

The last issue regards the interpretation of anatomopathological results. Over—but also under—diagnosis exists. Diagnosis of melanoma is very difficult to make on a single biopsy because there is a progression from atypical melanocytic hyperplasia and melanoma. There are also atypical melanocytic nevi of genital type. Repeat biopsies and discussions with the pathologist may be important.

Diagnosing Vulvar Melanoma: Breaking the Myths

- Although melanoma is thought to be an easy lesion to recognize as it is a dark lesion, it is missed frequently, for several reasons:
  - Vulvar inspection is rarely performed on a routine basis by gynecologists.
  - Vulvar pigmented lesions are common, but vulvar melanoma is extremely rare, even rarer than on the skin. It is important not to miss a melanoma but also not to worry when unnecessary. C-KIT mutations are usually found in mucosal melanomas. They are different from skin melanomas.
- Differential diagnosis of vulvar melanoma is difficult, as clinical features are often difficult to distinguish between melanocytic lesions (nevus and melanomas) or between melanocytic lesions and epithelial hyperpigmentation without melanocytic hyperplasia (vulvar melanosis, lentigines, post-inflammatory hyperpigmentation). Regarding the skin, the ABCDE criteria (asymmetry, irregular border, irregular color, diameter more than 6 mm, extension) may be helpful, but this algorithm does not work for mucous membranes, palms, or soles.
- Dermoscopy and confocal microscopy are important for diagnosing vulvar melanoma. However, they are carried out by experts, sometimes found only in referral hospitals.
- A biopsy for suspect melanoma should be performed with care:
  - For a single pigmented lesion: complete excision is recommended.
  - For flat multiple pigmented lesions, mostly post-inflammatory: a usual biopsy is performed.
  - For pigmented lesions, not thought to be post-inflammatory: several biopsies should be carried out, guided by dermoscopy.
  - For raised, multiple pigmented lesions, possibly HPV or vulvar high-grade squamous intraepithelial lesion (VHSIL)—a usual diagnostic biopsy is recommended.
- Histopathological over- and underdiagnoses of pigmented lesions may occur, especially with atypical melanocytic nevus of genital type (AMNGT). Therefore, repeated biopsy and discussion with the pathologist in these cases are recommended.

References

1. Moxley KM, Fader AN, Rose PG, Case AC, Mutch DG, Berry E. Malignant melanoma of the vulva: an extension of cutaneous melanoma? Gynecol Oncol. 2011;122:612–7.
2. Mihajlovic M, Vlajkovic S, Jovanovic P, Stefanovic V. Primary mucosal melanomas: a comprehensive review. Int J Clin Exp Pathol. 2012;5:739–53.
3. Weinstock MA. Malignant melanoma of the vulva and vagina in the United States: patterns of incidence and population based estimates of survival. Am J Obstet Gynecol. 1994;171:1225–30.
4. Rosamilia LL, Scwartz JL, Lowe L. Vulvar melanoma in a 10 years old girl in association with lichen sclerosus. J Am Acad Dermatol. 2006;54(suppl I):S52–3.
5. La Spina M, Meli MC, De Pasquale R, Perrotta RE. Vulvar melanoma associated with lichen sclerosus in a child: case report and literature review. Pediatr Dermatol. 2016;33:190–4.
6. Sugiyama VE, Chan JK, Shin JY, Berek JS, Osann K, Kapp DS. VUlvar melanoma: a multivariable analysis of 644 patients. Obstet Gynecol. 2007;110:296–301.
7. Omholt K, Grafstrom E, Kanter Lewenson L, Hansson J, Ragnarsson Olding BK. KIT pathway alterations in mucosal melanomas of the vulva and other sites. Clin Cancer Res. 2011;17:3933–42.

8. Yélamos O, Merkel EA, Sholl LM, Zhang B, et al. Nonoverlapping clinical and mutational patterns in melanomas from the female genital tract and atypical genital nevi. J Invest Dermatol. 2016;136(9):1858–65.
9. Carlson JA, Mu XC, Slominski A, Weismann K, Crowson AN, Malfetano J. Melanocytic proliferations associated with lichen sclerosus. Arch Dermatol. 2002;138:77–87.
10. Ragnarsson olding BK, Kanter Lewensohn LR, Lagerlof B, Nilsson BR, Ringborg UK. Malignant melanoma of the vulva in a nationwide, 25 year study of 219 swedish females: clinical observation and histopathologic features. Cancer. 1999;86:1273–84.
11. Kerley SW, Blute ML, Keeney GL. Multifocal malignant melanoma arising in vesicovaginal metastasis. Arch Pathol Lab. 1991;115:950–2.
12. Debarbieux S, Perrot JL, Erfan N, Ronger-Savlé S, Labeille B, Cinotti E, Depaepe L, Cardot-Leccia N, Lacour JP, Thomas L, Bahadoran P, Groupe d'Imagerie Cutanée non invasive de la Société Française de Dermatologie. Reflectance confocal microscopy of mucosal pigmented macules: a review of 56 cases including 10 macular melanomas. Br J Dermatol. 2014;170(6):1276–84.
13. Murzaku EC, Penn LA, Hale CS, Keltz Pomeranz M, Polsky D. Vulvar nevi, melanosis, and melanoma: an epidemiologic, clinical and histopathological review. JAAD. 2014;71:1241–9.
14. Mert I, Semaan A, Winer I, Morris RT, Ali Fehmi R. Vulvar/vaginal melanoma: an updated surveillance epidemiology and results database review, comparison with cutaneous melanoma and significance of racial disparities. Int J Gynecol Cancer. 2013;23:1118–25.
15. Spencer KR, Mehnert JM. Mucosal melanoma: epidemiology, biology and treatment. Cancer Treat Res. 2016;167:295–320.
16. De Hullu JA, Hollema H, Hoekstra HJ. Vulvar melanomas: is there a role for sentinel lymph node biopsy? Cancer. 2002;94:486–91.
17. Pstow MA, Hamid O, Carvajal RD. Mucosal melanoma: pathogenesis, clinical behavior, and management. Curr Oncol Rep. 2012;14:441–8.
18. Creasman WT, Phillips JL, Menck HR. A survey of hospital management practices for vulvar melanoma. J Am Coll Surg. 1999;188(6):670–5.
19. Larkin J, Hodi FS, Wolchok JD. Combined nivolumab and ipilimumab or monotherapy in untreated melanoma. N Engl J Med. 2015;373:23–34.

Part X

Vulvar Lesions: Blisters—Vesicles and Bullae

42 Herpesvirus Infections

Sarah Shaffer and Colleen K. Stockdale

42.1 Herpes Simplex

Herpes simplex virus (HSV) is a common sexually transmitted infection. Herpesviruses cause latent, recurring or lytic infections. Nine herpesvirus types are known to infect humans (Table 42.1). Of them HSV-1 and HSV-2, both can cause orolabial herpes and genital herpes. The duration, severity, and symptomatology may vary, but overall the visible manifestation of genital herpes simplex is painful, grouped vesicles that quickly erode to superficial, coalescing ulcers. Notable risk factors include a higher number of lifetime sexual partners.

There are initial infection with HSV is usually unrecognized, but the primary outbreak is often worse than recurrent outbreaks. The primary outbreak usually begins within a week of initial infection and is manifested by fever, malaise, and regional lymphadenopathy. A vesicular eruption occurs on the mucous membranes of the vulva and may extend to keratinized skin (Fig. 42.1). Small (1–3 mm) scattered or grouped vesicles are delicate and quickly evolve to well-demarcated erosions with crusting; the latter is the more common clinical finding (Figs. 42.2 and 42.3). Unusually large or long-standing lesions should raise suspicion of an associated HIV infection (Fig. 42.4). Lesions may take several weeks to heal completely; superinfection is a risk during this time. Other complications related to severe pain and/or edema can include dysuria, urinary retention, and dehydration. It should be

Table 42.1 Types of human herpes viruses

Herpes number	Name
HHV-1	Herpes simplex virus-1 (HSV-1)
HHV-2	Herpes simplex virus-2 (HSV-2)
HHV-3	Varicella zoster virus (VZV)
HHV-4	Epstein–Barr virus (EBV)
HHV-5	Cytomegalovirus (CMV)
HHV-6A and 6B	Roseolovirus, Herpes lymphotropic virus
HHV-7	
HHV-8	Kaposi's sarcoma-associated herpesvirus

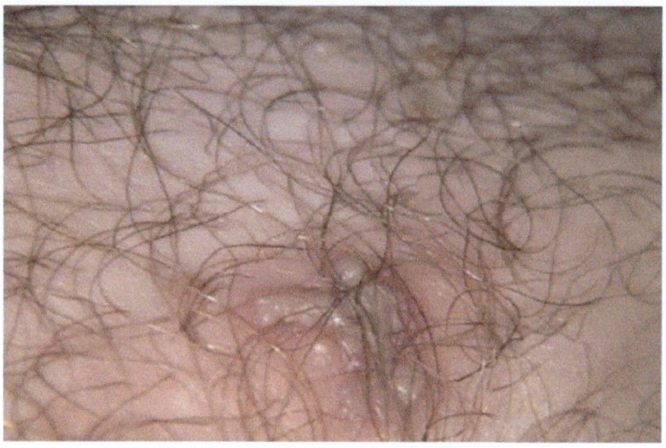

Fig. 42.1 Herpes genitalis covering the mons pubis, in a vesicular pattern. Courtesy of Professor Jacob Bornstein

S. Shaffer · C. K. Stockdale (✉)
Department of Obstetrics and Gynecology, University of Iowa, Iowa City, IA, USA
e-mail: colleen-stockdale@uiowa.edu

J. Bornstein (ed.), *Vulvar Disease*, https://doi.org/10.1007/978-3-319-61621-6_42

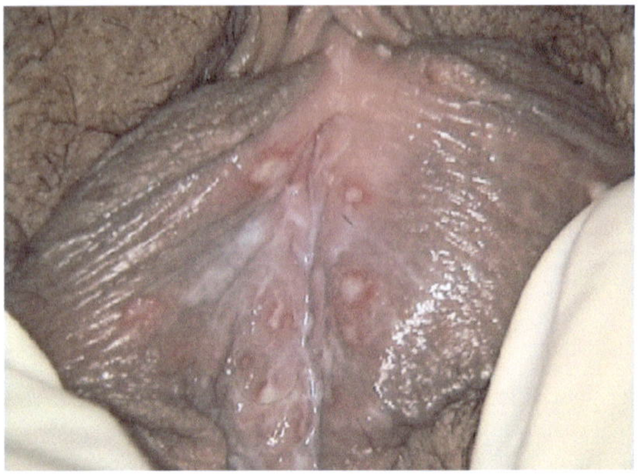

Fig. 42.2 Herpes genitalis, erosions developing on the labia minora and majora, where the vesicles rupture. Courtesy of Professor Jacob Bornstein

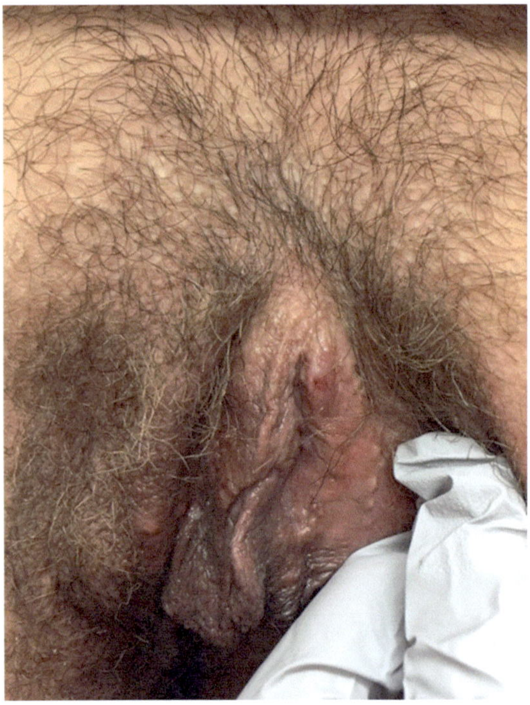

Fig. 42.3 Herpes genitalis, erosions on the labia minora and majora. Courtesy of Diane Elas

noted, however, that a primary outbreak may be mild enough to be subclinical; these patients may not be aware of their herpes simplex virus infection.

After initial infection and/or outbreak, HSV lies dormant in the dorsal root ganglion and will reactivate causing recurrent outbreaks that are usually milder and less symptomatic. A prodrome of paresthesia may be noted. Linear, fissure-like lesions or erosions without the red halo may be noted with recurrent outbreaks (Fig. 42.5). Lesions often resolve in a shorter time frame, usually 1–2 weeks.

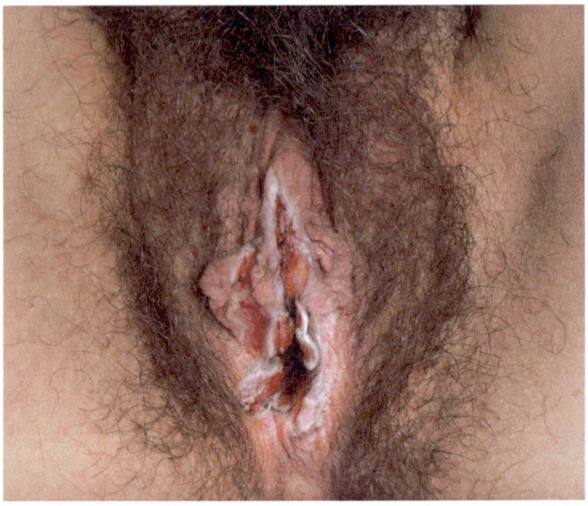

Fig. 42.4 Herpes genitalis. Large and long-standing erosions associated with HIV infection. Courtesy of Professor Jacob Bornstein

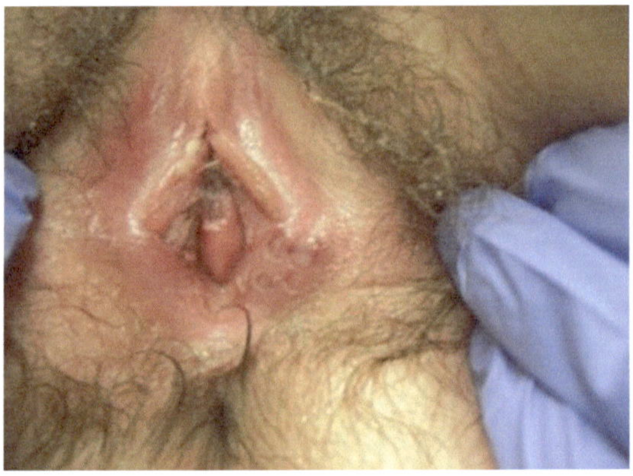

Fig. 42.5 Herpes genitalis erosions on the labia minora. Courtesy of Dr. Colleen Stockdale

Diagnosis should be made with laboratory testing. A viral culture is best obtained from the base of a vesicle or fresh erosion; collection from older lesions and/or delay in transport to the lab may cause a false-negative viral culture. A shave biopsy from a vesicle or ulcer edge can confirm herpes infection, but does not differentiate simplex from varicella-zoster. Polymerase chain reaction (PCR) testing is currently preferred for diagnosing genital HSV infection. Serology is not recommended to diagnose the cause of vulvar vesicles mainly because it cannot differentiate between the herpes simplex types. Human immunodeficiency virus (HIV) testing should be offered to all patients newly diagnosed with HSV as HIV acquisition is increased in patients who are infected with HSV type 2.

Primary and recurrent outbreaks can be treated with oral antiviral medications to decrease the duration and number of lesions, as well as the associated symptomatology. Oral antivirals are first-line therapy and usually well-tolerated; topical antiviral medications have not been shown to have a clinical benefit and are not used. Primary outbreaks can be treated with one of the following regimens: acyclovir 400 mg orally three times a day for 7–10 days, acyclovir 200 mg orally five times a day for 7–10 days, or valacyclovir 1000 mg orally twice a day for 7–10 days [1]. Episodic therapy for recurrent HSV outbreaks can be achieved with a variety of regimens. Suppressive therapy for recurrent genital HSV outbreaks may decrease the risk of transmission to sexual partners as well as the frequency of symptomatic recurrent outbreaks; it is also employed in the third trimester of pregnancy, albeit different dosing, to decrease vertical transmission and allow for vaginal delivery. Current CDC recommendations for suppressive therapy include acyclovir 400 mg orally two times a day, valacyclovir 500 mg or 1000 mg orally once a day, or famciclovir 250 mg orally twice a day [1]. Intravenous antiviral therapy is indicated for severe outbreaks with related complications as well as in some immunocompromised patients. Resistance to currently available antivirals has been documented in immunocompromised patients [2].

Management must also include nonjudgmental education and counseling. Patients should be encouraged to share their diagnosis with sexual partners. The occurrence of asymptomatic viral shedding must be mentioned along with the use of condoms to decrease transmission. Oral analgesic medications may be necessary with the pain of a primary outbreak; a short course of narcotics can be considered as can the short-term use of topical anesthetics (e.g., periurethral lesions). Oral antipruritic medications can also be of use, usually later in the course of healing crusted lesions. Care of the vulvar skin may include twice-daily sitz baths, use of peri-rinse bottle to decrease pain with urination, and a skin protectant like white petroleum applied several times a day once lesions have evolved beyond the vesicle stage. Good hand hygiene should be counseled when caring for acute lesions to decrease risk of autoinoculation of the oral or anal mucous membranes.

42.2 Herpes Varicella-Zoster

Varicella-zoster virus (VSV) is a herpesvirus that can cause two distinct diseases: varicella (also known as “chicken pox”) and zoster, more commonly referred to as “shingles” (Fig. 42.6). While these diseases have varying presentations, both can have manifestations localized to the vulva and should be considered in the differential diagnosis of vulvar vesicles and erosions/ulcers (Figs. 42.3 and 42.4).

Differentiating herpes simplex virus from VZV may be difficult. Varicella-zoster virus outbreaks often occur once or rarely in the immunocompetent patient, rather than recurrently as with herpes simplex virus. Varicella that initially presents on the vulva will manifest in other locations on the body thereafter; this most commonly

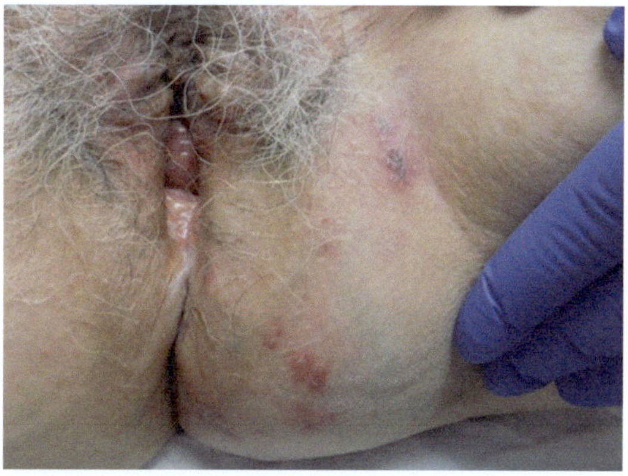

Fig. 42.6 Herpes zoster cluster on the buttocks. Courtesy of Diane Elas

occurs in children, although less frequently with increasing use of the varicella vaccination. Zoster outbreaks are more common in older patient and usually occur in a unilateral dermatomal distribution (i.e., including the medial thigh or buttock) rather than the bilateral vulvar structures (as in herpes simplex virus) or in multiple dissociated body locations (as in varicella).

Varicella usually presents in younger patients and can initially present in any location, although the mucous membranes including the vulva and vagina are common. Initial lesions appear as vesicles or red papules that present in various locations and then erode and crust; successive "crops" of lesions may appear [3] (Fig. 42.7). Constitutional symptoms are common including low-grade fever, malaise, fatigue, and anorexia. Formation of new lesions usually stops after 4 and 6 days; crusts tend to flake off in 1–2 weeks. Complications are rare but can include skin infection, encephalitis, and hepatitis. A small case series presented young children who, each after a routine course of the chicken pox, suffered acute worsening of genital condyloma attributed to the relative immunosuppression effected by the varicella infection [4]. The rare report of a pregnant patient with varicella outbreak at 41 weeks gestation described symptomatic vulvar and vaginal lesions which necessitated cesarean delivery. The patient did not suffer varicella pneumonia, another rare complication of varicella in adult patients [5].

Zoster is the reactivation of latent VZV from the dorsal root ganglia after a remote episode of varicella. After a prodrome of symptoms including localized aching and burning pain, zoster manifests as a localized eruption of red plaques with overlying clustered vesicles confined to a unilateral dermatome; the lesions usually do not cross the midline [6]. There are rarely any related constitutional symptoms once the rash presents. The vesicles will coalesce, erode, crust, and then heal over a period of weeks. Diagnosis is best made by PCR which can differentiate between herpes simplex virus and VZV [7]; viral culture and biopsy can also be considered, but the latter cannot differentiate the type of herpes virus. A host of rare complications has been reported including a variety of neuropathies as well as zoster cystitis with related urinary retention [8].

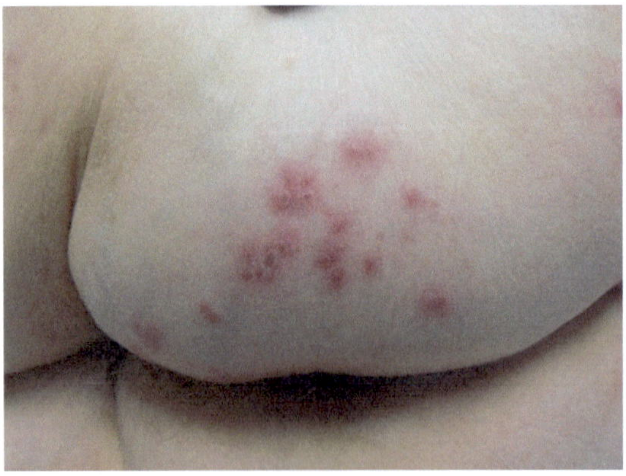

Fig. 42.7 Herpes zoster cluster on the breast. Courtesy of Diane Elas

The major complication of zoster is the development of postherpetic neuralgia (PHN), where chronic pain and paresthesia develop in the involved dermatome and may persist for years after. Zoster is now known to be more common in women, and in the USA there is a 30% lifetime risk of zoster with approximately 8% of cases involving the dermatomes that innervate the vulva. This neurocutaneous infection is likely an under-recognized source of vulvar and pelvic pain in women, both acute pain and PHN [9]. One study of genital viral specimens tested with PCR found zoster in 3% of samples [7]. Zoster involving the female genital dermatomes is more likely than varicella to leave pigmented scars of the genital mucosal tissues [9].

Treatment involves controlling pain, usually with narcotic pain medications, and starting oral antiviral medications. The earlier antiviral therapy is begun, the more likely it will mitigate duration and severity of symptoms; early antiviral therapy may also decrease the severity of PHN. Oral antiviral therapy options include acyclovir 800 mg five times a day, valacyclovir 1000 mg three times a day, or famciclovir 500 mg three times a day for 7 days [10]. Postherpetic neuralgia should be treated with medication to address the neuropathic component of pain—options include amitriptyline, nortriptyline, gabapentin, pregabalin, venlafaxine, or duloxetine [10]. The Federal Drug Administration-approved "shingles" vaccine is for all patients over the age of 50.

Herpes Virus Infections: Breaking the Myths

- The "classic" appearance of painful, grouped vesicles is very short-lived; hence they are seldom detected. The more common presentation is superficial, coalescing ulcers.
- Although the primary genital herpes outbreak is often worse than recurrent outbreaks, the initial infection with HSV is usually unrecognized.
- Women with genital herpes may not always be treated on an ambulatory basis. Those with urinary retention and dehydration should be hospitalized.
- The workup of a patient with herpes genitalis is not complete unless he or she is offered to be tested for human immunodeficiency virus (HIV), as HIV acquisition is increased in patients who are infected with HSV type 2.
- Although some clinicians offer topical antiviral medications for genital herpes infection, they have not been shown to have a clinical benefit. Oral antivirals are the recommended first-line therapy.
- Herpes genitalis may be infective even when there is no apparent lesion, as asymptomatic viral shedding is frequent, mainly during the first year after the primary infection.

References

1. CDC. 2015 sexually transmitted disease treatment guidelines – genital HSV infections. 2015.
2. Levin MJ, Bacon TH, Leary JJ. Resistance of herpes simplex virus infections to nucleoside analogues in HIV-infected patients. Clin Infect Dis. 2004;39(Suppl 5):S248–57.
3. Yurichisin MJ. Management quandary. J Pediatr Adolesc Gynecol. 1998;11:103–4.
4. Persaud DI, Squires J. Genital papillomavirus infection: clinical progression after varicella infection. Pediatrics. 1997;100(3 Pt 1):408–12.
5. Sites CK, Sherer DM, Gandell DL, Woods JR Jr. Extensive vulvar and vaginal varicella necessitating abdominal delivery. Am J Obstet Gynecol. 1990;163(5 Pt 1):1630–1.
6. Brown D. Herpes zoster of the vulva. Clin Obstet Gynecol. 1972;15(4):1010–4.
7. Birch AD, Druce JD, Catton MC, MacGregor L, Read T. Detection of varicella zoster virus in gential specimens using a multiplex polymerase chain reaction. Sex Transm Infect. 2003;79(4):298–300.
8. Julia JJ, Cholhan HJ. Herpes zoster-associated acute urinary retention: a case report. Int Urogynecol J Pelvic Floor Dysfunct. 2007;18(1):103–4.
9. Oaklander AL, Rissmiller JG. Postherpetic neuralgia after shingles: an under-recognized cause of chronic vulvar pain. Obstet Gynecol. 2002; 99(4):625–8.
10. Danby CS, Margesson LJ. Approach to the diagnosis and treatment of vulvar pain. Dermatol Ther. 2010;23(5):485–504.

43 Acute Eczema

Sarah Shaffer and Colleen K. Stockdale

43.1 Introduction

Eczema is an inflammatory skin condition with many causes and varying manifestations. In the acute phase, direct contact with an endogenous or exogenous irritant or allergen results in a vesicular eruption with associated erythema and localized edema. Stinging, burning, or profound pruritus are commonly described. Vesicles in the genital area are easily unroofed leaving erosions or ulcers.

43.2 Pathophysiology

Irritants are more common exposures than allergens, but the vulva is particularly susceptible to either. The barrier function of the vulvar skin is ever at risk for compromise by moisture, enzymes, friction, occlusion, and heat. Estrogen deficiency, urinary incontinence, and preexisting dermatoses, among other issues, can further weaken the vulvar skin barrier.

Both irritants and allergens can cause an acute eczematous eruption; subtle differences should be noted. Irritants are often associated with hygiene and may include topical medications or native fluids in contact with altered or damaged skin.

S. Shaffer · C. K. Stockdale (✉)
Department of Obstetrics and Gynecology, University of Iowa, Iowa City, IA, USA
e-mail: colleen-stockdale@uiowa.edu

43.3 Clinical Presentation

An acute reaction to an irritant is equivalent to a chemical burn with immediate sensation of burning or stinging preceding the rapid development of vesicles, erythema, and edema in the area of exposure (Fig. 43.1). Acute allergic eruptions occur when the skin is exposed to a substance to which the patient has a previously established hypersensitivity. One notable difference is the lack of immediate symptoms with application of the allergen. Likewise, the development of edema and confluent vesicles may take several days, although these appear in the area of contact (Figs. 43.2 and 43.3). In some cases, linear or geometric erythematous plaques extending away from the eruption can delineate where fingers or

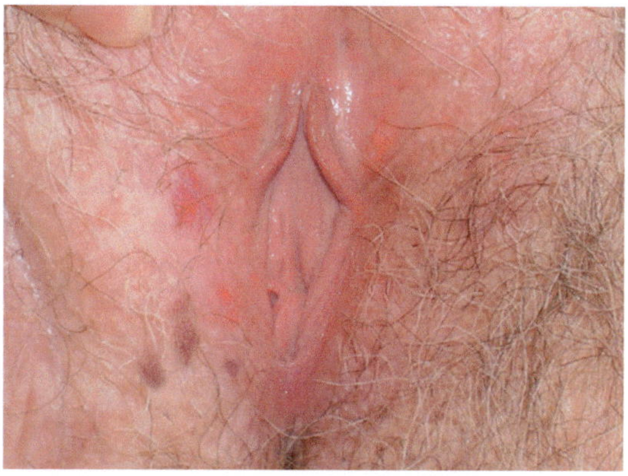

Fig. 43.1 Acute vulvar eczema. Several scaly lesions are noticed. Courtesy of Professor Jacob Bornstein

J. Bornstein (ed.), *Vulvar Disease*, https://doi.org/10.1007/978-3-319-61621-6_43

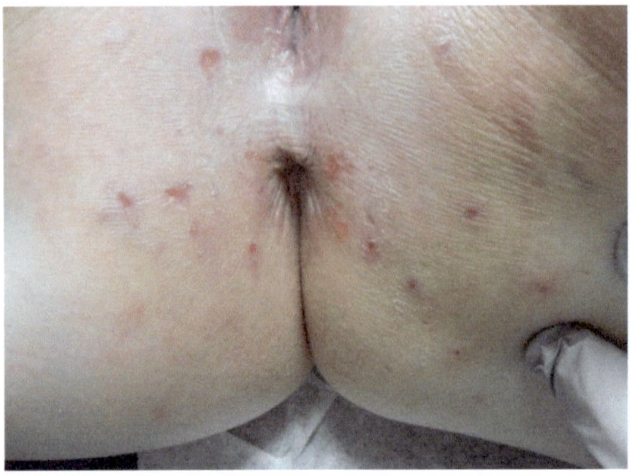

Fig. 43.2 Perineal and perianal acute eczema. A pruritic lesion composed of plaques and thickened patches. Small blisters were eroded. Courtesy of Dr. Colleen Stockdale

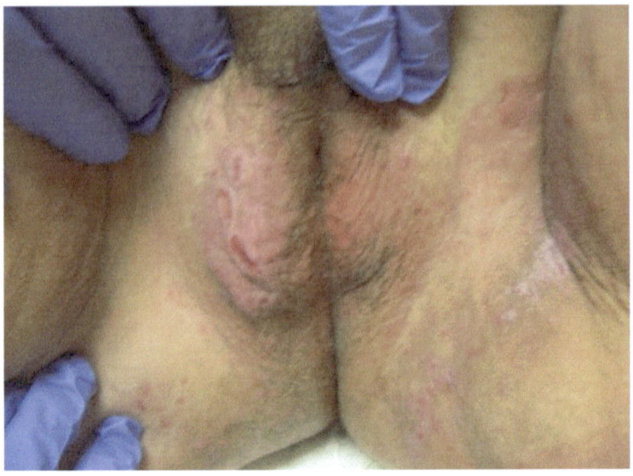

Fig. 43.4 Vulvar acute eczema. Red plaques with significant erosions, probably resulting from excoriation. Courtesy of Diane Elas

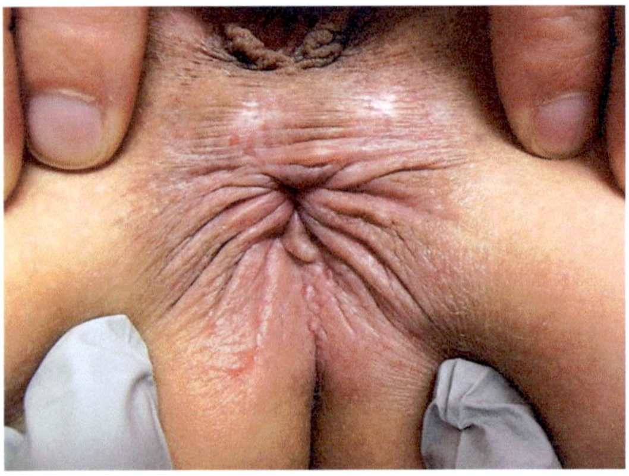

Fig. 43.3 Perineal and perianal acute eczema. A pruritic lesion composed of thickened skin. Excoriations are evident. Courtesy of Dr. Colleen Stockdale

skin folds contacted and spread the allergen (Figs. 43.4 and 43.5). Identification of an allergen can be more difficult with the slow onset of an acute allergic eczematous reaction, which mimics the more indolent onset of other blistering diseases of the vulva. Furthermore, an allergic reaction may manifest at a body site distant from the site of acute contact with a known allergen; this "recall" phenomenon can be quite confusing.

43.4 Treatment

The main therapeutic intervention is identification and discontinuation or elimination of the offending agent. Misguided, compulsive, or ritualistic hygiene practices may be to blame, and careful, nonjudgmental patient questioning is important. A thorough history must be obtained with careful inventory of all vulvar products including medications, contraceptives, and sexual products, inquiring also about products used by intimate partners [1]. Identifying the irritant or allergen, however, can be quite challenging. In some cases it is the binder or vehicle of a topical medication or other hygienic substances and not the medication itself. A biopsy is rarely necessary to make the diagnosis. The possibility of concomitant disease process should always be considered [2]. Patch testing is suggested for accurate identification of allergens with different sources making varying recommendations for useful series [1–3].

Treatment involves control of pruritus and scratching that can cause skin changes and symptoms more consistent with subacute and chronic eczema. Pruritus can be treated topically with cool compresses; heat should be avoided as it can increase histamine release worsening pruritus. Oral antihistamines are often helpful, especially to aid sleep and limit scratching during the night. A short course of oral corticosteroids may be required for treating the severe pruritus of acute eczema. In this situation, consider prophylaxis for candidiasis during the steroid course. Topical steroids are a standard part of the treatment plan, although they may not be utilized initially on significantly

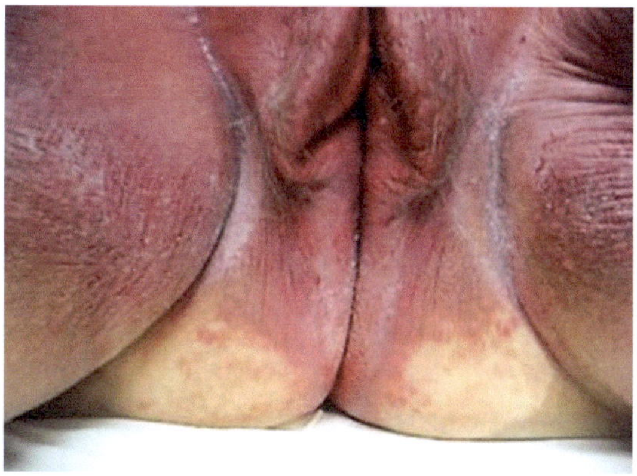

Fig. 43.5 Diffuse vulvar, perineal, and buttock acute eczema. Red plaques, covered by thickened skin. Courtesy of Diane Elas

eroded skin. An extended course of topical steroids with a slow taper may be required during prolonged healing. Oral analgesics are preferred over topical analgesics. Treatment to address estrogen deficiency should be considered, as should therapy to improve urinary or fecal incontinence. Secondary infections should be diagnosed accurately and treated [4].

Sitz baths and bathing in general for relief of pruritus and softening of scale must be limited as these can desiccate damaged skin. Urinating in water or diluting urine by pouring or spraying water on the vulva can relieve pain related to urine irritating damaged skin. Washcloths and other cleansing implements can damage delicate vulvar skin; only bare hands should be used during hygiene. Afterward, the vulvar skin should be patted dry or allowed to air dry. A skin protectant, white petroleum, for example, can provide hydration, lubrication, as well as a barrier function for damaged skin from other native irritants like urine and feces.

Acute Eczema: Breaking the Myths

- Although eczema is caused by irritants and allergens, the barrier function of the vulvar skin needs to be compromised before the lesion develops. This is caused by moisture, enzymes, friction, occlusion, heat, estrogen deficiency, urinary incontinence, and preexisting dermatoses.
- Although in the vulva a biopsy is frequently needed to establish a diagnosis, with eczema, biopsy is rarely necessary to make the diagnosis. However, patch testing is useful for accurate identification of allergens.
- Hot compresses should be avoided in eczema as they can increase histamine release and augment the pruritus. Use cold pad instead.

References

1. Schlosser BJ. Contact dermatitis of the vulva. Dermatol Clin. 2010;28(4):697–706.
2. Nardelli A, Degreef H, Goossens A. Contact allergic reactions of the vulva: a 14-year review. Dermatitis. 2004;15(3):131–6.
3. Bauer A, Rodiger C, Greif C, Kaatz M, Elsner P. Vulvar dermatoses--irritant and allergic contact dermatitis of the vulva. Dermatology. 2005; 210(2):143–9.
4. Carey E, Zedek D, Lewis J, Zolnoun D. Superimposed methicillin-resistant Staphylococcus aureus infection of vulvar eczematous dermatitis: a case report. J Reprod Med. 2013;58(5–6):261–3.

Lymphangioma Circumscriptum (Lymphangiectasia)

44

Sarah Shaffer and Colleen K. Stockdale

44.1 Introduction

Lymphangioma circumscripta (LC), lymphangiectasia, and superficial lymph vessel ectasia [1] are a few of the terms used to describe a rare but benign condition of dilatation of the dermal lymphatic vessels visible through the epidermis due to obstructed lymphatic return. A vascular malformation of the lymphatics may be superficial, located in the layers of the skin, or may include a deeper component causing an extensive area of grouped and/or multiloculated bulging lymphatic vessels. Congenital malformations or defects can cause LC in children. Acquired LC in adults can have many causes including trauma or localized radiation therapy; if lymphatic obstruction and chronic edema result, LC may develop (Fig. 44.1).

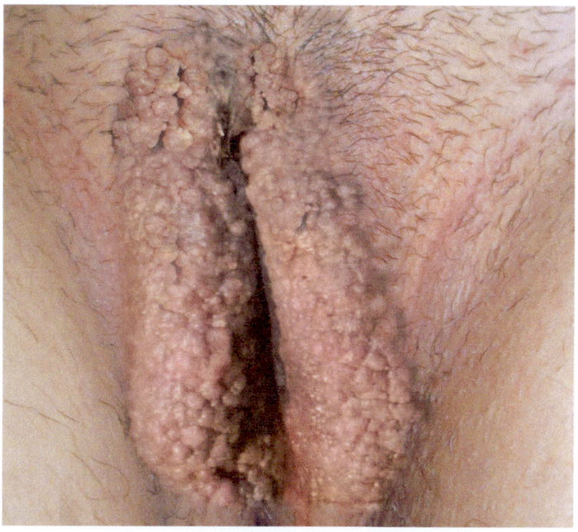

Fig. 44.1 Vulvar lymphangioma. The dilatation of the dermal lymphatic vessels is visible through the epidermis as vesicles or bullae. Courtesy of Professor Jacob Bornstein

44.2 Clinical Presentation

Lymphangioma circumscripta can occur anywhere on the body including intraperitoneal and retroperitoneal manifestations [2]. Skin manifestations are far more common, but vulvar LC is rare. The subepidermal vessels of LC can be mistaken for vasculature, vesicles, papules, angiokeratomas, and genital warts [2], among other vulvar pathologies. Color can vary from white to brown to purple and size can range up to 2 cm in diameter. Associated symptoms can include swelling, pain, or a sensation of heaviness. Patients may present after observing the lesions or with weeping of lymphatic fluid from disrupted lesions. The fluid is chylous and may appear milky or may be blood-tinged [1]. The amount of fluid lost from these lesions can be extensive in some situations. The lesions of LC, if disrupted, can become eroded and ulcerated and may become infected causing a secondary cellulitis. The appearance, the symptoms, or

S. Shaffer · C. K. Stockdale (✉)
Department of Obstetrics and Gynecology, University of Iowa, Iowa City, IA, USA
e-mail: colleen-stockdale@uiowa.edu

J. Bornstein (ed.), *Vulvar Disease*, https://doi.org/10.1007/978-3-319-61621-6_44

complications of vulvar LC can lead to alteration of sexual activity and psychosocial dysfunction [2].

44.3 Pathogenesis

History most often will elucidate a prolonged presence of the lesions with minimal symptoms. Considering causes of acquired vulvar LC, the most common predisposing condition in one review was radical surgery and/or radiation for cervical cancer and Hodgkin's lymphoma [2–4]. Malignancy-associated LC can demonstrate significant delay to onset [5] and may be accompanied by lymphedema of adjacent body regions causing a large amount of chylous discharge from the LC [1]. There are reports of LC related to fistulous Crohn's disease and tuberculous infection [3] as well as rare reports of pregnancy-induced LC [1, 3].

In addition to a careful history and physical examination, a biopsy may be helpful to exclude other causes of vesicles or ulcerations. The biopsy, however, may prove unhelpful if taken from an area of reactive epidermal change sufficient to mask an underlying vascular lymphatic abnormality [5]. Additional imaging should be obtained if there is any concern for a related malignancy or malignant source. Testing for systemic or localized infections may be indicated. Certain medications have also been identified as causing LC [1], and discontinuation is required to keep the disorder from worsening.

44.4 Treatment

Treatment may require CO_2 laser ablation to seal superficial lymphatic vessels [2, 6], although experience is limited. Other therapies that have been trialed for vulvar LC include sclerotherapy, electrocoagulation, and liquid nitrogen cryotherapy [2]. Surgical management has been the most successful treatment reported with wide superficial excision for smaller areas; larger areas may require flaps to be developed to minimize defects at risk for infections [1, 4, 6]. Recurrence is difficult to predict as identifying the damaged or malformed deeper communicating lymph channel or vasculature is not always possible; follow-up in most reports is limited, so duration of relief is truly unknown. Observation of an asymptomatic patient is entirely appropriate. Treatments to avoid include topical podophyllin, trichloroacetic acid, and imiquimod; these cause irritation of the already altered vulvar skin and can aggravate the disease process [1]. Consideration of treatment for related conditions, such as physiotherapy for related lymphedema, is also quite important [4]. Finally, vulvar skin care guidelines should be reviewed with the patient emphasizing the importance of soaks and skin barriers and minimizing extraneous contact irritants.

Lymphangioma Circumscriptum (Lymphangiectasia): Breaking the Myths

- Lymphangioma circumscriptum (LC) is frequently misdiagnosed as vulvar vesicles, papules, angiokeratomas, or genital warts.
- This is a rare but benign condition of obstruction of the dermal lymphatic vessels visible through the epidermis.
- LC affects more commonly the intraperitoneal cavity and retroperitoneal space.

References

1. Verma SB. Lymphangiectasias of the skin: victims of confusing nomenclature. Clin Exp Dermatol. 2009;34(5):566–9.
2. Vlastos AT, Malpica A, Follen M. Lymphangioma circumscriptum of the vulva: a review of the literature. Obstet Gynecol. 2003;101(5 Pt 1):946–54.
3. Chang MB, Newman CC, Davis MD, Lehman JS. Acquired lymphangiectasia (lymphangioma circumscriptum) of the vulva: clinicopathologic study of 11 patients from a single institution and 67 from the literature. Int J Dermatol. 2016;55(9):e482–7.
4. Vignes S, Arrault M, Trevidic P. Surgical resection of vulva lymphoedema circumscriptum. J Plast Reconstr Aesthet Surg. 2010;63(11):1883–5.
5. Stewart CJ, Chan T, Platten M. Acquired lymphangiectasia ('lymphangioma circumscriptum') of the vulva: a report of eight cases. Pathology. 2009;41(5):448–53.
6. Huilgol SC, Neill S, Barlow RJ. CO(2) laser therapy of vulval lymphangiectasia and lymphangioma circumscriptum. Dermatol Surg. 2002;28(7):575–7.

Immune Blistering Disorders

45

Sarah Shaffer and Colleen K. Stockdale

45.1 Introduction

Immune blistering diseases may involve the cutaneous or mucosal surfaces of the female genital structures. These noninfectious bullous disorders are characterized by autoantibodies to antigens that have a role in adherence of epidermis to dermis or epithelial cells to one another [1]. Antibodies affix to a target antigen, trigger complement activation, and attract eosinophils and neutrophils, which degranulate releasing proteolytic enzymes that cause blister formation in either a subepidermal or intraepidermal location. Cutaneous and mucosal tissue can be affected; blisters that form on mucosal surfaces erode quickly and appear more commonly as erosions. A biopsy taken from the edge of a blister or erosion should include a small sample of normal-appearing epithelium. Histology and direct immunofluorescence are necessary to diagnose and differentiate these diseases. Indirect immunofluorescence of serum for autoantibodies may also be considered.

Unless noted, both subepidermal and intraepidermal blistering diseases occur more commonly in the elderly, often peaking in or after the sixth decade of life. Diagnosis of immune blistering disorders requires a thorough history as well as a full examination of all cutaneous and mucosal sites to identify lesions that may be asymptomatic, healing, or hidden from view (i.e., vaginal vault). There is no proven link to malignancy demonstrated for any of the immune blistering diseases [2, 3].

Management principles and recommended medications overlap for many of the immune blistering diseases; where specific differences exist, notations are made with the description of the disease. The use of topical steroids is occasionally sufficient, but systemic steroids are often indicated and should be tapered with clinic response. Case reports or small case series exist for most of the immune bullous disorders for the following immune-suppressive medications: azathioprine (often noted to be the preferred immune-suppressive medication for an acceptable side effect profile), cyclophosphamide, mycophenolate mofetil (nonsteroidal option), methotrexate and thalidomide (beware the need for contraception if either is used in a reproductive-aged woman), cyclosporine, dapsone (screen for G6PD deficiency before use), rituximab, nicotinamide and tetracycline antibiotics, colchicine, antimalarial medications, plasmapheresis, and intravenous immunoglobulin (IVIG) [3–12]. When treating vulvovaginal manifestations of immune blistering disorders, topical steroid ointments are the predominant form of therapy.

Care of the vulvar skin should always include review of basic guidelines with emphasis on the use of soaks and addition of barriers

S. Shaffer · C. K. Stockdale (✉)
Department of Obstetrics and Gynecology, University of Iowa, Iowa City, IA, USA
e-mail: colleen-stockdale@uiowa.edu

J. Bornstein (ed.), *Vulvar Disease*, https://doi.org/10.1007/978-3-319-61621-6_45

or skin protectants. Minimizing the presence of contact irritants which often include bodily fluids and overzealous hygiene is also important [13]. Topical estrogen therapy may be warranted for those with deficiency and may benefit in patients with immune bullous disease after initial eruptions are adequately managed. With disorders that cause scarring, mechanical dilation of the vagina may be required [3]. Finally, close follow-up and examinations of cutaneous and mucosal surfaces are warranted for surveillance, early treatment of recurrences as well as identification of rare but associated conditions [14].

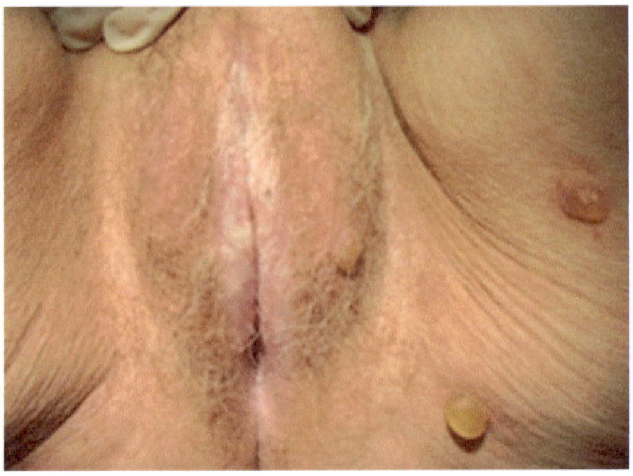

Fig. 45.1 Bullous pemphigoid—biopsy confirmed. Patient also has vulvar lichen sclerosus. Courtesy of Diane Elas

45.2 Pemphigoid Diseases or Subepidermal Blistering Diseases

45.2.1 Lack of Predominance of Mucosal Involvement

Bullous Pemphigoid The most common autoimmune blistering disease, bullous pemphigoid (BP), has a more indolent and prolonged onset than other similar blistering diseases. Bullous pemphigoid often arises spontaneously and less commonly has an identifiable instigating factor (e.g., medication use).

Pink or red plaques and significant pruritus may precede the manifestation of tense blisters which are rarely hemorrhagic (Figs. 45.1 and 45.2). Common locations include inner thighs, inguinal creases, and perineum. Involvement of keratinized epithelium is more common than involvement of mucous membranes; oral lesions are less common in this pemphigoid disease. Genital involvement occurs in approximately 10% of patients, with the vulva described as the most commonly affected site in both adults and children [13, 15–20]. The Nikolsky sign, slippage of the epithelium from the underlying skin layers with mild pressure from a finger or speculum, is absent with BP. Recently, associations of BP with neurologic disease have been reported [1].

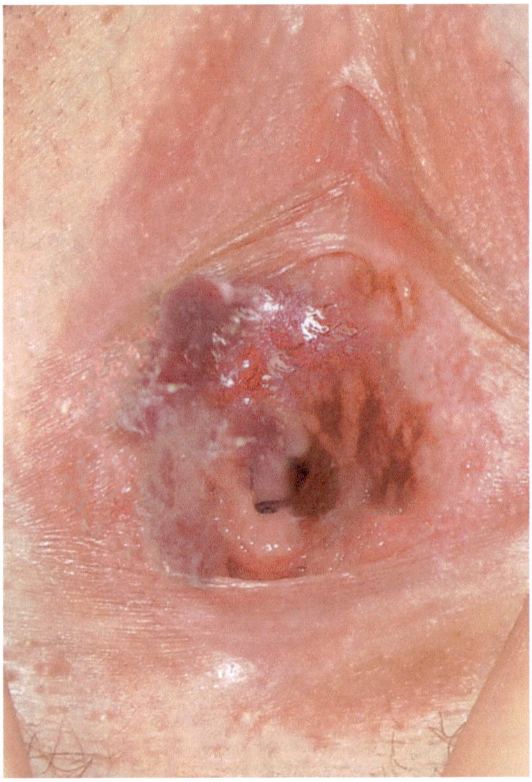

Fig. 45.2 Bullous pemphigoid. Erosions on the labia minora and vestibule. Courtesy of Professor Jacob Bornstein

Histology will show subepidermal blistering and dermal inflammatory infiltrate with prominent eosinophils. Direct immunofluorescence (DIF) demonstrates linear deposition of IgG

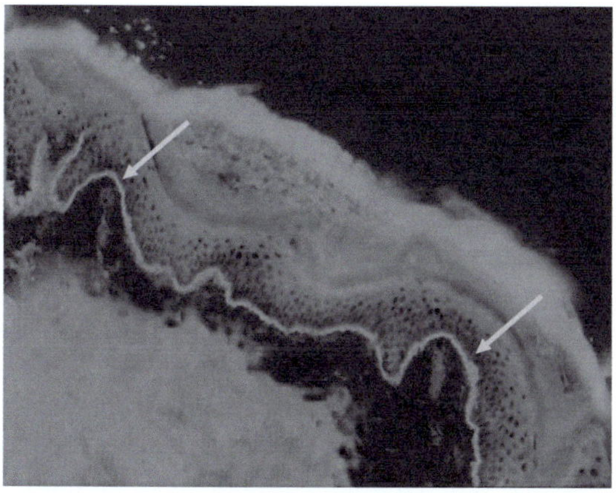

Fig. 45.3 Bullous pemphigoid. Indirect immunofluorescence showing linear deposition of IgG along the epidermal surface of the basement membrane zone. Courtesy of Professor Jacob Bornstein

(and, in some cases, complement 3, IgM, and IgA) along the epidermal surface of the basement membrane zone in an "n-serrated" pattern (Fig. 45.3). This pattern reveals IgG deposited at a higher layer in the skin than is evidenced by epidermolysis bullosa acquisita in particular (refer to Sect. 44.2.3). Indirect immunofluorescence (IIF) shows IgG bound to target antigens of the basement membrane zone.

The course of BP is self-limited with slow remission over several years in treated patients [21]. Recurrences are common but often milder than the initial manifestation. Scarring is rare, in contrast to several other pemphigoid diseases; scarring occurs more common in children and with secondary infection. Treatment has not been shown to decrease mortality but greatly improves quality of life.

Anti-p200/Anti-Laminin g1 Pemphigoid A rare disease that mimics bullous pemphigoid, anti-p200/anti-laminin g1 pemphigoid, is only currently noted to be distinctive in that it affects a younger population, has a defined association with psoriasis and reacts more favorably to treatment [1].

Linear IgA Disease Linear IgA disease is an acquired autoimmune blistering disorder that may be induced by use of certain medications; malignancies and environmental exposures have also been implicated. It can present at any age, but peak incidence is in the elderly. This disease is often referred to as "chronic bullous disease of childhood" in the literature.

A typical presentation is acute development of annular, erythematous, non-scaling plaques that form tense blisters at the periphery, a unique finding. The plaques become more generalized with time often resulting in post-inflammatory hyperpigmentation. Mucosal involvement and scarring may both occur. Perineal, genital, and perioral blistering are more common in children [21, 22]. Complaints of itching or burning are highly variable, while systemic symptoms including fever and anorexia are common.

Histology shows a subepidermal blister with neutrophilic infiltrate and often microabscesses, which are a unique feature. A linear band of IgA deposition (and possibly complement components) on the epidermal side of the basement membrane zone in "n-serrated" pattern is seen on DIF. Indirect immunofluorescence reveals IgA antibodies at the basement membrane zone.

Severe mucosal involvement appears to be associated with a lower likelihood of remission in children [22, 23] although the majority of children generally experience remission prior to puberty. Remission is common in adults. Pregnancy generally induces latency of the disease, but postpartum relapse is common.

Differentiating linear IgA disease from urticaria, bullous pemphigoid, and erythema multiforme may be challenging. Treatment with dapsone can be diagnostic as linear IgA disease tends to respond rapidly to this medication. Sulfonamides have also shown benefit.

45.2.2 Mucosal Involvement

Mucous Membrane Pemphigoid and Cicatricial Pemphigoid Mucous membrane pemphigoid (dropping the historic and inaccurate modifier "benign") is the recommended terminology for immune blistering disease that has predominantly mucosal involvement. Cicatricial

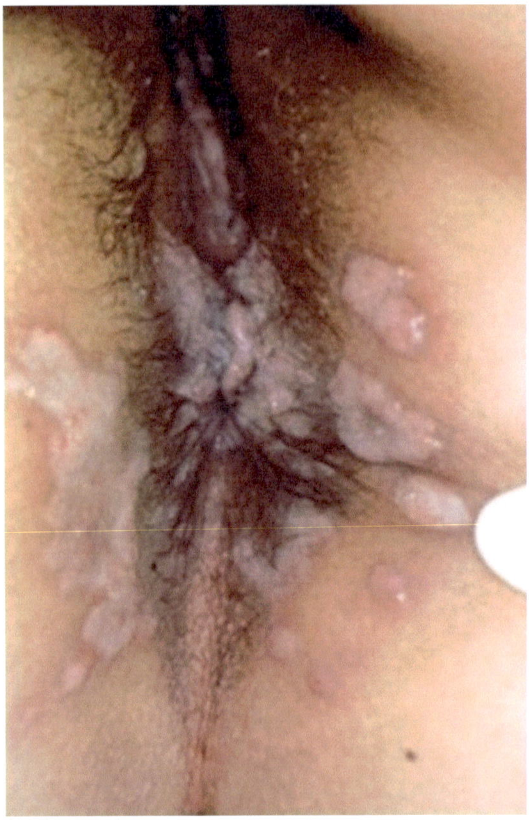

Fig. 45.4 Cicatricial pemphigoid. Courtesy of Professor Jacob Bornstein

pemphigoid is the term recommended for the rare clinical variant with minimal mucosal involvement and with scarring of affected skin [1, 24] (Fig. 45.4).

Mucous membrane pemphigoid (MMP) typically presents with irritation and pain accompanying mild blisters that may also appear as small pustules. The conjunctivae and nasal and oral mucosae are commonly affected; adhesions can form in the eye, and gingival tissue damage can lead to further dental disease. The genital mucosa is affected in 50% of cases with accompanying pain, pruritus, and dysuria [21]. Scarring of affected mucosal surfaces, including genitalia, is the rule and can occur rapidly after erosion of blisters [20]. Severe disease can result in stenosis of the urethra or vaginal introitus, phimosis of the clitoris, or fusion of the labia [3, 25]. These findings can make differentiation from lichen planus or lichen sclerosus difficult; the necessity of direct immunofluorescence (DIF) is noted as DIF is negative for both lichen planus and lichen sclerosus [25, 26]. The Nikolsky sign, slippage of the epithelium from the underlying skin layers with mild pressure from a finger or speculum, occurs in MMP (and pemphigus vulgaris) and not lichen planus or lichen sclerosus.

The histology for MMP is subepidermal blistering and dermal scarring, but no evidence of other similar disease (lichen planus, pemphigus vulgaris). The DIF and IIF findings often mimic bullous pemphigoid, so the clinical picture must be carefully considered. The presence of IgA antibodies detected with IIF is associated with severe disease.

Remission is rare, even with treatment; recurrence and progression are the rule. In addition to systemic therapy, potent topical steroids should be employed for vulvovaginal lesions as an adequate response is often noted, even in children [20, 27]. Topical steroids can be supplemented with an anti-inflammatory antibiotic (e.g., tetracycline).

45.2.3 Others

Epidermolysis Bullosa Acquisita Similar in clinical and histologic appearance to bullous pemphigoid due to a shared target antigen, epidermolysis bullosa acquisita (EBA) presents with skin fragility and trauma-induced blistering. Mucous membrane involvement occurs in half of cases [13]. Notable cutaneous effects include pigmentation changes, milia, and tapering of the fingers that can resemble scleroderma. Resultant scarring can significantly distort anatomy, especially on mucosal surfaces as well as alter urogenital function. The histology of EBA mimics bullous pemphigoid as does the IIF, although the latter is more commonly unreactive in EBA and therefore useless for diagnosis. Direct immunofluorescence reveals a "u-serrated" (versus "n-serrated" mentioned in Sect. 44.2.1) pattern of deposition of IgG along the basement membrane, which is unique revealing IgG deposited at a deeper layer in the skin than the majority of other subepidermal blistering diseases [1]. Treatment is difficult as this disease is particularly unresponsive to steroids and immune-suppressive medications.

Pemphigoid Gestationis Pemphigoid gestationis (PG; previously herpes gestationis) is a rare immune blistering disease that affects pregnant women exclusively. It occurs in the second or third trimester of pregnancy, the postpartum period, or in the setting of gestational trophoblastic neoplasia as a paraneoplastic manifestation [28]. A notable association with Grave's disease has been identified [29] as has a risk for fetal growth restriction and preterm birth [30]. The severity of PG increases with eruptions in subsequent pregnancies. Pruritic, pink, non-scaling plaques appear on the abdomen and progress to a generalized bullous eruption that can include the vulva but rarely involve mucous membranes. In some cases, pruritus is the only symptom or the onset may occur so late in gestation that bullae do not have time to develop [1]. A puerperal flare is common and neonates occasionally manifest mild cutaneous lesions. The condition resolves rapidly after delivery but has a significant rate of recurrence. Pemphigoid gestationis appears to be hormone-responsive as one in three patients experiences a flare of symptoms with combined oral contraceptive use or the onset of menses [28]. In 5% of cases, the disease persists, converting to bullous pemphigoid [1].

The histology of PG is subepidermal blister formation with mixed inflammatory infiltrate and papillary edema with eosinophils. The DIF shows complement 3 (C3) bound to the epidermal side at the basement membrane, with or without IgG, while IIF also shows C3 at the basement membrane. A newer diagnostic option is C4d immunohistochemistry to distinguish PG from other disorders [28].

Systemic steroids are safe in the latter half of pregnancy and can be used in combination with topical steroids, which may be sufficient alone. Control of pruritus is often paramount, and there are many medical options that are safe in pregnancy. When considering the use of various immune-suppressant medications, breastfeeding status must be considered. There are reports of IVIG employed during pregnancy as an emerging therapy with excellent outcomes [12]. Monitoring of maternal BP180 antibody levels can correlate with disease activity and assist with monitoring the effect of therapy [31].

Lichen Planus Pemphigoides Lichen planus pemphigoides (LPP) is a rare cause of bullous disease affecting adults and children diagnosed with lichen planus [1]. The average time from diagnosis of lichen planus to diagnosis of LPP is 8 months, and several cases note a medication as an instigating factor [32]. The bullae of LPP usually arise on lichenoid lesions, or locations of previous lichenoid lesions, but also may affect normal skin and bullous oral lesions may be identified. Clinically evident mucosal erosions can easily be confused with those of pemphigus vulgaris, while scarring of mucosal surfaces can appear similar to that with mucous membrane pemphigoid. Histology mimics bullous pemphigoid as do DIF and IIF; the clinical picture and past medical history are paramount. Most cases respond to systemic corticosteroids coupled with topical steroids [5]. There are reports of spontaneously resolution of the bullous lesions despite the persistence of lichen planus [32]. Recurrence is less common than with other bullous disorders.

45.2.4 Other Related Diseases (Not a Pemphigoid Disease [1])

Bullous Systemic Lupus Erythematosus Bullous systemic lupus erythematosus (BSLE) is a rare blistering disorder that occurs in approximately 5% of patients who meet criteria for systemic lupus erythematosus [33]. Diagnostic criteria specific to BSLE have been defined (Table 45.1) [7, 34]. BSLE most commonly presents in African-American women in their 20s–40s, although cases in children have been described [8]. It is considered a variant of lupus

Table 45.1 Diagnostic criteria for bullous systemic lupus erythematosus (BSLE)

(1) Diagnosis of systemic lupus erythematosus by American College of Rheumatology criteria
(2) Eruption of vesicles and/or bullae
(3) Histologic evidence of a subepidermal blister and a predominantly neutrophilic dermal infiltrate
(4) Direct immunofluorescence (DIF) microscopy demonstrating IgG with or without IgA and IgM deposits at the basement membrane zone
(5) Evidence of antibodies to type VII collagen via indirect immunofluorescence (IIF) on salt-split skin, immunoblotting, immunoprecipitation, enzyme-linked immunosorbent assay (ELISA), or immunoelectron microscopy or via DIF

and may be the initial presentation of lupus [7]. Subepidermal tense bullae develop on either normal or erythematous skin of the trunk, upper extremities, neck, and face; these may contain serous or hemorrhagic fluid. The mucous membranes are less commonly affected with the mouth and vermillion of the lips described most often and the vulva described rarely [35]. Bullae resolve without scarring or milia formation (in contrast to epidermolysis bullosa acquisita) but very often cause hypopigmentation of the affected area. Pruritus is usually mild.

The histology is similar to epidermolysis bullosa acquisita and/or dermatitis herpetiformis but often with the unique feature of large deposits of mucin. Direct immunofluorescence may show IgG, IgM, IgA, or complement components at dermo-epidermal junction in granular or linear pattern. In most cases, this disease responds well to dapsone, and several reports note discontinuation of this medication within a year without recurrence of BSLE [7].

All five criteria listed are needed to diagnose type 1 BSLE. Only the first four criteria are required to diagnose type 2 BSLE; antibodies to type VII collagen are absent with this type. The first four criteria are required for type 3 BSLE, and the presence of criterion 5 is variable [7, 34].

Dermatitis Herpetiformis Dermatitis herpetiformis (DH) is considered the cutaneous manifestation of celiac disease [6] which is a chronic, immune-mediated enteropathy precipitated by dietary gluten in genetically predisposed persons [36]. Dermatitis herpetiformis predominates in Caucasians and often presents in young adults, unlike many other bullous disorders. Intense pruritus usually accompanies eruption of symmetrical, small, grouped vesicles that arise on the elbows, knees, neck, face, back, and buttocks; these are quickly denuded due to scratching, and the surrounding skin is distorted by excoriations. Hyperpigmentation may result. Dermatitis herpetiformis rarely affects the vulva.

Subepidermal blistering with a neutrophilic (and occasionally eosinophilic) infiltrate at the papillary tips is noted on histology. Direct immunofluorescence requires a biopsy of perilesional, visibly uninvolved skin while on a normal, gluten-containing diet to demonstrate IgA deposits in a granular pattern in the dermal papillae or at the basement membrane.

An asymptomatic gluten-sensitive enteropathy is often identified with DH. Lifelong, strict adherence to a gluten-free diet is a main pillar of treatment for DH as well as the other manifestations of celiac disease. Gastrointestinal symptoms will typically resolve in 3–6 months, but DH skin lesions can take up to a year or more to clear when treating with dietary modification alone [6]. Recurrence of gastrointestinal symptoms and cutaneous lesions occurs within weeks of resuming gluten ingestion. This disease is also particularly responsive to dapsone and sulfasalazine [36]. These medications can be used during the early months of initiating a gluten-free diet [6].

45.3 Intraepidermal Blistering Diseases

Pemphigus Vulgaris Pemphigus vulgaris (PV) generally presents as a non-scarring blistering disease with involvement of the skin and the mucous membranes. The frequency of mucosal involvement is a distinctive characteristic for this disease, including the propensity of some mucosal surfaces (e.g., vagina) to scar. Childhood cases are rare but have been described. Without prompt and proper identification and treatment, this disease can be life-threatening and may result in death from related infection or other complications.

Flaccid blisters arise on non-inflamed keratinized epithelium. These rupture easily to leave large erosions that do not routinely scar once healed. The majority of cases initially manifest in the oral cavity [37, 38], and the Nikolsky sign is often positive. At least half of women with PV will have genital involvement, and more recent reports have found that genital lesions may be the only identifiable lesions [13, 39]. Vulvar lesions are the most common genital manifestation with 40–60% of women affected [37, 40]. Scarring can appear as partial or complete involution of the labia minora and clitoral hood. The distal one-third of the vagina is the most common vaginal location of PV; one report describes a case of profuse vaginal discharge eventually diagnosed as vaginal PV [41]. Urethral, cervical, and rectal involvements are rare [37]. Interestingly, regular penetrative vaginal intercourse has not been shown to affect the severity of disease [37].

Histology shows intraepidermal blistering that differentiates PV from the group of pemphigoid diseases, which produce subepidermal blisters. Pemphigus vulgaris exhibits loss of adhesion of the basal cells from the upper epidermis, so they remain attached to the basement membrane. Basal cells also lose attachment to adjacent cells creating a "tombstone" appearance. The DIF reveals IgG deposition at epidermal intracellular junctions and IIF also shows IgG antibodies directed against glycoproteins bound to the epidermal intracellular antigens.

Management of PV, including genital PV, often requires systemic therapy that will treat other affected areas. After initial control, oral steroids or other immune-suppressive medications can be tapered to minimum doses. Intralesional injection of genital lesions has also been reported [37]. Prevention and treatment of secondary infection are very important. Recurrence is common, but noted treatments have reduced mortality, which was historically quite high, to a mere 10%.

Consideration should be given to possible abnormalities on cervical cytology (Pap smear) specimens obtained from women with PV [13]. Two studies noted acantholysis on cervical cytology can be variously misinterpreted leading to additional testing and treatment [39]. Pathologists interpreting cervical cytology must be informed if the patient has a history of a mucocutaneous blistering disease. Finally, passage of pemphigus IgG antibody can cause neonatal pemphigus, a transient condition.

Benign Familial Pemphigus (Hailey-Hailey Disease) As the name implies, benign familial pemphigus (BFP) is not immune in nature but hereditary. It is transmitted in an autosomal dominant fashion; thus family history is often positive. The first manifestation of BFP is usually during adolescence with clusters of vesicles that form in intertriginous areas where heat, friction, and perspiration all contribute to epidermal separation from the dermis. Vesicles then rupture and coalesce into crusted plaques over time (Fig. 45.5). Short linear or angular fissures present in the plaques are a unique feature. Vulvar involvement has been described, while the mucous membranes are unaffected [42]. Chronic peripheral scaling can resemble a fungal infection. Secondary infection can occur with BFP including rare coinfection of lesions with herpes simplex virus which should be considered with refractory disease.

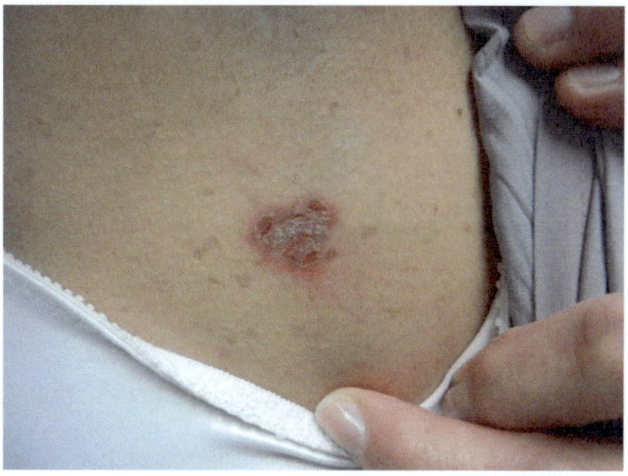

Fig. 45.5 Hailey-Hailey disease. Courtesy of Diane Elas

Diagnosis is made by history, physical examination, and biopsy; DIF and IIF are negative in this disease. Histology demonstrates intraepidermal blistering as well as partial separation from adjacent keratinocytes, termed acantholysis.

Attention to hygiene in affected areas and prompt treatment of any secondary infections are the mainstays of therapy for BFP. Suppression with oral or topical antibiotics can help control cutaneous lesions [42]. Retinoids may provide relief in some cases. Prescription strength antiperspirants can be used on skin that is not eroded or crusted.

Stevens-Johnson Syndrome and Fixed Drug Eruption Stevens-Johnson syndrome (SJS) is a bullous disorder in the spectrum of toxic epidermal necrosis caused by an aberrant immunologic reaction to medications or infection. Patients suffer acute, vigorous, widespread development of cutaneous lesions with associated bullae leading to epidermal necrosis (Fig. 45.6, 45.7, and 45.8). Hemorrhagic mucositis can also occur, and bullae on mucosal surfaces may heal with significant scarring. This disorder can affect patients of any age, and the primary treatment is cessation or elimination of the offending substance, as well as supportive care. While effects of SJS on the vulva and vagina are rarely reported, the results of post-eruption scarring can be devastating and may results in complete labial fusion and coaptation of the vaginal opening with blockage of vaginal and menstrual fluids [43]. These devastating alterations should be anticipated in a woman of any age who suffers SJS [44]. Supportive care of the vulva and vagina includes use of barriers and skin protectants as well as consideration of the need for vaginal dilation to maintain patency.

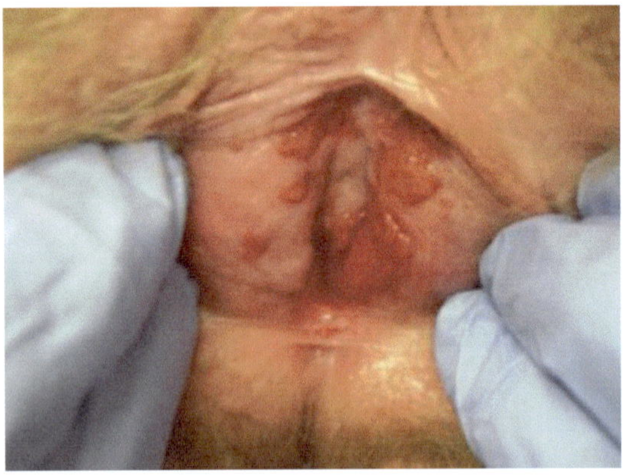

Fig. 45.6 Vulvar Stevens-Johnson syndrome. Bullae resulting in epidermal necrosis heal with significant scarring. It may also lead to labial fusion and coaptation of the vaginal opening with blockage. Courtesy of Dr. Colleen Stockdale

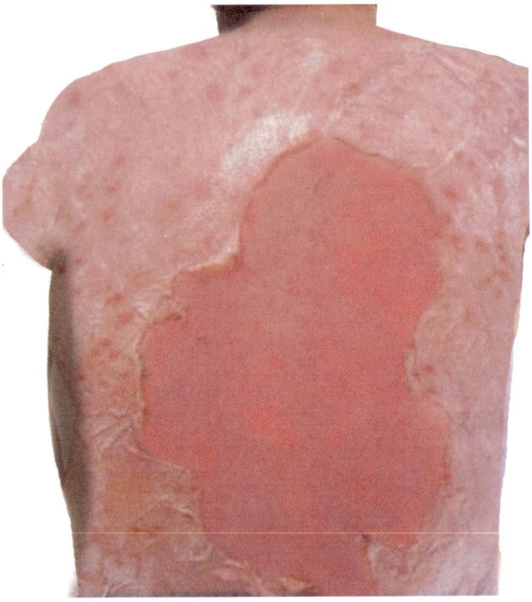

Fig. 45.7 Vulvar Stevens-Johnson syndrome. Courtesy of Dr. Colleen Stockdale

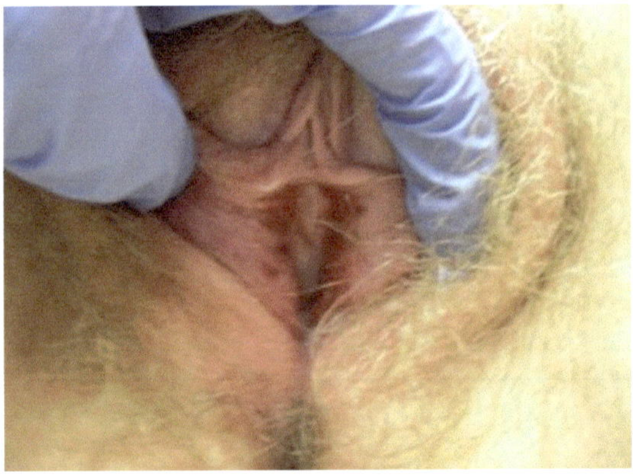

Fig. 45.8 Stevens-Johnson syndrome. Skin loss at the back. Multiple erythematous maculae. Courtesy of Professor Jacob Bornstein

Fixed drug eruption represents 0.5% of all drug-related skin rashes. It manifests as a localized area of acute pruritus, pain, and erythematous plaques with central blister formation that develop in response to use of a medication. This reaction can occur anywhere on the body and has been described to affect the vulva [45, 46]. Post-inflammatory hyperpigmentation may result, especially with recurrent episodes. Recurrence is common, possibly with extension to adjacent or additional body sites. Misdiagnosis is common, and treatment is identification and discontinuation of the instigating medication or substance. Patch testing is not useful. An oral provocation test is gold standard but not often recommended as a thorough history and clinical evaluation usually suffice.

Immune Blistering Disorders: Breaking the Myths

- Most probably, blisters cannot be found in immune blistering disorders, because on mucosal surfaces they erode quickly and appear more commonly as erosions.
- Although differentiating between the various immune blistering disorders is desired, the management overlaps for many of them: use of soaks, addition of barriers or skin protectants, minimizing the presence of contact irritants, topical steroid ointments, and sometimes systemic steroids. Immune-suppressive medications, mainly azathioprine, are the second line of treatment.
- Although considered to be associated with lichen sclerosus—pruritus, phimosis of the clitoris or fusion of the labia—may develop in cicatricial pemphigoid as well.

References

1. Schmidt E, Zillikens D. Pemphigoid diseases. Lancet. 2013;381(9863):320–32.
2. Bifulco G, Mandato VD, Piccoli R, Giampaolino P, Mignogna C, Mignogna MD, et al. Early invasive vulvar squamous cell carcinoma arising in a woman with vulvar pemphigus vulgaris and systemic lupus erythematosus. BMC Cancer. 2010;10:324.
3. Goldstein AT, Anhalt GJ, Klingman D, Burrows LJ. Mucous membrane pemphigoid of the vulva. Obstet Gynecol. 2005;105(5 Pt 2):1188–90.
4. Huilaja L, Makikallio K, Hannula-Jouppi K, Vakeva L, Hook-Nikanne J, Tasanen K. Cyclosporine treatment in severe gestational pemphigoid. Acta Derm Venereol. 2015;95(5):593–5.
5. Malakar S, Saha A. Successful treatment of resistant Lichen Planus Pemphigoides with cyclosporine: a new hope. Indian J Dermatol. 2016;61(1):112–4.
6. Antiga E, Caproni M. The diagnosis and treatment of dermatitis herpetiformis. Clin Cosmet Investig Dermatol. 2015;8:257–65.
7. Contestable JJ, Edhegard KD, Meyerle JH. Bullous systemic lupus erythematosus: a review and update to diagnosis and treatment. Am J Clin Dermatol. 2014;15(6):517–24.
8. Barbosa WS, Rodarte CM, Guerra JG, Maciel VG, Fleury Junior LF, Costa MB. Bullous systemic lupus erythematosus: differential diagnosis with dermatitis herpetiformis. An Bras Dermatol. 2011;86(4 Suppl 1):S92–5.
9. Lebeau S, Mainetti C, Masouye I, Saurat JH, Borradori L. Localized childhood vulval pemphigoid treated with tacrolimus ointment. Dermatology. 2004;208(3):273–5.
10. Gunther C, Wozel G, Meurer M, Pfeiffer C. Topical tacrolimus treatment for cicatricial pemphigoid. J Am Acad Dermatol. 2004;50(2):325–6.
11. Howell E, Johnson SM. Venous thrombosis occurring after initiation of thalidomide for the treatment of cicatricial pemphigoid. J Drugs Dermatol. 2004;3(1):83–5.
12. Nguyen T, Alraqum E, Razzaque Ahmed A. Positive clinical outcome with IVIg as monotherapy in recurrent pemphigoid gestationis. Int Immunopharmacol. 2015;26(1):1–3.
13. Pipkin C. Erosive diseases of the vulva. Dermatol Clin. 2010;28(4):737–51.
14. Lebeau S, Braun RP, Masouye I, Perrinaud A, Harms M, Borradori L. Acquired melanocytic naevus in childhood vulval pemphigoid. Dermatology. 2006;213(2):159–62.
15. Urano S. Localized bullous pemphigoid of the vulva. J Dermatol. 1996;23(8):580–2.
16. Levine V, Sanchez M, Nestor M. Localized vulvar pemphigoid in a child misdiagnosed as sexual abuse. Arch Dermatol. 1992;128(6):804–6.
17. Stage AH, Humeniuk JM, Easley WK. Bullous pemphigoid of the vulva: a case report. Am J Obstet Gynecol. 1984;150(2):169–70.
18. Ridley CM. Cicatricial pemphigoid of the vulva. Am J Obstet Gynecol. 1985;152(7 Pt 1):916–7.
19. Leonard N, Biswas A, Hickey S, Bell H. Eosinophilic spongiosis in a case of lichen sclerosus: a marker for

superimposed bullous pemphigoid? Histopathology. 2008;52(7):885–7.
20. Farrell AM, Kirtschig G, Dalziel KL, Allen J, Dootson G, Edwards S, et al. Childhood vulval pemphigoid: a clinical and immunopathological study of five patients. Br J Dermatol. 1999;140(2):308–12.
21. Marren P, Wojnarowska F, Venning V, Wilson C, Nayar M. Vulvar involvement in autoimmune bullous diseases. J Reprod Med. 1993;38(2):101–7.
22. Wojnarowska F, Marsden RA, Bhogal B, Black MM. Chronic bullous disease of childhood, childhood cicatricial pemphigoid, and linear IgA disease of adults. A comparative study demonstrating clinical and immunopathologic overlap. J Am Acad Dermatol. 1988;19(5 Pt 1):792–805.
23. Edwards S, Wojnarowska F, Armstrong LM. Chronic bullous disease of childhood with oral mucosal scarring. Clin Exp Dermatol. 1991;16(1):41–3.
24. Chan LS, Ahmed AR, Anhalt GJ, Bernauer W, Cooper KD, Elder MJ, et al. The first international consensus on mucous membrane pemphigoid: definition, diagnostic criteria, pathogenic factors, medical treatment, and prognostic indicators. Arch Dermatol. 2002;138(3):370–9.
25. Edwards L, Hays S. Vulvar cicatricial pemphigoid as a lichen sclerosus imitator. A case report. J Reprod Med. 1992;37(6):561–4.
26. Marren P, Walkden V, Mallon E, Wojnarowska F. Vulval cicatricial pemphigoid may mimic lichen sclerosus. Br J Dermatol. 1996;134(3):522–4.
27. Hoque SR, Patel M, Farrell AM. Childhood cicatricial pemphigoid confined to the vulva. Clinical. Dermatology. 2005;31:63–4.
28. Sadik CD, Lima AL, Zillikens D. Pemphigoid gestationis: toward a better understanding of the etiopathogenesis. Clin Dermatol. 2016;34(3):378–82.
29. Jenkins RE, Hern S, Black MM. Clinical features and management of 87 patients with pemphigoid gestationis. Clin Exp Dermatol. 1999;24(4):255–9.
30. Chi CC, Wang SH, Charles-Holmes R, Ambros-Rudolph C, Powell J, Jenkins R, et al. Pemphigoid gestationis: early onset and blister formation are associated with adverse pregnancy outcomes. Br J Dermatol. 2009;160(6):1222–8.
31. Sitaru C, Powell J, Messer G, Brocker EB, Wojnarowska F, Zillikens D. Immunoblotting and enzyme-linked immunosorbent assay for the diagnosis of pemphigoid gestationis. Obstet Gynecol. 2004;103(4):757–63.
32. Zaraa I, Mahfoudh A, Sellami MK, Chelly I, El Euch D, Zitouna M, et al. Lichen planus pemphigoides: four new cases and a review of the literature. Int J Dermatol. 2013;52(4):406–12.
33. Petri M, Orbai AM, Alarcon GS, Gordon C, Merrill JT, Fortin PR, et al. Derivation and validation of the systemic lupus international collaborating clinics classification criteria for systemic lupus erythematosus. Arthritis Rheum. 2012;64(8):2677–86.
34. Camisa C. Vesiculobullous systemic lupus erythematosus. A report of four cases. J Am Acad Dermatol. 1988;18(1 Pt 1):93–100.
35. Miziara ID, Mahmoud A, Chagury AA, Alves RD. Bullous systemic lupus Erythematosus: case report. Int Arch Otorhinolaryngol. 2013;17(3):344–6.
36. Pinto-Sanchez MI, Bercik P, Verdu EF, Bai JC. Extraintestinal manifestations of celiac disease. Dig Dis. 2015;33(2):147–54.
37. Malik M, Ahmed AR. Involvement of the female genital tract in pemphigus vulgaris. Obstet Gynecol. 2005;106(5 Pt 1):1005–12.
38. Lopez-Jornet P, Bermejo-Fenoll A. Gingival lesions as a first symptom of pemphigus vulgaris in pregnancy. Br Dent J. 2005;199(2):91–2.
39. Fairbanks Barbosa ND, de Aguiar LM, Maruta CW, Aoki V, Sotto MN, Labinas GH, et al. Vulvo-cervico-vaginal manifestations and evaluation of Papanicolaou smears in pemphigus vulgaris and pemphigus foliaceus. J Am Acad Dermatol. 2012;67(3):409–16.
40. Kavala M, Topaloglu Demir F, Zindanci I, Can B, Turkoglu Z, Zemheri E, et al. Genital involvement in pemphigus vulgaris (PV): correlation with clinical and cervicovaginal pap smear findings. J Am Acad Dermatol. 2015;73(4):655–9.
41. Batta K, Munday PE, Tatnall FM. Pemphigus vulgaris localized to the vagina presenting as chronic vaginal discharge. Br J Dermatol. 1999;140(5):945–7.
42. Wieselthier JS, Pincus SH. Hailey-Hailey disease of the vulva. Arch Dermatol. 1993;129(10):1344–5.
43. de Jesus LE, Dekermacher S, Manhaes CR, Faria LM, Barros ML. Acquired labial sinechiae and hydrocolpos secondary to Stevens-Johnson syndrome. Urology. 2012;80(4):919–21.
44. Ting HC, Adam BA. Stevens-Johnson syndrome. A review of 34 cases. Int J Dermatol. 1985;24(9):587–91.
45. Wain EM, Neill S. Fixed drug eruption of the vulva secondary to fluconazole. Clin Exp Dermatol. 2008;33(6):784–5.
46. Fischer G. Vulvar fixed drug eruption. A report of 13 cases. J Reprod Med. 2007;52(2):81–6.

Part XI

Vulvar Lesions: Blisters—Pustules

46 Methicillin-Resistant *Staphylococcus aureus*

Sara Wood

46.1 Introduction

Methicillin-resistant *Staphylococcus aureus* (MRSA) infections relevant to the women's health care provider include skin and soft tissue infections (SSTIs) and abscesses at the vulva, vagina, groin, breast, and postoperative wounds. MRSA infections commonly exhibit purulence and abscess formation due to virulence factors which inhibit phagocytosis and destroy neutrophils [1–3]. The genital region is particularly predisposed to MRSA colonization and infection due to practices of hair removal via shaving/waxing, sexual relations with other MRSA carriers, sharing of personal hygiene products, or poor hygiene practices due to obesity or immobility [3].

In two of the largest cohort studies of women with vulvar abscess, nearly two-thirds of cultures revealed MRSA [2, 3]. Thus, culture should be obtained in cases of a vulvar abscess, and empiric treatment with coverage for MRSA is recommended. Further directed antibiotic therapy is based on the results of culture sensitivities. Incision and drainage (I&D) with disruption of any loculation followed by dressing with clean, dry bandages is important in the treatment of abscesses, furuncles, and carbuncles within the vulva [4, 5].

Studies have revealed that trimethoprim-sulfamethoxazole (TMP-SMX) is largely effective against MRSA along with other common vulvar abscess microbes, such as *Proteus*, *Escherichia coli*, and group B streptococcus [2, 3, 5]. Other antibiotic options include tetracyclines (i.e., doxycycline or minocycline), clindamycin, or linezolid [4–6]. However, local antibiotic resistance patterns should be taken into account during antibiotic selection as studies have reported significant resistance to clindamycin in up to 65% of isolates [2, 6]. Treatment courses are dependent on the resolution of symptoms [4, 5].

A careful history may reveal comorbidities that may indicate whether inpatient hospitalization is necessary. An outpatient course of oral antibiotic treatment in addition to I&D in the presence of an abscess with serial examination is appropriate in patients with risk factors, such as diabetes mellitus, obesity, immunosuppression, pregnancy, trauma, or iatrogenic trauma [5]. Hospitalization has been proposed for patients with an abscess of greater than 5 cm or blood glucose levels greater than 200 with appropriate surgical and antibiotic interventions as displayed in Table 46.1 [3, 7].

Recurrence of MRSA abscess or SSTI should prompt investigation into predisposing conditions, such as improper wound care, poor personal hygiene, sharing or reusing of personal

S. Wood (✉)
Division of Female Pelvic Medicine and Reconstructive Surgery, Department of Obstetrics and Gynecology, Mercy Hospital St. Louis, St. Louis, MO, USA

J. Bornstein (ed.), *Vulvar Disease*, https://doi.org/10.1007/978-3-319-61621-6_46

Table 46.1 Intravenous antibiotics for purulent vulvar infections

Moderate infection[a]	MRSA: TMP/SMX MSSA: Dicloxacillin or cephalexin
Severe infection[b]	MRSA: Vancomycin or daptomycin or linezolid MSSA: Nafcillin or cefazolin

Reproduced with permission from Wood [7]
MRSA methicillin-resistant *Staphylococcus aureus*, *MSSA* methicillin-sensitive *Staphylococcus aureus*, *TMP/SMX* trimethoprim-sulfamethoxazole
[a]Purulent infection with systemic signs
[b]Purulent infection that has previously failed antibiotics with systemic signs

items, and insufficient cleansing of areas frequently touched by bare skin within the household [4, 5]. If possible, these risk factors should be addressed and eliminated. Decolonization of the patient and roommates may be considered in cases of recurrent MRSA infection despite remedying the above risk factors [4]. Decolonization includes two main steps: nasal decolonization with twice daily mupirocin and topical body decolonization with skin disinfectants: chlorhexidine for 5–14 days or dilute bleach baths for 15 min twice a week for 3 months (1/4 cup per ¼ tub of water) [4]. Oral antibiotics for decolonization have not been shown to be efficacious unless an active infection is present [4].

Vulvar MRSA: Breaking the Myths

- Although vulvar colonization with MRSA is considered to be rare, it is the cause of nearly two-thirds of vulvar abscesses.
- Decolonization of MRSA by oral antibiotics is useless. Instead, nasal decolonization with mupirocin and skin wash with disinfectants, such as chlorhexidine, is helpful.

References

1. Gordon R, Lowy F. Pathogenesis of methicillin-resistant *Staphylococcus aureus* infection. Clin Infect Dis. 2008;46:S350–9.
2. Kilpatrick C, Alagkiozidis I, Orejuela F, et al. Factors complicating surgical management of the vulvar abscess. J Reprod Med. 2010;55(3–4):139–42.
3. Thurman A, Satterfield T, Soper D. Methicillin-resistant *Staphylococcus aureus* as a common cause of vulvar abscesses. Obstet Gynecol. 2008;112(3):538–44.
4. Liu C, Bayer A, Cosgrove S, et al. Clinical practice guidelines by the Infectious Diseases Society of America for the treatment of methicillin-resistant *Staphylococcus aureus* infections in adults and children: executive summary. Clin Infect Dis. 2011; 52(3):285–92.
5. Stevens D, Bisno A, Chambers H, et al. Practice guidelines for the diagnosis and management of skin and soft tissue infections: 2014 update by the Infectious Diseases Society of America. Clin Infect Dis. 2014;59(2):e10–52.
6. Breen J. Skin and soft tissue infections in immunocompetent patients. Am Fam Physician. 2010;81(7):893–9.
7. Wood S. Clinical manifestations and therapeutic management of vulvar cellulitis and abscess: methicillin-resistant Staphylococcus aureus, necrotizing fasciitis bartholin abscess, crohn disease of the vulva, hidradenitis suppurativa. Clin Obstet Gynecol. 2015;58(3):503–11.

Necrotizing Fasciitis

47

Sara Wood

47.1 Introduction

Necrotizing fasciitis (NF) of the female vulva and perineum is a life-threatening soft tissue infection that necessitates immediate multidisciplinary coordinated care to limit morbidity and mortality. The contiguous nature of the vulvar fascia and associated adipose tissue facilitates rapid spread of NF and leads to widespread destruction of tissue and systemic infection. Perineal NF carries a twofold increase in mortality compared to NF originating in the limbs with reported mortality rates ranging from 14% to 48% [1–6]. Delays in diagnosis and debridement likely represent two of the greatest factors responsible for even higher rates of mortality, underscoring the prompt multidisciplinary efforts needed for treatment [2, 7].

47.2 Risk Factors

Risk factors for necrotizing fasciitis include diabetes mellitus, obesity, immunosuppression, intravenous drug and alcohol abuse, trauma, and iatrogenic causes from postoperative surgical wounds [7–10]. These severe infections have also been reported after routine obstetric and gynecologic procedures, such as vaginal and cesarean delivery, episiotomy, marsupialization of Bartholin's gland, mid-urethral sling, and hysterectomy [7, 11–15]. Providers caring for women with wound infections in the postpartum setting should be particularly astute to the possibility and risk of group A streptococcus (GAS) and its associated severe systemic illness [7, 16].

47.3 Pathophysiology and Microbiology

The pathophysiology of NF is complex. Microbial invasion commonly begins through superficial skin trauma or perforation of the lower gastrointestinal tract or urogenital organs [8]. As bacteria spread along the fascia, virulence factors (i.e., endo- or exotoxins, surface proteins, and superantigens) are produced allowing for evasion of host immune factors and cause activation of host inflammatory and coagulation cascades [17–19]. Ultimately, tissue edema and impaired capillary blood flow lead to tissue necrosis, subsequent shock, and multi-organ system failure with possible death [18–20].

Although NF is most commonly polymicrobial, single-pathogen NF also occurs, particularly in the obstetric setting [8]. Polymicrobial infections include gram-positive cocci (*Staphylococcus aureus* and *Streptococcus*),

S. Wood (✉)
Division of Female Pelvic Medicine and Reconstructive Surgery, Department of Obstetrics and Gynecology, Mercy Hospital St. Louis, St. Louis, MO, USA

J. Bornstein (ed.), *Vulvar Disease*, https://doi.org/10.1007/978-3-319-61621-6_47

gram-negative rods (*Klebsiella*, *Escherichia coli*, and *Bacteroides*), anaerobes, and less frequently gram-positive rods (*Clostridia* species) [8, 10, 21–23]. Monomicrobial NF infections caused by group A streptococcus (GAS) are unique due to the potential for associated toxic shock syndrome and the ability of GAS to survive within macrophages, thereby evading antibiotic treatment [8, 17].

47.4 Clinical Presentation

Multiple studies have shown that there is a direct correlation between a delayed diagnosis and/or initiation of therapy and increased mortality [9, 21–23]. Clinicians must have a high index of suspicion for timely diagnosis to be made. Clinical manifestations of NF can be vague, such as tissue erythema, edema, and pain/tenderness out of proportion to clinical exam, and initial misdiagnosis frequently occurs [22, 24, 25]. These manifestations comprise a differential that includes cellulitis, abscess, erysipelas, or even noninfectious inflammatory conditions of the skin or subcutaneous tissue [22, 26].

The characteristic exam finding is extensive necrosis of the fascial layer with a lack of tissue resistance upon probing and significant undermining of the tissue [2, 5–7]. Crepitus, skin necrosis, anesthesia, and skin discoloration are rarely present on initial evaluation and are considered late findings once extensive tissue damage has already occurred [7, 22, 24, 27].

The diagnosis of NF is largely clinical, and therefore radiologic imaging is of little use nor should its use delay treatment and initiation of surgical debridement. Fascial edema and increased enhancement, when contrast is used, are findings identified by CT scan, which have higher sensitivity but less specificity in the diagnosis NF [28, 29]. The finding of subcutaneous air is highly specific for NF but rarely seen [26, 28, 29]. Although studies have shown that MRI has high sensitivity for detecting NF, the use of this imaging modality may delay treatment and is therefore not recommended [8, 30]. As NF progresses, shock and multi-organ damage are reflected on laboratory studies including elevated inflammatory markers, anemia, electrolyte disturbances, renal failure, and hyperglycemia [31, 32].

47.5 Treatment

Early consultation between multiple disciplines including infectious disease and surgical specialists is imperative in the management of NF [4]. The two main pillars of NF therapy are prompt surgical debridement and antibiotics. Because of the poor blood flow within the capillaries of tissue affected by NF, antibiotics cannot reach sufficient levels to eradicate causative bacteria [33, 34]. Removing all devitalized tissue, even when large surface areas need to be resected, is the only way that antibiotics can be fully effective [8] (Figs. 47.1 and 47.2). Hence, delayed or inadequate debridement has been directly correlated with increasing mortality [9, 22]. Often, multiple debridement procedures are necessary [35–37].

While local debridement focuses on controlling the source of NF, antibiotics help control systemic spread of infection [33]. Broad-spectrum antibiotics, which cover methicillin-resistance *Staphylococcus aureus*, should be initiated and tailored as cultures result as noted in Table 47.1 [38]. Electrolyte replacement and fluid resuscitation should be proactively managed with frequent reassessment of serum fluctuations to assess insensible fluid losses and hemodynamic instability. Intensive critical care settings are the preferred units for these patients with care delivered by providers experienced in the treatment of severely ill patients.

Due to extensive debridement, wounds may be quite large and difficult to heal, and thus consultation of wound care providers is important to the recovery process. Adjunctive therapies such as wound vacuums and hyperbaric oxygen therapy may assist with healing of large wounds and rehabilitation to resume normal activities of daily living may be necessary in those with large functionally limiting lesions [5, 7, 36].

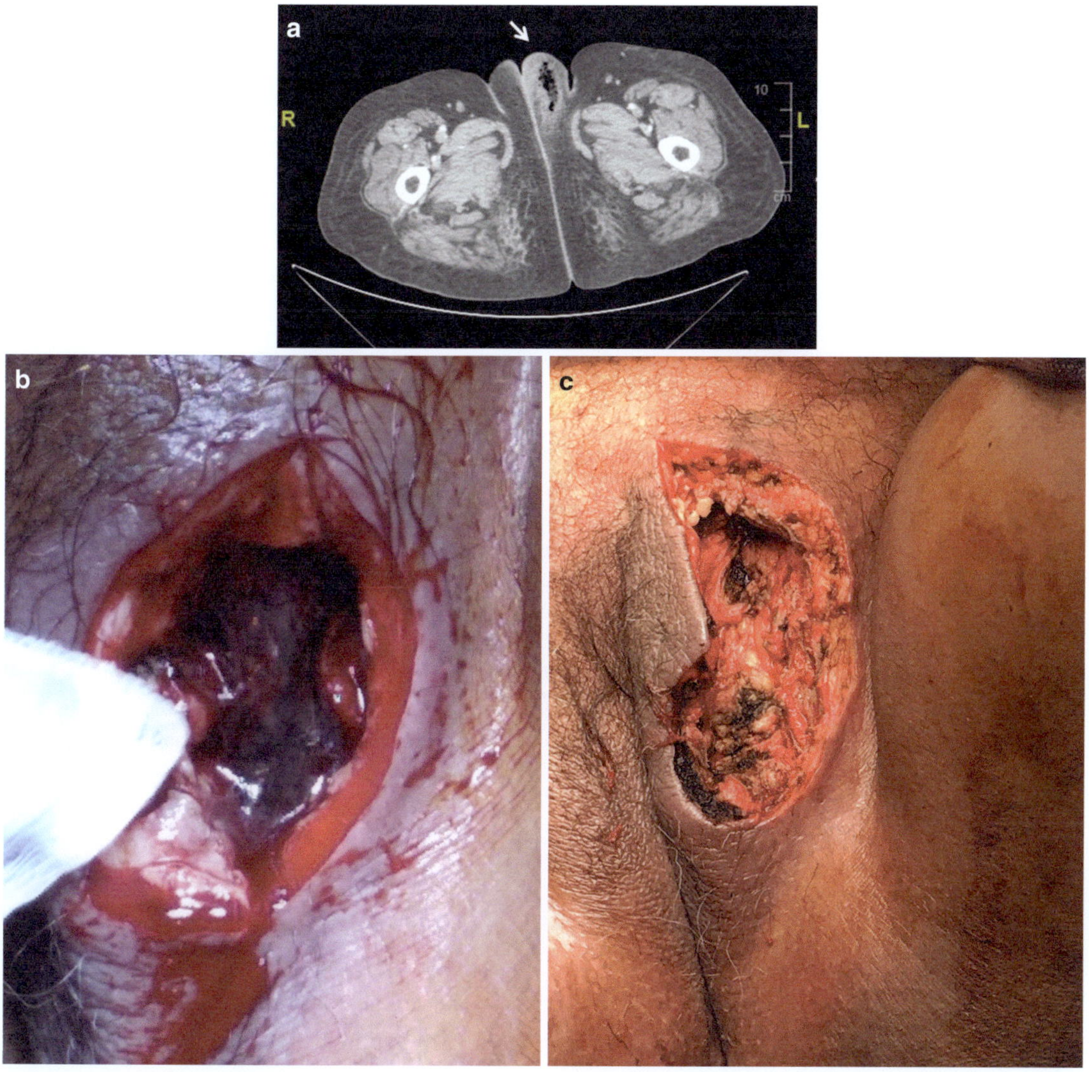

Fig. 47.1 62 year old patient with end-stage kidney disease, undergoing hemodialysis. Presented with pain, diffuse erythema and edema of the left labia majora, quickly spreading to the pubis. (**a**) Pelvic CT scan. Arrow points to left labia majora where air is located inside the labia, a sign of necrotizing Fasciitis. The right labia majora is normal. (**b**) Deep labial incision reveals necrosis of the subcutaneous tissues, muscles and fascia. (**c**) Debridement and removal of devitalized tissues was repeated the next day and followed with chlorine soaks. Granulation slowly develops. Courtesy of Professor Jacob Bornstein

Necrotizing Soft Tissue Infection: Breaking the Myths

- Although rarely seen in the gynecological practice, necrotizing fasciitis in the perineum carries a twofold increase in mortality compared to that originating in the limbs. Mortality ranges from 14% to 48%.
- Surgery is not the only causative procedure of necrotizing fasciitis. Normal vaginal delivery may also initiate it.

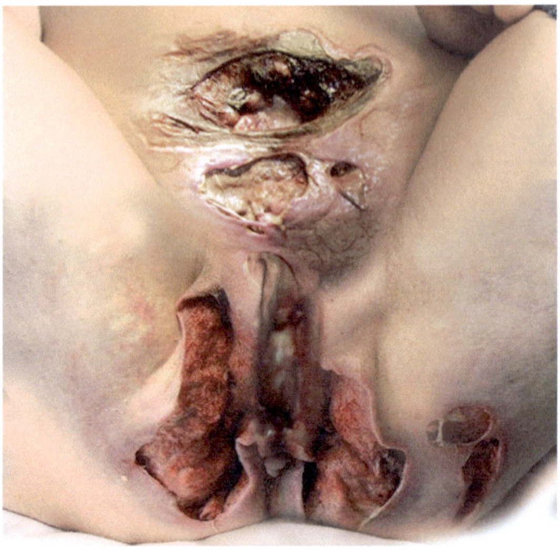

Fig. 47.2 Necrotizing fasciitis. Procedure including debridement and removing devitalized tissue

Table 47.1 Intravenous antibiotic therapy for necrotizing fasciitis

Polymicrobial	*Staphylococcus* species	*Streptococcus* species	*Clostridium* species
Piperacillin/tazobactam + vancomycin	Penicillin + clindamycin	Nafcillin	Clindamycin + penicillin
Clindamycin or metronidazole + aminoglycoside or fluoroquinolone (if penicillin hypersensitivity)	Vancomycin Linezolid	Oxacillin	
		Cefazolin	
		Vancomycin (if MRSA)	

Reproduced with permission from Wood [38]
MRSA methicillin-resistant *Staphylococcus aureus*

References

1. Nolan T, King L, Smith R, et al. Necrotizing surgical infection and necrotizing fasciitis in obstetric and gynecologic patients. South Med J. 1993;86:1363–7.
2. Stephenson H, Dotters D, Katz V, et al. Necrotizing fasciitis of the vulva. Am J Obstet Gynecol. 1992;166:1324–7.
3. Gallup D, Freedman M, Meguiar R, et al. Necrotizing fasciitis in gynecologic and obstetric patients: a surgical emergency. Am J Obstet Gynecol. 2002;187:305–10.
4. Courtney-Brooks M, Scalici J, Henretta M, et al. Vulvar necrotizing soft tissue infection: a review 73 of a multidisciplinary surgical emergency and management in the modern era. Gynecol Oncol Case Rep. 2013;5:6–9.
5. Thompson C, Brekken A, Kutteh W. Necrotizing fasciitis: a review of management guidelines in a large obstetrics and gynecology teaching hospital. Infect Dis Obstet Gynecol. 1993;1:16–22.
6. Rea W, Wyrick W. Necrotizing fasciitis. Ann Surg. 1970;172:957–64.
7. Faro S, Faro J. Necrotizing soft-tissue infections in obstetric and gynecologic patients. Clin Obstet Gynecol. 2012;55(4):875–87.
8. Sarani B, Strong M, Pascual J, et al. Necrotizing fasciitis: current concepts and review of the literature. J Am Coll Surg. 2009;208(2):279–88.
9. Voros D, Pissiotis C, Georgantas D. Role of early and extensive surgery in the treatment of severe necrotizing soft tissue infection. Br J Surg. 1993;80(9):1190–1.
10. Childers B, Potyondy L, Nachreiner R, et al. Necrotizing fasciitis: a fourteen-year retrospective study of 163 consecutive patients. Am Surg. 2002;68:109–16.
11. Schorge J, Granter S, Lerner L. Postpartum and vulvar necrotizing fasciitis. J Reprod Med. 1998;43(7):586–90.
12. Morris M, Aru M, Gaugler A, et al. Necrotizing fasciitis of the perineum associated with a bartholin abscess. Surg Infect. 2014;15(2):131–3.
13. Lynch C, Pinelli D, Cruse C, et al. Maternal death from postpartum necrotizing fasciitis arising in an episiotomy: a case report. Infect Dis Obstet Gynecol. 1997;5:341–4.

14. Flam F, Boijsen M, Lind F. Necrotizing fasciitis following transobturator tape treated by extensive surgery and hyperbaric oxygen. Int Urogynecol J Pelvic Floor Dysfunct. 2009;20(1):113–5.
15. Mahal A, Bradley C. Necrotizing postsurgical infection complicating midurethral sling procedure with unrecognized cystotomy. Female Pelvic Med Reconstr Surg. 2012;18:183–5.
16. Rimawi B, Soper D, Eschenbach D. Group A streptococcal infections in obstetrics and gynecology. Clin Obstet Gynecol. 2012;55(4):864–74.
17. Thulin P, Johansson L, Low D, et al. Viable Group A streptococcus in macrophages during acute soft tissue infection. PLoS Med. 2006;3(3):e53.
18. Wartha F, Beiter K, Normark S, et al. Neutrophil extracellular traps: casting the net over pathogenesis. Curr Opin Microbiol. 2007;10:52–6.
19. Hackett S, Stevens D. Streptococcal toxic shock syndrome: synthesis of tumor necrosis factor and interleukin-1 by monocytes stimulated with pyrogenic exotoxin A and streptolysin O. J Infect Dis. 1992;165(5):879–85.
20. Salcido R. Necrotizing fasciitis: reviewing the causes and treatment strategies. Adv Skin Wound Care. 2007;20(5):288–93.
21. McHenry C, Piotrowski J, Petrinic D, et al. Determinants of mortality for necrotizing soft-tissue infections. Ann Surg. 1995;221(5):558–63.
22. Wong C, Chang H, Pasupathy S, et al. Necrotizing fasciitis: clinical presentation, microbiology, and determinants of mortality. J Bone Joint Surg. 2003;85(8):1454–60.
23. Bilton B, Zibari G, McMillan R. Aggressive surgical management of necrotizing fasciitis serves to decrease mortality: a retrospective study. Am Surg. 1998;64(5):397–400.
24. Elliott D, Kufera J, Myers R. Necrotizing soft tissue infections: risk factors for mortality and strategies for management. Ann Surg. 1996;224(5):672–83.
25. Haywood C, McGeer A, Low D. Clinical experience with 20 cases of Group A streptococcus necrotizing fasciitis and myonecrosis: 1995–1997. Plast Reconstr Surg. 1999;103(6):1567–73.
26. Beauchamp N, Scott W, Gottlieb L. CT evaluation of soft tissue muscle infection and inflammation: a systematic compartmental approach. Skeletal Radiol. 1995;24:317–24.
27. Wang Y, Wong C, Tay Y. Staging of necrotizing fasciitis based on the evolving cutaneous features. Int J Dermatol. 2007;46:1036–41.
28. Wysoki M, Santora T, Shah R, et al. Necrotizing fasciitis: CT characteristics. Radiology. 1997;203:859–63.
29. Becker M, Zbaren P, Hermans R, et al. Necrotizing fasciitis of the head and neck: role of CT in diagnosis and management. Radiology. 1997;202:471–6.
30. Schmid M, Kossmann T, Duewell S. Differentiation of necrotizing fasciitis and cellulitis using MR imaging. AJR Am J Roentgenol. 1998;170:615–20.
31. Anaya D, McMahon K, Nathens A, et al. Predictors of mortality and limb loss in necrotizing soft tissue infections. Arch Surg. 2005;140:151–7.
32. Wong C, Khin L, Heng K, et al. The LRINEC (laboratory risk indicator for necrotizing fasciitis) score: a tool for distinguishing necrotizing fasciitis from other soft tissue infections. Crit Care Med. 2004;32(7):1535–41.
33. Cainzos M, Gonzalez-Rodriguez F. Necrotizing soft tissue infections. Curr Opin Crit Care. 2007;13:433–9.
34. Hsiao G, Chang C, Hsiao C. Necrotizing soft tissue infections: surgical or conservative treatment. Dermatol Surg. 1998;24:243–8.
35. Goh T, Goh L, Ang C, et al. Early diagnosis of necrotizing fasciitis. Br J Surg. 2014;101:e119–25.
36. Czymek R, Kujath P, Bruch H, et al. Treatment, outcome, and quality of life after Fournier's gangrene: a multicentre study. Colorectal Dis. 2013;15:1529–36.
37. Chawla S, Gallop C, Mydlo J. Fournier's gangrene: an analysis of repeated surgical debridement. Eur Urol. 2003;43:572–5.
38. Wood S. Clinical manifestations and therapeutic management of vulvar cellulitis and abscess, methicillin-resistant Staphylococcus aureus, necrotizing fasciitis, bartholin abscess, crohn disease of the vulva, hidradenitis suppurativa. Clin Obstet Gynecol. 2015;58(3):503–11.

48 Hidradenitis Suppurativa

Jacob Bornstein

48.1 Introduction

Hidradenitis suppurativa (HS) is a chronic, follicular, occlusive, inflammatory skin condition. It is also called "acne inversa" and "Verneuil's disease" [1].

HS affects the intertriginous skin areas of the axillary, groin, perianal, perineal, and inframammary regions. It presents as recurrent, inflamed nodules and abscesses, draining sinus tracts and bands of severe scar formation. It is associated with pain, bad odor, discharge, and disfigurement [2]. Its prevalence is 1–4% [3]; most cases are mild. It usually begins before age of 40, in women twice as much as men.

48.2 Pathogenesis

Past theory assumed that apocrine glands are involved. Currently follicular occlusion or rupture with an associated immune response is thought to cause the disease. There is a genetic susceptibility: 40% of patients with HS have an affected first-degree family member [4]. A candidate locus for HS is at chromosome 1p21.1–1q25.3.

Other risk factors are pressure and friction on intertriginous skin, obesity, and smoking. Despite abscess formation, the early, unruptured HS lesions are sterile. Older and ruptured lesions and sinuses may grow staphylococci, streptococci, Gram-negative rods, anaerobic bacteria, and coagulase-negative staphylococci. Positive cultures may represent contaminants from normal skin flora or secondary infection. Oral contraceptives containing androgenic progestins, intramuscular medroxyprogesterone acetate, or levonorgestrel intrauterine device may precipitate or worsen HS [5]. Paradoxically, HS has been reported as an adverse effect of anti-TNF-alpha therapies and other biologic treatments given for other chronic inflammatory diseases.

48.3 Clinical Presentation

HS develops in intertriginous areas: the axillae, inguinal area, inner thighs, perianal and perineal areas, mammary and inframammary regions, buttocks, pubic region, scrotum, vulva, and trunk. The primary lesions are inflammatory nodules, sometimes with suppurative discharge. Sinus formation, clusters of open comedones and scar formation are seen in

J. Bornstein (✉)
Department of Obstetrics and Gynecology Galilee Medical Center, Bar-Ilan University Faculty of Medicine, Nahariya, Israel

J. Bornstein (ed.), *Vulvar Disease*, https://doi.org/10.1007/978-3-319-61621-6_48

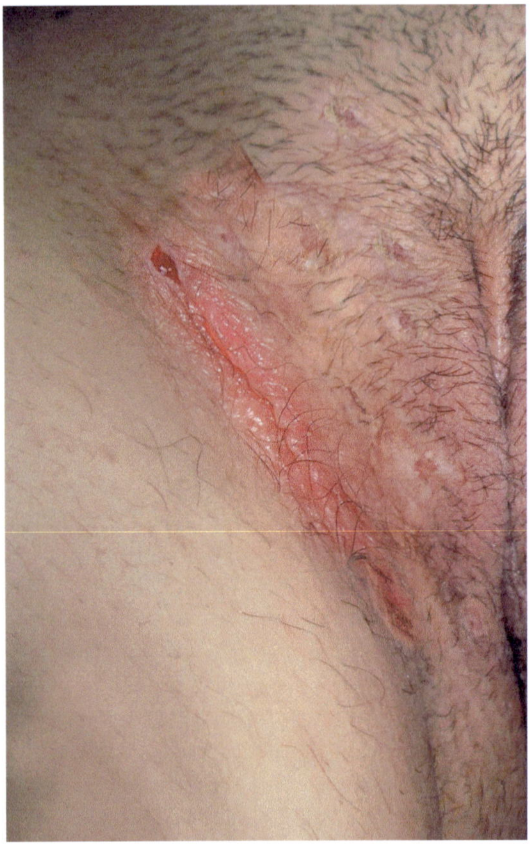

Fig. 48.1 Severe hidradenitis suppurativa (Hurley stage III)—inflammatory nodules, draining sinuses, and scars, in the right side of the mons pubis, labia majora, and labiocrural fold

recurrent or persistent disease (Fig. 48.1). HS is painful and a major cause of disability [6] with resultant depression.

HS may be staged clinically according to the Hurley staging system [7]: *stage I*, abscesses without sinus tracts or scarring; *stage II*, recurrent abscesses with sinus tracts and scarring; and *stage III*, diffuse disease, with connecting sinus tracts and abscesses.

48.4 Comorbidities

HS may be associated with metabolic syndrome and inflammatory bowel disease, including Crohn's disease and acne vulgaris.

48.5 Histopathology

Early lesions have characteristics of follicular hyperkeratosis, plugging, follicular dilation, and lymphocytic perifolliculitis [8]. Established areas of disease demonstrate also psoriasiform hyperplasia of the interfollicular epithelium [8] or a dense, mixed inflammatory infiltrate in the dermis. In addition, chronic abscesses, sinus tracts, and granulation tissue—sometimes with foreign body giant cells—may be seen. Destruction of folliculo-pilosebaceous units and fibrosis are characteristics of advanced disease.

48.6 Diagnosis

The diagnosis of HS is made by revealing the characteristic history and location of the lesions—in the axillae or groin, usually bilateral, with the lesions being multiple, deep, and inflamed. In addition, the presence of comedones, sinus tracts, abscesses, and scars is typical. Frequent recurrence also contributes to diagnosis.

48.7 Laboratory Work-Up

A skin biopsy is needed only where the diagnosis is not clear or vulvar carcinoma is suspected. Bacterial cultures are not necessary unless infection is probable. To delineate the extensions of the disease before surgery is undertaken, ultrasound or MRI imaging may be carried out.

48.8 Long-Term Sequelae

Urethral, bladder, rectum, and peritoneum fistulae may develop, although they raise the possibility of coexistent Crohn's disease. Tissue deformation and contractions may cause lymphedema in long-standing disease. Lumbosacral abscess, sacral osteomyelitis, and squamous cell carcinoma are also considered complications of HS. Systemically, HS may lead to malaise and depression, anemia, hypoproteinemia, and amyloidosis.

48.9 Differential Diagnosis

Other diseases that may look like HS are—other types of abscesses, the sexually transmitted infections—lymphogranuloma venereum or granuloma inguinale, Crohn's disease, and pilonidal sinus.

48.10 Treatment

The patient should be instructed to avoid skin trauma, to stop smoking, and to lose weight. She needs to use antiseptics for washing the affected area.

Management of pain may start with local anesthetic for mild HS (stage I). Clindamycin cream, topical resorcinol, and intralesional corticosteroid injections are second line treatment options. Sometimes oral tetracyclines help. For HS stage II, oral treatment by tetracyclines, clindamycin, and rifampin are indicated. In resistant cases, dapsone, erythromycin, or cephalosporins may be used for prolonged time [9].

Other systemic medications that have been used, although infrequently, are retinoids and antiandrogenic pills—including cyproterone acetate, oral contraceptive pills, spironolactone, and finasteride.

48.10.1 Surgery

Cold knife or CO_2 laser excision of lesions may be used for nodules and sinus tracts. "Punch debridement" is unroofing of lesions, nodules, or sinuses. For HS stage III, wide excision is appropriate. Extensive excisions with skin grafts are also used, with a good chance of cure. However, it is difficult to obtain a good cosmetic outcome of surgery in the genital and perineal areas. Following surgery, medical therapy could prevent recurrences. Other treatments for severe disease are systemic glucocorticoids, cyclosporine, or the TNF-alpha inhibitors—adalimumab and infliximab [10].

Limited experience exists with the use of the interleukin 12/23 inhibitor, ustekinumab [11], and with anakinra—an antagonist of the IL-1 receptor.

Overall, about one third of the patients subsequently get cured. The others suffer exacerbations of the disease or remain at the same stage of HS for years.

Hidradenitis Suppurativa: Breaking the Myths

- Although Hidradenitis Suppurativa presents with abscesses and inflammatory nodule, the lesions are sterile
- Positive cultures, if obtained in Hidradenitis Suppurativa, represent contamination from normal skin flora, or secondary infection
- Paradoxically, although Hidradenitis Suppurativa may respond and improve with anti-TNF-alpha therapy, it has been reported as an adverse effect of anti-TNF-alpha administration for other chronic inflammatory diseases
- Surgical treatment of Hidradenitis Suppurativa is a good option for treating advanced "stage III" disease. However, radical excision of the lesions is rarely necessary. Instead, "Punch debridement" is a method of surgically unroofing lesions, nodules, or sinuses, with favorable outcome.

References

1. Sellheyer K, Krahl D. "Hidradenitis suppurativa" is acne inversa! An appeal to (finally) abandon a misnomer. Int J Dermatol. 2005;44:535.
2. Kouris A, Platsidaki E, Christodoulou C, et al. Quality of life and psychosocial implications in patients with hidradenitis suppurativa. Dermatology. 2016;232:687.
3. Garg A, Kirby JS, Lavian J, et al. Sex- and age-adjusted population analysis of prevalence estimates for hidradenitis suppurativa in the United States. JAMA Dermatol. 2017;153:760.
4. von der Werth JM, Williams HC. The natural history of hidradenitis suppurativa. J Eur Acad Dermatol Venereol. 2000;14:389.
5. Faivre C, Villani AP, Aubin F, et al. Hidradenitis suppurativa (HS): an unrecognized paradoxical effect of biologic agents (BA) used in chronic inflammatory diseases. J Am Acad Dermatol. 2016;74:1153.

6. Riis PT, Vinding GR, Ring HC, Jemec GB. Disutility in patients with hidradenitis suppurativa: a cross-sectional study using EuroQoL-5D. Acta Derm Venereol. 2016;96:222.
7. Hurley HJ. Axillary hyperhidrosis, apocrine bromhidrosis, hidradenitis suppurativa, and familial benign pemphigus: surgical approach. In: Roenigk RK, Roenigk HH, editors. Dermatologic surgery. New York: Marcel Dekker; 1989. p. 729.
8. von Laffert M, Stadie V, Wohlrab J, Marsch WC. Hidradenitis suppurativa/acne inversa: bilocated epithelial hyperplasia with very different sequelae. Br J Dermatol. 2011;164:367.
9. Danby FW, Margesson LJ. Hidradenitis suppurativa. Dermatol Clin. 2010;28:779.
10. Shuja F, Chan CS, Rosen T. Biologic drugs for the treatment of hidradenitis suppurativa: an evidence-based review. Dermatol Clin. 2010;28:511.
11. Blok JL, Li K, Brodmerkel C, et al. Ustekinumab in hidradenitis suppurativa: clinical results and a search for potential biomarkers in serum. Br J Dermatol. 2016;174:839.

Part XII

Vulvar Lesions: Erosions

Vulvar Erosions: Excoriations, Erosive Lichen Planus, and Fissures

49

Veronika Suzuki, Veronica Maldonado, and Silvio Tatti

49.1 Introduction

A meticulous vulvar examination and the correct description of the findings are fundamental in the study of vulvar diseases. Also, recognizing the normal vulva with its variants is very important to be able to differentiate normal structures from abnormal findings. The morphology, configuration, and distribution of the lesions may guide us to the presumptive diagnosis.

Erosions, ulcers, excoriations, and fissures are among the secondary morphology presentations in the IFCPC clinical terminology of the vulva. Erosions are superficial defects in the skin surface with loss of the epidermis while the dermis remains intact; *ulcers* are deep defects in the skin surface with absence of the epidermis and/or dermis too. Some of them may appear necrotic at the base with white or yellow fibrinous material, e.g., syphilis, Behcet's disease, Crohn's disease, and vulvar aphthae [1]. Large, deep, or long-standing ulcers may heal with scarring, while erosions heal without scar. Vasculopathy pattern is characterized histologically by bloody vessel damage occurring in the setting of widespread dermal inflammation. The resultant deprivation of oxygen and nutrient flow generally lead to erosion or ulceration [2].

V. Suzuki (✉) · V. Maldonado · S. Tatti
Hospital de Clinicas "Jose de San Martin", University of Buenos Aires, Buenos Aires, Argentina

49.2 Erosions

Excoriations are erosions or ulcers caused by scratching; they are often linear or angular in configuration. *Fissures* are thin linear erosions of the skin surface [3]. Many conditions can cause scratching, resulting in excoriations in the vulvar skin, such as the cycle of itching-scratching-rubbing-itching that ends up in lichen simplex chronicus (LSC), a morphologic condition resulting from scratching and rubbing, also called eczema. LSC can be related to an allergic contact dermatitis or an irritant contact dermatitis. Excoriations can also be found in patients with candidiasis, psoriasis, other vulvar dermatoses like lichen sclerosus or lichen planus, or any other vulvar condition that causes itching and scratching, for example, a bacterial infection or scabies. The rest of the vulvar skin needs to be examined to see if there is edema, erythema, scales, papules, or pustular lesions in the adjacent skin.

49.3 Lichen Planus

Lichen planus (LP) is a chronic inflammatory mucocutaneous disease of unknown etiology.

49.3.1 Pathogenesis

Although it probably has an immunological cause, genetic predisposition has also been dis-

J. Bornstein (ed.), *Vulvar Disease*, https://doi.org/10.1007/978-3-319-61621-6_49

cussed, with an association between the DRB1*0101 allele and the cutaneous LP. The DRB1*0102 allele has been detected in 90% of vulvovaginal-gingival LP [4]. There are also other studies that have demonstrated an association between LP with autoimmune diseases like thyroiditis and vitiligo [5]. Other autoimmune disorders that were significantly more prevalent in erosive LP other than thyroid disease were alopecia areata and celiac disease [6].

49.3.2 Clinical Presentation

LP can affect the vulva as well as the vagina, producing erosions, adhesions, and scarring, which can result in complete closure of the vagina. It tends to occur in perimenopausal and postmenopausal women, appearing in the sixth decade with increased frequency [4]. Patients present with vaginal discharge, soreness, burning, itching, pain, or bleeding with sexual intercourse. This happens mainly when the vagina is affected, and adhesions develop. Bleeding with intercourse, pain, and sexual difficulties are common complaints. There are different clinical presentations of LP. Classic LP developing on the skin consists of small violet papules with a reticulated pattern (Fig. 49.1). Hypertrophic LP can affect perianal and perineal regions. The erosive LP mainly affects the labia minora, vestibule, and the vagina (Figs. 49.2 and 49.3) [7, 8]. The vulvovaginal-gingival syndrome affects the oral mucosa, vagina, and vulva. Approximately 65% of patients with cutaneous involvement may have oral lesions.

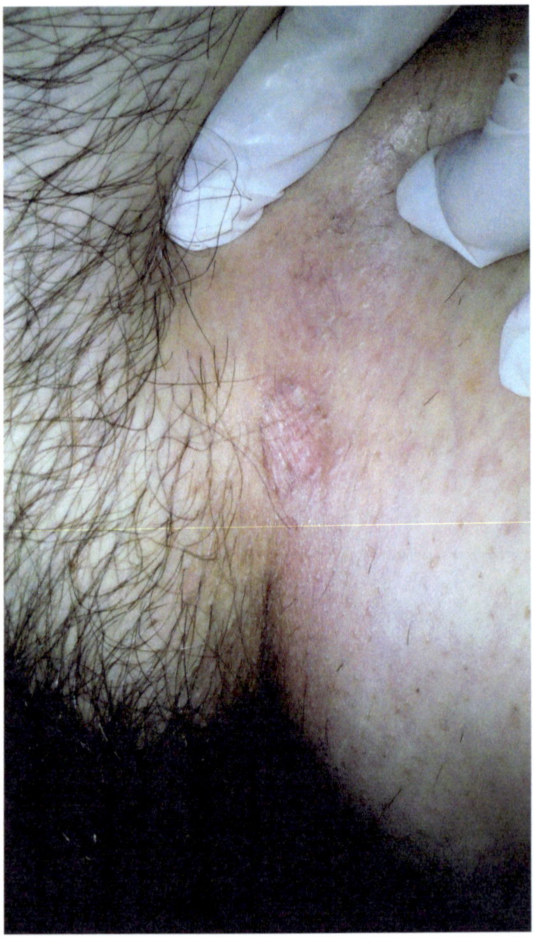

Fig. 49.1 Lichen planus on the skin. It consists of small violet papules with a reticulated pattern

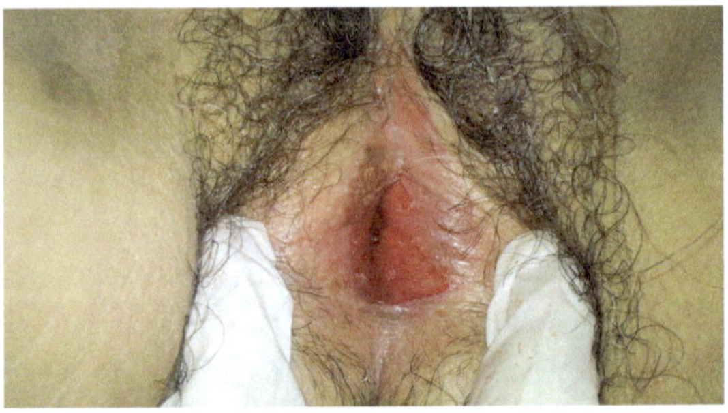

Fig. 49.2 Vulvovaginal erosive lichen planus in the labia minora, vestibule, and vagina

49.3.3 Treatment

Treatment often consists of topical immunosuppressive therapy and vaginal dilators. At times, vulvovaginal surgery is required to release adhesions in patients with LP. First-line therapy is clobetasol dipropionate 0.05% ointment to the vestibule and intravaginal steroids, managed according to each patient's symptoms and clinical findings [9, 10]. Vulvovaginal surgery for LP (lysis of vulvovaginal adhesions) consists of opening the adhesions under anesthesia, followed by long-term vaginal dilation and application of topical and intravaginal steroids, for example, hydrocortisone acetate 25 mg [11]. In these cases,

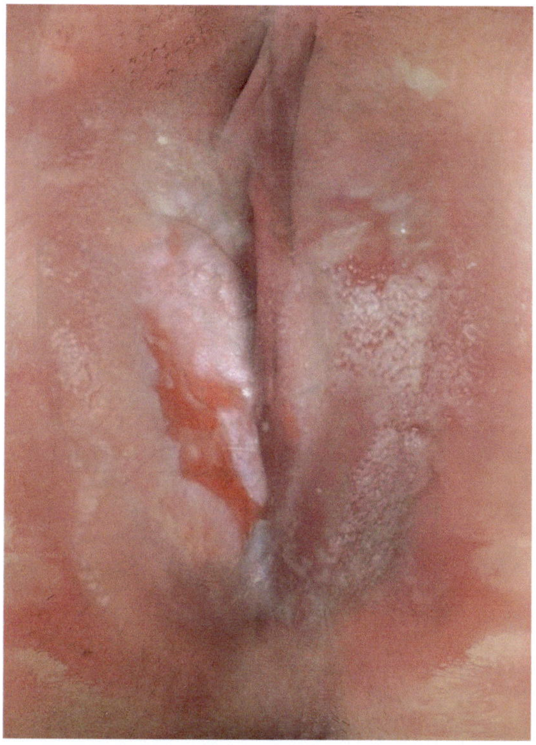

Fig. 49.3 Vulvovaginal erosive and hypertrophic lichen planus. The border is hyperkeratotic and the lesion is erythematous and sharply demarcated

intravaginal steroid is indicated along with regular use of vaginal dilators to decrease inflammation and hence increase the likelihood of preventing recurrence of adhesions.

Other treatments that can be considered are the calcineurin inhibitors: pimecrolimus 1% cream or tacrolimus 0.03% and 0.1% ointment. There are severe cases of LP that require oral steroids or systemic immunosuppressive treatment. During follow-up, if there are hyperkeratotic lesions that arise, symptoms that don't respond to the treatment, or any suspicious lesion appears, a new biopsy is considered mandatory because of the possible association of vulvar lichen planus with the development of invasive vulvar carcinoma.

49.4 Fissures

Fissures are thin linear erosions of the skin surface [1] that are sometimes too narrow to be easily identified as such and very often, they are characterized only by a red line. They feel like a "paper cut" pain and may cause bleeding with intercourse or dyspareunia. The most frequent localization is the posterior fourchette, but they can also be found in skin folds and creases (Fig. 49.4). Recurrent superficial splitting of the mucosa can occur with severe pain with intercourse and vaginal examination.

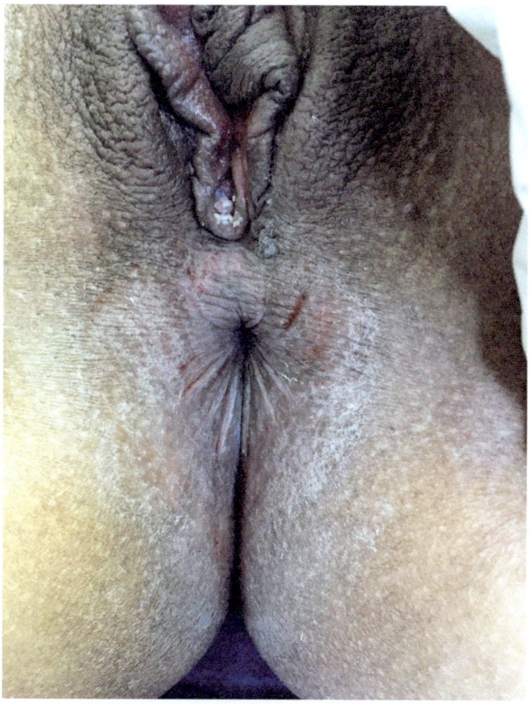

Fig. 49.4 Fissure affecting the perineum

Fissures may be caused by inflammation, trauma with vaginal penetration—intercourse or vaginal examination, infections (i.e., candida vulvovaginitis, bacterial infection, herpes simplex), dermatoses (lichen sclerosus, lichen simplex chronicus), genitourinary syndrome of menopause (formerly—vulvovaginal atrophy), malignancies (HSIL, differentiated VIN, Carcinoma), and systemic diseases with vulvar involvement.

Fibrosis is a significant finding when reviewing histologic specimens with recurrent posterior fourchette fissures, but chronic inflammation—predominantly submucosal—hyperkeratosis, and parakeratosis appear to be the only common, although nonspecific, histopathologic findings. Thus, supporting that although vulvar fissures are common with some vulvar dermatoses, they may develop as a primary nonspecific change [12].

Treatment varies acording to the specific causative lesion. However, general measures of vulvar care apply, and include elimination of any underlying infection, topical corticosteroid ointment if there vulvar dermatoses related, or perineoplasty in other cases. Women should avoid irritant products, and moisture the skin with lubricants and natural emollients. Olive oil or petrolatum and topical estrogen treatment are recommended for women with genitourinary syndrome of menopause [13].

Erosions: Breaking the Myths

- Lichen planus (LP), a chronic inflammatory disease, is not only a keratinized skin condition but may develop on the vulva and vagina, causing erosions and ulcers.
- Although LP probably has an immunological cause, genetic predisposition has also been discussed, as the DRB1*0102 was detected in 90% of vulvovaginal-gingival LP.
- Biopsy of an erosion seems important to many clinicians. However, the histopathologic finding is frequently nonspecific, including chronic submucosal inflammation, hyperkeratosis, and parakeratosis.
- Treatment of lichen planus is not different than of the other two lichens—lichen sclerosus and lichen simplex chronicus, i.e., topical superpotent steroid, systemic steroids, and calcineurin inhibitors.

References

1. Lynch PJ, Moyal-Barracco M, Scurry J, Stockdale C. 2011 ISSVD terminology and classification of vulvar dermatological disorders: an approach to clinical diagnosis. J Low Genit Tract Dis. 2012;16(4):339–44.
2. Lynch PJ, Moyal-Barracco M, Bogliatto F, Micheletti L, Scurry J. 2006 ISSVD classification of vulvar dermatoses: pathologic subsets and their clinical correlates. J Reprod Med. 2007;52(1):3–9.
3. Bornstein J, Sideri M, Tatti S, Walker P, Prendiville W, Haefner HK, Nomenclature Committee of International Federation for Cervical Pathology and Colposcopy. 2011 terminology of the vulva of the International Federation for Cervical Pathology and Colposcopy. J Low Genit Tract Dis. 2012;16(3):290–5.
4. Lewis FM. Vulval lichen planus. Br J Dermatol. 1998;138(4):569–75.
5. McPherson T, Cooper S. Vulval lichen sclerosus and lichen planus. Dermatol Ther. 2010;23(5):523–32.
6. Cooper SM, Ali I, Baldo M, Wojnarowska F. The association of lichen sclerosus and erosive lichen planus of the vulva with autoimmune disease: a case-control study. Arch Dermatol. 2008;144(11):1432–5.
7. Kirtschig G, Wakelin SH, Wojnarowska F. Mucosal vulval lichen planus: outcome, clinical and laboratory features. J Eur Acad Dermatol Venereol. 2005;19:301–7.
8. Moyal-Barracco M, Edwards L. Diagnosis and therapy of anogenital lichen planus. Dermatol Ther. 2004;17:38–46.
9. Cooper SM, Haefner HK, Abrahams-Gessel S, Margesson LJ. Vulvovaginal lichen planus treatment: a survey of current practices. Arch Dermatol. 2008;144:1520–1.
10. Anderson M, Kutzner S, Kaufman RH. Treatment of vulvovaginal lichen planus with vaginal hydrocortisone suppositories. Obstet Gynecol. 2002;100:359–62.
11. Stalburg CM, Haefner HK. Vaginal stenosis in lichen planus: surgical treatment tips for patients in whom conservative therapies have failed. Female Pelvic Med Reconstr Surg. 2008;14:193–8.
12. Kennedy CM, Manion E, Galask RP, Benda J. Histopathology of recurrent mechanical fissure of the fourchette. Int J Gynaecol Obstet. 2009;104(3):246–7.
13. Portman DJ, Gass ML, Vulvovaginal Atrophy Terminology Consensus Conference Panel. Genitourinary syndrome of menopause: new terminology for vulvovaginal atrophy from the International Society for the Study of Women's Sexual Health and the North American Menopause Society. Menopause. 2014;21(10):1063–8.

Paget's Disease of the Vulva

50

Mila Pontremoli Salcedo
and Kathleen M. Schmeler

50.1 Introduction

Mammary Paget's disease involving the nipple and areola was first described in 1874 by Sir James Paget [1]. It was later noted that other (extramammary) anatomic sites could be affected including the vulva, perineal, perianal, scrotal, and penile skin [2]. The first case of extramammary Paget's disease was described in 1889 affecting the scrotum and penis [3]. The first case of Paget's disease of the vulva was reported in 1901 by Dubreuilh [4]. It is now estimated that Paget's disease of the vulva is the most frequent site of extramammary site, accounting for 65% of all cases [5].

50.2 Clinical Presentation

Paget's disease of the vulva is a rare vulvar neoplasm most commonly seen in postmenopausal women. The mean age at diagnosis has been reported to range from 50 to 80 years, and it is most common in Caucasian women [2, 6–9]. Paget's disease of the vulva can have a variety of clinical presentations [7]. Women commonly have a well-demarcated pink eczematous lesion with white islands of hyperkeratosis ("icing cake effect"), often accompanied by pruritus [2] (Figs. 50.1 and 50.2). Vulvar pain and erythema may also be part of the clinical presentation. However, many women are asymptomatic, and

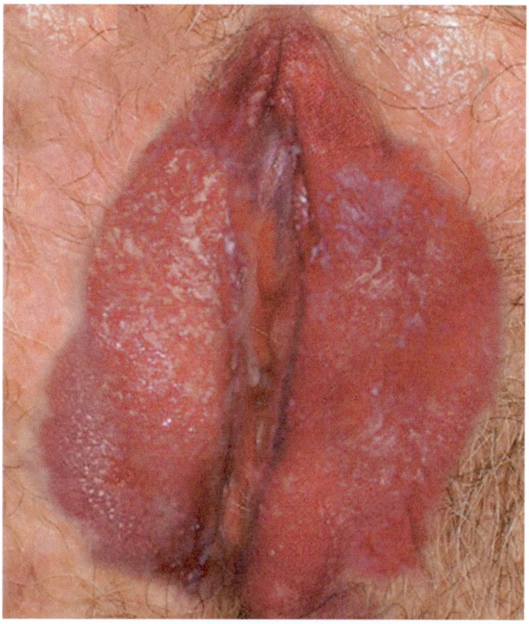

Fig. 50.1 Vulvar Paget's disease on both vulvar labia, perineum. Eczematous bright red patch with excoriation erosions and exudation. Courtesy of Professor Jacob Bornstein

M. Pontremoli Salcedo
Federal University of Health Sciences Porto Alegre (UFCSPA)/Irmandade Santa Casa de Misericordia de Porto Alegre, Porto Alegre, Brazil
e-mail: MPSalcedo@mdanderson.org

K. M. Schmeler (✉)
Department of Gynecologic Oncology and Reproductive Medicine, The University of Texas MD Anderson Cancer Center, Houston, TX, USA
e-mail: kschmele@mdanderson.org

J. Bornstein (ed.), *Vulvar Disease*, https://doi.org/10.1007/978-3-319-61621-6_50

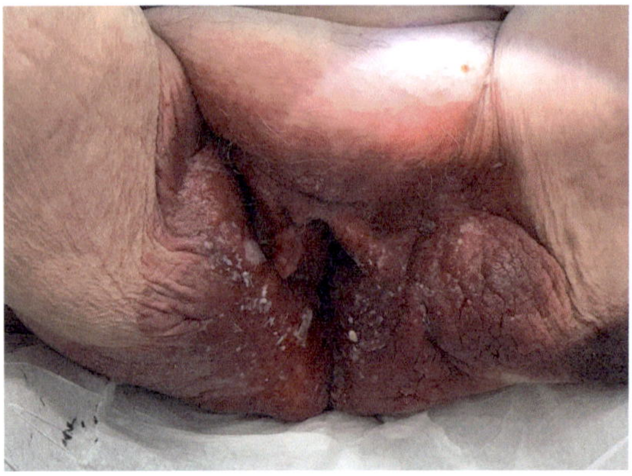

Fig. 50.2 A diffuse vulvar Paget's disease spreading to the labiacrural folds, lower abdomen, and perianal area. The lesion is red and eczematous with white islands of hyperkeratosis. Courtesy of Professor Jacob Bornstein

Paget's disease is present for many years before diagnosis [5, 10]. A confirmed diagnosis with biopsy and histopathology is often delayed due to non-specific clinical findings. The differential diagnosis can also be difficult as is often misdiagnosed as Lichen Simplex Chronicus, basal cell carcinoma, squamous cell carcinoma, condylomata accuminata, Crohn's disease, or hidradenitis suppurativa [2, 5, 11].

50.3 Histopathology

Paget's disease of the vulva is often limited to the epidermis and mucosa without invasion [7, 11]. It appears that the risk of invasive disease is low, with underlying adenocarcinoma reported to occur in approximately 4% of cases [12]. The most established classification system was described by Wilkinson and Brown who classify Paget's disease into two types based on histologic origin. Type 1 is a primary cutaneous form and is further classified into subtypes: intraepithelial Paget's disease (1a), intraepithelial disease with invasion (1b), and intraepithelial Paget's disease with underlying adenocarcinoma of a skin appendage or subcutaneous gland (1c). Type 2 is a non-cutaneous form representing metastasis from underlying malignancy of the gastrointestinal tract (2a), urogenital tract (2b), or adenocarcinoma originating elsewhere (2c) [13]. Patients with Paget's disease of the vulva have a high incidence of secondary synchronous or metachronous malignancies [2, 5, 10]. These include colorectal adenocarcinoma, cervical adenocarcinoma, carcinoma of the transitional epithelium from the renal pelvis to urethra, and/or breast carcinoma [7, 14].

50.4 Treatment

The optimal management of Paget's disease of the vulva remains unclear and challenging. A systematic review was unable to define a superior treatment for this disease [15]. Regardless of treatment, 12–62% [7, 12, 16] of patients develop recurrent disease.

Surgical excision is usually the primary and mainstay therapy; however, the histological disease often extends past clinically apparent borders resulting in positive margins, and surgical excision is limited by the anatomy of the vulva. In addition, the disease is often multifocal [7, 12, 17]. Many patients require multiple excisions resulting in significant morbidity [7, 18]. The surgical options include wide local excision, Moh's microsurgery, simple vulvectomy, and radical vulvectomy based on the extent of disease [12]. Many studies have been demonstrated a high rate of positive margins despite radical surgery [9, 12, 19]. Lymphadenectomy is performed if invasive disease is noted [11].

Several alternative treatments have been proposed including radiotherapy, photodynamic therapy, laser therapy, and topical chemotherapy with fluorouracil and bleomycin [7, 10, 12, 15]. A more recent approach is the use of imiquimod, a topical immune response modifier that is commonly used to treat genital warts, vulvar dysplasia, superficial basal cell carcinoma, and actinic keratosis. Although the data for imiquimod use in Paget's disease of the vulva are limited, it has shown efficacy in some women. Dogan et al. [20] performed a systematic review of 70 patients with Paget's disease of the vulva and reported a complete remission rate of 71% and a partial remission rate of 16%. A systematic review of the literature by Machida et al. [19] showed imiquimod to have a response in some women, especially in those with recurrent disease after surgery or in those unable to undergo a surgery. The most commonly recommended regimen is to apply imiquimod cream (5%), with a frequency of 3–4 times/week and a duration of approximately 4 months. If severe burning or other adverse events are noted, it is recommended to stop treatment until resolution and then decrease the number of treatments per week to one or two [19, 21, 22].

Our group previously performed a retrospective analysis of 89 patients with Paget's disease of the vulva [18]. The primary treatment was surgery for 74 (83.1%) patients, with positive margins noted in 70.1% of cases. Five patients (5.6%) underwent topical treatment with imiquimod and/or 5-fluorouracil, one patient (1.1%) underwent laser ablation, and treatment was unknown in nine patients (10.1%). The majority of patients had multiple recurrences. There were no significant differences in recurrence rates between patients who underwent surgery and those who did not. Furthermore, there was no association between positive margins following primary surgery and recurrence. Seven patients (7.9%) were found to have invasive vulvar cancer with 1 mm or more depth of invasion, but none of the patients died of Paget's disease or associated vulvar/vaginal cancer. Our findings suggest that the majority of patients with Paget's disease of the vulva develop multiple recurrences regardless of treatment modality or margin status.

50.5 Surveillance

It is recommended that women undergo long-term follow-up due to the high risk of recurrence [2, 16]. Paget's disease can recur more than 15 years after initial treatment. Follow-up should include regular inspection of the vulva every 6–12 months. Biopsy should be done of any suspicion lesions [2, 12]. Given the high risk of other malignancies, women with Paget's disease of the vulva should undergo routine screening with colonoscopy, Pap/HPV testing, and mammogram.

Paget's Disease of the Vulva: Breaking the Myths

- Although Paget's disease is an intraepithelial neoplasia, most cases recur even after surgery.
- Long-term follow-up should be very long term: Paget's disease can recur more than 15 years after initial treatment.
- Radical surgery is never radical with Paget's disease; many studies have demonstrated a high rate of positive margins despite radical surgery.

References

1. Paget J. On disease of the mammary areola preceding cancer of the mammary gland. Bartholomew's Hosp Rep. 1874;10:87–9.
2. Shepherd V, Davidson EJ, Davies-Humphreys J. Extramammary Paget's disease. BJOG. 2005; 112(3):273–9.
3. Crocker HR. Paget's disease, affecting the scrotum and penis. Trans Pathol Soc Lond. 1889;40:187–91.
4. Dubreuilh W. Paget's disease of the vulva. Br J Dermatol. 1901;13:403–13.
5. Delport ES. Extramammary Paget's disease of the vulva: an annotated review of the current literature. Australas J Dermatol. 2013 Feb;54(1):9–21. https://doi.org/10.1111/j.1440-0960.2012.00898.x.
6. Kay JM, Southwood WF. Paget's disease of the vulva associated with an unusual bladder tumour. Br J Cancer. 1964;18:233–7.
7. Preti M, Micheletti L, Ghiringhello B, Privitera S, Condello V, Chieppa P, et al. Vulvar Paget's disease. Clinico-pathologic review of the literature. Minerva Ginecol. 2000;52(5):203–11.
8. Tebes S, Cardosi R, Hoffman M. Paget's disease of the vulva. Am J Obstet Gynecol. 2002;187(2):281–3.
9. Black D, Tornos C, Soslow RA, Awtrey CS, Barakat RR, Chi DS, et al. The outcomes of patients with positive margins after excision for intraepithelial Paget's disease of the vulva. Gynecol Oncol. 2007;104(3):547–50.
10. Parashurama R, Nama V, Hutson R. Paget's disease of the vulva: a review of 20 years' experience. Int J Gynecol Cancer. 2017;27:791–3.
11. Borghi C, Bogani G, Ditto A, Martinelli F, Signorelli M, Chiappa V, et al. Invasive Paget disease of the vulva. Int J Gynecol Cancer. 2018;28(1):176–82.

12. Nitecki R, Davis M, Watkins JC, Wu YE, Vitonis AF, Muto MG, et al. Extramammary Paget disease of the vulva: a case series examining treatment, recurrence, and malignant transformation. Int J Gynecol Cancer. 2018;28(3):632–8. https://doi.org/10.1097/IGC.0000000000001189.
13. Wilkinson EJ, Brown HM. Vulvar Paget disease of urothelial origin: a report of three cases and a proposed classification of vulvar Paget disease. Hum Pathol. 2002;33(5):549–54.
14. Feuer GA, Shevchuk M, Calanog A. Vulvar Paget's disease: the need to exclude an invasive lesion. Gynecol Oncol. 1990;38(1):81.
15. Edey KA, Allan E, Murdoch JB, Cooper S, Bryant A. Interventions for the treatment of Paget's disease of the vulva. Cochrane Database Syst Rev. 2013;10:CD009245.
16. Fanning J, Lambert L, Hale TM, Morris PC, Schuerch C. Paget's disease of the vulva: prevalence of associated vulvar adenocarcinoma, invasive Paget's disease, and recurrence after surgical excision. Am J Obstet Gynecol. 1999;180(1 Pt 1):24–7.
17. Parker LP, Parker JR, Bodurka-Bevers D, Deavers M, Bevers MW, Shen-Gunther J, Gershenson DM. Paget's disease of the vulva: pathology, pattern of involvement, and prognosis. Gynecol Oncol. 2000;77:183–9.
18. Onaiwu CO, Salcedo MP, Pessini SA, Munsell MF, Euscher EE, Reed KE, Schmeler KM. Paget's disease of the vulva: a review of 89 cases. Gynecol Oncol Rep. 2016;19:46–9.
19. Machida H, Moeini A, Roman LD, Matsuo K. Effects of imiquimod on vulvar Paget's disease: a systematic review of literature. Gynecol Oncol. 2015;139:165–71.
20. Dogan A, Hilal Z, Krentel H, Cetin C, Hefler LA, Grimm C, et al. Paget's disease of the vulva treated with imiquimod: case report and systematic review of the literature. Gynecol Obstet Investig. 2017;82(1):1–7.
21. Hatch KD, Davis JR. Complete resolution of Paget disease of the vulva with imiquimod cream. J Low Genit Tract Dis. 2008;12(2):90–4.
22. Luyten A, Sörgel P, Gieseking F, Maass-Poppenhusen K, Lellé RJ, Harter P, et al. Treatment of extramammary Paget disease of the vulva with imiquimod: a retrospective, multicenter study by the German Colposcopy Network. J Am Acad Dermatol. 2014;70(4):644–50.

Part XIII

Vulvar Lesions: Ulcers

51 Aphthous Ulcers: Lipschütz Ulcer, Syphilis and Other STI

Jacob Bornstein

51.1 Introduction

The presentation of a patient with vulvar ulcer is often dramatic, especially when it is associated with acute or chronic pain.

Of all causes of vulvar cancers, herpes genitalis is the most frequent one. Indeed, most genital ulcers are caused by sexually transmitted infections (STIs) (Table 51.1).

There are approaches to differentiate vulvar ulcers according to their presentation, for example, the ulcer being acute, recurrent, or chronic (Table 51.2).

The patient with vulvar ulcer: Table 51.3 illustrates the workup of a patient with genital ulcer. Not all tests need to be performed. Target the evaluation according to the presumed etiology.

51.2 Significant Questions to Consider in Evaluating a Genital Ulcer [1–4]

- *Is the ulcer painful?* Painful ulcers tend to be more typical of HSV and chancroid, while ulcers associated with syphilis, LGV, and granuloma inguinale are usually painless. Pruritus may be the presenting symptom in intraepithelial neoplasia.
- *Is dysuria present?* Dysuria or urinary retention is sometimes caused by urine touching the urethral meatus or vestibular ulcer. Many patients are referred to urine analysis or treated unnecessarily by antibiotics with the empiric diagnosis of urinary tract infection [1]. However, chlamydia and gonorrhea infections may cause urethritis.
- *Does the episode recur frequently?* Frequent breakouts are typical of HSV infection. Less common recurrences occur in Behcet's syndrome or fixed drug eruption.
- *Are there multiple ulcers?* If they are, they may be due to HSV or *H. ducreyi* (chancroid). Syphilis usually presents as a single lesion.
- *Is the lesion presenting first as a vesicle?* Vesicles that rupture and turn into erosions or ulcers are typical of HSV.
- *How are the lesions arranged?* If they are grouped in a serpentine line, they are typical of HSV (hence the origin of the name "herpes").
- *Is there a halo around the lesion?* An erythematous halo is typical of HSV.

J. Bornstein (✉)
Department of Obstetrics and Gynecology Galilee Medical Center, Bar-Ilan University Faculty of Medicine, Nahariya, Israel

J. Bornstein (ed.), *Vulvar Disease*, https://doi.org/10.1007/978-3-319-61621-6_51

Table 51.1 Causes of vulvar ulcers

Infectious causes		Noninfectious causes	
Sexually transmitted infections	Nonsexually transmitted infections	Nonneoplastic diseases	Neoplastic disease
• Genital herpes simplex, type 1 or type 2 or herpes zoster	• Tuberculosis	• Lipschütz ulcer	• Vulvar intraepithelial Neoplasia
• Syphilis (caused by *Treponema pallidum*)	• Ecthyma	• Behcet's syndrome	• Vulvar carcinoma
• Chancroid (caused by *Haemophilus ducreyi*)	• Vulvovaginal candidiasis	• Reiter's disease	
• Lymphogranuloma venereum (LGV) (caused by *Chlamydia trachomatis* serovars L1–3	• Extraintestinal *Entamoeba histolytica*—Amebiasis	• Crohn's disease	
• Granuloma inguinale (donovanosis) (caused by *Klebsiella granulomatis*)	• Cutaneous leishmaniasis	• Systemic lupus erythematosus	
• Human immunodeficiency virus (HIV) infection		• Erosive lichen planus	
• Epstein-Barr virus infection		• Vesiculobullous disease	
		• Fixed drug eruption	

Table 51.2 Vulvar ulcers—mode of appearance

Characteristic	Acute	Recurrence	Long-lasting
Infectious	Sexually transmitted infections: *syphilis, lymphogranuloma inguinale, and chancroid*	Herpes genitalis	
Noninfectious	Lipshütz ulcer	Behcet's syndrome	Crohn's disease Neoplasia

Table 51.3 Vulvar ulcer—workup

History
• Systemic symptoms (fever, malaise, headache, GI symptoms, respiratory symptoms, and myalgia)
• Past oral ulcers, skin lesions, and ocular symptoms
• Sexual activity
• A family history of autoimmune disorders
Examination
• Oral ulcers
• Uveitis (Behcet's syndrome)
• Skin inspection (eczema, rash, other ulcers, or bullae)
• Lymphadenopathy (cervical, inguinal/femoral)
• Size, shape, and location of the vulvar ulcer
Laboratory tests
• *Specimen from the ulcer*: HSV 1 and 2, varicella zoster: PCR or culture
• Gram stain and bacterial culture
• Yeast culture
• *Serology*: HSV-1/HSV-2; EBV (IgM and IgG); CMV and mycoplasma
• CRP and ESR
• ANA and consider HLA-B51 if Behcet's disease is a possibility
• *Urine*: pregnancy test, PCR for chlamydia and gonorrhea
• *Serology*: RPR for syphilis, HIV
• *Biopsy from the edge of the lesion if chronic or nonhealing*

51.3 Specific Etiologies of Vulvar Ulcer

51.3.1 Infectious Etiology

- *Syphilis*: The primary lesion in a syphilitic infection, the chancre, begins as a papule, which is typically painless. In that it is different from herpes genitalis. This papule ulcerates to produce the classic chancre of primary syphilis, a 1–2 cm ulcer on the vulva with a raised, indurated margin (Fig. 51.1). The ulcer has a non-exudative base and is associated with mild to moderate bilateral lymphadenopathy that is often bilateral. The chancre heals spontaneously within 3–6 weeks even without treatment. Since the ulcer is painless, many patients fail to resort to medical attention. The syphilitic spirochete spread and become systemic. This dissemination may be associated with systemic symptoms (secondary). Late syphilis includes neurosyphilis. Serologic testing for syphilis should be performed during the initial evaluation of a patient who presents with a genital ulcer. However, serologies may be negative in up to 25% of primary syphilis. Treponemal tests are more sensitive than nontreponemal tests for primary syphilis, and it is recommended to start by a *T. pallidum* antibody screen. If positive, a nontreponemal test, such as a rapid plasma regain should be performed.

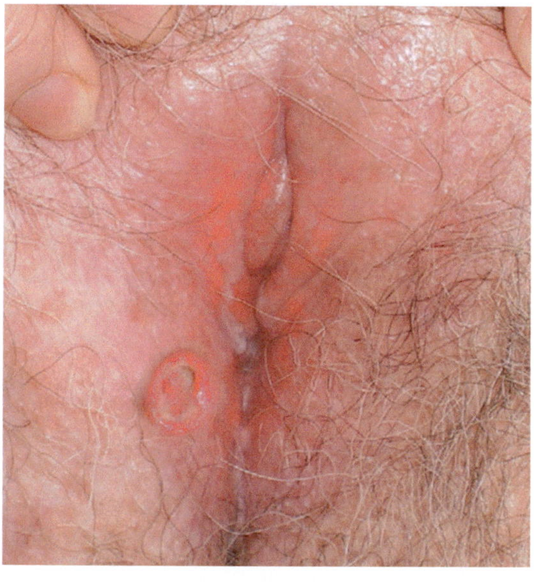

Fig. 51.1 Chancre—the primary lesion in syphilis. It is indurated

- Dark-field microscopy to visualize *T. pallidum* is rarely carried out. PCR tests for the detection of *T. pallidum* DNA are not commercially available. Direct fluorescent antibody tests for *T. pallidum* may be available.
- Treatment of syphilis: The drug of choice for primary syphilis is a single intramuscular (IM) dose of penicillin G benzathine (2.4 million units). Prior to initiating treatment, all patients should have serologic testing. If the nontreponemal tests are positive, they should be used to monitor the response to therapy.
- *Lymphogranuloma venereum (LGV)*: A nucleic acid amplification test for chlamydia is sensitive for the presence of LGV. Additional tests must be used to differentiate LGV from non-LGV *C. trachomatis*. Serologic testing can also be helpful in making the diagnosis of LGV [4].
- Empiric treatment for LGV is doxycycline 100 mg orally twice daily for 21 days.
- *Granuloma inguinale*: A biopsy specimen of the ulcer demonstrating Donovan bodies are diagnostic of granuloma inguinale. Treatment should be by azithromycin for at least 3 weeks, preferably until the lesions have completely disappeared [4]. Other options are doxycycline, ciprofloxacin, erythromycin, or trimethoprim-sulfamethoxazole [4, 5]. For a nonresponder, add aminoglycoside [4]. Erythromycin or azithromycin should be given for pregnant women.
- *Chancroid*: Specialized cultures can be used to diagnose chancroid. Some laboratories have developed locally validated PCR tests for chancroid as well.

Treatment of chancroid, azithromycin (1 g orally), or ceftriaxone (250 mg IM) can be used. The patient should be treated for syphilis as well.

51.3.2 Noninfectious Etiology of Vulvar Ulcers

51.3.2.1 Lipschütz Ulcer

A painful ulcer, or a cluster of vulvar ulcers, (Figs. 51.2 and 51.3). Prodrome is frequent with fever and malaise. The condition is synonymous with "nonsexually acquired acute genital ulceration" (NAGU). It is an immune response to a recent infection (e.g., EBV, cytomegalovirus, mycoplasma) [6, 7], although the exact etiology is unknown. This condition occurs most often in adolescent girls and young women [8, 9].

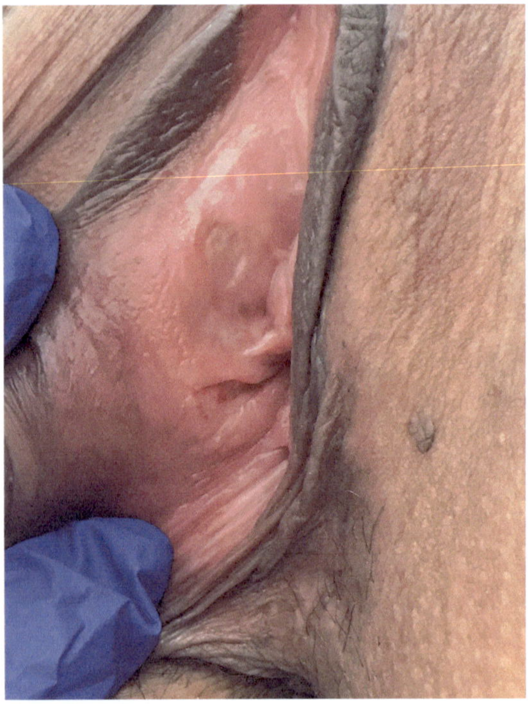

Fig. 51.2 Vulvar Lipschütz ulcers. The lesions are shallow

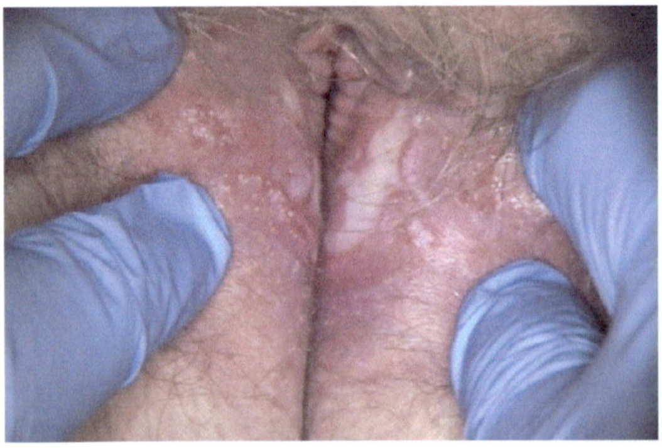

Fig. 51.3 Vulvar Lipschütz ulcers. The lesion on the patient's left is large and deep. More ulcers are seen on the right labia

Since it has been associated with acute Epstein-Barr virus (EBV) infection or other viral and bacterial infections [10, 11], when suspecting a Lipshütz ulcer, serology for EBV, cytomegalovirus (CMV), and mycoplasma pneumoniae should be taken [12].

The histopathologic findings in acute genital ulcerations are nonspecific and include necrosis of the epithelium with a polymorphic dermal infiltrate of neutrophils and CD8+ mononuclear cells [8].

Clinically, several vulvar ulcers usually develop. They may be large, red, and deep, with a necrotic base. Mostly they develop in the labia minora but can be found in the labia majora, perineum, vestibule, and lower vagina. They may involve both sides of the vulva and be associated with edema and inguinal lymphadenopathy.

A prodrome is frequently experienced by the patients, consisting of dysuria and flu-like symptoms. Infrequently, oral aphthosis may be present, mimicking Behcet's syndrome [12].

Evaluation of a patient with suspect Lipshütz ulcer should include, besides the workup for vulvar ulcer (Table 51.3), also bacterial cultures. Biopsy may be indicated to rule out vesiculobullous disease.

The treatment should include reassurance, as many of these ulcers regress spontaneously. In addition, local hygiene should be kept using sitz baths with plain warm water where gentle debridement of the ulcers may be carried out. Pain control is of special significance. It should start with topical anesthetics such as lidocaine 2% especially before micturition, then oral analgesics and even narcotics may be needed. In addition, steroids such as the potent clobetasol propionate 0.05% ointment or fluocinonide 0.1% ointment may be applied. If that does not cause any relief, then oral corticosteroids should be started with prednisone at the dose of 0.5–1.0 mg/kg per day may be given for 7–10 days and then tapered down over the following 2 weeks.

Patients with suspected bacterial superinfection or cellulitis should be treated with systemic antibiotics.

51.3.2.2 Behcet's Syndrome

Behcet's syndrome is a multisystem disorder. The classic triad includes recurrent vulvar ulcers, uveitis, and oral aphthae, but there are more symptoms and signs. The appearance is not different from other recurrent aphthae, but the ulcer is usually very deep and may fenestrate the labia (Fig. 51.4). Its development may be associated with headache, weakness, anorexia, lymphadenopathy, arthralgia, and sore throat. The full-blown syndrome may deteriorate to thromboembolism, vascular aneurisms, and encephalitis.

As there are many similar features with other aphthae, diagnosis should be strict according to the International Study Group for Behcet's Disease [14] (Table 51.4), requiring the presence of recurrent oral aphthous ulceration at least three times in 12 months plus two of the other criteria.

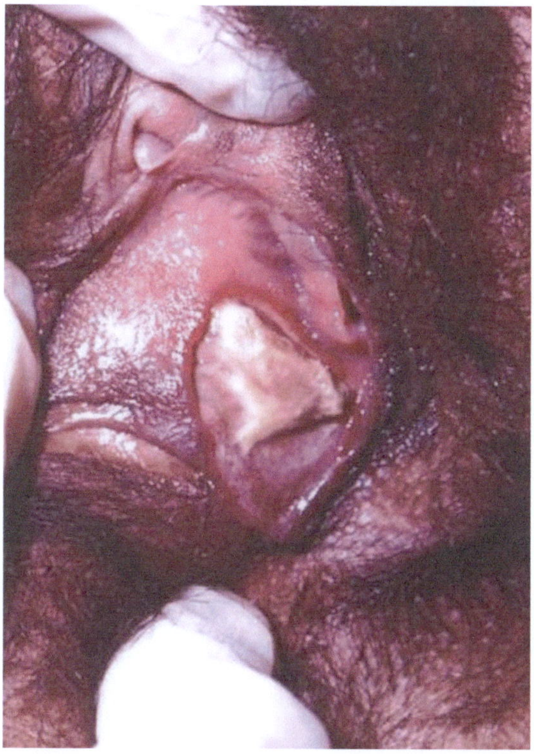

Fig. 51.4 Behcet's disease: The ulcer is very deep, painful, and hard to treat

It may be caused by an immune response to infection. The people of the Mediterranean and Middle and Far East are mostly affected by this syndrome. HLA-B51/B5 allele presence raises the risk of developing the condition [13].

Biopsy of Behcet's disease depicts vasculitis involving all size of vessels, endothelial swelling, extravasation of red blood cells and neutrophils. Thromboembolism may develop due to infiltration of the vessels by lymphocytes.

Treatment of Behcet's disease should start with topical therapy and gradually changing to systemic. See Table 51.5 for treatment options.

Other types of vulvar ulcers can be found in the following chapters.

Table 51.4 International Study Group for Behcet's Disease [14]—diagnosis criteria

Location	Criteria
Oral (major)	Recurrent vulvar ulcers
Vulvar (minor)	Recurrent vulvar/vaginal ulceration or aphthae
Ocular (minor)	At least three recurrences of ulcers or aphthae in 1 year
Dermatological (minor)	Erythema nodosum or acne post-adolescence
Pathergy test positive (minor)	Erythema of more than 2 mm 48 h post 20 gauge needle prick

Table 51.5 Treatments for Behcet's syndrome and other aphthous diseases

Treatment option	Details of treatment
Topical treatment	Clobetasol propionate, fluocinolone acetonide
	Topical anesthetic: lidocaine gel
	Topical antibiotics: tetracyclines
	Topical antiseptics
	Hyaluronic acid gel
Systemic preparations	Colchicine
	Multivitamins
	Corticosteroids
	Tetracyclines
	Dapsone
	Zinc sulfate
	Thalidomide

Vulvar Ulcers: Breaking the Myths

- If you are not sure what is the cause of a vulvar ulcer, think about herpes genitalis. It is the most frequent etiology.
- In addition, most genital ulcers are caused by sexually transmitted infections.
- Important questions that help us to differentiate between the various causes of a vulvar ulcer are: Is the ulcer painful? Does the episode recur frequently? How are the lesions arranged, and is there a halo around the lesion?
- Lipschütz ulcer and Behcet's syndrome are more frequent causes of vulvar ulcers than appreciated.

References

1. Tomas ME, Getman D, Donskey CJ, Hecker MT. Overdiagnosis of urinary tract infection and underdiagnosis of sexually transmitted infection in adult women presenting to an emergency department. J Clin Microbiol. 2015;53:2686.
2. Morshed MG, Singh AE. Recent trends in the serologic diagnosis of syphilis. Clin Vaccine Immunol. 2015;22:137.
3. O'Farrell N. Donovanosis. Sex Transm Infect. 2002;78:452.
4. Workowski KA, Bolan GA, Centers for Disease Control and Prevention. Sexually transmitted diseases treatment guidelines. MMWR Recomm Rep. 2015;64:1–137.
5. Mertz KJ, Weiss JB, Webb RM, et al. An investigation of genital ulcers in Jackson, Mississippi, with use of a multiplex polymerase chain reaction assay: high prevalence of chancroid and human immunodeficiency virus infection. J Infect Dis. 1998;178:1060–6.
6. Sehgal VN, Pandhi D, Khurana A. Nonspecific genital ulcers. Clin Dermatol. 2014;32:259.
7. Finch JJ, Wald J, Ferenczi K, et al. Disseminated Lyme disease presenting with nonsexual acute genital ulcers. JAMA Dermatol. 2014;150:1202.
8. Farhi D, Wendling J, Molinari E, et al. Non-sexually related acute genital ulcers in 13 pubertal girls: a clinical and microbiological study. Arch Dermatol. 2009;145:38.
9. Vieira-Baptista P, Lima-Silva J, Beires J, Martinez-de-Oliveira J. Lipschütz ulcers: should we rethink this? An analysis of 33 cases. Eur J Obstet Gynecol Reprod Biol. 2016;198:149.
10. Jerdan K, Aronson I, Hernandez C, et al. Genital ulcers associated with Epstein-Barr virus. Cutis. 2013;91:273.
11. Sárdy M, Wollenberg A, Niedermeier A, Flaig MJ. Genital ulcers associated with Epstein-Barr virus infection (ulcus vulvae acutum). Acta Derm Venereol. 2011;91:55.
12. Lehman JS, Bruce AJ, Wetter DA, et al. Reactive nonsexually related acute genital ulcers: review of cases evaluated at Mayo Clinic. J Am Acad Dermatol. 2010;63:44.
13. Calamia KT, Wilson FC, Icen M, et al. Epidemiology and clinical characteristcs of Behçet's disease in the US: a population-based study. Arthritis Rheum. 2009;61:600–4.
14. International Study Group for Behçet Disease. Criteria for diagnosis of Behçet's disease. International study Group for Behçet disease. Lancet. 1990;335:1078–80.

52 Crohn's Disease of the Vulva

Darion Rowan

52.1 Introduction

Crohn's disease is an idiopathic chronic relapsing inflammatory bowel disease first described by Crohn, Ginzberg, and Oppenheimer in 1932. Any segment of the gastrointestinal tract can be affected, but most often it affects the terminal ileum and colon. Symptoms are intermittent severe abdominal pain, recurrent diarrhea with blood and mucus, and weight loss. The disease has a major impact on a person's well-being.

The incidence is increasing worldwide but varies from country to country. For example, in recent years Australia had 29.3 cases/100,000, whereas northern Europe had 10 cases/100,000. There is a lower incidence in developing countries.

It is more common in those with a family history of Crohn's disease and slightly more frequent in females than males. It usually develops in the second and third decades of life, but children can be affected. It results in a higher mortality rate than in the unaffected population.

Causes of the increase in incidence may be due to improved diagnostic techniques, urbanization, environmental factors including change in diet, and alterations in gut flora with resultant abnormal immune responses to both commensal and pathogenic organisms. Mycobacterium avium paratuberculosis may play a role. Mutations in CARD genes could be pathogenic.

There is defective innate and adaptive intestinal immunity resulting in increased tumor necrosis factor (TNF) α and interleukin 1β, which lead to a chronic inflammatory response.

The diagnosis is based on clinical features together with investigations: a. laboratory: raised inflammatory markers, low serum iron levels and nutritional deficiencies, ASCA (anti-*Saccharomyces cerevisiae* antibody), and fecal calprotectin; b. radiological: CT (computed tomography) and MRI (magnetic resonance imaging); and c. endoscopic: ileocolonoscopy which reveals discontinuous inflammation or ulceration and rectal sparing.

52.2 Histopathology of Crohn's Disease

There are focal or patchy areas of chronic inflammation, focal crypt irregularity, and granulomas.

D. Rowan (✉)
Omnicare Womenâ€™s Health,
Auckland, New Zealand

J. Bornstein (ed.), *Vulvar Disease*, https://doi.org/10.1007/978-3-319-61621-6_52

Skin lesions develop in up to 44% of patients with Crohn's disease and, most often (80%), develop after the diagnosis has been made. However 20% develop before gastrointestinal Crohn's disease has been recognized.

52.3 Classification of Skin Lesions in Crohn's Disease

1. Crohn's-specific—involving a mechanism identical to that occurring in the gut
2. Reactive—which arise by a distinct pathogenic mechanism and include erythema nodosum, pyoderma gangrenosum, and Sweet's syndrome
3. Associated but distinct disorders such as palmoplantar pustulosis, psoriasis, clubbing, vitiligo, and palmar erythema

52.3.1 Vulval Metastatic Crohn's Disease

Vulval metastatic Crohn's disease was first reported in 1965, and 90% of vulval disease is metastatic so that it is not contiguous with the bowel. More than half of all cases of metastatic disease affect the vulva, and one quarter is present before bowel Crohn's disease develops. Most Crohn's disease affects the proximal gastrointestinal tract, but in patients with vulval metastatic disease, the colon is affected.

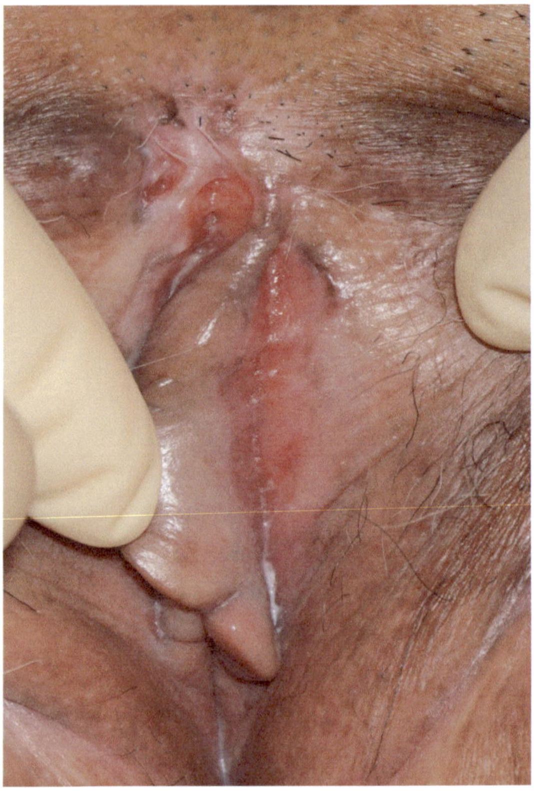

Fig. 52.1 Inflamed "knifelike" fissures of anterior vulva

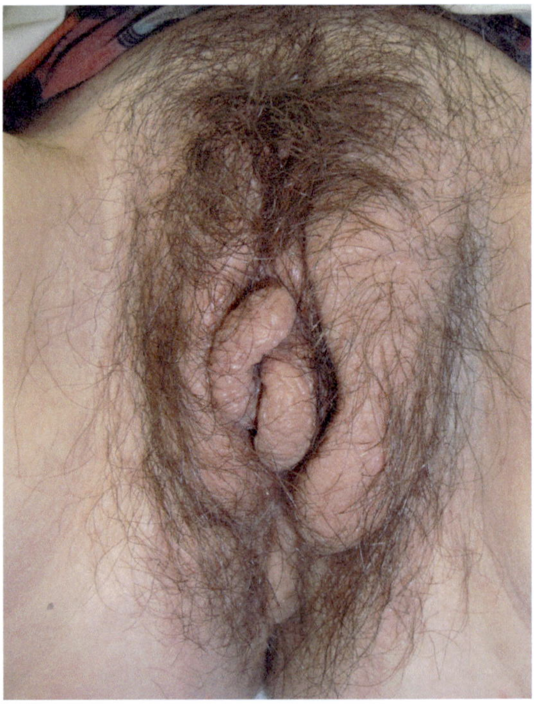

Fig. 52.2 Long-standing generalized edema of vulva in a patient with Crohn's disease

52.3.2 Clinical Presentation

Clinically vulval Crohn's disease is often painful, and the features are of ulceration, flexural fissures which are described as knifelike (Fig. 52.1) diffuse edema (Fig. 52.2), and erythema. Less common there may be condyloma-like papules, plaques, isolated lymphedema, or lymphangiectasia (Fig. 52.3).

Metastatic Crohn's disease in children is most common on the genital skin, and most children do not have intestinal Crohn's disease diagnosed at the time of presentation, but it develops up to 6 years later.

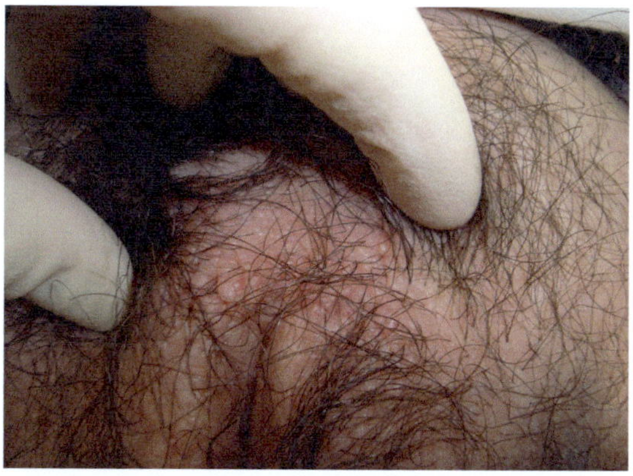

Fig. 52.3 Lymphangiectasia of anterior vulva in the same patient as in Fig. 52.2 who presented with "leaking" from her vulva

52.3.3 Specific Cutaneous Crohn's Disease

There are three types:

1. The most common are lesions that are a direct extension from Crohn's disease affecting the bowel. This results in abscesses, fistulae, and ulcers which may be perianal or peristomal. Most often they are located in the anogenital area, but they tend to spare the vulva. Fistulae may extend from the skin into the rectum, colon, or vagina [1–7].
2. Oral Crohn's disease manifests as labial or gingival swelling, a cobblestone appearance of the mucosa, ulcers, and nodules. Granulomatous cheilitis may be a manifestation of Crohn's disease.
3. Metastatic Crohn's disease can affect any area of the skin and appears to have a similar pathogenesis to bowel disease.

Metastatic Crohn's disease is rare and is defined as granulomatous skin lesions which are noncontiguous with gastrointestinal disease. Most often they develop after the bowel disease, and they may be multiple or single. The condition is less common in children than in adults, and the lesions may be genital or extragenital. They occur mainly in patients with colon Crohn's disease, and the disease activity is not related to the activity of the bowel disease.

52.3.4 Differential Diagnosis

The differential diagnosis of cutaneous Crohn's disease includes infections especially tuberculosis, sarcoidosis, hidradenitis suppurativa, neoplasm, or lymphedema.

52.3.5 Histopathology of Metastatic Crohn's Disease

Microscopic examination of metastatic Crohn's disease shows nonsuppurative granulomatous dermatitis where the granulomas are composed of epithelioid eosinophils. Langhans' giant cells are common, and the infiltrate is often both superficial and deep. It may encroach the epidermis. Less common features are lichenoid inflammation, ulceration, granulomatous vasculitis (or perivasculitis), and massive edema. The histopathological differential diagnosis includes sarcoidosis, mycobacterium infection, rheumatoid arthritis, foreign body reaction, and superficial granulomatous pyoderma.

52.3.6 Treatment

There are many treatments used in vulval Crohn's disease. Topical corticosteroids and tacrolimus may be therapeutic in mild cases, but systemic therapy is often required. This includes metronidazole, sulfasalazine, systemic steroids, and steroid-sparing agents such as azathioprine, six mercaptopurine, mycophenolate mofetil, and cyclosporine. Nutritional deficiencies must be corrected.

For severe cases biologic agents especially TNFα inhibitors, infliximab, and adalimumab are often effective.

Surgery is a last resort as poor healing is expected in the majority with subsequent recurrence of lesions. Debridement, local excision, or vulvectomy with skin grafts if required may be successful, but surgery is best used in combination with medical treatments.

Vulvar Crohn's Disease: Breaking the Myths

- Most children do not have intestinal Crohn's disease diagnosed at the time of presentation, and it develops up to 6 years later.
- Vulvar Crohn's disease is most unusual—presenting as painful, knife-like ulcerations.

References

1. Andreani SM, et al. Crohn's disease of the vulva. Int J Surg. 2010;8:2–5.
2. Eames T, Landthaler M, Karrer S. Crohn's disease: an important differential diagnosis of granulomatous skin diseases. Eur J Dermatol. 2009;19:360–4.
3. Emanuel PO, Phelps RG. Metastatic Crohn's disease: a histopathological study of 12 cases. J Cutan Pathol. 2008;35:457–61.
4. Ishida M, et al. Metstatic Crohn's disease accompanying granulomatous vasculitis and lymphangitis in the vulva. Int J Clin Exp Pathol. 2013;6:2263–6.
5. Kurtzman DJB, Jones T, Lian F, Peng LS. Metastatic Crohn's disease: a review and approach to therapy. J Am Acad Dermatol. 2014;71:804–8013.
6. Leu S, et al. Clinical spectrum of vulva metastatic Crohn's disease. Dig Dis Sci. 2009;54:1565–71.
7. Sides C, Trinidad MC, Heitlinger L, Anasti J. Crohn's disease and the gynecologic patient. Obstet Gynecol Surv. 2013;68:51–61.

Part XIV

Vulvar Lesions: Edema

53 Vulvar Edema

Jacob Bornstein

53.1 Introduction

Edema is defined as a palpable swelling produced by expansion of the interstitial fluid volume. Vulvar edema is composed of plasma or lymph. Most cases involve the labia minora, which is composed of loose connective tissue, lymphatics, and blood vessels. Edema may affect one or both sides of the vulva [1, 2].

The approach to the management of vulvar edema is by defining the type and the source of the edema present: it could be of either acute or chronic type and primary or secondary.

Acute versus chronic vulvar edema: acute edema develops mainly due to allergy and contains plasma. It develops within hours from the contact with the allergen but may appear within minutes or later, after a few days. Chronic edema is the accumulation of lymph in the vulva. The vulvar tissue is firmer in chronic edema than in acute edema. Another way to differentiate between the types is that in acute edema, there is pitting after pressure is applied to the edematous area for at least 5 seconds. Pitting reflects movement of the excess interstitial water in response to pressure. Non-pitting edema suggests chronic-lymphatic edema.

J. Bornstein (✉)
Department of Obstetrics and Gynecology Galilee Medical Center, Bar-Ilan University Faculty of Medicine, Nahariya, Israel

Primary versus secondary source of vulvar edema: primary edema is defined when it is a fundamental part of a specific disease. Secondary vulvar edema when edema accompanies a specific disease or condition.

53.2 Acute Vulvar Edema: Primary Source

Acute allergic angioedema: Vulvar angioedema results from allergy to latex, semen, or vulvovaginal candidiasis. In addition to the vulva, it usually affects the lips, eyelids, or the larynx. Acute allergic angioedema is usually IgE mediated and may deteriorate to anaphylactic shock. The color of the edematous vulva is usually pink or skin colored. It develops within minutes and subsides spontaneously after several hours. Prevention is possible by reducing the use of latex, which may be found in examination gloves and in condoms and contraceptive vaginal diaphragms. Semen allergy may also cause this condition. It develops after exposure to the seminal plasma. It may be confirmed—and prevented—by the use of condoms. In vivo patch and prick tests or blood test (radioallergosorbent test—RAST) are available for confirmation and grading the severity of the specific allergy. Allergy to candidiasis may also cause this type of allergic angioedema. Prevention of both semen and candida allergies should involve graded intravaginal exposure challenge.

J. Bornstein (ed.), *Vulvar Disease*, https://doi.org/10.1007/978-3-319-61621-6_53

Allergic contact dermatitis: to topical deodorants, perfumes, detergents, and antibiotics. This condition is not IgE mediated but rather cell-mediated immune reaction. It usually starts only days after the exposure to the allergen. It is red and eczematous. The edema usually subsides when the dermatitis is taken care of.

53.3 Acute Vulvar Edema: Secondary Origin

Systemic allergic angioedema: may develop from hypersensitivity to certain ingested foods such as shell fish and peanuts. It is IgE mediated. Antihistamines and steroids are useful. Complete avoidance of any contact with these foods is necessary to prevent this life threatening condition.

Hereditary angioedema: vulvar edema due to C1 inhibitor deficiency is usually a part of a systemic reaction.

Trauma: a ruptured blood vessel after an acute trauma to the vulva may lead to edema. In addition, local pressure from a fall or bicycle or horseback riding may also lead to vulvar edema, mostly in the clitoris.

Perineal necrotizing fasciitis (Fournier's gangrene): results of spreading bacterial infection in diabetic or immune-suppressed patient. It is accompanied with fever, chills, and leukocytosis. Edema accompanies the process.

Hydrostatic vulvar edema: edema resulting from increased hydrostatic pressure, such as with peritoneal dialysis.

Edema due to pregnancy: Several causes of edema may involve pregnancy. Pressure by the enlarging uterus on blood vessels may cause edema. The birth itself may be associated with local trauma and edema. Tears and incisions to the perineum and vagina may be a reason to development of edema. Preeclampsia may cause edema in all body parts. Local compresses with diluted magnesium sulfate help to absorb the vulvar edema.

Edema due to infection: Vulvar cellulitis may cause vulvar edema. Other causes are genital herpes, Bartholin's gland duct abscess, and vulvovaginal candidiasis. The edema remains many days after the infection has been treated.

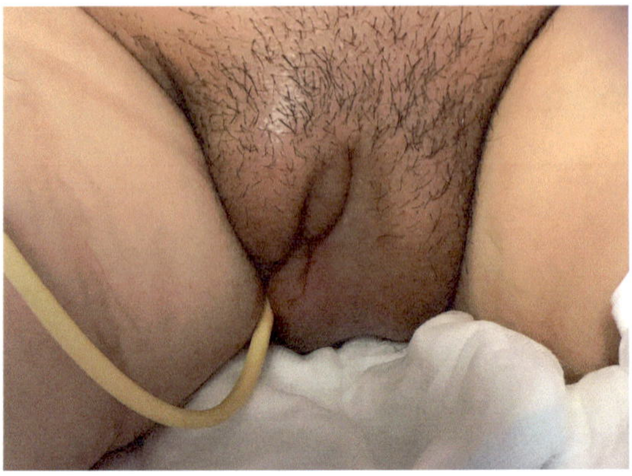

Fig. 53.1 Acute secondary vulvar edema in a patient hospitalized in the intensive care unit

"Systemic" causes of vulvar edema: hypoproteinemia, ovarian hyper-stimulation syndrome, ascites, congestive heart failure, and nephrotic syndrome may lead to edema, mainly in the lower half of the body.

Postsurgical and postradiation edema may be caused by pelvic and mainly inguinal lymph node dissection.

Immobility and hospitalization, such as in the intensive care unit, may lead to vulvar edema (Fig. 53.1).

53.4 Chronic Vulvar Edema: Primary Origin

Melkersson-Rosenthal syndrome: this is a granulomatous disease associated with chronic edema that affects the face and the vulva. The edema is usually unilateral and may precede or accompany Crohn's disease. Treatment is with intralesional injections of steroids as well as oral dapsone, metronidazole, or methotrexate.

Congenital localized lymphangioma: develops as a result of abnormal lymph vessel formation at the genital area.

Idiopathic vulvar edema: the cause is not clear, but experts believe that it results from an unrecognized underlying infection.

53.5 Chronic Vulvar Edema: Secondary Origin

Chronic bacterial infection: the edema of chronic bacterial infection results from blockage or even destruction of the draining lymphatic vessels, especially if recurrent infection or if cellulitis develops. This is in contrast to short-term infections that cause acute edema. Antibiotic treatment sometimes should be given for a long time to prevent recurrences. Rare infections that may cause chronic edema are *Klebsiella*, *Chlamydia*, and *Wuchereria bancrofti*—a parasitic roundworm leading to elephantiasis. Postinfectious edema may follow bacterial infection and develops after the infection resolves. This is consequent to damage of the lymphatic system.

Crohn's disease: Edema here can develop without clear lesions, but usually edema accompanies the Crohn's vulvar ulcer. This condition is detailed elsewhere in this book.

Hidradenitis suppurativa: vulvar edema may precede the lesions. This condition is detailed elsewhere in this book.

Milroy disease: (primary or hereditary lymphedema type 1A or early onset lymphedema) this disease results from a disruption of the normal drainage of lymph. It leads to fluid accumulation and hypertrophy of soft tissues, including the vulva. The condition develops after birth and is associated with firm vulvar edema. Milroy's disease is an autosomal dominant condition caused by a mutation in the FLT4 gene which encodes of the vascular endothelial growth factor receptor 3 (VEGFR-3) gene located on the long arm (q) on chromosome 5 (5q35.3).

Neoplasia: vulvar neoplasia may be associated with malignant lymphatic spread. Lymphatic drainage is therefore halted and edema results. Treatment of the primary tumor may relieve the edema.

Summary: In most cases vulvar edema results from an underlying condition. Treatment consists of reversal of the primary disorder. However, vulvar edema may present as primary.

Vulvar Edema: Breaking the Myths

- Many clinicians cannot identify the cause of vulvar edema. However, in most cases vulvar edema results from an underlying condition and treatment consists of reversal of the primary disorder. Rarely, vulvar edema presents as primary.
- The approach to the management of vulvar edema is by defining the type and the source of the edema present: it could be of either acute or chronic type, and primary or secondary.
- Acute edema develops mainly due to allergy and contains plasma. It may be caused by acute allergic angioedema or allergic contact dermatitis, and the edema is pitting, as pressure causes movement of the excess interstitial water.
- Chronic edema includes lymph and is firmer than in acute edema.

References

1. Amankwah Y, Haefner H. Vulvar edema. Dermatol Clin. 2010;28:765.
2. Pinto e Silva MP, Bassani MA, Miquelutti MA, Marques Ade A, do Amaral MT, de Oliveira MM, Ferreira Nde O. Manual lymphatic drainage and multilayer compression therapy for vulvar edema: a case series. Physiother Theory Pract. 2015;31(7):527–31.

Part XV

Vulvar Pain and Vulvodynia

54 Vulvar Pain and Vulvodynia

Jacob Bornstein

54.1 Introduction

Vulvar pain is an enigma. Its etiology, pathophysiology, and treatment have not yet been elucidated. The most perplexing presentation is pain during intercourse, sometimes prevents the possibility to have intercourse.

Around the enigma of vulvar pain, myths about its causes and treatments emerged. Most of these treatment myths have not been proven to be effective. Consequently, they also lead to unnecessary treatments and despair on the side of the patients. In 2015, an evidence-based consensus terminology has been introduced by the scientific organizations dealing with vulvar disease ("2015 terminology") [1], giving clear definition and understanding of vulvar pain. Consequently, a new paradigm to the treatment of vulvar pain can now be formed [2], making it an etiology-based.

Electronic Supplementary Material The online version of this chapter (doi:10.1007/978-3-319-61621-6_54) contains supplementary material, which is available to authorized users.

J. Bornstein (✉)
Department of Obstetrics and Gynecology Galilee Medical Center, Bar-Ilan University Faculty of Medicine, Nahariya, Israel

54.2 "Vulvar Pain," "Vulvodynia," or "Dyspareunia"?

Why are we talking about "vulvar pain," although the most common and disturbing presenting symptom is introital pain during intercourse, i.e., superficial dyspareunia? Dyspareunia is one of the most common complaints associated with sexual dysfunction. There are several reasons to that. One is the attempt of the ISSVD to broaden the terminology so that it involves pain in general and not only pain during intercourse. An additional reason is to move away from the limited psycho-sexual connotation of "dyspareunia" that prevailed years ago.

Here again, the significance of the 2015 consensus terminology of "persistent vulvar pain and vulvodynia" [1] is depicted (Table 54.1). That terminology has been created by three international societies: the ISSVD, the International Society for The Study of Women's Sexual Health (ISSWSH), and the International Pelvic Pain Society (IPPS). The 2015 terminology divides "persistent vulvar pain" into two categories: vulvar pain that its cause is known (e.g., inflammatory, neoplastic, traumatic, infection-related, neurologic, traumatic, iatrogenic, and hormonal) and "vulvodynia.". The new definition of vulvodynia is "vulvar pain of at least three months' duration, without clear identifiable cause, which may have potential associated factors." The 2015 terminology further characterizes vulvodynia based on location (vestibulodynia, cliterodynia, generalized, mixed), provocation (upon contact

J. Bornstein (ed.), *Vulvar Disease*, https://doi.org/10.1007/978-3-319-61621-6_54

Table 54.1 2015 Consensus terminology and classification of persistent vulvar pain and vulvodynia

A. Vulvar pain caused by a specific disorder[a]
• Infectious (e.g., recurrent candidiasis, herpes)
• Inflammatory (e.g., lichen sclerosus, lichen planus, immunobullous disorders)
• Neoplastic (e.g., Paget disease, squamous cell carcinoma)
• Neurologic (e.g., post-herpetic neuralgia, nerve compression or injury, neuroma)
• Trauma (e.g., female genital cutting, obstetrical)
• Iatrogenic (e.g., post-operative, chemotherapy, radiation)
• Hormonal deficiencies (e.g., genito-urinary syndrome of menopause [vulvo-vaginal atrophy], lactational amenorrhea)
B. Vulvodynia—Vulvar pain of at least 3 months' duration, without clear identifiable cause, which may have potential associated factors
Descriptors:
• Localized (e.g., vestibulodynia, clitorodynia) <u>or</u> generalized <u>or</u> mixed (localized and generalized)
• Provoked (e.g., insertional, contact) <u>or</u> spontaneous <u>or</u> mixed (provoked and spontaneous)
• Onset (primary or secondary)
• Temporal pattern (intermittent, persistent, constant, immediate, delayed)

[a]Women may have both a specific disorder (e.g., lichen sclerosus) and vulvodynia

or spontaneous), temporal pattern (intermittent or constant), and onset (primary or secondary). Lastly, the most important innovation of the 2015 terminology is in the appendix table (Table 54.2) with a list of potential associated factors (musculoskeletal, neuroproliferation, associated co-morbidities, psychosocial factors, etc.) acknowledging that vulvodynia is likely not a single condition, but several diseases. Only few recognize the significance of that "appendix" to the consensus terminology, but these "potential associated factors" are helpful in identifying possible etiologies of vulvodynia. So far, no etiology of vulvodynia has been recognized by the ISSVD. Hence, the new terminology revolutionized the approach to the study and management of vulvodynia, which now needs to be individualized, according to the associated factor.

Table 54.2 2015 Consensus terminology and classification of persistent vulvar pain and vulvodynia

Appendix: Potential factors associated with vulvodynia[a]
• Co-morbidities and other pain syndromes (e.g., painful bladder syndrome, fibromyalgia, irritable bowel syndrome, temporomandibular disorder) [level of evidence 2]
• Genetics [level of evidence 2]
• Hormonal factors (e.g., pharmacologically induced) [level of evidence 2]
• Inflammation [level of evidence 2]
• Musculoskeletal (e.g., pelvic muscle overactivity, myofascial, biomechanical) [level of evidence 2]
• Neurologic mechanisms:
– Central (spine, brain) [level of evidence 2]
– Peripheral—neuroproliferation [level of evidence 2]
• Psychosocial factors (e.g., mood, interpersonal, coping, role, sexual function) [level of evidence 2]
• Structural defects (e.g., perineal descent) [level of evidence 3]

[a]The factors are ranked by alphabetical order

54.3 Descriptors of Vulvodynia

Of the various descriptors that are included in the 2015 terminology, the most important is its localization (localized or generalized) and relation to provocation (provoked and spontaneous) of vulvodynia. Generalized vulvodynia (formerly termed "essential" or "dysesthetic" vulvodynia) affects the whole vulva and is usually spontaneous [3]. It is regarded as a neuropathic pain and affects postmenopausal women mainly. The definitions of these descriptors are presented in Table 54.3.

In addition, the onset of vulvodynia significantly matters to treatment outcome [4, 5]. LPV that has been present since the first attempt of vaginal penetration is termed primary. If LPV started after a period of pain-free intercourse, it is named "secondary" LPV. Several researchers believe that primary LPV is more difficult to treat than secondary LPV [4].

Table 54.3 Definitions of the descriptors of vulvar pain and vulvodynia—addendum to the 2015 ISSVD, ISSWSH, and IPPS consensus terminology and classification of persistent vulvar pain and vulvodynia

Descriptor	Definition
Localized	Involvement of a portion of the vulva, such as the vestibule (vestibulodynia) and clitoris (clitorodynia)
Generalized	Involvement of the whole vulva
Provoked	The discomfort is provoked by physical contact. Such contact may be sexual, non-sexual, or both, i.e., vaginal penetration, clothing, pressure tampon insertion, cotton-tipped applicator pressure, fingertip pressure, etc.
Spontaneous	The symptoms occur without any provoking physical contact
Primary	Onset of the symptoms occurs with first provoking physical contact (i.e., tampon placement, intercourse, vaginal penetration), or: The symptoms are present since first recollection
Secondary	Onset of the symptoms did not occur with first provoking physical contact, or: The symptoms have not always been present
Persistent	The condition persists over a period of at least 3 months (symptoms can be constant or intermittent). Synonym—chronic (condition)
Constant	The symptoms are always present
Intermittent	The symptoms are not always present
Immediate	The symptoms occur during the provoking physical contact
Delayed	The symptoms occur after the provoking physical contact

54.4 How Frequent Is Vulvar Pain?

Vulvar pain is a condition that women frequently conceal, because they are ashamed to admit to it, and thus, vulvar pain was considered to be rare. But this is not the case. The prevalence of vulvar pain is currently found to be 14–34% in young women and 6.5–45% in old women [6]. In the USA 30% of women reported pain during vaginal penetration. In the National Health and Social Life Survey, complaints of "physical pain during intercourse during the past 12 months" were 21% in 18–19 year olds, 13% in women aged 30–39 years, and 13% and 8% in women of 40–49 and 50–59, respectively. Another study found that 17% of postmenopausal women suffer from vulvodynia. Women of Hispanic origin were more likely to develop vulvar pain symptoms as compared to Caucasian [7–12].

54.5 How to Evaluate a Patient with Vulvar Pain?

The woman with vulvar pain usually goes through years of endless visits to health care providers without achieving any significant improvement. This leads to depression and suspicion in the capability of anybody to cure her. This condition preoccupies her thoughts and negatively affects her whole life. Therefore, the approach should be very empathic. We suggest to use a structured questionnaire (Table 54.4) to obtain the following information.

54.6 Essentials of Medical History

1. Pain characteristics, such as time since onset, temporal pattern, duration, location, quality, what elicits it, the intensity, and whether the pain is primary or secondary.
2. Musculoskeletal conditions, such as a history of surgery or injury affecting the lumbo-pelvic-hip region and sacrum.
3. Bowel and bladder function history; disturbances may be associated with pelvic floor dysfunction.
4. Sexuality: is there a desire, is an orgasm reached, frequency of sex; this is a good measure of the severity of the condition.
5. Coexistence of "comorbidities"—other medical or mental health conditions and treatments.
6. Previous treatments of vulvar pain and the outcome.
7. Childhood trauma including abuse and neglect, and any adult negative sexual experience.

Table 54.4 Useful questions to ask when obtaining a sexual pain history. "Do you have a history of"

• Physical, sexual, and emotional abuse or anxiety?
• Low back or hip pain?
• Urinary urgency, frequency, hesitancy, or incomplete emptying?
• Chronic constipation or rectal fissures?
• Oral contraceptive pill use (especially HCPs with 20 µg of ethyl estradiol, or the progestins, norgestimate or drospirenone) preceding or during onset of symptoms?
• Ovarian suppression by Lupron, Depo-Provera?
• Decreased libido or decreased vaginal lubrication prior to the onset of dyspareunia?
• Peri-menopausal or menopausal symptoms such as hot flashes and night sweats?
• Contact allergies or skin sensitive to chemicals?
• Recurrent (culture positive) yeast infections?
• Persistent yellowish vaginal discharge?
• Persistent white vaginal discharge?
• Severe burning or an allergic reaction to a topical medication on the vulva or vagina?
• Burning after intercourse?
• Pain since first attempt at intercourse without any pain-free sex?
• Pain with first tampon use?
• Increased sensitivity of the umbilicus?
• Postcoital spotting or bleeding?
• Vulvar itching?
• Night-time scratching?
• Diarrhea?
• Mid-cycle spotting or pain?
• Pain is worse in sexual position with deep thrusting?
• Vulvar ulcerations, tears, fissures?
• Painful periods?
• Chronic pelvic pain?
• Feeling of an obstruction in the vagina?
• Pain beginning after childbirth?
• Dribbling after urination?
• Changes in coloration or architecture of the labia or vulva?
• Decreased clitoral sensation?
• Frequent bicycle riding?
• Aggressive abdominal muscle strengthening or Pilates?
• Pain mainly at clitoris?
• Pain during intercourse began, has there been any pain-free intercourse?
• Oral lesions or bleeding gums?
• A history of high-risk human papilloma or cervical dysplasia?

Table 54.5 Recommended core and secondary outcome measures of vulvovaginal pain characteristics in provoked vulvodynia clinical trials, part of IMMPACT

Pain characteristic	Core outcome measures	Secondary outcome measures
Pain intensity	11-point NRS during sexual activities	
Pain quality and affect	Short-form McGill pain questionnaire	
Pain temporality		Specific activities that might provoke the pain of PVD

8. In a research setting, use the "Initiative on Methods, Measurement, and Pain Assessment in Clinical Trials (IMMPACT)" series of questionnaires [13] (Table 54.5).

54.7 Examining the Vestibule

54.7.1 Cotton-Swab Test

The cotton-swab test, also named Q-tip test, is the most commonly used clinical test for diagnosing localized provoked vulvodynia (LPV, vestibulodynia) (Video 54.1). Its significance originates from the fact that at this time, a biopsy is not required in order to make a diagnosis of vulvodynia. Hence, we rely on the clinical diagnosis. The cotton-swab test involves pressing on foci throughout the vestibule with a cotton-tipped applicator [14]. Some recommend that the cotton tip be moist to avoid the dryness sensation. I suggest pressing in a nonconsecutive order on vestibular foci in the following seven vestibular foci, according to clock's position: 1, 2, 4 (Fig. 54.1), 6 (Fig. 54.2), 8 (Fig. 54.3), 10, 11 (Fig. 54.4), and 12 o'clock (Fig. 54.5). Foci 1 and 11 are located on both sides of the urethra. In addition to the vestibule, the surrounding tissues in the labia majora, perineum, and clitoris should also be touched with the cotton swab. The resultant pain is scored by a visual analog score

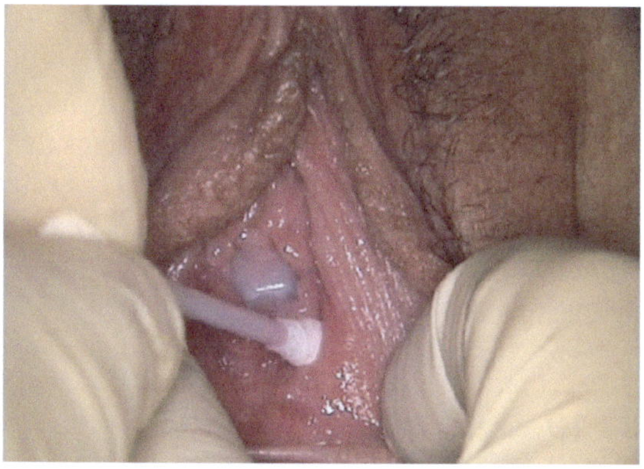

Fig. 54.1 The cotton-swab test, pressing on the 4 o'clock focus in the vestibule

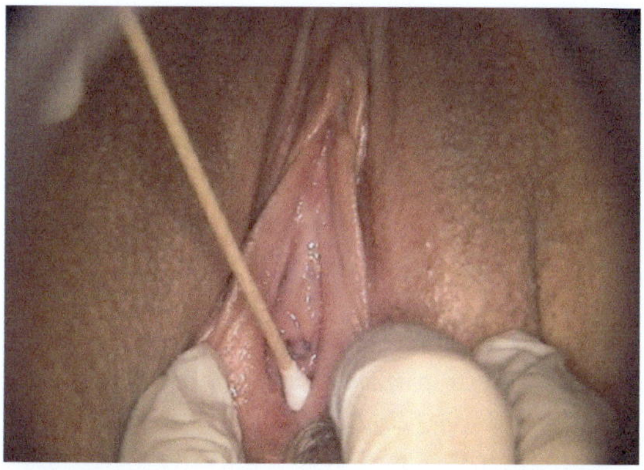

Fig. 54.2 The cotton-swab test, pressing on the 6 o'clock focus in the vestibule

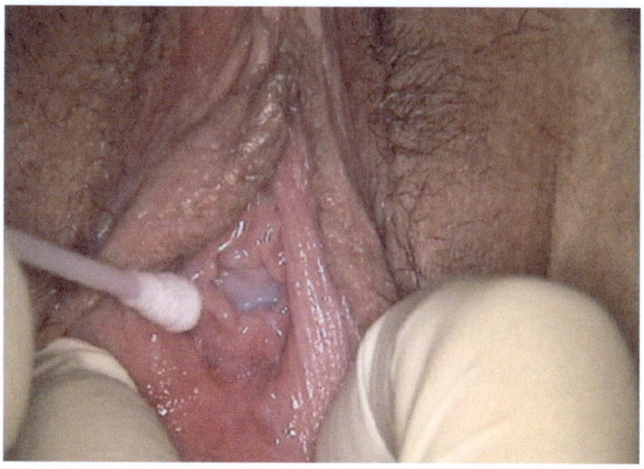

Fig. 54.3 The cotton-swab test, pressing on the 8 o'clock focus in the vestibule

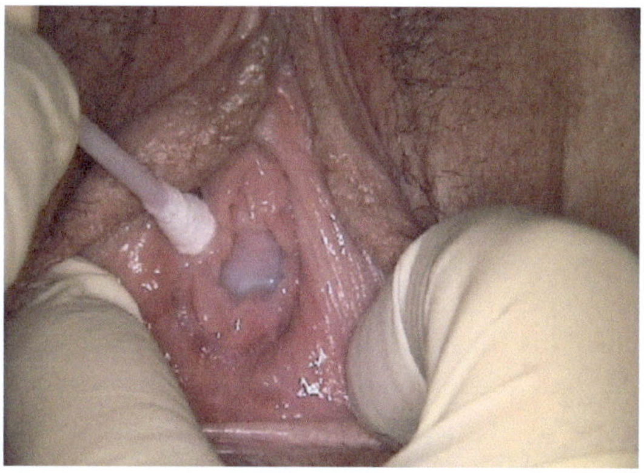

Fig. 54.4 The cotton-swab test, pressing on the 11 o'clock focus in the vestibule

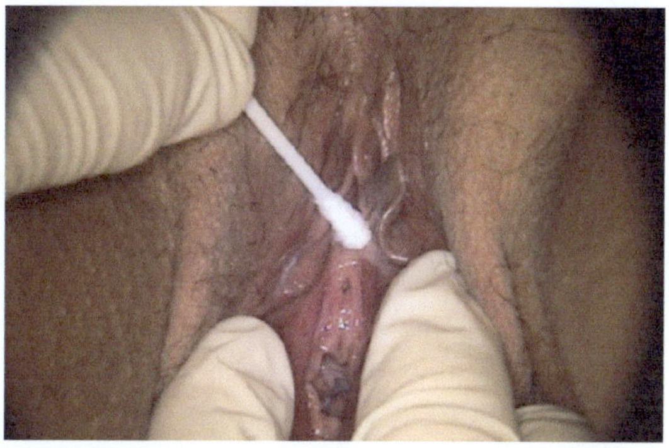

Fig. 54.5 The cotton-swab test, pressing on the 12 o'clock focus in the vestibule

(VAS) by observing the patient's reactions or asking her to rate the intensity of the pain on a numerical rating scale of 0–10 or alternatively 0–3. This test, however, is imperfect: It depends not only on the patient's tenderness but also on the amount of pressure exerted by the examiner [15, 16]. In addition, the openings of the Skene's glands (lateral to the urethra) and of the Bartholin's glands may be sensitive even in women without LPV.

Location of the sensitivity, posterior versus anterior vestibular portion: One of the myths associated with the location of the sensitivity in LPV is that in most cases it is only the posterior portion of the vestibule which is affected. This is not true. The majority of the women with posterior vestibular sensitivity develop anterior soreness as well. The involvement of the anterior vestibular part may develop at a later date. Because of this myth, during many surgical procedures for LPV, only the posterior part is excised, and the sensitivity later extends to the anterior part, rendering the procedure as a failure. This inadequate technique is the cause of the bad reputation of vestibulectomy, in the past.

An additional myth is that if the sensitivity is extensive throughout the entire vestibule—it resulted from neuroproliferation and if it is confined to the posterior vestibule—the etiology is musculoskeletal [17]. In my experience there is no association between the localization and the etiology.

54.8 Vulva Algesiometer

A vulva algesiometer measures the amount of pressure causing pain, applied to the vestibule in the cotton-topped test, allowing to standardize it [17] (Fig. 54.6). The foci pressed may be the same as recommended with the Q-tip test.

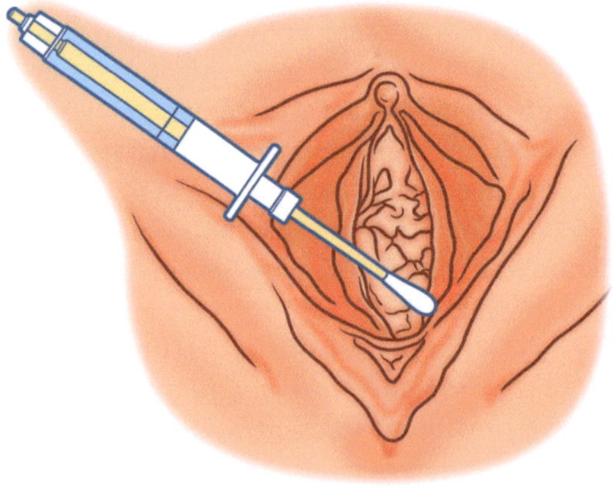

Fig. 54.6 A drawing depicting the vulvar algesiometer. It is composed of a cotton-swab applicator, connected to a spring manometer, measuring the pressure applied. Here pressing on the 5 o'clock area

54.9 Characteristics of the Pain

Pain may present in a few forms: as allodynia—perception of pain resulting from a stimulus that normally is not painful, such as a cotton-swab; hyperalgesia—perception of extreme pain to a stimulus that is usually causing pain; hyperpathia—pain provoked by very light touch [18].

54.10 Determining Severity

The severity of LPV is determined by the patient's level of pain during vaginal intercourse (dyspareunia), using the Marinoff criteria [19]:

Level 1: dyspareunia causes discomfort but does not prevent sexual intercourse;
Level 2: dyspareunia sometimes prevents sexual intercourse;
Level 3: dyspareunia completely prevents sexual intercourse.

However, when intercourse is not practiced, a tampon insertion may be used to determine the severity of LPV [20].

Although this is a very subjective determination, it affects the choice of treatment: In level 1 cases, treatment should not involve surgery. Unfortunately, in many cases there is deterioration of LPV severity with time, and LPV that was evaluated as level 1 may become level 2 or 3 in severity. Less frequently, a level 3 LPV will spontaneously resolve or become a level 1 in severity [21, 22]. Response to treatment should be measured by the degree of reduction of the level of sensitivity.

54.11 Association with Vulvovaginal Infection

Many women with LPV have been diagnosed with vulvovaginal candidiasis (VVC). In the past, this co-occurrence originated a theory that VVC causes LPV [23]. Interestingly, in mice, repeated vulvar applications of a yeast allergen (zymosan) caused in a few neuroproliferation and local sensitivity

[24, 25], serving as an animal model for LPV. However, prolonged treatment with oral fluconazole has not been shown to cure LPV [26]. Actually, the association between VVC and LPV is a myth. It is not a causal association. We suspect that the frequent diagnosis of VVC made in women with LPV results from a missed diagnosis of LPV by the health care provider, so that while examining a woman with dyspareunia, every slight vaginal discharge receives the presumed diagnosis of VVC. The woman then believes that every time she experiences pain during intercourse, she actually suffers from a breakout of VVC. This leads to repeated cycles of topical therapy with imidazole preparations against VVC, with no real response in pain level. Obviously, there are times when a woman with LPV does suffer from VVC. However, the VVC is incidental, and after treatment by imidazole, the LPV persists and the woman continues to suffer from dyspareunia.

This chain of events (dyspareunia—“diagnosis” of VVC—treatment by topical azoles—persistent dyspareunia) has even led to a hypothesis that it is the therapy of VVC—repeatedly administered, rather than the VVC—that causes LPV, via an allergic reaction [27, 28]. Currently, it seems that this theory is also a myth, resulting from over-diagnosis of VVC and repeated imidazole treatment rather than diagnosing LPV, in women with vulvar discomfort and pain, in an attempt to provide a possible explanation for the pain, by a health care provider who is not acquaint with the condition of LPV.

54.12 Hormonal Contraception and LPV

Hormonal oral contraceptive pills have been claimed to be associated with an increase in the LPV incidence and severity [29]. A suggested pathophysiologic mechanism will be discussed later. In some cases, this association holds true, but more than 100 million women use hormonal oral contraception, and the majority practice painless intercourse. Furthermore, many women with level 3 LPV are not using HCP.

54.13 Physical Examination

Vulvar conditions that may cause vulvar pain and dyspareunia are detailed in part A of the 2015 terminology [1]. Accordingly, the genital examination of a woman with vulvar pain should rule out Candida and bacteriologic vaginal infections, dermatoses, deformities, birth lacerations, and past trauma as causes of vulvar pain.

54.14 Colposcopic Examination

Experts of vulvar disease differ in opinions as to whether colposcopic examination of the vulva, commonly referred to as “vulvoscopy,” should be a part of a vulvar examination. The traditional aim of colposcopy—after acetic acid application—is used on the cervix for the evaluation of abnormal Pap test, looking for intraepithelial neoplasia. On the vulva, naked eye examination may suffice in many cases. However, colposcopy is applied by many experts to magnify the vestibule and look for vulvar lesions in cases of suspect LPV. The exact painful foci can be localized with the aid of the colposcope, and a fissure may be seen in the posterior fourchette. We have found that when women with level 3 (severe) LPV attempt intercourse, the forced penile insertion leads many times to an erosion (Fig. 54.7) or ulcer (Figs. 54.8) in the fourchette. Sometimes this fissure is the most disturbing painful area, and the presenting symptom of LPV.

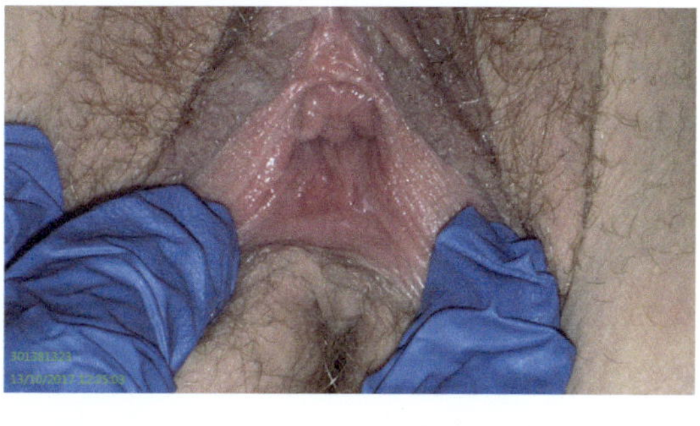

Fig. 54.7 An erosion in the 6 o’clock area of the vestibule. It is frequently caused by forceful intercourse in women with LPV. It may bleed and hurt for a few days

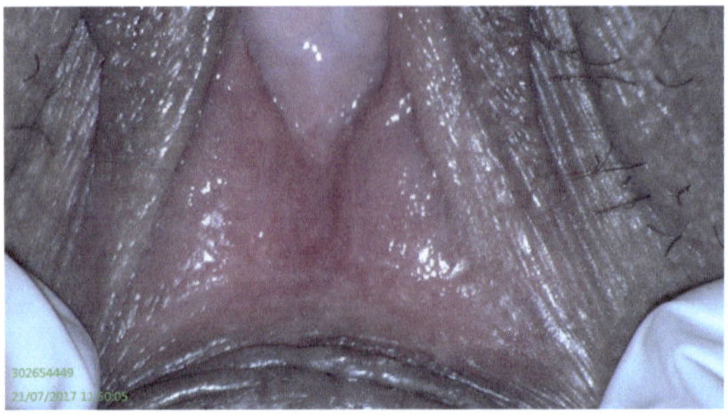

Fig. 54.8 An ulcer in the 6 o'clock area of the vestibule. It is frequently caused by forceful intercourse in women with LPV. It may bleed and hurt for a few days

In addition, colposcopic magnification can aid in excluding the presence of intraepithelial neoplasia, inflammation, infection, or any other dermatologic disease of the vulva. Erythema is a nonspecific finding, and should not be used as a criterion for diagnosing LPV.

54.15 Speculum Examination

It is usually difficult or impossible to carry out a speculum examination of the vagina because of the entry sensitivity. It may be deferred until after the patient is more relaxed or improved with treatment. If a speculum examination was carried out, any abnormal discharge should be evaluated for vaginitis. Women who are lactating, are on birth control pills or are menopausal may have atrophic vaginal mucosa which may be sensitive and cause or exacerbate vestibular sensitivity. However, it should be kept in mind that the presence of any vaginal infection or atrophy does not exclude LPV. They may coexist with LPV, rather than being the cause of it.

The speculum examination may be deferred to a later visit because at the initial visit its insertion may cause excruciating vestibular pain. However, pelvic manual examination is essential for initial evaluation because it will help to determine which associated factor is present and needs to be taken care of. Inserting one finger to the vagina is less painful than two, and it can suffice to perform the evaluation of the vagina, cervix, uterus, bladder, and pelvic musculoskeletal structures.

The digital pelvic examination is very important and should include:

- A gentle palpation of the urethra and bladder trigone. Tenderness of the bladder may be suggestive of either a urinary tract infection, a painful bladder syndrome (PBS, formerly—interstitial cystitis), or endometriosis infiltration.
- Palpation of the deep pelvic musculoskeletal structures for the presence of tender points and hypertonicity. If these are detected, a hypertonic pelvic floor muscle dysfunction may be suspected, and a referral to pelvic floor assessment and possibly rehabilitative physical therapy is recommended.
- The area around the ischial spine should be touched to detect the pudendal nerve. Tenderness of the pudendal nerve may suggest that the reason for the pain is pudendal neuralgia or pudendal nerve entrapment.
- The uterus and adnexa are palpated and moved to rule out pelvic inflammatory disease.
- If endometriosis is suspected, a recto-vaginal examination may reveal nodularity and sensitivity of endometriosis.
- Repaired lacerations or episiotomies should be examined for sensitivity that may result from traumatic neuromas that can also be a source of pain in women who have had prior vaginal surgery. However, the notion that birth lacerations and episiotomy scars are a cause of dyspareunia is a myth. Post-partum dyspareunia results from the new onset of LPV, while the scar tissue itself is not sensitive at all, because in these foci the nerve nociceptors have been teared and destroyed.

54.16 Pathology of LPV

A biopsy is not required for making the diagnosis of vestibulodynia; however, there are three pathological features typical for vestibulodynia in biopsy:

- Stromal hyperinnervation: the stromal nerve cell surface area was found to be ten times that of controls ($p = 0.01$) [30].
- Intraepithelial innervation: PGP 9.5 immunoreactive stain shows intraepithelial nerve fibers only in women with LPV. The fibers penetrate the basal membrane and continue vertically for more than half the distance to the epithelial surface [31] (Figs. 54.9 and 54.10).
- Stromal inflammation, localized around the minor vestibular minor glands (Fig. 54.11)
- Increased number of stromal mast cells; in one study an ROC analysis showed that 90% of patients with vestibulitis showed more than eight mast cells per high power field [30]. Mast cells may be depicted using a Giemsa staining (Fig. 54.12) or immunohistochemistry detecting CD117 (c-kit) antigen (Figs. 54.13 and 54.14)

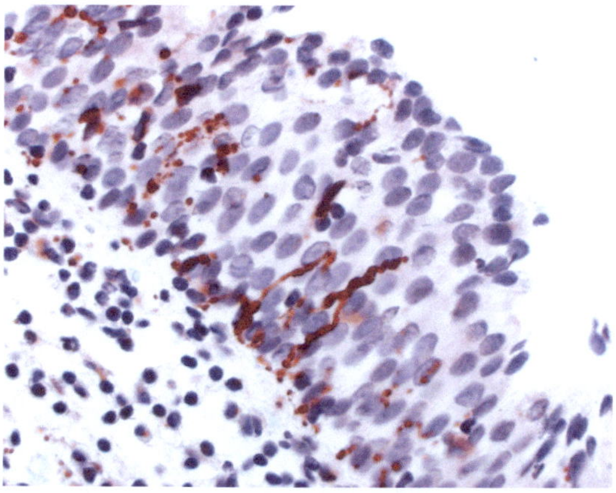

Fig. 54.9 Nerve fibers intruding into the vestibular epithelium, in a case of LPV (PGP9.5 staining ×400 magnification) [31]

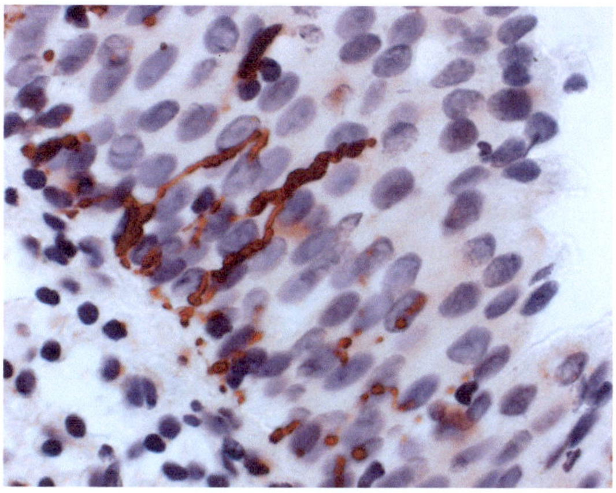

Fig. 54.10 Nerve fibers intruding into the vestibular epithelium, in a case of LPV (PGP9.5 staining ×600 magnification) [31]

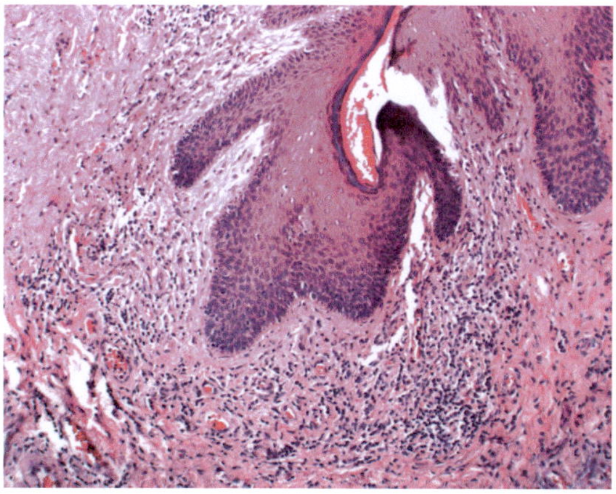

Fig. 54.11 Stromal inflammation, localized around a metaplastic minor vestibular gland, in a case of LPV H&E stain ×100

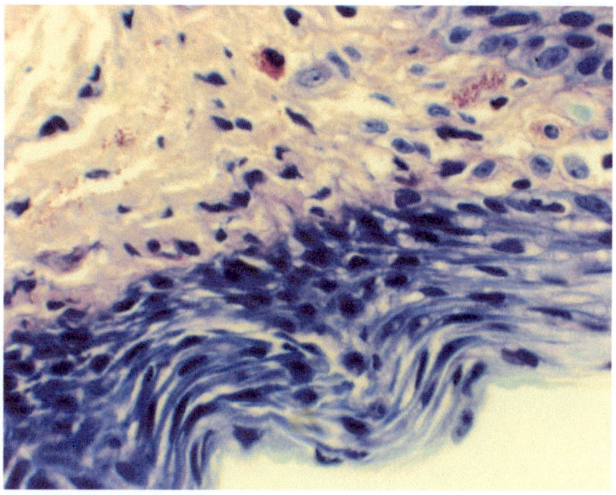

Fig. 54.12 Mast cells located subepithelially, among other inflammatory cells in a case of LPV. Giemsa stain ×200

54.17 Serum Testing

Serum hormone testing is not required to rule out or rule in LPV. In women with one of the conditions associated with vulvar pain with a

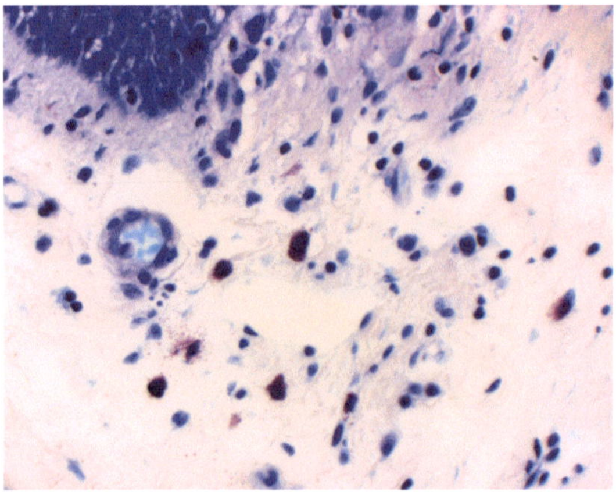

Fig. 54.13 Mast cells located subepithelially, among other inflammatory cells in a case of LPV. CD117 (C-kit) stain ×400

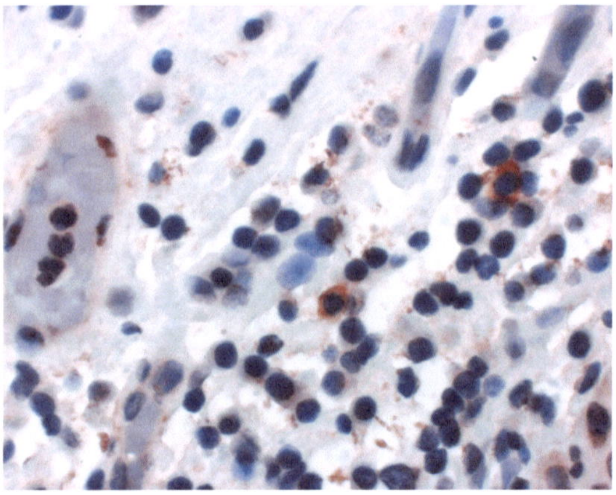

Fig. 54.14 Mast cells located subepithelially, among other inflammatory cells in a case of LPV. CD117 (C-kit) stain ×300

specific disorder—genito-urinary syndrome of the menopause (GUSM, formerly: atrophic vaginitis), a decreased serum estradiol and a high level of follicular stimulating hormone (FSH) may be found. Elevated serum hormone binding globulin (SHBG) and decreased free testosterone and estradiol may be detected in women with vestibulodynia associated with hormonal contraceptives [29]. However, the presence of GUSM may coexist with vulvodynia of other causes, such as LPV.

54.18 Is Any Additional Testing Required?

In most cases the vestibular examination is sufficient and no other test is required to diagnose LPV. However, additional testing may be needed in the following women:

- In women with associated deep dyspareunia or deep pelvic pain, vaginal ultrasound examination should be carried out to diagnose endometriosis.
- Diagnostic laparoscopy may be necessary if there is significant evidence of deep endometriosis.
- If nerve entrapment or compression is suspected, Tesla 3 magnetic resonance imaging using "nerve protocol" may be contributory.
- Colonoscopy and CT scan with orally ingested contrast material may be used to rule out pathology of the lower gastrointestinal tract.
- Cystoscopy may be done to diagnose painful bladder syndrome (interstitial cystitis) if LPV is associated with lower abdominal pain, dysuria, etc.
- An electromyogram may be utilized to assess the tone and strength of the levator ani muscles when, upon pelvic examination, there is evidence of hypertonic pelvic floor dysfunction.

54.19 Assessment of the Pelvic Floor Musculature

Some women with LPV may have an increase in pelvic floor muscle tone [32]. Interestingly, when the patient is asked to contract the introitus during a pelvic examination, the examiner hardly feels any contraction of the introital muscles, e.g., the bulbocavernosus muscle. The exact mechanism by which the increase in pelvic floor musculature is associated with LPV has not been elucidated. Perhaps pressure is applied by the contracted muscles on the pudendal nerve fibers entering the pelvis, leading to allodynia. Nevertheless, detecting a musculoskeletal factor associated with LPV calls for a physical therapy rehabilitation of the pelvic floor muscles.

54.20 Associated Factors

54.20.1 Neuroproliferation or Hyperinnervation (Table 54.2)

An increase in the density of nerve endings in the vestibular stroma of women with LPV as compared to controls has been repeatedly documented [33–37] (Figs. 54.9 and 54.10). These nerve endings have been shown to be nociceptors [34] and have an increased density of the vanilloid receptor VR1 (TRPV1) [38]. We have shown that the increased density of nerve fibers in women with LPV was ten times greater than in non-affected women, and was associated with significant increase in the number of mast cells and degranulated mast cells within the vestibular mucosa [30] (Figs. 54.12, 54.13, and 54.14). We then demonstrated an increased subepithelial heparanase activity (degranulated from the aforementioned mast cells) in the vestibular mucosa [31] (Figs. 54.15 and 54.16). We further postulated that histamine, leukotrienes, and nerve growth factor—which are released from the degranulated mast cell—can cause nociceptor nerve fibers proliferation and sensitization. In addition, the heparanase, which can degrade the vestibular stroma, allows these activated and proliferating nociceptors to penetrate through the basement membrane into the superficial mucosal epithelium of the vestibule (Figs. 54.9 and 54.10). It has been theorized by many groups that certain genetic polymorphisms may predispose affected women with LPV to have an exaggerated inflammatory response or chronic infection, which leads to mast cell activation and subsequent nociceptor proliferation [39].

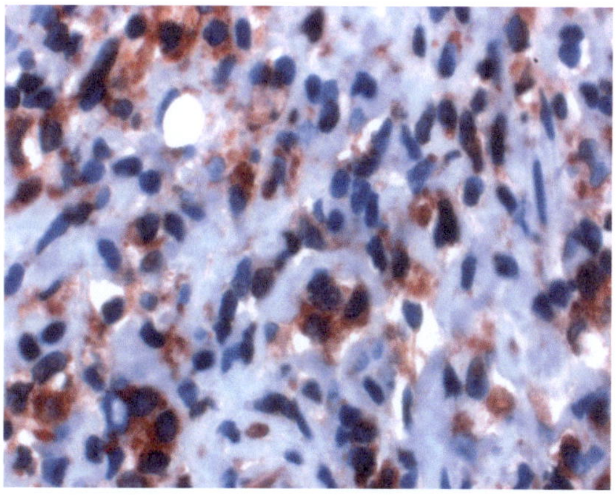

Fig. 54.16 Cytoplasmic heparanase expression in the subepithelial layer of a patient with LPV. Immunohistostaining with antihuman heparanase monoclonal antibody 92.4 ×600

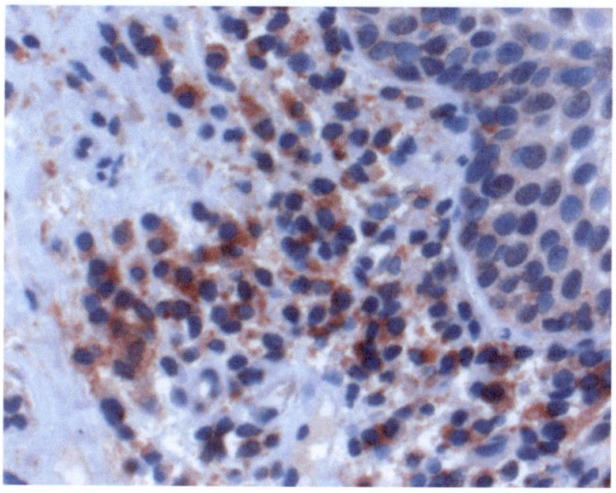

Fig. 54.15 Cytoplasmic heparanase expression in the subepithelial layer of a patient with LPV. Immunohistostaining with antihuman heparanase monoclonal antibody 92.4 ×400

54.20.2 Central Nervous System Involvement in Vulvodynia

Central nervous system alterations as a cause of vulvodynia has been suspected. Several mechanisms have been proposed:

- Altered central nervous system processing [40];
- Global sensitization of nociceptive transmission [41];
- Activation of the hypothalamic pituitary adrenal (HPA) axis via chronic stress;
- Visceromotor responses to vaginal distension [42];

54.20.3 Genetic Predisposition of Vulvodynia

Genetic studies have focused on two mechanisms:

- An inability to end an infection or inflammation [43];
- An increased susceptibility to hormonal changes caused by oral contraceptive pills [44].

Women with LPV were likely to have the less effective polymorphism of mannose-binding lectin (MBL) [45]. MBL is a major component of antimicrobial innate immunity, thus leading to an increased rate of infections.

Furthermore, Foster and colleagues [46] showed the presence of a loss-of-function mutation in the melanocortin-1 receptor (MC1R)—which carries anti-inflammatory effects, in women with LPV. Additional risk may be caused by a loss-of-function mutation in the MC1R gene with a variant allele of the IL-1B receptor antagonist gene.

54.20.4 Musculoskeletal Factors

The association between LPV and the pelvic floor muscle overactivity may work both ways. The dyspareunia frequently results in reflex pelvic muscles contractions and subsequently an involuntary increased muscle tone. On the other hand, increased muscle tension may press on fibers of the pudendal nerve and pelvic trauma may lead to nerve damage, myofascial trigger points, and pain [47]. Furthermore, it was hypothesized that myofascial tissue reflexes activate nociceptive and visceral neurons [47].

54.20.5 Hormonal Factors

A controversy exists as to whether combined oral hormonal contraceptives pills (HCP) play a role in the development of LPV. Against that association is that of the millions of women taking HCP, only a slight fraction suffers from LPV.

Indeed, three studies have failed to show an association between HCPs and vulvodynia: Studies by Reid et al. [48] and Arnold et al. [27] showed no association. Foster and Woodruff [49] showed in a case control study that HCPs decreased the risk of vestibulodynia.

Nevertheless, some women with LPV describe an improvement with cessation of the HCP, and other studies depicted association of vestibulodynia with HCP [50–54]. Goldstein et al. [44] identified a polymorphism in the androgen receptor that significantly increased the risk of developing HCP-induced LPV in affected women.

We suggest that with prolonged use of HCP, the net effect is progestogenic, so that the estrogen influence on the vestibule and vagina is reduced. This leads to diminished lubrication and decreased elasticity, causing increased friability and epithelial damage with vaginal intercourse. Later, allodynia and burning may occur [55].

54.20.6 Embryological/Congenital Factors

Vulvodynia is sometimes associated with painful bladder syndrome (interstitial cystitis) and with periumbilical hypersensitivity. This association originates in the embryo development period; the vestibule develops from the urogenital sinus, which is contiguous with the allantois, which later differentiates to the urachus and the umbilicus.

54.20.7 Inflammatory Factors

Women with vulvodynia are more likely to have a history of allergic rashes [56]. This is in accordance with the finding of excess of mast cells in the stroma of women with LPV. Mast cells have a known role in allergy and anaphylaxis, and are found significantly more in cases with LPV compared to controls [30, 36, 37, 57, 58] (Figs. 54.12, 54.13, and 54.14). Mast cell produced tumor necrosis factor (TNF) which has been associated with nerve fiber elongation in animal models of contact hypersensitivity [59].

54.20.8 Psychological Factors

54.20.8.1 Changes in Mood

We doubt that mood changes precede and cause LPV and believe that it develops in response to the extreme inconvenience and difficulties of LPV.

Similarly, women with vulvodynia report significantly less sexual desire, arousal and satisfaction, difficulty in reaching orgasm, a lower frequency of intercourse, more negative attitudes toward sexuality, and more sexual distress than pain-free controls [6]. Here also, these psychosexual changes are thought by some investigators to be the initiating factor of LPV. Again, we suspect that they may be consequent to the persistent pain associated with vaginal penetration.

Another controversial issue is whether childhood victimization may be a risk factor for the development of sexual pain [60–62].

Many women with vulvar pain report feelings of shame and low self-esteem [63, 64].

54.21 Multidisciplinary Approach

Managing vulvodynia requires a unique cooperation of the specialties. Not surprisingly, the combination of chronic genital pain and sexual dysfunction might amplify the difficulty that health professionals—and patients—have in raising the issue of sexuality for discussion. Indeed, many women with chronic vulvar pain are silent sufferers, with only about 60% of them consult health care professionals [27]. More than half of the sufferers consult three or more physicians before receiving a diagnosis [65].

54.22 Treatment

54.22.1 What You Should Do

- Prepare a treatment plan. Rather than prescribing the patient one treatment at a time, give her a multi-step plan. Explain that you arrange it from easy to difficult treatments. This is the key to obtaining patient's compliance.
- Determine the "associated factors": Prepare the treatment plan only after you determined the associated factors of LPV for the specific woman. This is a new paradigm in the approach to patients with vulvar pain. The 2015 consensus terminology [1], in addition to introducing the updated terminology, has actually led to a novel approach to the management of LPV [2]; In the past, a random choice of treatment has been made per the therapist choice or expertise. Alternatively, treatment was based on "trial and error" [66]; Now the treatment should be targeted per the presumed factor that has caused, or at least is associated with, LPV.
- For each treatment plan, it is preferable that the first line of treatment is non-surgical, leaving surgery for last resort. However, surgery (vestibulectomy) may sometimes be the only indicated treatment, for example, in patients who have a neuroproliferative LPV with no associated musculo-skeletal, psychological, or neuropathic factors. Therefore, the myth that surgery should be carried out only when all other treatments fail should, in our opinion, be broken.
- For patients who are anxious to complete treatment as soon as possible, several therapies may be tried concomitantly, rather than one after the other.
- Do not refer a patient to surgery only because she has been suffering from LPV for many years. She should first try the treatment that is tailored to her associated factor.

54.22.2 What You Shouldn't Do

- Do not tell the patient that "it is all in her head," although there is a large body of evidence that vulvodynia may be associated with an emotional impairment. However, it is not clear if emotional factors cause vulvodynia, and it may well be that the direction is opposite, and the presence of vulvodynia is the cause of emotional disability. Be that as it may, emphasizing the psycho-sexual association may stigmatize the patient as a psychiatric case.
- It is important to spend a long time with the patient, discussing what in her mind caused the vulvar pain, what her concerns and fears are. However, the main message in the visit is that the condition is a physical, and that there

are successful treatments. Also, that the emotional burden will be relieved once the patient realizes that the pain is gone.

- Do not criticize previous misdiagnoses and treatments, although it is sometimes very clear that the patient had vulvodynia all the years, and her health care providers constantly missed it. Common diagnoses mistakenly given to women with vulvodynia are: chronic, recurrent vulvovaginitis, recurrent herpes, lichen sclerosus, and more. Common wrong medications prescribed are: Clobetasol dipropionate (Dermovate) topical treatment for presumed lichen sclerosus, prolonged antibiotic administration, ablative laser treatment, etc.

54.22.3 Initial Approach

A frequent question asked by women with vulvodynia is if the condition might resolve spontaneously. Indeed, each year, roughly 10% of women with vulvodynia experience symptom remission [8].

Traditionally, treatments were presented as medical or surgical. However, some treatments may include a combination of both approaches, such as surgical excision of the posterior vestibule and Interferon injections in the anterior vestibule [67]. Interferon injections are not used any more.

Should the approach to primary LPV be different than that of secondary LPV? Most experts believe that having primary LPV lowers the success rate of surgical treatment [68, 69]. However, the response to all treatments is lower in women with primary LPV versus secondary LPV [36, 37]; So, the type of LPV should not affect the treatment choice.

54.22.4 General Vulvar Care

There are a few general steps that may lower the pain and burning:

- For immediate relief of vulvar burning and pain, use ice packs, with caution.
- Use water to clean the vulva after urination, and then dry immediately. Soap should be used as little as possible.
- Avoid synthetic pads and underwear, use only cotton.
- Do not apply vulvar irritants such as strong soaps.
- To avoid drying, use an emollient without preservative.
- Use lubrication during intercourse.

54.22.5 Treating Vulvodynia: The New Paradigm

The treatments should be planned according to the associated factor, as per the 2015 consensus terminology (Table 54.2). For details on the dosages and scheduling of topical treatment, see Table 54.6. For oral neuropathic treatment, see Table 54.7.

54.22.6 Approach to Treatment of a Patient with Hormonal Factors

In women where the initiation of oral contraceptive pills was associated with the onset of LPV, the pills may be discontinued for 3 months, and a non-hormonal contraception be used at that time.

Table 54.6 Topical medications used to treat vulvodynia

Topical medication	Dosage	Side effects
5% lidocaine ointment	Apply to skin as needed; dispense 30-g tube	Erythema or edema. Rare cases of purpura. If ointment is present on skin during intercourse, the partner may experience numbness
EMLA cream (lidocaine 2.5% and prilocaine 2.5%; AstraZeneca Pharmaceuticals LP, Wilmington, DE)	Apply to skin PRN	Paleness, erythema, and swelling

Table 54.7 Oral neuropathic treatments of vulvodynia

Medication	Dose/Mode of application	Very common (>10%) side effects
Amitriptyline or desipramine tablet 10 mg or 25 mg	Start with 5 mg (1/2 a tablet) before bed time, increase by 5 mg q 1 week Cease increasing the dose when resolution of vulvodynia is achieved Maximum dose 100 mg qd. Decrease amount and discontinue after 3 months	Drowsiness, confusion, dizziness, dry mouth, constipation, tachycardia
Gabapentin (Neurontin) tablet 300–800 mg	Start with 100–300 mg hs and increase until resolution of vulvodynia or until intolerance Divide dose bid to tid Maximum 3600 mg	Dizziness, fatigue, drowsiness, ataxia, peripheral edema, nystagmus, tremor
Pregabalin (Lyrica) tablet 50–300 mg	Start with 50–75 mg Maximum 600 mg bid	Dizziness, drowsiness

If LPV is not improved by the break, the pills can be started again. Although it is controversial if oral contraception plays any role in the pathogenesis of LPV, the hormonal contraception has a net progestogenic effect, causing vaginal atrophy. There are two options of overcoming this atrophying effect: one, as suggested earlier, is to discontinue the hormonal contraceptive pills and the other option is to continue the use of the hormonal contraception, but apply a topical estradiol cream to the vestibule and vagina. Adding testosterone 0.1% may further reduce the sensitivity.

54.23 Approach to Treatment of a Patient with Inflammation

54.23.1 Cutaneous Fibroblast Lysate

This topical cream reduced 20–30% of pain in women with LPV. It contains human cytokines that may interfere with the inflammatory process and promote tissue healing.

54.23.2 Corticosteroids

The rationale to using corticosteroids was that they reduce the production of IL1 [70], which is significantly higher in the hymen region of the vestibule of women with LPV [46]. However, topical and intravestibular injections of corticosteroids have not been found to be significantly effective in treating LPV.

54.23.3 Interferon

We have been involved in several studies of treating LPV with Interferon (INF). Initially IFN was used when LPV was presumed to be caused by human papillomavirus (HPV). LPV was then named "condylomatous vulvitis" [71]. A very high response rate was reported after injecting 12 million units of Interferon alfa to the vestibule, one million units each time to a different focus on the vestibule. Later it was shown that IFN downregulates the expression of proinflammatory cytokines [72] which are very high in the hymeneal region of the vestibule of LPV patients [73]. Additionally, INF is a potent mast cell inhibitor. Mast cells have a role in the initiation of LPV [30].

Early studies have shown a considerable success of Interferon in treating LPV [74–77]. However, recurrences were frequent.

54.23.4 Other Medications

Cromolyn cream, a mast cell stabilizer [78] has not been shown to be more effective than placebo in LPV.

Subcutaneous enoxaparin administration, a low molecular weight heparin with anti-heparanase properties [58] has been effective in a subgroup of women with LPV, who had a high level of tissue heparanase, a mast cell product.

54.23.5 Approach to Treatment in a Patient with Musculoskeletal Factors

54.23.5.1 Vaginal Diazepam Insertion

Vaginal diazepam use has been reported for vulvar pain with musculoskeletal factors [79]. However, because diazepam is a benzodiazepine with a central nervous system depressant effect, patients should be cautioned that they may reach systemic therapeutic levels after vaginal administration and that benzodiazepines are addictive.

54.23.5.2 Botulinum Type A

Botulinum Type A (Botox®) is used for disorders with hypertonicity. In cases of LPV it was presumed that botulinum toxin reduces hypertonicity of the pelvic floor muscles and peripheral neuropathy through both peripheral and central nervous mechanisms. It also inhibits the release of glutamate and substance-P from nociceptive neurons [80]. However, one RCT of Botulinum Type A showed no improvement as compared to placebo [81], while non-controlled studies have shown significant efficacy [82–85].

54.23.5.3 Pelvic Floor Physiotherapy (Physical Therapy)

Pelvic floor physiotherapy treatment for LPV has developed over the years and employs several techniques, including visceral (vaginal and rectal) mobilization and trigger point release. Biofeedback and electrical stimulation are also used [86].

54.23.5.4 Transcutaneous Electrical Nerve Stimulation (TENS)

The TENS has been effective in several chronic pain conditions. In cases with LPV, the results were inconsistent [87, 88].

54.23.5.5 Complementary and Alternative Therapies

Women with LPV, before resorting to medical consultation, use acupuncture, various diets, and homeopathic medications. Many do not disclose their experience with alternative medicine. Results of these treatments have been variable. I do not discourage patients from using complementary medicine, as I have seen, although rarely, good response with these treatments.

54.23.6 Approach to Treatment in a Patient with Neurologic Mechanisms

54.23.6.1 Central

Antidepressants

Oral tricyclic antidepressants are a common treatment for vulvar pain, although not evidence based. With both tricyclic antidepressants and anticonvulsants, the dose is gradually increased to lower side effects. Once the pain is controlled, there is no need to further increasing the dose, and the same dose should be maintained for three more months, then gradually decreased and discontinued.

I found the antidepressants helpful in cases of generalized, spontaneous vulvodynia. I usually start with amitriptyline. In these cases, they offer a quick relief of the pain. The dosing information is given in Table 54.7. Excessive alcohol consumption is prohibited, and should be limited to one drink daily. Contraception should be provided to women of reproductive age. Side effects can be troublesome and include constipation, dry mouth, and floating sensation.

Anticonvulsants

In cases where amitriptyline fails, I usually use gabapentin (Table 54.7). Its success rates ranged from 50 to 82%. Lamotrigine was used in one study; satisfaction was reported in 82%. The dosage is in table B. Adverse effects include sedation, constipation, dry mouth, and cognitive dysfunction. Carbamazepine, another anticonvulsant, may also be used.

Neuromodulation

There are sporadic reports of successful vulvodynia treatment using peripheral subcutaneous and transcranial neuromodulation [89, 90].

54.23.7 Peripheral: Neuroproliferation

54.23.7.1 Anti-Nociceptive Agents: Local Anesthetics

Topical lidocaine 5% ointment is the most common anesthetic prescribed in the treatment of vulvodynia [91], but lidocaine creams (3%, 4%, and 5% strengths) are also used. EMLA® cream (comprised of lidocaine 2.5% and prilocaine 2.5%, Watson, Inc.) is useful as well. Ointment is the preferred topical preparation, as creams contain more irritants [91]. We have found that the recommendation to apply a local anesthetic before intercourse is a myth: in fact, the use of local anesthetics before intercourse might be troublesome as the partner receives the topical anesthetic on his genitalia, causing him a loss of sensation and numbness leading to prolonged intercourse. The woman consequently suffers from significant burning and pain after intercourse.

Lidocaine has also been prescribed for continuous overnight use [92]. By placing a cotton ball generously coated with the 5% lidocaine ointment on the vestibule to assure overnight contact with the area (for 8 h or more).

Topical application of lidocaine may initially cause burning and stinging that usually subsides within a short time. After applying lidocaine, partners should avoid oral contact. It is important to use caution in using excessive amounts of lidocaine and other topical anesthetics because of the potential for toxicity and sensitization.

Although nightly application of lidocaine 5% reduced dyspareunia in a prospective cohort [93, 94], in a randomized, placebo-controlled trial, lidocaine 5% cream was found to be successful in only 20% [95].

Other topical agents found to be no more effective than placebo include cromolyn 4% and nifedipine. Despite a case series demonstrating benefit, the topical application of cromolyn 4% applied locally in a placebo-controlled randomized, double-blind study demonstrated no statistically significant difference in symptom reduction (54% reduction) compared with placebo use (38% reduction) [78]. Likewise, the effectiveness of topical nifedipine 0.2% and 0.4% did not exceed placebo in a double-blind study of 30 women with vulvodynia [96]. Other compounded topical agents were found to reduce vulvodynia, e.g., gabapentin, 2% amitriptyline, and 2% baclofen, nitroglycerine, capsaicin, estrogen [97]. Several other topical therapies have not been shown to have significant benefit to patients with vulvodynia, including topical corticosteroids, topical testosterone, and topical antifungal medications [97].

Note that a compounding pharmacy may be needed to formulate topical medications. Choosing the proper vehicle for topical medications is important because creams contain more preservatives and stabilizers and often produce burning on application, whereas ointments are usually better tolerated [98].

No difference was found between topical 5% lidocaine cream, oral desipramine, lidocaine + desipramine, in an RCT in pain reduction on the tampon test or algesiometer, during intercourse, or during 24-h pain [95, 99].

In a placebo-controlled study conducted to estimate the effectiveness of enoxaparin in treating 40 women with vestibulodynia, 15 of 20 enoxaparin-treated women reported more than 20% pain reduction compared with 5 of 18 women in the placebo group [58]. Enoxaparin was used because of the presence of heparanase in the vestibule of women with vulvodynia [31].

54.23.7.2 Capsaicin

After the hyperesthesia caused by the initial exposure, capsaicin produces a long-lasting desensitization to burning and pain [100]. Capsaicin is available as cream over the counter.

54.23.7.3 Vestibulectomy

The success rate for vestibulectomy ranges between 60% and 90% compared with 40–80% for nonsurgical interventions [101]. However, there is no consensus or standardized definition of "successful" treatment and methods for evaluation of outcomes between studies. As noted previously, surgical management frequently becomes a treatment option of last resort for patients with vestibulodynia [102].

Sexual counseling may enhance post-operative improvement by reducing vaginismus and poor sexual arousal, which can develop after long-standing dyspareunia [103].

Regarding the surgical technique, vestibuloplasty, consisting of undercutting the vestibular tissue and re-suturing it, without any tissue excision, has been noted to be ineffective [104].

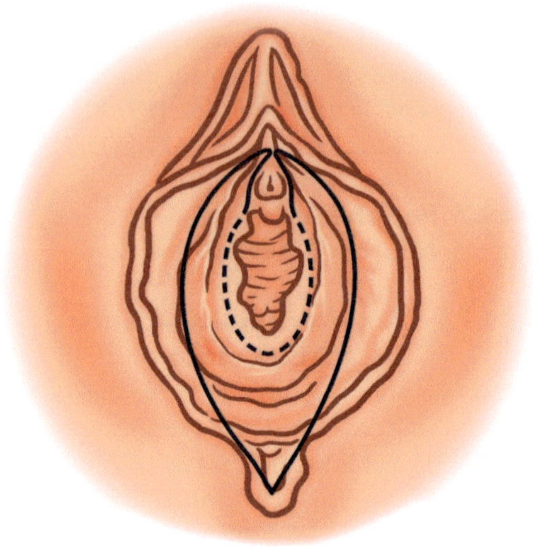

Fig. 54.17 Vestibulectomy in cases of LPV consists of excising a semicircular segment of perineal skin, the mucosa of the posterior and anterior vulvar vestibule, including the hymeneal ring

54.23.8 Predicting the Outcome of Vestibulectomy

There may be subsets of patients more likely to experience a benefit from vestibulectomy surgery. Patients with secondary dyspareunia have odds of improvement greater than those of patients with primary dyspareunia; those with constant pain in addition to dyspareunia are more likely to fail from improving their pain after surgery [105].

Long-term outcomes at means of 2.8–3.4 years after vestibulectomy for provoked vestibulodynia showed 35–68% complete cure or major improvement, and 24–56% reporting a partial response [106]. Women with secondary vestibulodynia were more likely to report a complete cure than those with primary vestibulodynia [107] (56% vs 17% in one study).

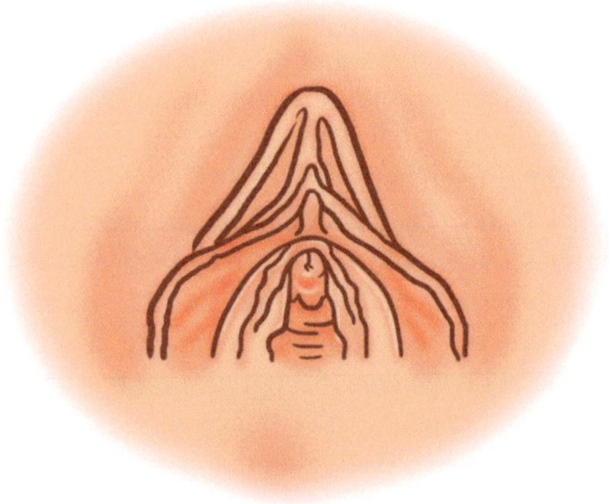

Fig. 54.18 Vestibulectomy in cases of LPV should include the anterior vestibule as well as the posterior, to prevent recurrence

It has been well established that surgical treatment of LPV is the most effective medical strategy to reduce the pain. In 1983, Woodruff and Parmley were the first authors to describe vulvar vestibulectomy [108]. The operation consisted of excising a semicircular segment of perineal skin, the mucosa of the posterior vulvar vestibule, and the posterior hymeneal ring (Fig. 54.17). The anterior vestibule needs to be removed as well, to avoid recurrence (Fig. 54.18). The Bartholin's glands are excised if identified, to prevent a later formation of Bartholin's duct cyst from occlusion the duct during repair of the excision, and to remove the pudendal nerve branch fibers traversing through the Bartholin's gland (Fig. 54.19). Three centimeters of the vaginal mucosa is then undermined and approximated to the perineum. In the fourchette, the vaginal flap is advanced to half way between the introitus and the anus (Fig. 54.20). This is done to move the mucosal-skin new scar line from the introitus, where constant friction may occur during intercourse.

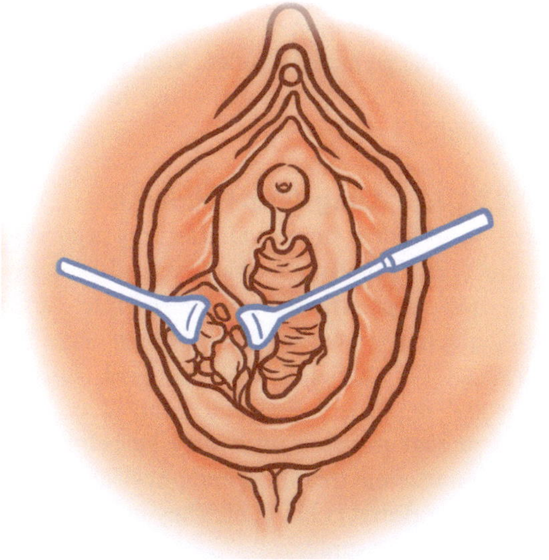

Fig. 54.19 Vestibulectomy in cases of LPV may include the Bartholin's glands if identified

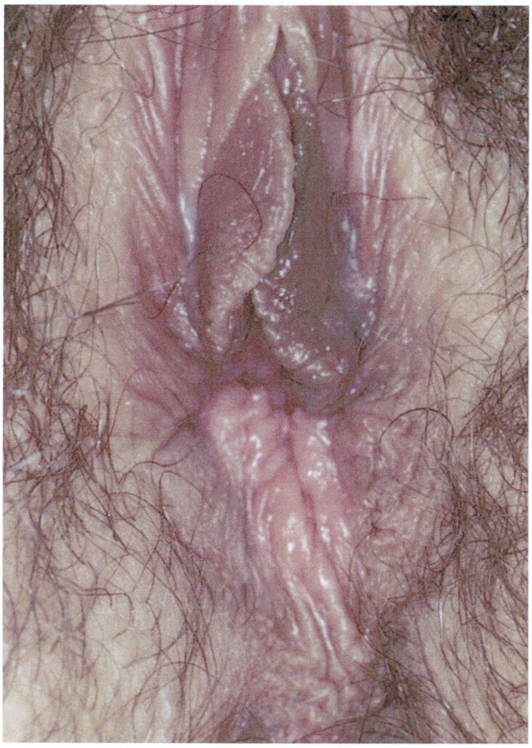

Fig. 54.20 Vestibulectomy in cases of LPV—after excising the vestibule, the vaginal flap should be advanced to half way between the introitus and the anus

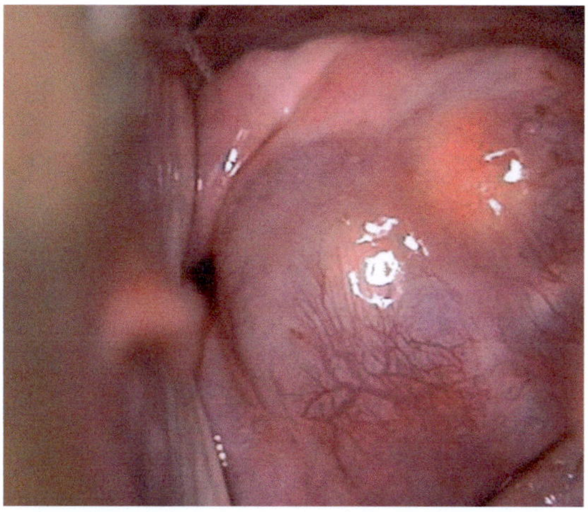

Fig. 54.21 A complication of vestibulectomy in 5% of patients is the formation of a Bartholin's duct cyst

Several variations of this procedure have since been described to decrease complications, such as dehiscence of the vaginal advancement flap, as well as to improve operative success. A complete vulvar vestibulectomy with vaginal advancement includes the excision of the mucosa of the entire vulvar vestibule including the mucosa adjacent to the urethra, while a modified vestibulectomy limits excision of the mucosa to the posterior vestibule [105]. However, it is important to note that studies of surgical techniques are difficult to compare, and they are typically not controlled. Complications of vestibulectomy include bleeding, infection, increased pain, hematoma, wound dehiscence, scar tissue formation, and Bartholin's cyst formation [19] (Fig. 54.21).

Surgical management of LPV results in success rates of 60–90% [105], in women with LPV1 having lower success rates than those with LPV2 [4]. Many have questioned, why surgery which is the most successful treatment of LPV is often used as a "last-resort," that is, only after other "less invasive" (i.e., conservative) treatment options failed.

Failures of vestibulectomy may occur when the anterior part of the vestibule has not been resected. In 5% of surgeries, a Bartholin's duct cyst is formed (Fig. 54.21), resulting in vestibular pain, which may be regarded by patients as a sign of recurrent vestibulitis. This cyst should be treated by incision and drainage, and rarely by enucleation of the cyst. When possible, I recommend removing the Bartholin's gland at the primary vestibulectomy. This will prevent the post-operative formation of a cyst and delete a few additional sensitive nerve fibers.

54.23.9 Parturition After Vestibulectomy

One small cohort study included 44 women having at least one-term pregnancy after vestibulectomy [109]. Cesarean section was performed in 21 cases and vaginal delivery in 23 cases (one of which sustained a fourth degree perineal laceration). Although the study did not address recurrent vulvar pain after delivery, the authors found that vaginal delivery after vulvar vestibulectomy seems to be a safe option, with no increase in perineal morbidity greater than that reported in the general population [109]. In my experience, tears are rarely encountered after vestibulectomy, as the perineal tissue is removed during vestibulectomy, so that there is no tension on the tissues.

54.23.10 Approach to Treatment in a Patient with Psychosocial Factors

54.23.10.1 Psychological Interventions

Currently, cognitive-behavioral therapy (CBT) is used mostly. It is more effective than other forms of psychological therapy [110] and comparable with surgery in a prospective, randomized study [107]. Self-exploration of the genitals and localization of the pain are included. With the partner, the therapist works on strengthening the relationship bond.

54.23.10.2 Long-Term Follow-Up

Long-term follow-up is available only after vestibulectomy. No adverse effect on vaginal delivery has been noted. Success rate after vestibulectomy has been shown to last for decades. For patients with surgical failure, pudendal nerve isolation and removal of neuroma or scar pressing on it may be helpful. In addition, medical treatment and physical therapy should be offered [111, 112]. They may be more successful after surgery.

54.23.10.3 Concluding Remarks

Vulvar pain and vulvodynia have been recognized since the first century AD. However, there were periods when these conditions disappeared from the medical literature, for example, from 1928 to 1976. Possibly, failure to resolve vulvar pain and vulvodynia led to disregarding them. Health care givers felt helpless, and patients—desperate. Suffering from a painful condition that maimed women and caused the loss of femininity leads to misery on their side. The condition has changed names and terminologies, as the understanding of its nature evolved (Table 54.8). Only recently, the medical community resumed interest and initiated significant research into its etiology, pathogenesis, and possible treatments. I hope that this chapter succeeded in elucidating them.

Table 54.8 Historic descriptions and terminologies of idiopathic vulvar pain[a]

Period, author	Term or terminology
First century AD, Soranus	Satyriasis in females
1880, Thomas	Excessive hypersensibility of the nerves
1889, Kellogg	Sensitive points
1889, Skene	Super-sensitiveness of the vulva
1928, Kelly	Exquisitely sensitive in hymeneal ring
1976, Weisfogel	The burning vulva
1976, ISSVD	The burning vulva syndrome

Period, author	Term or terminology
1978, Dodson and Friedrich	Psychosomatic vulvovaginitis
1978, Tovell and Young	Vulvodynia or pudendagra
1983, ISSVD task force	Vulvodynia or burning vulva syndrome
1983, Friedrich	Vestibular adenitis
1983, Woodruff and Parmley	Infection of the minor vestibular glands
1986, Peckham	Focal vulvitis
1987, Friedrich	Vulvar vestibulitis syndrome
1988, McKay	Classification: vestibulitis and dysesthetic vulvodynia
1997, Bornstein	Vestibulodynia
1999, ISSVD	Terminology: generalized and localized vulvar dysesthesia
2001, ISSVD	Terminology: provoked and spontaneous vulvar dysesthesia, each has subsets of generalized and localized
2003, ISSVD	2003 ISSVD terminology
2015, ISSVD, IPPS, ISSWSH	2015 consensus terminology

ISSVD International Society for the Study of Vulvovaginal Disease, *PPS* International Pelvic Pain Society, *ISSWSH* International Society for the Study of Women's Sexual Health
[a]Based on Ref. [1]

Vulvar Pain and Vulvodynia: Breaking the Myths

- Vulvar experts still believe that localized provoked vulvodynia (previously—vestibulitis) (LPV) usually involves only the posterior portion of the vestibule. This is not true. Most of the women with posterior vestibular sensitivity later develop anterior soreness as well
- Determining the etiology by the LPV localization is still used: Some believe that if the sensitivity is extensive throughout the entire vestibule, it resulted from neuroproliferation; and if it is confined to the posterior vestibule, the etiology is musculoskeletal. This has not been proven
- Several texts associate vulvovaginal candidiasis (VVC) and LPV. However, this is not a causal association. We suspect that the frequent diagnosis of VVC made in women with LPV results from misdiagnosing LPV as VVC
- This chain of events (dyspareunia–"diagnosis" of VVC–treatment by topical azoles–persistent dyspareunia) has even led to a hypothesis that it is the therapy of VVC that causes LPV, via an allergic reaction. This hypothesis has not been proven
- Post-partum dyspareunia has been thought to result from birth lacerations and sloppy repair of episiotomy. In fact, the woman suffers from a new onset of LPV, while the scar tissue itself is not sensitive at all, because in these foci the nerve nociceptors have been teared and destroyed.
- Surgery for LPV—vestibulectomy—is considered a treatment of last resort. However, It may sometimes be the only indicated treatment, for example in patients who have a neuroproliferative LPV with no

associated musculoskeletal, psychological, or neuropathic factors
- Some patients receive a recommendation to apply topical anesthetic before intercourse. However, this might be troublesome as it causes loss of sensation to the partner with resultant prolongation of the intercourse. The woman consequently suffers from significant burning and pain after intercourse.

References

1. Bornstein J, Goldstein AT, Stockdale CK, Bergeron S, Pukall C, Zolnoun D, Coady D. 2015 ISSVD, ISSWSH, and IPPS consensus terminology and classification of persistent vulvar pain and vulvodynia. J Low Genit Tract Dis. 2016;20:126–30.
2. Bogliatto F, Miletta M. Vulvodynia: when a paradigm challenges the management. J Low Genit Tract Dis. 2017;21:85–6.
3. McKay M. Dysesthetic ("essential") vulvodynia: treatment with amitriptyline. J Reprod Med. 1993;38:9–13.
4. Bornstein J, Maman M, Abramovici H. Primary versus secondary vestibulitis - one disease, two variants. Am J Obstet Gynecol. 2001;184:28–31.
5. Sutton K, Pukall C, Chamberlain S. Pain, psychosocial, sexual, and psychophysical characteristics of women with primary vs. secondary provoked vestibulodynia. J Sex Med. 2009;6:205.
6. van Lankveld JJDM, Granot M, Weijmar Schultz WCM, et al. Women's sexual pain disorders. J Sex Med. 2010;7:615.
7. Reed BD, Harlow SD, Sen A, et al. Prevalence and demographic characteristics of vulvodynia in a population-based sample. Am J Obstet Gynecol. 2012;206:170.e1.
8. Reed BD, Haefner HK, Sen A, et al. Vulvodynia incidence and remission rates among adult women: a 2-year follow-up study. Obstet Gynecol. 2008;112:231.
9. Reed BD, Crawford S, Couper M, et al. Pain at the vulvar vestibule: a web-based survey. J Low Genit Tract Dis. 2004;8:48.
10. Harlow BL, Stewart EG. A population-based assessment of chronic unexplained vulvar pain: have we underestimated the prevalence of vulvodynia? J Am Med Womens Assoc. 2003;58:82.
11. Arnold LD, Bachmann GA, Rosen R, et al. Assessment of vulvodynia symptoms in a sample of US women: a prevalence survey with a nested case control study. Am J Obstet Gynecol. 2007;196:128.e1.
12. Harlow B, Kunitz C, Nguyen R, et al. Prevalence of symptoms consistent with a diagnosis of vulvodynia: population-based estimates from 2 geographic regions. Am J Obstet Gynecol. 2014; 210:40.e1.
13. Turk DC, Galer BS, Hewitt DJ, et al. Core outcome domains for chronic pain clinical trials: IMMPACT recommendations. Pain. 2003;106:337–45.
14. Friedrich EG. Vulvar vestibulitis syndrome. J Reprod Med. 1987;32:110.
15. Goldfinger C, Pukall CF, Gentilcore-Saulnier E, et al. A prospective study of the effectiveness of pelvic floor physical therapy: pain and psychosexual outcomes in provoked vestibulodynia. J Sex Med. 2009;6:1955–68.
16. King M, Rubin R, Goldstein AT. Current uses of surgery in the treatment of genital pain. Curr Sex Health Rep. 2014;6:252.
17. Pukall CF, Binik YM, Khalifé S. A new instrument for pain assessment in vulvar vestibulitis syndrome. J Sex Marital Ther. 2004;30:69.
18. Pukall CF, Binik YM, Khalifé S, et al. Vestibular tactile and pain thresholds in women with vulvar vestibulitis syndrome. Pain. 2002;96:163.
19. Marinoff SC, Turner ML. Vulvar vestibulitis syndrome. Dermatol Clin. 1992;10:435–44.
20. Foster D, Kotok M, Huang L, et al. The tampon test for vulvodynia treatment outcomes research reliability, construct validity, and responsiveness. Obstet Gynecol. 2009;113:825–32.
21. Reed BD, Harlow SD, Plegue MA, Sen A. Remission, relapse, and persistence of vulvodynia: a longitudinal population-based study. J Womens Health (Larchmt). 2016;25:276–83.
22. Reed BD, Plegue MA, Harlow SD, Haefner HK, Sen A. Does degree of vulvar sensitivity predict vulvodynia characteristics and prognosis? J Pain. 2017;18:113–23.
23. Smith EM, Ritchie JM, Galask R, Pugh EE, Jia J, Ricks-McGillan J. Case-control study of vulvar vestibulitis risk associated with genital infections. Infect Dis Obstet Gynecol. 2002;10(4):193–202.
24. Farmer MA, Taylor AM, Bailey AL, et al. Repeated vulvovaginal fungal infections cause persistent pain in a mouse model of vulvodynia. Sci Transl Med. 2011;3:101–91.
25. Foster DC, Falsetta ML, Woeller CF, et al. Site-specific mesenchymal control of inflammatory pain to yeast challenge in vulvodynia-afflicted and pain-free women. Pain. 2015;156:386–96.
26. Bornstein J, Livnat G, Stolar Z, Abramovici H. Pure versus complicated vulvar vestibulitis: a randomized trial of fluconazole treatment. Gynecol Obstet Invest. 2000;50(3):194–7.

27. Arnold LD, Bachmann GA, Rosen R, et al. Vulvodynia: characteristics and associations with comorbidities and quality of life. Obstet Gynecol. 2006;107:617.
28. Marinoff SC, Turner ML. Hypersensitivity to vaginal candidiasis or treatment vehicles in the pathogenesis of minor vestibular gland syndrome. J Reprod Med. 1986;31(9):796–9.
29. Burrows LJ, Basha M, Goldstein AT. The effects of hormonal contraceptives on female sexuality: a review. J Sex Med. 2012;9:2213.
30. Bornstein J, Goldshmid N, Sabo E. Hyperinnervation and mast cell activation may be used as histopathologic diagnostic criteria for vulvar vestibulitis. Gynecol Obstet Invest. 2004;58:171–8.
31. Bornstein J, Zarfati D, Sela S, Cohen Y, Ophir E. Involvement of heparanase in the pathogenesis of localized vulvodynia. Int J Gynecol Pathol. 2008;27(1):136–41.
32. Morin M, Bergeron S, Khalifé S, et al. Morphometry of the pelvic floor muscles in women with and without provoked vestibulodynia using 4D ultrasound. J Sex Med. 2014;11:776–85.
33. Westrom LV, Willen R. Vestibular nerve fiber proliferation in vulvar vestibulitis syndrome. Obstet Gynecol. 1998;91:572–6.
34. Bohm-Starke N, Hilliges M, Falconer C, Rylander E. Neurochemical characterization of the vestibular nerves in women with vulvar vestibulitis syndrome. Gynecol Obstet Invest. 1999;48:270–5.
35. Bohm-Starke N, Hilliges M, Brodda-Jansen G, Rylander E, Torebjörk E. Psychophysical evidence of nociceptor sensitization in vulvar vestibulitis syndrome. Pain. 2001;94:177–83.
36. Leclair CM, Goetsch MF, Korcheva VB, et al. Differences in primary compared with secondary vestibulodynia in immunohistochemistry. Obstet Gynecol. 2011;117:1307.
37. Goetsch MF, Morgan TK, Korcheva VB, et al. Histologic and receptor analysis of primary and secondary Vestibulodynia and controls: a prospective study. Am J Obstet Gynecol. 2010;202:614.e1.
38. Tympanidis P, Casula MA, Yiangou Y, Terenghi G, Dowd P, Anand P. Increased vanilloid receptor VR1 innervation in vulvodynia. Eur J Pain. 2004;8(2):129–33.
39. Gerber S, Bongiovanni AM, Ledger WJ, et al. Defective regulation of the proinflammatory immune response in women with vulvar vestibulitis syndrome. Am J Obstet Gynecol. 2002;186:696.
40. Pukall CF, Cahill CM. New developments in the pathophysiology of genital pain: the role of central sensitization. Curr Sex Health Rep. 2014;6:11.
41. Willis WD. Role of neurotransmitters in sensitization of pain responses. Ann N Y Acad Sci. 2001;933:142–56.
42. Pierce AN, Zhang Z, Fuentes IM, Wang R, Ryals JM, Christianson JA. Neonatal vaginal irritation results in long-term visceral and somatic hypersensitivity and increased hypothalamic-pituitary-adrenal axis output in female mice. Pain. 2015;156(10):2021–31.
43. Gerber S, Bongiovanni AM, Ledger WJ, et al. Interleukin-1b gene polymorphism in women with vulvar vestibulitis syndrome. Eur J Obstet Gynecol Reprod Biol. 2003;107:74.
44. Goldstein AT, Belkin ZR, Krapf JM, et al. Polymorphisms of the androgen receptor gene and hormonal contraceptive induced provoked vestibulodynia. J Sex Med. 2014;11:2764.
45. Babula O, Linhares IM, Bongiovanni AM, Ledger WJ, Witkin SS. Association between primary vulvar vestibulitis syndrome, defective induction of tumor necrosis factor-alpha, and carriage of the mannose-binding lectin codon 54 gene polymorphism. Am J Obstet Gynecol. 2008;198(1):101.e1–4.
46. Foster DC, Sazenski TM, Stodgell CJ. Impact of genetic variation in interleukin-1 receptor antagonist and melanocortin-1 receptor genes on vulvar vestibulitis syndrome. J Reprod Med. 2004;49:503.
47. FitzGerald MP, Kotarinos R. Rehabilitation of the short pelvic floor. I: background and patient evaluation. Int Urogynecol J. 2003;14:261–8.
48. Reed B, Harlow S, Legocki L, et al. Oral contraceptive use and risk of vulvodynia: a population-based longitudinal study. BJOG. 2013;120:1678.
49. Foster DC, Woodruff JD. Case-control study of vulvar vestibulitis syndrome. J Womens Health. 1995;4:677.
50. Bazin S, Bouchard C, Brisson J, et al. Vulvar vestibulitis syndrome: an exploratory case-control study. Obstet Gynecol. 1994;83:47.
51. Bouchard C, Brisson J, Fortier M, et al. Use of oral contraceptive pills and vulvar vestibulitis: a case-control study. Am J Epidemiol. 2002;156:254.
52. Harlow BL, Vitonis AF, Stewart EG. Influence of oral contraceptive use on the risk of adult-onset vulvodynia. J Reprod Med. 2008;53:102.
53. Greenstein A, Ben-Aroya Z, Fass O, et al. Vulvar vestibulitis syndrome and estrogen dose of oral contraceptive pills. J Sex Med. 2007;4:1679.
54. Burrows LJ, Goldstein AT. The treatment of Vestibulodynia with topical estradiol and testosterone. Sex Med. 2013;1:30.
55. Kingsberg S, Kellogg S, Krychman M. Treating dyspareunia caused by vaginal atrophy: a review of treatment options using vaginal estrogen therapy. Int J Womens Health. 2010;1:105–11.
56. Harlow BL, He W, Nguyen RHN. Allergic reactions and risk of vulvodynia. Ann Epidemiol. 2009;19:771.
57. Chaim W, Meriwether C, Gonik B, et al. Vulvar vestibulitis subjects undergoing surgical intervention: a descriptive analysis and histopathological correlates. Eur J Obstet Gynecol. 1996;68:165.
58. Farajun Y, Zarfati D, Abramov L, Livoff A, Bornstein J. Enoxaparin treatment for vulvodynia: a randomized controlled trial. Obstet Gynecol. 2012;120(3):565–72.

59. Kakurai M, Monteforte R, Suto H, Tsai M, Nakae S, Galli SJ. Mast cell-derived tumor necrosis factor can promote nerve fiber elongation in the skin during contact hypersensitivity in mice. Am J Pathol. 2006;169(5):1713–21.
60. Harlow B, Stewart E. Adult-onset vulvodynia in relation to childhood violence victimization. Am J Epidemiol. 2005;161:871.
61. Khandker M, Brady SS, Stewart EG, et al. Is chronic stress during childhood associated with adult-onset vulvodynia? J Womens Health. 2014;23:649.
62. Leclerc B, Bergeron S, Binik YM, et al. History of sexual and physical abuse in women with dyspareunia: association with pain, psychosocial adjustment, and sexual functioning. J Sex Med. 2010;7:971.
63. Ayling K, Ussher JM. "If sex hurts, am I still a woman?" The subjective experience of vulvodynia in hetero-sexual women. Arch Sex Behav. 2008;37:294.
64. Desrochers G, Bergeron S, Khalifé S, et al. Fear avoidance and self-efficacy in relation to pain and sexual impairment in women with provoked vestibulodynia. Clin J Pain. 2009;25:520–7.
65. Nguyen RHN, Turner RM, Rydell SA, et al. Perceived stereotyping and seeking care for chronic vulvar pain. Pain Med. 2013;14:1461.
66. Landry T, Bergeron S, Dupuis M, et al. The treatment of provoked vestibulodynia: a critical review. Clin J Pain. 2008;24:155–71.
67. Bornstein J, Abramovici H. Combination of subtotal perineoplasty and interferon for vulvar vestibulitis - a comparative study. Gynecol Obstet Invest. 1997;44:53–4.
68. Bornstein J, Goldik Z, Stolar Z, et al. Predicting the outcome of surgical treatment of vulvar vestibulitis. Obstet Gynecol. 1997;89:695–8.
69. Heddini U, Bohm-Starke N, Nilsson KW, et al. Provoked vestibulodynia—medical factors and comorbidity associated with treatment outcome. J Sex Med. 2012;9:1400–6.
70. Snyder DS, Unanue ER. Corticosteroids inhibit murine macrophage 1a expression and interleukin 1 production. J Immunol. 1982;129:1803–5.
71. Horowitz BJ. Interferon therapy for condylomatous vulvitis. Obstet Gynecol. 1989;73(3 Pt 1):446–8.
72. Kieseier BC. The mechanism of action of interferon-β in relapsing multiple sclerosis. CNS Drugs. 2011;25(6):491–502.
73. Foster DC, Hasday JD. Elevated tissue levels of interleukin-1b and tumor necrosis factor-a in vulvar vestibulitis. Obstet Gynecol. 1997;89:291–6.
74. Bornstein J, Pascal B, Abramovici H. Intramuscular beta interferon treatment for severe vulvar vestibulitis. J Reprod Med. 1993;38:117–20.
75. Bornstein J, Pascal B, Abramovici H. Long term follow up of patients treated for severe vulvar vestibulitis by intramuscular interferon beta administration. Isr J Obstet Gynecol. 1994;5:146–8.
76. Marinoff S, Turner M, Hirsch R, Richard G. Intralesional alpha interferon. Cost-effective therapy for vulvar vestibulitis syndrome. J Reprod Med. 1993;38:19–24.
77. Kent HL, Wisniewski PM. Interferon for vulvar vestibulitis. J Reprod Med. 1990;35:1138–40.
78. Nyirjesy P, Sobel JD, Weitz MV, et al. Cromolyn cream for recalcitrant idiopathic vulvar vestibulitis: results of a placebo controlled study. Sex Transm Infect. 2001;77:53–7.
79. Crisp CC, Vaccaro CM, Estanol MV, Oakley SH, Kleeman SD, Fellner AN, Pauls RN. Intra-vaginal diazepam for high-tone pelvic floor dysfunction: a randomized placebo-controlled trial. Int Urogynecol J. 2013;24:1915–23.
80. Cui M, Khanijou S, Rubino J, Aoki KR. Subcutaneous administration of botulinum toxin A reduces formalin-induced pain. Pain. 2004;107:125–33.
81. Petersen CD, Giraldi A, Lundvall L, Kristensen E. Botulinum toxin type A e a novel treatment for provoked vestibulodynia? Results from a randomized, placebo controlled, double blinded study. J Sex Med. 2009;6:2523–37.
82. Pelletier F, Parratte B, Penz S, et al. Efficacy of high doses of botulinum toxin A for treating provoked vestibulodynia. Br J Dermatol. 2011;164:617–22.
83. Dystra DD, Presthus J. Botulinum toxin type A for the treatment of provoked vestibulodynia: an open-label pilot study. J Reprod Med. 2006;51:467–70.
84. Romito S, Bottanelli M, Pellegrini M, et al. Botulinum toxin for the treatment of genital pain syndromes. Gynecol Obstet Invest. 2004;58:164–7.
85. Brown CS, Glazer HI, Vog V, Menkes D, Bachmann G. Subjective and objective outcomes of botulinum toxin type A treatment in vestibulodynia: pilot data. J Reprod Med. 2006;51:635–41.
86. Hartmann D, Strauhal MJ, Nelson CA. Treatment of women in the United States with localized, provoked vulvodynia: practice survey of women's health physical therapists. J Reprod Med. 2007;52:48.
87. Vallinga MS, Spoelstra SK, Hemel IL, van de Wiel HB, Weijmar Schultz WC. Transcutaneous electrical nerve stimulation as an additional treatment for women suffering from therapy-resistant provoked vestibulodynia: a feasibility study. J Sex Med. 2015;12(1):228–37.
88. Murina F, Graziottin A, Felice R, Radici G, Tognocchi C. Vestibulodynia: synergy between palmitoylethanolamide + transpolydatin and transcutaneous electrical nerve stimulation. J Low Genit Tract Dis. 2013;17(2):111–6.
89. Cecilio SB, Zaghi S, Cecilio LB, Correa CF, Fregni F. Exploring a novel therapeutic approach with noninvasive cortical stimulation for vulvodynia. Am J Obstet Gynecol. 2008;199(6):e6–7.
90. Morin A, Léonard G, Gougeon V, Cyr MP, Waddell G, Bureau YA, Girard I, Morin M. Efficacy of transcranial direct-current stimulation in women with provoked vestibulodynia. Am J Obstet Gynecol. 2017;216(6):584.e1–584.e11.
91. Haefner HK, Collins ME, Davis GD, Edwards L, Foster DC, Hartmann ED, Kaufman RH, Lynch

PJ, Margesson LJ, Moyal-Barracco M, Piper CK, Reed BD, Stewart EG, Wilkinson EJ. The vulvodynia guideline. J Low Genit Tract Dis. 2005;9(1):40–51.
92. Zolnoun DA, Hartmann KE, Steege JF. Overnight 5% lidocaine ointment for treatment of vulvar vestibulitis. Obstet Gynecol. 2003;102:84–7.
93. Goetsch MF, Lim JY, Caughey AB. Locating pain in breast cancer survivors experiencing dyspareunia: a randomized controlled trial. Obstet Gynecol. 2014;123(6):1231–6.
94. Rapkin AJ, McDonald JS, Morgan M. Multilevel local anesthetic nerve blockade for the treatment of vulvar vestibulitis syndrome. Am J Obstet Gynecol. 2008;198(41):e1–5.
95. Foster DC, Kotok MB, Huang L, et al. Oral desipramine and topical lidocaine for vulvodynia: a randomized controlled trial. Obstet Gynecol. 2010;116:583–93.
96. Bornstein J, Tuma R, Farajun Y, Azran A, Zarfati D. Topical nifedipine for the treatment of localized provoked vulvodynia: a placebo-controlled study. J Pain. 2010;11(12):1403–9.
97. Goldstein AT, Pukall CF, Brown C, Bergeron S, Stein A, Kellogg-Spadt S. Vulvodynia: assessment and treatment. J Sex Med. 2016;13(4):572–90.
98. Stockdale CK, Lawson HW. 2013 vulvodynia guideline update. J Low Genit Tract Dis. 2014;18(2):93–100.
99. Danielsson I, Torstensson T, Brodda-Jansen G, et al. EMG biofeedback versus topical lidocaine gel: a randomized study for the treatment of women with vulvar vestibulitis. Acta Obstet Gynecol Scand. 2006;85:1360–7.
100. Baron R. Capsaicin and nociception: from basic mechanism to novel drug. Lancet. 2000;356:785–6.
101. Andrews JC. Vulvodynia interventions--systematic review and evidence grading. Obstet Gynecol Surv. 2011;66(5):299–315.
102. Bornstein J, Zarfati D, Goldik Z, Abramovici H. Vulvar vestibulitis: physical or psychosexual problem. Obstet Gynecol. 1999;93:876–80.
103. Har-Toov J, Militscher I, Lessing JB, Abramov L, Chen J. Combined vulvar vestibulitis syndrome with vaginismus: which to treat first? J Sex Marital Ther. 2001;27:521–3.
104. Bornstein J, Zarfati D, Goldik Z, Abramovici H. Perineoplasty versus vestibuloplasty for severe vulvar vestibulitis: a randomized comparison. Br J Obstet Gynecol. 1995;102:652–5.
105. Bornstein J, Goldik Z, Stolar Z, Zarfati D, Abramovici H. Predicting the outcome of surgical treatment for vulvar vestibulitis. Obstet Gynecol. 1997;89:695–8.
106. Tommola P, Unkila-Kallio L, Paavonen J. Surgical treatment of vulvar vestibulitis: a review. Acta Obstet Gynecol Scand. 2010;89:1385–95.
107. Bergeron S, Khalifé S, Glazer HI, et al. Surgical and behavioral treatments for vestibulodynia: two-and-one-half year follow-up and predictors of outcome. Obstet Gynecol. 2008;111:159–66.
108. Woodruff JD, Parmley TH. Infection of the minor vestibular gland. Obstet Gynecol. 1983;62(5):609–12.
109. Burrows LJ, Sloane M, Davis G, Heller DS, Brooks J, Goldstein AT. Parturition after vestibulectomy. J Sex Med. 2011;8:303–5.
110. Corsini-Munt S, Bergeron S, Rosen NO, et al. Feasibility and preliminary effectiveness of a novel cognitive behavioral couple therapy for provoked vestibulodynia: a pilot study. J Sex Med. 2014;11:2515–27.
111. Wan EL, Goldstein AT, Tolson H, Dellon AL. Injury to perineal branch of pudendal nerve in women: outcome from resection of the perineal branches. J Reconstr Microsurg. 2017;33:395–401.
112. Bornstein J, Goldik Z, Alter Z, Zarfati D, Abramovici H. Persistent vulvar vestibulitis- the continuing challenge. Obstet Gynecol Surv. 1997;53:39–44.

Part XVI

Neoplastic and Pre-neoplastic Vulvar Conditions

Vulvar Intraepithelial Neoplasia 55

Fabrizio Bogliatto

55.1 Introduction

Vulvar intraepithelial neoplasia (VIN) is a premalignant vulvar skin disorder that often causes severe and long-lasting pruritus, pain, and psychosexual dysfunction. The incidence of this disorder is increasing, particularly in young women. Recent surveillance data from the United States shows the incidence has increased more than fourfold in 30 years [1]. While spontaneous regression may occur in a subset of those with this condition, vulvar intraepithelial lesions should be considered a precancerous disease. It is impressive that in a case series of 405 women with VIN [2], 10 untreated cases progressed to invasion in a mean of 3.9 years. In addition, it is noteworthy that an occult invasive cancer was reported in 3% of women undergoing surgery for VIN [3]. The annual incidence of vulvar intraepithelial lesions (from 1999–2004) has been reported as 1.2/100,000 with a peak in women aged 45–49 years [4]. The overall human papilloma virus (HPV) prevalence in vulvar intraepithelial lesions is 80.4% with HPV 16 the most common subtype (71.2%) followed by HPV 33 [5]. The clinical characteristics, the outcome following surgical treatment, and the natural history of VIN, and consequently the terminology, began to be clarified in the 1980s, along with the identification of the HPV infection.

55.2 Historical Background

In 1912, John Bowen [6] described for the first time in a young man a precancerous dermatosis on the gluteal region that, even if it recurred several times after local therapy, never progressed to invasive cancer. In 1922, Hudelo [7] described, for the first time in a woman, a similar multifocal lesion on the vulva. Until 1943, in the literature 31 cases of the so-called Bowen's disease of the vulva have been described. The first series of Bowen's disease of the vulva was described by Knight and co-workers in 1943 [8]. From that time, more than ten different names have been used to describe this vulvar disease, such as erythroplasia of Queyrat, bowenoid papulosis, bowenoid dysplasia, hyperplastic dystrophy with atypia, condylomatous dysplasia, carcinoma simplex, dysplasia, or carcinoma in situ. This confusion was principally due to the fact that the vulva is approached by different medical specialists (gynecologists, dermatologists, pathologists) with their own set of terminologies and classifications and to the fact that vulvar intraepithelial neoplasia had a lack of specific macroscopical features, the histopathological aspect of the lesion did not correlate with a specific histological pattern, and both the macroscopic aspect and histology did not correlate with the prognosis.

F. Bogliatto (✉)
Department of Obstetrics and Gynaecology, Lower Female Anourogenital Tract Network, Chivasso Civic Hospital, Turin, Italy

J. Bornstein (ed.), *Vulvar Disease*, https://doi.org/10.1007/978-3-319-61621-6_55

This lack of definition has also led to consider as vulvar intraepithelial neoplasia some non-neoplastic epithelial disorders, leading to unnecessary surgery for that vulvar benign diseases. The first important step to separate non-neoplastic from neoplastic vulvar disorders was by Raymond Kaufman in 1965, who tried to define a group of “precancerous lesions” [9]. Many researches were conducted on vulvar intraepithelial neoplasia in order to clarify its origin; during the years, the term “dystrophy” was felt to have no precise meaning and was thus inadequate; moreover it appeared that lesions with atypia really belong to the neoplasia rather than benign disease; in 1982, for the first time, HPV DNA was detected in vulvar carcinoma in situ specimen; in the same years, Friedrich and Wilkinson (founding fathers of the ISSVD) published a paper entitled “Carcinoma in situ of the vulva: a continuing challenge” [10].

55.3 Terminology Evolution

In 1986 the ISSVD Task Force agreed upon a modified nomenclature for the uniform classification of “vulvar intraepithelial neoplasia (VIN),” to be intended as a single diagnostic category [11].

The 1986 classification graded vulvar atypia in a manner similar to that commonly used for intraepithelial neoplasia of the cervix. VIN was thus classified as (1) *squamous* (may include HPV change), (a) VIN 1 (showing mild atypia), (b) VIN 2 (moderate atypia), and (c) VIN 3 (severe atypia, carcinoma in situ), and (2) *non-squamous*, (a) Paget’s disease and (b) melanoma in situ.

In this classification, vulvar intraepithelial neoplasia included all the precancerous lesions of the vulva, squamous and non-squamous. This simplification carried the advantage of a clear identification of the lesions at risk for invasive cancer development but implied the inclusion under the same diagnostic term of different clinical entities which are deeply different in biology and oncological potential.

During the years, studies on vulvar cancer and precancer demonstrated there are two types of disease: one HPV related and one occurring in the absence of HPV, but usually related to dermatoses such as lichen sclerosus or lichen planus. This observation has led to the definition of two different types of squamous VIN, related and unrelated to HPV, respectively.

Recently, the ISSVD terminology for vulval intraepithelial lesions has been modified to include the Lower Anogenital Squamous Terminology (LAST) [12] keeping in mind that not all vulvar intraepithelial lesions are caused by HPV.

This 2015 ISSVD terminology for vulval intraepithelial lesions [13] is the following:

- Low-grade squamous intraepithelial lesions (L-SIL) [flat condyloma or HPV effect]
- High-grade squamous intraepithelial lesions (H-SIL) [VIN usual type]
- Differentiated type VIN (dVIN)

Since the majority of these lesions are HPV related, the knowledge of the biology and natural history of HPV has recently led to prefer the term “squamous intraepithelial lesion (SIL)” instead of “neoplasia.” This definition is not applicable to non-HPV-related differentiated lesion of the vulva (dVIN) because it has a different pathogenesis.

55.4 Pathogenesis

The identification of two histological subtypes of VIN, one primarily linked to infection with high-risk types of HPV and the other independent from HPV infection but usually found in a background of lichen sclerosus, has permitted a better understanding of the VIN natural history.

Regarding the first pathway, persistence of HPV infection can result in neoplastic changes of the anogenital tract. Although most infections are asymptomatic and the host immune system eliminates the HPV virus, in some cases the immune response may be inadequate [14]. Particularly, an immunosuppressed state of the epidermis has been observed in HPV-related H-SIL, showing a reduction of immature myeloid dendritic cells and CD8+ T cells.

Regarding differentiated VIN developmental pathway, it is commonly assumed it arises in the absence of HPV, on a background of chronic inflammation. Lichen sclerosus was the underlying inflammatory condition in the majority of HPV-negative cancers. Lichen sclerosus with characteristics mimicking differentiated VIN (dyskeratosis and parakeratosis, hyperplasia, and/or basal cellular atypia) should be kept under close surveillance, as these lesions are at higher risk to progress to squamous cancer [15–17].

55.5 Histopathology

Vulvar L-SIL is actually a flat condyloma or an HPV change. It is characterized (Fig. 55.1) by:

- Nuclear pleomorphism and hyperchromasia (low third of the epithelium)
- Increased mitotic activity in the lower third
- Koilocytic changes

Vulvar H-SIL, formerly usual VIN, is characterized (Fig. 55.2) by:

- Nuclear pleomorphism and hyperchromasia (low 2/3 of the thickness of the epithelium or the entire thickness of the epithelium).
- Binucleate or multinucleate cells are present.
- Atypical mitotic figures are identifiable.
- Koilocytic changes may be seen within or adjacent to the lesion.

The abnormal cell maturation is characterized by multinucleation and abnormal mitotic figures. The rete ridges are wide and deep, often reaching close to the surface.

The epithelium is thickened with a relatively flat and non-papillomatous surface. The epidermis consists of a monotonous proliferation of relatively uniform undifferentiated cells with a basaloid appearance. In either case, the intraepithelial neoplastic process may involve the underlying skin appendages.

Differentiated VIN (dVIN) is characterized (Fig. 55.3) by prematurely differentiated keratinocytes containing large vesicular nuclei and prominent nucleoli. Eosinophilic cells are located in the basal and parabasal area, often with keratin formation or "pearl-like" changes within the rete ridges.

The high degree of cellular differentiation and absence of widespread architectural disarray render this VIN difficult to diagnose and easily

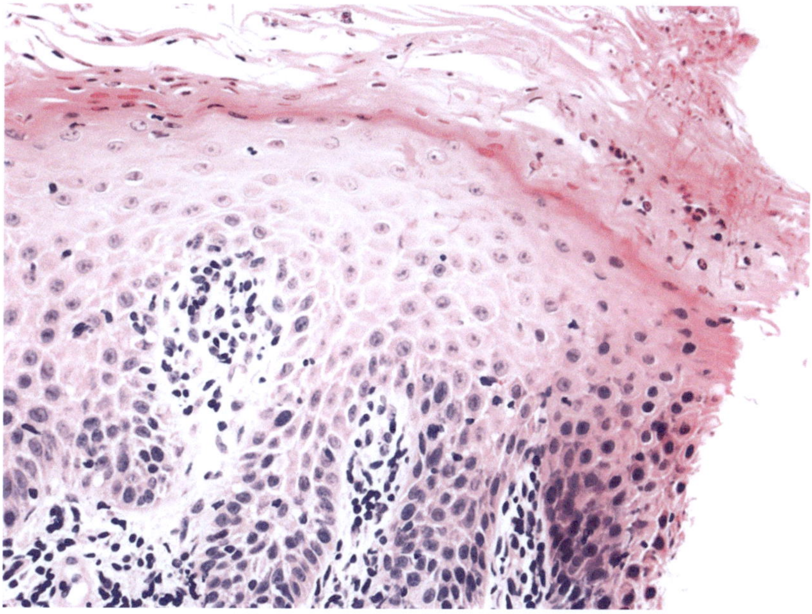

Fig. 55.1 Vulvar L-SIL. Nuclear pleomorphism and hyperchromasia (low third of the epithelium). Increased mitotic activity in the lower third. Koilocytic changes

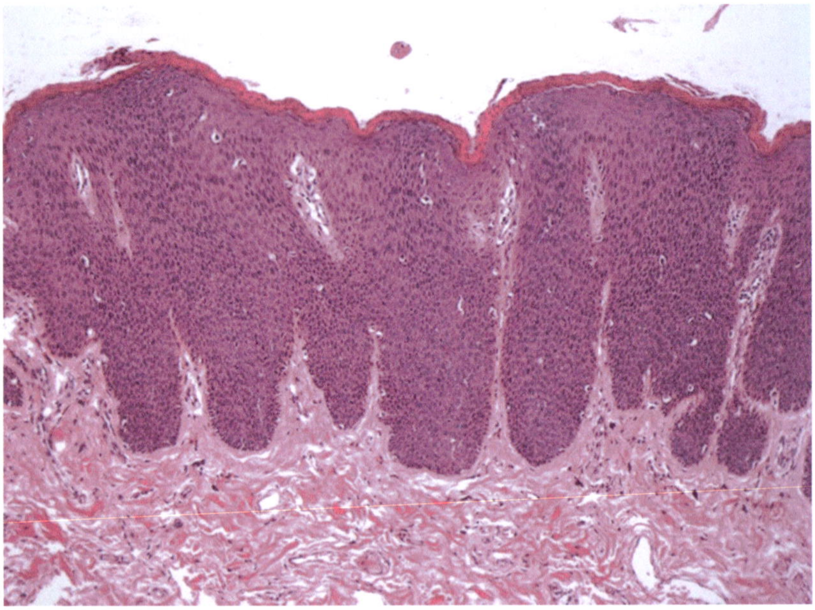

Fig. 55.2 Vulvar H-SIL. Nuclear pleomorphism and hyperchromasia (low 2/3 or the entire thickness of the epithelium) Binucleate or multinucleate cells are present. Atypical mitotic figures are identifiable. Koilocytic changes may be seen within or adjacent to the lesion

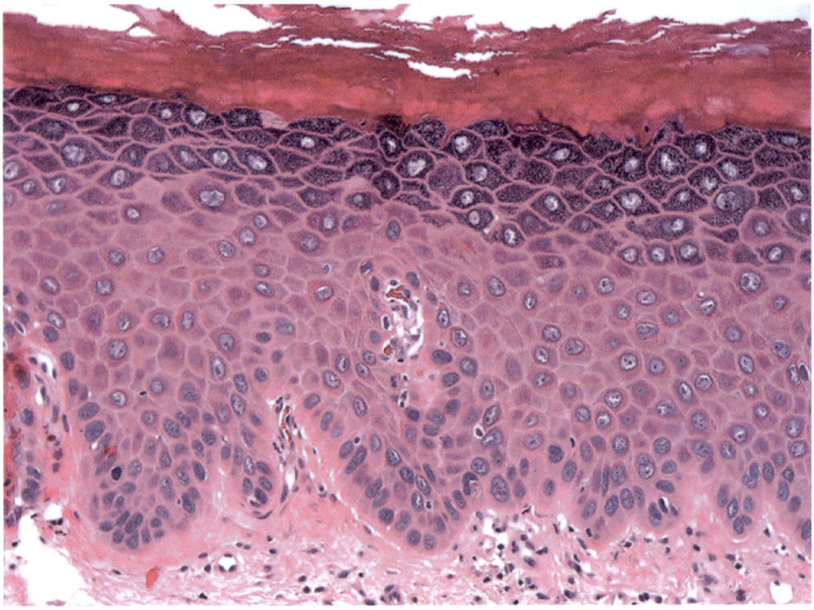

Fig. 55.3 Differentiated VIN. Differentiated keratinocytes containing large vesicular nuclei and prominent nucleoli. Eosinophilic cells are located in the basal and parabasal area, often with keratin formation or "pearl-like" changes within the rete ridges

mistaken for a benign lesion. Immunohistological staining may be useful.

55.6 Clinical Presentation

There is no single pathognomonic feature that can facilitate the diagnosis of VIN. On examination, a visible lesion is noted. It can occur on any location of the vulva but have been described most frequently on the lower border of the labium major. Lesions are variable in appearance; they can be brown, white, gray, or red in color. Elevated, white, irregular lesions are at highest risk for VIN. Pruritus is a common complaint, although the patient may also present with no symptoms and the lesion noted on routine examination. Other common symptoms include vulvar itching, burning, pain, and dyspareunia. VIN can appear at any time and under any circumstance.

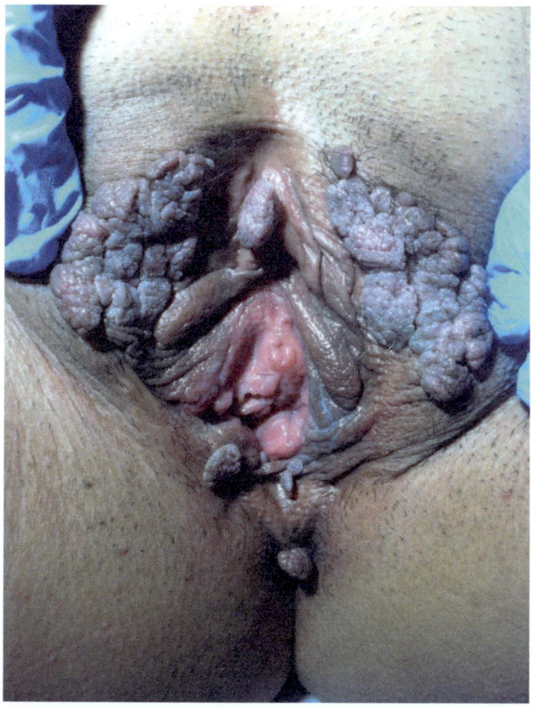

Fig. 55.4 Vulvar H-SIL

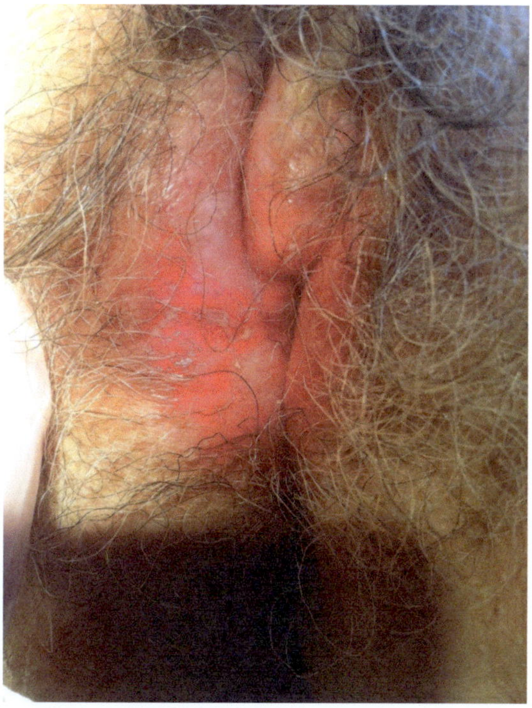

Fig. 55.5 Differentiated VIN

Vulvar H-SIL appears as white or erythematous papules or macules that frequently coalesce or demonstrate a verrucous appearance. Approximately 10–15% of the lesions are hyperpigmented. Two thirds of cases are multifocal at initial presentation (Fig. 55.4). Differentiated VIN appears as ill-defined white plaques or discrete elevated nodules but is typically less bulky than vulvar H-SIL. Vulvar lichen sclerosus may be associated (Fig. 55.5).

55.7 Diagnostic Evaluation

Diagnosis requires direct visual examination with biopsy and histologic examination. The use of colposcope as a magnification tool may help in the diagnosis. Acetic acid application is not necessary, similarly toluidine blue test. Biopsy of the suspected area, using a scalpel, a Keyes punch, or a punch biopsy, is mandatory. A complete evaluation includes a colposcopic assessment of cervix, vagina, and perianal areas due to the frequency of multifocal/concomitant disease. Vulvar H-SIL may be found in association with vulvar carcinoma; therefore this must be ruled out by biopsy prior to treatment for VIN.

55.8 Treatment (See Also Dedicated Chapters Following)

There are few high-quality studies to guide the choice of treatment. Excision is the gold standard as it provides further histology to evaluate for occult cancer. However, other interventions appear to be similarly effective and with same rates of recurrence. Vulvar H-SIL should be treated as condylomatous lesions.

55.8.1 Treatment: Vulvar H-SIL

55.8.1.1 Medical Therapy

- Imiquimod: The role of the immune system in HPV-related VIN provides the opportunity to employ an immune response modifier with antiviral and antitumor properties. The first results of immunomodulator therapy involved treatment of VIN on four patients with imiquimod and were reported in 2000 [18]. Imiquimod acts on dendritic cells, initiating intracellular signaling cascades that activate the innate and adaptive immune responses. Topical treatment with imiquimod is effective in stimulating cell-mediated immunity against different types of HPV including HPV-related VIN.

- Randomized controlled trials have demonstrated that the application of topical imiquimod 5% is effective for the treatment of VIN [19, 20]. However, it is not approved by the US Food and Drug Administration for this purpose. After 4 weeks of treatment, immune cell counts and p16 (INK4a) expression normalized in vulvar tissues, indicating that imiquimod-induced clearance of HPV is strongly correlated with histologic regression of the disease [21]. Published regimens include three times weekly application for 12–20 weeks, with clinical reevaluation at 4–6-week intervals. Residual lesions require surgical treatment. Erythema and vulvar pain may limit use. In a recent study [22] of 5% imiquimod on 62 women, 47 (76%) showed a complete response, 12 (19%) a partial response, 2 (3%) a weak partial response, and 1 did not respond. While 5% imiquimod cream is an alternative to ablative treatment of VIN, patient age, HPV status, and adverse effects may influence treatment outcomes.
- Topical 5-fluorouracil cream has a limited role in the treatment of vulvar intraepithelial lesions due to poor patient tolerance from the chemical desquamation despite reported response rates of 75% [23, 24].
- Cidofovir 1% gel has been compared with imiquimod in a randomized, phase 2 trial [25]. Results for a complete response were comparable in both groups (46% in each group). Adverse events were reported in 37% in the cidofovir group and 46% in the imiquimod group.
- Photodynamic therapy: topical or systemic application of 5-aminolevulinic acid (ALA) followed by application of nonthermal light from a laser constitutes photodynamic therapy. The light interacts with protoporphyrin IX resulting in generation of radicals capable of producing a local cytotoxic effect. This procedure may be performed in the outpatient setting. Findings in one retrospective study report complete response in 52% of patients receiving photodynamic therapy; however 48% had recurrence [26].

55.8.1.2 Surgical Therapy

Extensive surgery, such as vulvectomy, is no longer advisable for VIN. Rather, standard therapy for patients with VIN consists of surgical removal of only the visible lesions to relieve symptoms and prevent development of invasive disease. In 1995, Kaufman [27] outlined the importance of individualizing surgical treatment with the goals of preserving normal anatomy and function of the vulva, while avoiding psychosexual distress due to extensive surgical mutilation. Surgical treatment can be performed using cold knife or CO2 laser vaporization as single techniques or in combination. When representative biopsies have been taken beforehand, vaporization may be considered effective treatment especially in non-hair-bearing areas. A normal skin margin of 5–10 mm is desirable.

A retrospective review by Modesitt [28] found that 66% of women treated with surgical excision had positive margins. Of those patients with positive margins, 46% suffered recurrence, compared to 17% with negative margins. Margin negativity conferred a three-time lower risk of recurrence as well as a longer disease-free interval. An occult squamous cancer was found at the time of initial treatment in 22% of patients. These that were missed had ablation or medical therapy been performed, which emphasizes caution in patient selection for nonsurgical therapy. Skinning vulvectomy (removal of all vulvar skin) is rarely indicated, although it may be useful in cases of confluent multifocal lesions, which can occur in immunocompromised women.

A recent study quotes recurrence-free survival rates at 5 years among 50 women treated for VIN was 91.0% for surgery and 51.3% for the laser vaporization. This indicates that recurrence after CO_2 laser vaporization is more common and requires regular, close, and extended monitoring [29].

In hair-bearing areas, laser procedures must ablate hair follicles, which can contain VIN and extend into the subcutaneous tissue for 3 mm or more. This depth of ablation might lead to scarring. Therefore, in the case of large VIN lesions over hair-bearing areas, other therapeutic modalities are preferred. Ablation for non-hair-bearing VIN should not extend through the dermis (up to 2 mm) to avoid skin retraction and hypertrophic scarring. A power setting of 750–1250 W/cm^2 is required to avoid deep coagulation injury.

55.8.1.3 Therapeutic Vaccine

A recent study evaluated imiquimod treatment followed by therapeutic HPV vaccination (TA-CIN, fusion protein HPV16 E6E7L2) for patients with VIN. The hypothesis involves combining the effect of local immunomodulatory treatment, plus creation of an immunological platform for therapeutic HPV vaccination with the goal to achieve an enhanced and durable response. Immunomodulation was observed only in imiquimod treatment lesion responders, who showed increased local infiltration of CD8 and CD4 T cells [30]. Lack of immunomodulation in non-responder lesions may be due to CD4 T cell secretion of high levels of IL10 in response to imiquimod application, which prevents generation of CD4 and CD8 effector T cells able to migrate to the tumor site to suppress tumor cells [31]. Further studies are necessary to establish the role of IL10 at the time of imiquimod application in order to improve efficacy of the combined medical and vaccination treatment.

55.8.2 Treatment: Differentiated VIN

Treatment of dVIN should be surgical excision because of the high risk of SCC. The rate of progression of dVIN to vulval SCC is much higher than with undifferentiated VIN [32]. In a study of patients with lichen sclerosus that progressed to SCC, the median time to the development of malignancy in those with LS and dVIN was much shorter than in those with LS alone (28 months as compared to 84 months) [33].

Vulvar Intraepithelial Neoplasia: Breaking the Myths

- Although vulvar intraepithelial lesion is a precancerous disease, spontaneous regression may occur.
- Excision is the gold standard treatment of vulvar intraepithelial lesion as it provides tissue for histological evaluation for occult cancer. However, other interventions appear to be similarly effective and with same rates of recurrence.
- Treatment of differentiated VIN should be surgical excision, and not medical, because of the high risk of developing SCC.

References

1. Judson PL, Habermann EB, Baxter NN, Durham SB, Virnig BA. Trends in the incidence of invasive and in situ vulvar carcinoma. Obstet Gynecol. 2006;107:1018–22.
2. Jones RW, Rowan DM, Stewart AW. Vulvar intraepithelial neoplasia: aspects of the natural history and outcome in 405 women. Obstet Gynecol. 2005;106:1319–26.
3. van Seters M, van Beurden M, de Craen AJ. Is the assumed natural history of vulvar intraepithelial neoplasia III based on enough evidence? A systematic review of 3322 published patients. Gynecol Oncol. 2005;97:645–51.
4. Watson M, Saraiya M, Wu X. Update of HPV-associated female genital cancers in the United States, 1999–2004. J Womens Health. 2009;18(11):1731–8.
5. Smith JS, Backes DM, Hoot BE, et al. Human papillomavirus type-distribution in vulvar and vaginal cancers and their associated precursors. Obstet Gynecol. 2009;113(4):917–24.
6. Bowen JT. Precancerous dermatoses: a study of two cases of chronic atypical epithelial proliferation. J Cutan Dis. 1912;30:241–55.
7. Hudelo ML, Cailliau O. Dyskeratose erythroplasiforme de la muquese vulvaire. Bull Soc Fr Dermatol Syphiligr. 1922;29:139–42.
8. van Dyck Knight R. Bowen's disease of the vulva. Am J Obstet Gynecol. 1943;46:514–24.

9. Kaufman R, Gardner H. Intraepithelial carcinoma of the vulva. Clin Obstet Gynecol. 1965;8:1035–50.
10. Friedrich EG Jr, Wilkinson EJ, Fu YS. Carcinoma in situ of the vulva: a continuing challenge. Am J Obstet Gynecol. 1980;136:830–43.
11. ISSVD. New nomenclature for vulvar disease. Obstet Gynecol. 1976;47:122–4.
12. Darragh TM, Colgan TJ, Cox J, et al. Anogenital squamous terminology standardization project for HPV-associated lesions: background and consensus recommendations from the College of American Pathologists and the American Society for Colposcopy and Cervical Pathology. J Low Genit Tract Dis. 2012;16:205–42.
13. Bornstein J, Bogliatto F, Haefner HK, Stockdale CK, Preti M, Bohl TG, Reutter J, ISSVD Terminology Committee. The 2015 International Society for the Study of Vulvovaginal Disease (ISSVD) terminology of vulvar squamous intraepithelial lesions. Obstet Gynecol. 2016;127:264–8.
14. van Seters M, Beckmann I, Heijmans-Antonissen C, van Beurden M, Ewing PC, Zijlstra FJ, Helmerhorst TJ, Klein Jan A. Disturbed patterns of immunocompetent cells in usual-type vulvar intraepithelial neoplasia. Cancer Res. 2008;68:6617–22.
15. Del Pino M, Rodriguez-Carunchio L, Ordi J. Pathways of vulvar intraepithelial neoplasia and squamous cell carcinoma. Histopathology. 2013;62:161–75.
16. Kokka F, Singh N, Faruqi A, Gibbon K, Rosenthal AN. Is differentiated vulval intraepithelial neoplasia the precursor lesion of human papillomavirus-negative vulval squamous cell carcinoma? Int J Gynecol Cancer. 2011;21:1297–305.
17. van Seters M, ten Kate FJ, van Beurden M, Verheijen RH, Meijer CJ, Burger MP, Helmerhorst TJ. In the absence of (early) invasive carcinoma, vulvar intraepithelial neoplasia associated with lichen sclerosus is mainly of undifferentiated type: new insights in histology and aetiology. J Clin Pathol. 2007;60:504–9.
18. Davis G, Wentworth J, Richard J. Self-administered topical imiquimod treatment of vulvar intraepithelial neoplasia. A report of four cases. J Reprod Med. 2000;45:619–23.
19. Van Seters M, van Beurden M, ten Kate FJ, et al. Treatment of vulvar intraepithelial neoplasia with topical imiquimod. N Engl J Med. 2008;358:1465.
20. Mathiesen O, Buus SK, Cramers M. Topical imiquimod can reverse vulvar intraepithelial neoplasia: a randomized, double-blinded study. Gynecol Oncol. 2007;107:219–22.
21. Terlou A, van Seters M, Kleinjan A, Heijmans-Antonissen C, Santegoets LA, Beckmann I, van Beurden M, Helmerhorst TJ, Blok LJ. Imiquimod-induced clearance of HPV is associated with normalization of immune cell counts in usual type vulvar intraepithelial neoplasia. Int J Cancer. 2010;127:2831–40.
22. Westermann C, Fischer A, Clad A. Treatment of vulvar intraepithelial neoplasia with topical 5% imiquimod cream. Int J Gynaecol Obstet. 2013;120:266–70.
23. Sillman FH, Sedlis A, Boyce JG. A review of lower genital intraepithelial neoplasia and the use of topical 5-fluorouracil. Obstet Gynecol Surv. 1985;40:190.
24. Krupp PJ, Bohm JW. 5-flurouracil topical treatment of in situ vulvar cancer. A preliminary report. Obstet Gynecol. 1978;51:702.
25. Tristram A, Hurt CN, Madden T, et al. Activity, safety and feasibility of cidofovir and imiquimod for treatment of vulval intraepithelial neoplasia (RT3VIN): a multicenter, open-label, randomized phase 2 trial. Lancet Oncol. 2014;15:1361–8.
26. Hillemanns P, Wang X, Staehle S, et al. Evaluation of different treatment modalities for vulvar intraepithelial neoplasia (VIN): CO2 laser vaporization, photodynamic therapy, excision and vulvectomy. Gynecol Oncol. 2006;100:271–5.
27. Kaufman RH. Intraepithelial neoplasia of the vulva. Gynecol Oncol. 1995;56:8–21.
28. Modesitt SC, Waters AB, Walton L, et al. Vulvar intraepithelial neoplasia III: occult cancer and the impact of margin status on recurrence. Obstet Gynecol. 1998;92(6):962.
29. Leufflen L, Baermann P Jr, Rauch P, Routiot T, Bezdetnava L, Guillemin F, Desandes E, Marchal F. Treatment of vulvar intraepithelial neoplasia with CO2 laser vaporization and excision surgery. J Low Genit Tract Dis. 2013;17:446–51.
30. Daayana S, Elkord E, Winters U, Pawlita M, Roden R, Stern PL, Kitchener HC. Phase II trial of imiquimod and HPV therapeutic vaccination in patients with vulval intraepithelial neoplasia. Br J Cancer. 2010;102:1129–36.
31. Liu XS. Non-responders to topical imiquimod followed by vaccination therapy in VIN patients may be due to the level of IL10. Br J Cancer. 2010;103:595–6.
32. Yang B, Hart WR. Vulvar intraepithelial neoplasia of the simplex (differentiated) type: a clinicopathological study including analysis of HPV infection and p53 expression. Am J Surg Pathol. 2000;24:429–41.
33. Van de Nieuwenhof HP, Bulten J, Hollema H, et al. Differentiated VIN is often found in lesions, previously diagnosed as lichen sclerosus, which have progressed to vulvar squamous cell carcinoma. Mod Pathol. 2011;24:297–305.

56 Anal Squamous Intraepithelial Neoplasia

Silvio Tatti, Veronica Suzuki, and Laura Fleider

56.1 Epidemiology

Anal squamous intraepithelial lesions (ASILs) are part of the multicentric infection of the lower genital tract caused by the human papillomavirus (HPV). The term anal squamous intraepithelial lesions correlates with the Bethesda classification used for cervical lesions and is also subdivided into high-grade and low-grade lesions—this also applies using the LAST terminology, a unified and standardized nomenclature recommended for all HPV-associated squamous lesions of the lower anogenital tract [1].

The exact natural history of ASIL is not known, but it is widely believed that high-grade ASILs are considered potentially malignant and can progress to anal carcinoma, similar to the natural history of high-grade cervical lesions that can progress to cervical cancer [2, 3]. There are biological, epidemiological, and histological similarities between anal cancer and cervical cancer. Etiopathogenic characteristics include the association with an infection caused by the HPV, especially HPV16. Eighty-eight percent of anal carcinomas are associated with some type of HPV infection (73% HPV16 and 7% HPV18) [4, 5]. The cervix and anus both have a transformation zone where the squamous and columnar epithelium joins. The mucosa of the anal canal joins the squamous epithelium in the dentate line where we can find more intraepithelial lesions [6].

The rate of anal cancer during 2004–2008 in the United States among females was 1.8 per 100,000 and 1.2 per 100,000 among males [7]. Anal carcinoma and their precursor lesions have increased in the last decades, especially among men who have sex with men (MSM), renal transplant, and other causes of immunosuppression. Women with human immunodeficiency virus (HIV) infection have a higher risk compared to the general population. When highly active antiretroviral therapy (HAART) was introduced in 1996, the incidence did not decrease [8].

56.2 Risk Factors

The main risk factors described for HPV infection include multiple viral types involved and high oncogenic risk HPV, also HIV infection and low CD4+ count, history of genital warts, and anal sexual intercourses. Other risk factors include smoking, chronic immunosuppression such as receiving treatment with high-dose corticosteroids or solid organ transplants, or presence of other anogenital HPV lesions [9–14]. Men who have sex with men (MSM) and HIV-positive patients constitute a risk group. Non-immunosuppressed women with lower genital tract disease may also have ASIL.

S. Tatti (✉) · V. Suzuki · L. Fleider
Argentina Hospital de Clinicas "Jose de San Martin", University of Buenos Aires, Buenos Aires, Argentina

J. Bornstein (ed.), *Vulvar Disease*, https://doi.org/10.1007/978-3-319-61621-6_56

Regarding the association between ASIL and other intraepithelial lesions of the lower genital tract, Scholefield et al. described 29 (19%) of 152 women with cervical intraepithelial neoplasia grade III who had histological evidence of anal intraepithelial neoplasia. Fifty-seven percent (21/37) of those with more than one focus of intraepithelial neoplasia (cervix plus vulva, vagina, or both) had anal lesions [15]. Holly et al. studied 251 HIV-positive women and 68 HIV-negative. HIV-positive group had higher risk for abnormal anal cytologies than HIV-negative patients. They had 2% high-grade AIN and 8% of abnormal anal cytologies in HIV-negative women [16]. Moscicki et al. studied young women between 22.5 ± 2.5 years old. Seventeen of 410 (4%) had abnormal cytological results [17]. Zbar et al. described 17% of high-grade AIN in HIV-negative patients [18]. Santoso et al. showed a prevalence of 12.2% of anal intraepithelial neoplasia in women with cervical, vulvar, and vaginal intraepithelial neoplasia [19]. Tatti et al. published a study including 481 patients where 83% were immunocompetent women. 134 (27.86%) of 481 women with cervical, vaginal, or vulvar intraepithelial neoplasia had anal intraepithelial neoplasia. Twenty-eight (5.82%) of 481 had HG-AIN and 106 (22%) of 481 had LG-AIN. Women with cervical high-grade intraepithelial neoplasia (i.e., CIN-2,3) had higher risk of developing AIN. They found statistical significant difference between the frequency of vulvar and anal lesions. Women with vulvar condylomata and vulvar intraepithelial neoplasia (VIN) were more likely to develop AIN [20].

56.3 Diagnosis

The patient may be in left lateral decubitus position, while samples for anal cytology are collected. Subsequently, digital rectal examination (DRE) is performed to palpate any mass and ulcers and to recognize any tender area. Then, high-resolution anoscopy (HRA) is recommended: a disposable anoscope is inserted into the anal canal, and a gauze soaked in 5% acetic acid is placed inside. The anoscope is removed leaving the gauze for 2 min in the anal canal, and then the gauze is removed, and the anoscope is inserted again to perform the HRA. A colposcope with a 16×–25× magnification is used to examine the anal canal, the anal transformation zone, the dentate line, and the margin and perianal skin (Fig. 56.1). A biopsy is taken with small biopsy forceps of any suspicious colposcopic images like leukoplakia, acetowhite changes, mosaicism, punctuation, or irregular vessels using local anesthesia with lidocaine 2% for all biopsies distal to the dentate line. Monsel (ferric subsulfate) solution may be used for hemostasis. The anal cytology is classified according to the 2014 Bethesda system for cervical cytology, and histologic samples are classified as normal, low-grade ASIL (i.e., AIN-1) or high-grade ASIL (i.e., AIN 2/3) (Fig. 56.2).

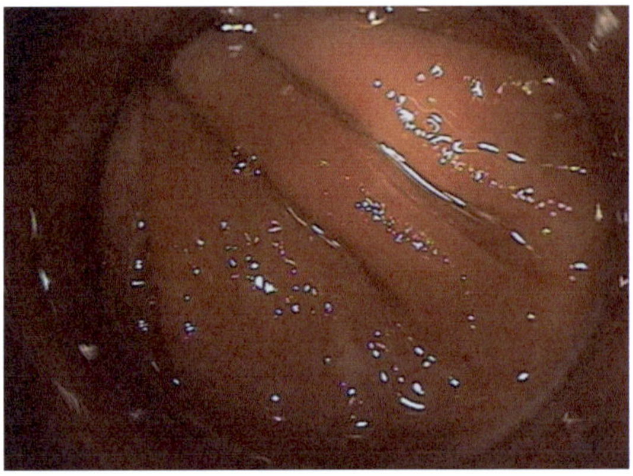

Fig. 56.1 Normal anal transformation zone

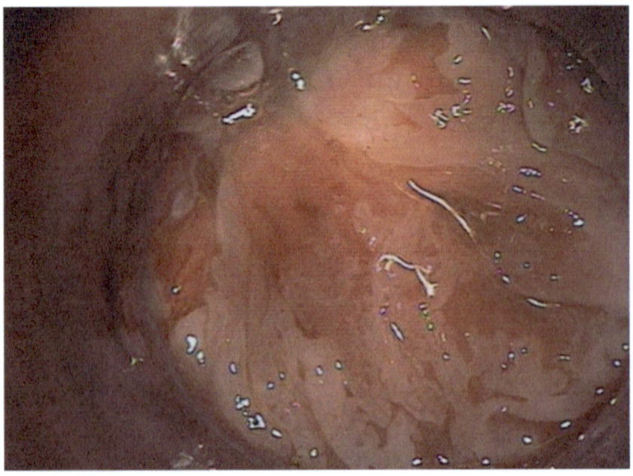

Fig. 56.2 Anal high-grade ASIL

The sensitivity of anal cytology is similar to cervical cytology—between 50% and 70% [21]. In HIV-positive patients, the sensitivity is 81% and the specificity is 63%. In HIV-negative patients, the sensitivity is 50% and the specificity is 92% [22]. It should be noted that anal cytology may be limited by fewer cells or contamination with feces [18].

We recommend performing anal cytology to screen for anal cancer among high-risk populations [23] (e.g., persons with HIV infection, MSM, and history of receptive anal intercourse), followed by high-resolution anoscopy (HRA) for those with abnormal cytologic results (e.g., ASC-US or worse). Although controversial, the New York State AIDS Institute does recommend that clinicians should obtain anal cytology at baseline and annually in the following HIV-infected populations: MSM, any patient with a history of anogenital condyloma, and women with abnormal cervical and/or vulvar histology [24]. Table 56.1 summarizes some of the indications for anal cytology and HRA.

56.4 Treatment

As there are no randomized controlled studies that could tell which the best option of treatment is, the treatment of ASIL is challenging, especially since many patients are immunosuppressed having recurrent disease. Treatments include application of trichloroacetic acid, imiquimod 5%, infrared coagulation, laser CO_2, and surgery. It will depend on the immune status of the patient and the extension of its disease. The aim is to perform its treatment under colposcopic assessment.

Table 56.1 Recommendations for anal cytology and high-resolution anoscopy (HRA)

Who?
1. Men who have sex with men (MSM)
2. HIV-infected men and women
3. High-grade squamous intraepithelial lesions in the lower genital tract
4. Cervical, vaginal, or vulvar cancer
5. Anogenital warts
6. Organ transplant
7. Autoimmune disease (systemic lupus erythematosus; Crohn disease)
How?
1. Digital anal rectal examination (DARE)
2. Anal cytology
3. High-resolution anoscopy (HRA)
4. HRA-guided biopsies of abnormal colposcopic images

Note: Some of them are not yet standard of care—see text

About vaccination, there are three vaccines worldwide to prevent HPV infection. Bivalent HPV vaccine, Cervarix, was approved by the US Food and Drug Administration for the prevention of cervical cancer, cervical intraepithelial neoplasia (CIN) grade 2 or worse and adenocarcinoma in situ, and cervical intraepithelial neoplasia (CIN) grade 1, caused by oncogenic human papillomavirus (HPV) types 16 and 18, in females 9 through 25 years of age.

In December 2010 the US Food and Drug Administration approved the quadrivalent vaccine Gardasil (qHPV) for the prevention of anal cancer and associated precancerous lesions due to human papillomavirus (HPV) types 6, 11, 16, and 18 in people ages 9 through 26 years. In December 2014, Gardasil 9 (Human Papillomavirus 9-valent Vaccine, Recombinant) (9vHPV) was approved for use in the United States by the Food and Drug Administration, and in March 2015, it was included in the CDC vaccination guidelines. It has 96.7% of efficacy and 95% confidence interval of 80.9–99.8 to prevent infection and disease related to HPV6, 11, 16, 18, 31, 33, 45, 52, and 58 [25]. Adverse events profile of this vaccine is similar to that reported by the quadrivalent HPV vaccine supporting its safety profile for its recommendation. The most common adverse events were related to local site injection (pain, swelling, erythema) which were described more common in the 9vHPV group than in the qHPV group and systemic symptoms like headache or pyrexia [26].

56.5 Conclusions

Generally, anal squamous intraepithelial lesions have no early symptoms so we could be warned of these findings. Most of these lesions are subclinical and the diagnosis is histological.

However, knowing that the anal and perianal regions are affected by the HPV and that immunocompetent women with cervical, vaginal, or vulvar intraepithelial neoplasia may also present with high-grade or low-grade anal intraepithelial lesions, we should consider ASIL as part of a multicentric disease of the lower genital tract and be aware when a patient has CIN, VIN, and VAIN that they could have anal intraepithelial lesions.

Anal Squamous Intraepithelial Lesions (ASIL): Breaking the Myths

- The anus is more similar to the cervix than the vagina: both have a transformation zone where the squamous and columnar epithelium joins.
- Eighty-eight percent of ASILs are associated with HPV infection, especially HPV16 and 18.
- To diagnose ASIL one needs a high index of suspicion. Women with cervical high-grade intraepithelial neoplasia, vulvar condylomata, and vulvar intraepithelial neoplasia (VIN) had high risk of developing ASIL.
- Obtaining a cytology smear is not the end of the screening procedure for detecting ASIL. A digital rectal examination and high-resolution anoscopy should also be done.

References

1. Darragh TM, Colgan TJ, Cox JT, Heller DS, Henry MR, Luff RD, McCalmont T, Nayar R, Palefsky JM, Stoler MH, Wilkinson EJ, Zaino RJ, Wilbur DC, Members of LAST Project Work Groups. The Lower Anogenital Squamous Terminology Standardization Project for HPV-Associated Lesions: background and consensus recommendations from the College of American Pathologists and the American Society for Colposcopy and Cervical Pathology. J Low Genit Tract Dis. 2012;16(3):205–42.
2. Scholefield JH, Harris D, Radcliffe A. Guidelines for management of anal intraepithelial neoplasia. Color Dis. 2011;13(Suppl 1):3–10.
3. Palefsky J, Holly E. Molecular virology and epidemiology of human papillomavirus and cervical cancer. Cancer Epidemiol Biomark Prev. 1995;4:415–28.
4. Frisch M, Fenger C, van den Brule AJ, et al. Variants of squamous cell carcinoma of the anal canal and perianal skin and their relation to human papillomaviruses. Cancer Res. 1999;59:753–7.
5. Daling JR, Madeleine MM, Johnson LG, et al. Human papillomavirus, smoking, and sexual practices in the etiology of anal cancer. Cancer. 2004;101:270–80.
6. Varnai AD, Bollmann M. HPV in anal squamous cell carcinoma and anal intraepithelial neoplasia (AIN). Impact of HPV analysis of anal lesions on diagnosis and prognosis. Int J Color Dis. 2006;21:135–42.
7. SEER Cancer Statistics Factsheets: Anal Cancer. http://seer.cancer.gov/statfacts/html/anus.html.
8. Palefsky JM, Holly EA, Ralston ML, Da Costa M, Greenblatt RM. Prevalence and risk factors for anal human papillomavirus infection in human immunodeficiency virus (HIV)-positive and high-risk HIV-negative women. J Infect Dis. 2001;183(3):383–91.
9. Moscicki AB, Hills NK, Shiboski S, Darragh TM, Jay N, Powell K, Hanson E, Miller SB, Farhat S, Palefsky J. Risk factors for abnormal anal cytology in young heterosexual women. Cancer Epidemiol Biomark Prev. 1999;8(2):173–8.
10. Palefsky JM, Rubin M. The epidemiology of anal human papillomavirus and related neoplasia. Obstet Gynecol Clin North Am. 2009;36:187–200.
11. Palefsky JM, Holly EA, et al. Virologic, immunologic and clinical parameters in the incidence and progression of anal squamous intraepithelial lesions in HIV positive and HIV negative homosexual men. J Acquir Immune Defic Syndr Hum Retrovirol. 1998;17(4):314–9.
12. Palefsky JM, Holly EA, Ralston ML, Arthur SP, Jay N, Berry JM, DaCosta MM, Botts R, Darragh TM. Anal squamous intraepithelial lesions in HIV-positive and HIV-negative homosexual and bisexual men: prevalence and risk factors. J Acquir Immune Defic Syndr Hum Retrovirol. 1998;17(4):320–6.
13. Palefsky JM, Shiboski S, et al. Risk factors for anal human papillomavirus infection and anal cytologic abnormalities in HIV-positive and HIV-negative homosexual men. J Acquir Immune Defic Syndr. 1994;7:599.
14. Welton ML, Sharkey FE, Kahlenberg MS. The etiology and epidemiology of anal cancer. Surg Oncol Clin N Am. 2004;13:263–75.
15. Scholefield JH, Hickson WGE, Smith JHF, et al. Anal intraepithelial neoplasia: part of a multifocal disease process. Lancet. 1992;340:1271–3.
16. Holly EA, Ralston ML, Darragh TM, et al. Prevalence and risk factors for anal squamous intraepithelial lesions in women. J Natl Cancer Inst. 2001;93:843–9.
17. Moscicki AB, Hills NK, Shiboski S, Darragh TM, et al. Risk factors for abnormal anal cytology in young heterosexual women. Cancer Epidemiol Biomarkers Prev. 1999;8:173–8.

18. Zbar AP, Fenger C, Efron J, et al. The pathology and molecular biology of anal intraepithelial neoplasia: comparisons with cervical and vulvar carcinoma. Int J Color Dis. 2002;17:203–15.
19. Santoso JT, Long M, Crigger M, Wan JY, Haefner HK. Anal intraepithelial neoplasia in women with genital intraepithelial neoplasia. Obstet Gynecol. 2010;116(3):578–82.
20. Tatti S, Suzuki V, Fleider L, Maldonado V, Caruso R, Tinnirello Mde L. Anal intraepithelial lesions in women with human papillomavirus-related disease. J Low Genit Tract Dis. 2012;16(4):454–9.
21. Bean SM, Chhieng DC. Anal-rectal cytology: a review. Diagn Cytopathol. 2010;38(7):538–46.
22. Abbasakoor F, Boulos PB. Anal intraepithelial neoplasia. Br J Surg. 2005;92(3):277–90.
23. HIV Clinical Resource at http://www.hivguidelines.org/.
24. Moscicki AB, Darragh TM, Berry-Lawhorn JM, et al. Screening for anal cancer in women. J Low Genit Tract Dis. 2015;19(3 Suppl 1):S27–42.
25. Joura EA, Giuliano AR, et al. A 9-valent HPV vaccine against infection and intraepithelial neoplasia in women. N Engl J Med. 2015;372(8):711–23.
26. Moreira ED Jr, Block SL, Ferris D, Giuliano AR, et al. Safety profile of the 9-valent HPV vaccine: a combined analysis of 7 phase III clinical trials. Pediatrics. 2016;138(2):e20154387.

Nonsurgical Treatment of Preneoplastic Vulvar Conditions

57

Mario Preti, Gianluigi Radici,
and Leonardo Micheletti

57.1 Introduction

Using the keywords "vulvar intraepithelial neoplasia" or "VIN" and "treatment" or "therapy" for PubMed search, we found at February 1, 2018, more than 1200 articles.

In this chapter, we report the guiding principles and comments on the most relevant publications.

The recent ISSVD classification [1], includes the following three conditions:

- Low-grade squamous intraepithelial lesions (L-SIL) [flat condyloma or HPV effect]
- High-grade squamous intraepithelial lesions (H-SIL) [VIN usual type]
- Differentiated type VIN (dVIN)

It allows us to consider for treatment only the lesions for which a risk of neoplastic progression is demonstrated: vulvar high-grade squamous intraepithelial lesion (VHSIL) and differentiated vulvar intraepithelial neoplasia (dVIN). The classification clearly highlights that there are two vulvar preneoplastic conditions. They have different oncogenic pathways, separated by etiology, epidemiology, and pathogenesis: HPV related (VHSIL) and not HPV related (dVIN) [1].

Vulvar low-grade squamous intraepithelial lesions (VLSIL-flat condyloma or HPV effect) do not have a malignant potential. This condition should be observed or treated only if symptomatic.

Because of the different pathogenetic mechanisms behind VHSIL and dVIN (Table 57.1, Figs. 57.1 and 57.2), we can consider nonsurgical therapies only for VHSIL (Figs. 57.3 and 57.4) [2].

dVIN (Fig. 57.5) is difficult to diagnose, due to the high degree of cellular differentiation and absence of widespread nuclear pleomorphism and atypia.

If a dVIN is suspected in a field of chronic dermatosis, we must biopsy and communicate to the pathologist our suspicion. Due to the short intraepithelial phase of dVIN and its rapid progression to VSCC. Its genesis, its risk of progression to invasive carcinoma, and its risk to harbor, in some parts of the lesion, invasive lesions missed at initial biopsy, this lesion is not appropriate to medical treatment. These concepts are underlined in Table 57.1.

57.2 Assessment of Coexistent Invasion

Five to eighteen percent of biopsies of vulvar intraepithelial lesions can have unsuspected stromal invasion on the final specimen. Therefore we must exclude any focus of invasion before

M. Preti (✉) · G. Radici · L. Micheletti
Department of Gynecology and Obstetrics, University of Torino, Torino, Italy

J. Bornstein (ed.), *Vulvar Disease*, https://doi.org/10.1007/978-3-319-61621-6_57

Table 57.1 Characteristics to consider in VHSIL and dVIN treatment planning

Patient/lesion characteristic	VHSIL	dVIN
Age	<50 years	>50 years
Comorbidity	Not frequent	Frequent
Symptoms	Frequent	Almost always
Smoking	Frequent	Rare
HIV positivity	Possible	Rare
Etiology	High-risk HPV	Chronic dermatoses
Size of lesion	Variable	Usually small
LSA on adjacent pathology	Rare	Frequent
HPV on adjacent pathology	Frequent	Very rare
Multifocality	Frequent	Very rare
Synchronous or metachronous VaIN or CIN or AIN	Possible	Very rare
Unrecognized invasive carcinoma	≈10%	≈40%
Recurrence	≈25%	≈40%
Risk of progression to invasive carcinoma	7–15%	35–40%
Not surgical therapies	Admitted in referral centers	Contraindicated

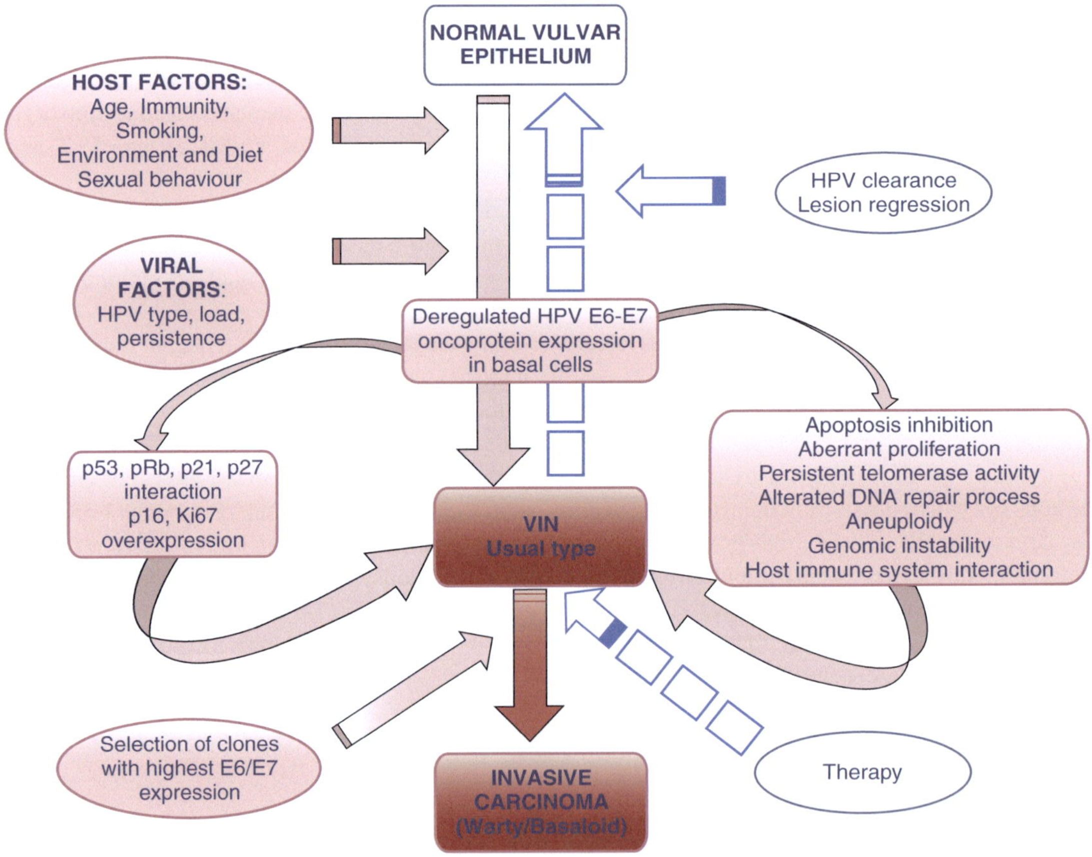

Fig. 57.1 A pathogenetic mechanism of vulvar high-grade squamous intraepithelial lesions (VHSIL, VIN usual)

Fig. 57.2 A pathogenetic mechanism of differentiated vulvar intraepithelial neoplasia (dVIN)

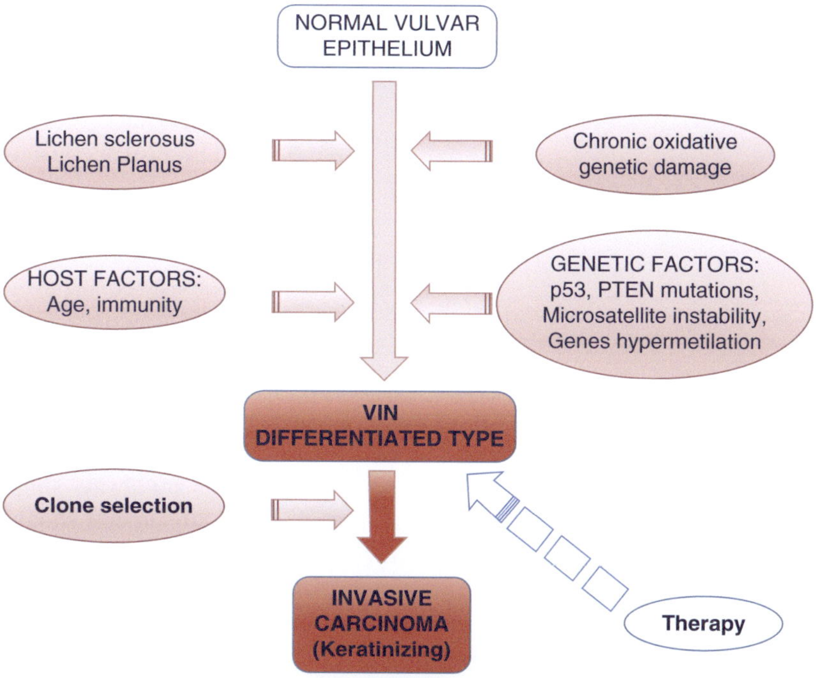

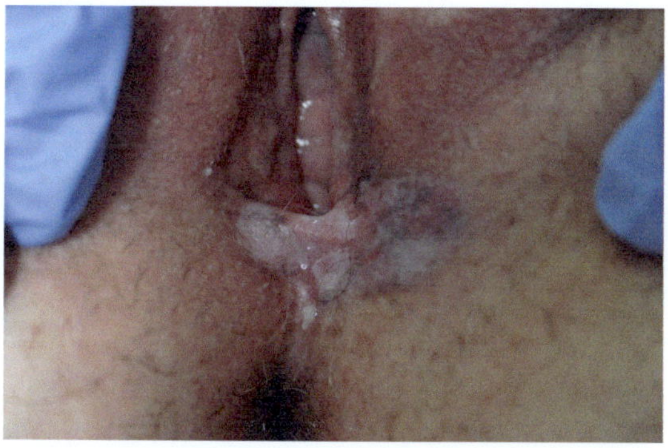

Fig. 57.3 Vulvar high-grade squamous intraepithelial lesions (VHSIL, VIN usual). Hyperkeratotic white patch in the perineum

nonsurgical therapy (Fig. 57.5). Correct sectioning of the specimens is of utmost importance, as tangential cut of the rete ridges can mimic invasion. Furthermore, where involvement of hair-bearing skin and its skin appendages is present, exclusion of stromal invasion can be harder to achieve if there are any technical difficulties in slides preparation.

In a recent paper on 216 VSHIL, Preti et al. [3] detected stromal invasion in 11% of excisional specimens with a median depth of 0.5 mm. In multivariate analysis, the risk of

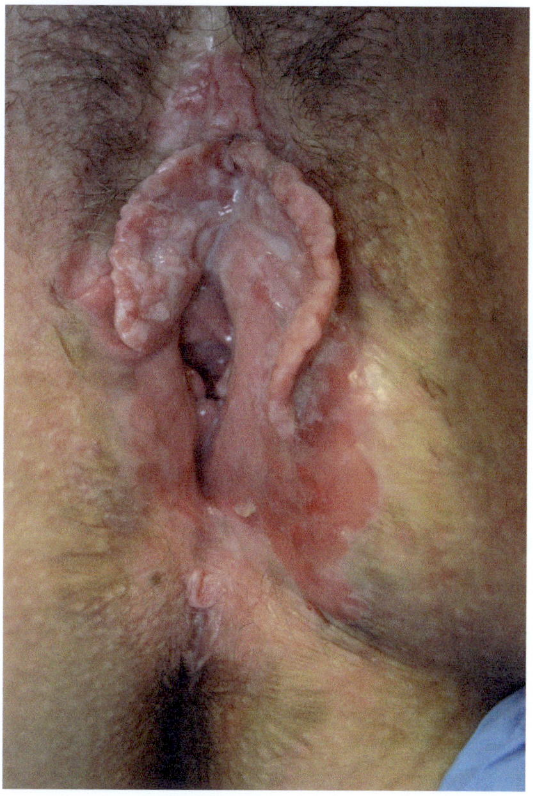

Fig. 57.4 Vulvar high-grade squamous intraepithelial lesions (VHSIL, VIN usual). Red erosion and white hyperkeratotic patches covering the vulva

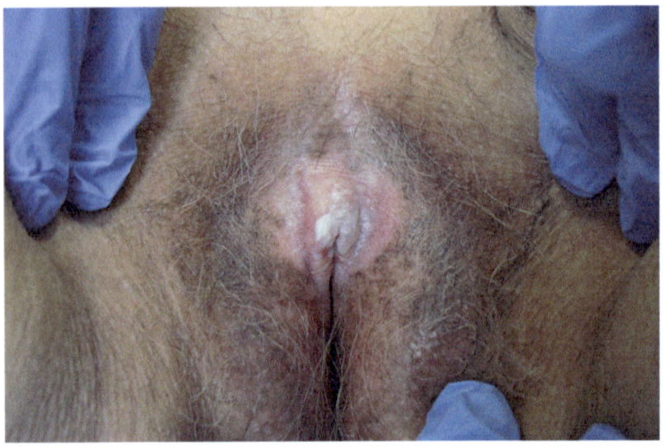

Fig. 57.5 Vulvar high-grade squamous intraepithelial lesions (VHSIL, VIN usual). Hyperkeratotic patches on the clitoris

detection of invasive carcinoma was significantly greater in patients in the highest tertile of age, in patients with a lesion ≥20 mm in size and in patients with clitoral involvement. This invasion risk must be considered when nonsurgical therapies are applied. In addition, the incidence of periclitoral invasive vulvar carcinomas have increased in recent decades with larger tumor size, deeper stromal invasion, and more frequent spread to lymph nodes. Therefore, extreme caution with nonsurgical therapies in this area is recommended.

Age represents also a risk factor for the increased incidence of VSCC during the follow-up of VHSIL-treated patients [4]. The risk of a subsequent diagnosis of VSCC is reported to be threefold higher for the group >75 years of age (8.5%) than <30 years, and 30% of all VSCC are diagnosed within 1 year of follow-up after the diagnosis of VHSIL. This underlines how crucial is follow-up in managing VHSIL [5].

57.3 Principles of Nonsurgical Treatment

In the above reported context, nonsurgical therapies for VHSIL must be individualized.

Three main aspects lead us in managing VHSIL [2]:

1. The *lesion* (its size, configuration, location, multifocality, and multicentricity)
2. The *patient* (her age, general condition, symptomatology, associated disease, psychologic issues, work environment, and reliability to follow-up)
3. The available *resources* and medical skills

Unfortunately, no single treatment resolves symptomatology, excludes invasion, preserves vulvar aspect, and avoids recurrences [6, 7].

The American College of Obstetricians and Gynecologists (ACOG) recommends treatment for all women with VIN. It underlines that "medical therapy could be adopted when occult invasion is not a concern" [7]. As previously affirmed this is not always simple to achieve, and nonsurgical treatments should be utilized only in referral centers with rigorous follow-up.

Medical treatments generally require prolonged treatment time, sometimes being associated with distressing treatment-related side effects [8].

To date, no medical therapy is approved neither by the Food and Drug Administration (FDA) nor by European Medicines Agency (EMA) for VHSIL treatment.

57.4 Imiquimod

Imiquimod is a non-nucleoside heterocyclic amine: it acts as immune-response modifier with antiviral and antitumor activity. Imiquimod activates Toll-like receptor 7 (TLR7) stimulating the synthesis of pro-inflammatory cytokines, in particular interferon-α, tumor necrosis factor-α, and interleukin-6, with enhanced cell-mediated cytolytic activity against viral targets. Imiquimod-induced clearance of HPV is associated with normalization of immune cell count in VHSIL [9].

Imiquimod 5% cream should be applied on the lesion two or three times a week for a period of 12–16 weeks. In case of severe side effects (intense local inflammatory reaction, itching, burning, and flu-like systemic signs), application could be reduced or leave treatment-free period. Patients must be monitored for efficacy of treatment, symptoms, and side effects.

The first randomized controlled trial of medical interventions for VHSIL is the work by van

Seters et al. [8]. This trial demonstrates the effectiveness of imiquimod in the treatment of VHSIL during an observation period of 1 year: lesion size was reduced by more than 25% in 81% of patients treated with imiquimod and in none of those treated with placebo ($P < 0.001$). The subsequent study of the same group [10] followed up for at least 5 years the complete responder women in the imiquimod arm, suggesting that imiquimod is effective in the long-term.

A meta-analysis of randomized controlled studies, assessing 104 participants, confirmed these findings [6], and there were 36/62 and 0/42 complete responders in the topical imiquimod and placebo groups, respectively.

The reported progression to vulvar cancer at 12 months after randomization [8] underlines the need to strictly follow up patients treated by imiquimod.

57.5 Cidofovir

Cidofovir is an acyclic nucleoside phosphonate that selectively targets and inhibits cytomegalovirus (CMV) DNA polymerase, and it is licensed for intravenous use in the treatment of CMV retinitis in HIV patients. HPV does not have a DNA polymerase as it uses the host enzyme: cidofovir can only work in HPV-transformed cells with compromised DNA repair and mediates its effect by causing apoptosis of HPV-infected cells [11, 12].

Apoptosis induction and S-phase arrest are concentration and time dependent. In a pilot study with cidofovir 1% [12], 12 women with VHSIL were treated with topical cidofovir, three times a week for 16 weeks. The intense sometimes painful ulcerative reaction was limited to the site of disease. Four of the ten women had a complete regression of disease with histological clearance and viral clearance. Three women had a partial response, two did not respond, and one woman progressed to invasive disease in spite of symptoms resolution.

High levels of DNA methylation of the HPV E2 gene, depicted in pretreatment biopsies from patients with VHSIL, demonstrated to be a predictive biomarker of response to treatment with 88.2% sensitivity and 84.6% specificity [13].

The most recent published RCT study on cidofovir and imiquimod enrolled 180 participants. At the posttreatment assessment visit, a complete proven histological response had been achieved by 46% of patients on both cidofovir and imiquimod [14]. At 18 months, 71.6% of imiquimod complete responders and 94.0% of cidofovir complete responders remained VHSIL-free [15].

Cidofovir is considerably more expensive than imiquimod and currently has to be individually formulated for patients.

57.6 Photodynamic Therapy

Photodynamic therapy (PDT) is an FDA-approved treatment option for the elimination of some early-stage malignancies in dermatology, gynecology, lung diseases, ophthalmology, liver and oral disease, and urology. PDT consists of three elements: photosensitizer, light, and oxygen. In this photoactivated chemotherapy, the photosensitizer, e.g., 5-aminolaevulinic acid (ALA), selectively accumulates in abnormal tissues without damaging healthy cells and minimizing undesired side effects. The exposure to a light of an appropriate wavelength activates the photosensitizer molecule and produces reactive oxygen species resulting in directed tumor cell death [16]. Microvascular disruption and local acute inflammation (with T cell activation) are secondary events that contribute to long-term tumor control combining both ablative and immunogenic modes of action [17].

In the works of Hillemanns [18] and Fehr [19], clearance rates ranged from 40% to 60%. Hillemanns [20] showed similar efficacy and recurrences in the PDT group compared to laser vaporization and local excision.

The combination of immunotherapy and PDT seems to be superior to single therapy alone [21].

Poor tolerability and need for opioids or spinal or general anesthesia to relieve the pain must be considered. Patient selection is essential, and due to design limitations of some studies, more trials are needed to evaluate efficacy and safety [22].

57.7 Therapeutic HPV Vaccination

There are hopes that therapeutic vaccination could be the new approach to VHSIL.

The current commercial available prophylactic HPV vaccines do not control established infections or treat HPV-related lesions. These vaccines, using virus-like particles, target L1 and/or L2 capsid proteins to stimulate production of neutralizing antibodies against HPV and establish protective immunity through.

Therapeutic vaccines need to generate T cell-mediated immunity targeting HPV early antigens: E6 and E7 proteins represent two ideal therapeutic HPV vaccine targets. E6 and E7 expression is preserved in persistent HPV infection and in its malignant transformation [23, 24]. According to these principles, the current development of therapeutic HPV vaccines focuses on activating T cells specific for the HPV E6 and E7 antigens. The activation of antigen-presenting cells (APCs), as dendritic cells (DCs), leads to amplification of specific helper CD4+ T cells, cytotoxic T lymphocytes (CTLs) that mediate the antigen-specific killing of tumor cells.

The route of HPV therapeutic vaccine administration to enhance antigen uptake by DCs and T cell-mediated immune response remain another crucial point in this field. Subdermal administration of a gene gun directly into immature DCs located under the skin or via IM injection encapsulated in microspheres seems to be promising.

57.8 Follow-Up

The need for long-term follow-up will never be stressed enough: treatment for preinvasive vulvar pathology requires lifelong follow-up.

Vulvoscopy is recommended every 3–4 months during the first 2–3 years after therapy when the risk of recurrence is greater and, then, in the absence of symptoms or lesions, every 6 months.

Women treated for VHSIL are at risk for coexisting cervical or vaginal disease and should be screened with cervical/vaginal cytology. Immunosuppression remains a statistically significant risk factor for high-grade cervical cytology in VHSIL-treated patients [25].

Nonsurgical Treatment of Preneoplastic Vulvar Conditions: Breaking the Myths

- Non-surgical treatment is not appropriate for the differentiated type of VIN (dVIN). This is because dVIN may rapidly progressed to vulvar squamous cell carcinoma, and therefore dVIN requires exclusively excisional treatment.
- The clinician should be very careful about choosing cases for non-surgical management. 5–18% of biopsies of vulvar intraepithelial lesions can have unsuspected stromal invasion on the final specimen.

References

1. Bornstein J, Bogliatto F, Haefner HK, et al. The 2015 International Society for the Study of Vulvovaginal Disease (ISSVD) terminology of vulvar squamous intraepithelial lesions. Obstet Gynecol. 2016;127:264–8.
2. Preti M, Scurry J, Marchitelli CE, et al. Vulvar intraepithelial neoplasia. Best Pract Res Clin Obstet Gynaecol. 2014;28:1051–62.
3. Preti M, Bucchi L, Ghiringhello B, et al. Risk factors for unrecognized invasive carcinoma in patients with vulvar high-grade squamous intraepithelial lesion at vulvoscopy-directed biopsy. J Gynecol Oncol. 2017;28:e27.
4. Van de Nieuwenhof HP, Massuger LF, van der Avoort IA, et al. Vulvar squamous cell carcinoma development after diagnosis of VIN increases with age. Eur J Cancer. 2009;45:851–6.
5. Jones RW, Rowan DM, Stewart AW. Vulvar intraepithelial neoplasia: aspects of the natural history and outcome in 405 women. Obstet Gynecol. 2005;106:1319e26.
6. Lawrie TA, Nordin A, Chakrabarti M, et al. Medical and surgical interventions for the treatment of usual-type vulval intraepithelial neoplasia. Cochrane Database Syst Rev. 2016;1:5.
7. American College of Obstetrics and Gynecologists Committee. Opinion summary number 675: management of vulvar intraepithelial neoplasia. Obstet Gynecol. 2016;128:937–8.

8. van Seters M, van Beurden M, ten Kate FJ, et al. Treatment of vulvar intraepithelial neoplasia with topical imiquimod. N Engl J Med. 2008;358:1465e73.
9. Terlou A, van Seters M, Kleinjan A, et al. Imiquimod-induced clearance of HPV is associated with normalization of immune cell counts in usual type vulvar intraepithelial neoplasia. Int J Cancer. 2010;127:2831–40.
10. Terlou A, van Seters M, Ewing PC, et al. Treatment of vulvar intraepithelial neoplasia with topical imiquimod: seven years median follow-up of a randomized clinical trial. Gynecol Oncol. 2011;121:157–62.
11. Stern PL, van der Burg SH, Hampson IN, et al. Therapy of human papillomavirus-related disease. Vaccine. 2012;20(30 Suppl 5):F71–82.
12. Tristram A, Fiander A. Clinical responses to cidofovir applied topically to women with high grade vulval intraepithelial neoplasia. Gynecol Oncol. 2005;99:652–5.
13. Jones SEF, Hibbitts S, Hurt CN, et al. Human papillomavirus DNA methylation predicts response to treatment using cidofovir and imiquimod in vulval intraepithelial neoplasia 3. Clin Cancer Res. 2017;23:5460–8.
14. Tristram A, Hurt CN, Madden T, et al. Activity, safety, and feasibility of cidofovir and imiquimod for treatment of vulval intraepithelial neoplasia (RT^{3}VIN): a multicentre, open-label, randomised, phase 2 trial. Lancet Oncol. 2014;15:1361–8.
15. Hurt CN, Jones SEF, Madden TA, et al. Recurrence of vulval intraepithelial neoplasia following treatment with cidofovir or imiquimod: results from a multicentre, randomised, phase II trial (RT3VIN). BJOG. 2018. https://doi.org/10.1111/1471-0528.15124.
16. Dougherty TJ, Gomer CJ, Henderson BW, Jori G, Kessel D, Korbelik M, Moan J, Peng Q. Photodynamic therapy. J Natl Cancer Inst. 1998;90:889–905.
17. Abdel-Hady ES, Martin-Hirsch P, Duggan-Keen M, et al. Immunological and viral factors associated with the response of vulval intraepithelial neoplasia to photodynamic therapy. Cancer Res. 2001;61:192–6.
18. Hillemanns P, Untch M, Dannecker C, et al. Photodynamic therapy of vulvar intraepithelial neoplasia using 5-aminolevulinic acid. Int J Cancer. 2000;85:649–53.
19. Fehr MK, Hornung R, Degen A, et al. Photodynamic therapy of vulvar and vaginal condyloma and intraepithelial neoplasia using topically applied 5-aminolevulinic acid. Lasers Surg Med. 2002;30:273–9.
20. Hillemanns P, Wang X, Staehle S, et al. Evaluation of different treatment modalities for vulvar intraepithelial neoplasia (VIN): CO(2) laser vaporization, photodynamic therapy, excision and vulvectomy. Gynecol Oncol. 2006;100:271–5.
21. Winters U, Daayana S, Lear JT, et al. Clinical and immunologic results of a phase II trial of sequential imiquimod and photodynamic therapy for vulval intraepithelial neoplasia. Clin Cancer Res. 2008;14:5292–9.
22. Tosti G, Iacobone AD, Preti EP, et al. The role of photodynamic therapy in the treatment of vulvar intraepithelial neoplasia. Biomedicine. 2018;2:6.
23. Yang A, Jeang J, Cheng K, et al. Current state in the development of candidate therapeutic HPV vaccines. Expert Rev Vaccines. 2016;15:989–1007.
24. Cheng MA, Farmer E, Huang C, et al. Therapeutic DNA vaccines for human papillomavirus and associated diseases. Hum Gene Ther. 2018;9. https://doi.org/10.1089/hum.2017.197.
25. Kuroki LM, Frolova AI, Wu N, Liu J, Powell M, Thaker PH, Massad LS. Yield of cytology surveillance after high-grade vulvar intraepithelial neoplasia or cancer. J Low Genit Tract Dis. 2017;21:193–7.

Vulvar Carcinoma: Diagnosis, Staging, and Treatment

58

Anne-Floor W. Pouwer, Nienke C. te Grootenhuis, Maaike H. M. Oonk, and Joanne A. de Hullu

58.1 Introduction

Vulvar cancer is the fourth most common gynecologic cancer after endometrial, ovarian, and cervical cancer. It accounts for only 5% of all gynecologic cancers with an incidence rate of 2.4 per 100,000 women [1]. The most common histological type of vulvar cancer is vulvar squamous cell carcinoma (VSCC), which accounts for around 80% of all cases. Other histological types of vulvar cancer are basal cell carcinoma, melanoma, adenocarcinoma, and extremely rare types such as sarcoma and lymphoma [2].

VSCC mostly affects elderly women, with more than half of the patients aged above 70 years at the time of diagnosis [3]. Over the past few decades, the incidence of VSCC increased both in the younger and elderly population. This increase of incidence rate in younger patients is probably related to human papillomavirus (HPV), while the increase in the elderly population is due to aging.

A.-F. W. Pouwer · J. A. de Hullu (✉)
Department of Obstetrics and Gynaecology, Radboud University Medical Center Nijmegen, Nijmegen, The Netherlands
e-mail: Anne-Floor.W.Pouwer@radboudumc.nl; joanne.dehullu@radboudumc.nl

N. C. te Grootenhuis · M. H. M. Oonk
Academic Medical Centre Groningen, UMCG Groningen, Groningen, The Netherlands
e-mail: n.c.te.grootenhuis@umcg.nl; m.h.m.oonk@umcg.nl

In this chapter, we will discuss the pathogenesis, diagnosis, staging, and treatment of VSCC.

58.2 Pathogenesis

There are two different types of VSCC with their own associated premalignant lesions (Fig. 58.1). The most common type occurs in elderly women and leads to mostly differentiated keratinizing VSCC, in a background of lichen sclerosus (LS) and often differentiated vulvar intraepithelial neoplasia (dVIN) [4] (Fig. 58.2). dVIN is underreported, has a relatively brief intraepithelial phase before progression to invasive carcinoma, and is a difficult clinical and histological diagnosis. The second type of VSCC consists of mainly nonkeratinizing carcinomas, primarily affecting younger women. This type of VSCC is caused by an infection with high-risk HPV, predominantly HPV 16 and 18. These HPV-associated high-grade squamous intraepithelial lesions (HSIL) are seen adjacent to approximately 30% of the VSCC [5].

58.3 Clinical Presentation

The majority of VSCC are diagnosed in the seventh decade [3]. Patients' and doctors' delay in diagnosis is frequent. Most patients with VSCC present with a vulvar mass, although there is often a long history of pruritus or discomfort.

J. Bornstein (ed.), *Vulvar Disease*, https://doi.org/10.1007/978-3-319-61621-6_58

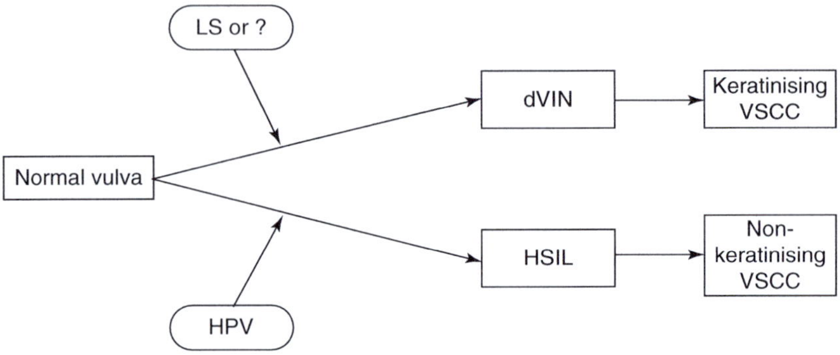

Fig. 58.1 A drawing of the pathogenesis of VSCC. *LS* lichen sclerosus, *?* unknown, *HPV* human papillomavirus, *dVIN* differentiated vulvar intraepithelial neoplasia, *HSIL* high-grade squamous intraepithelial lesion, *VSCC* vulvar squamous cell carcinoma

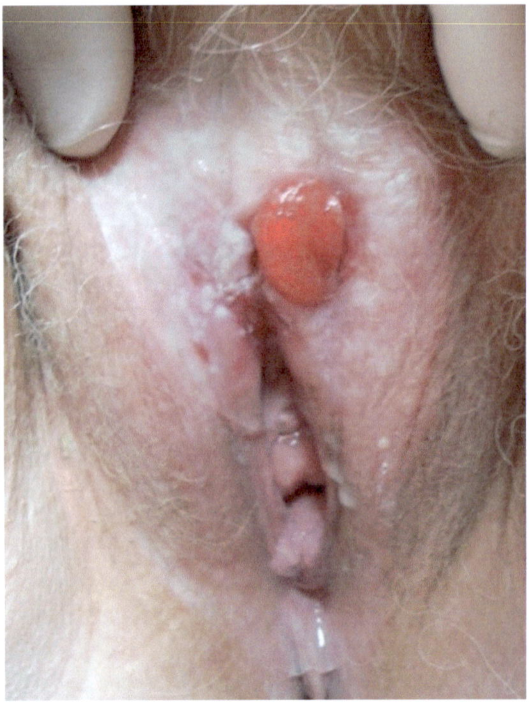

Fig. 58.2 Squamous cell carcinoma of the vulva on the left side with dVIN and lichen sclerosus around the tumor

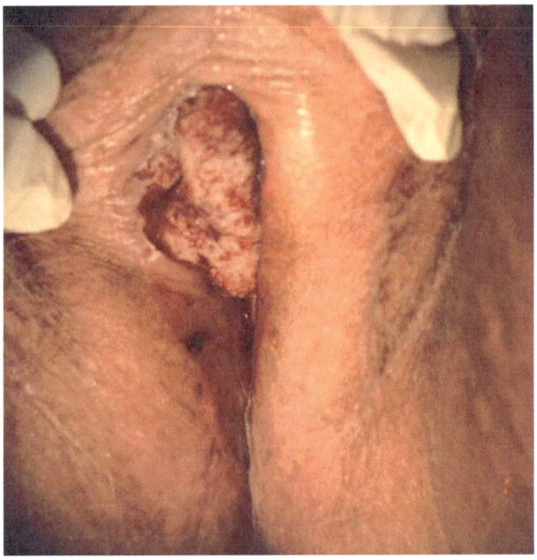

Fig. 58.3 Squamous cell carcinoma of the vulva (HPV related), on the clitoris. Courtesy of Professor Jacob Bornstein

Less common presenting symptoms include vulvar bleeding, pain, or dysuria. Besides obtaining patient history, physical examination of the vulva and both groins should be performed. On physical examination, an ulcer, a red macule or papule, or a white hyperkeratotic (warty) plaque can be seen.

The diagnosis of VSCC should be confirmed histologically, preferably by a punch biopsy that should be taken from the most suspicious part of the lesion or, in case of an ulcer, from the edge of the lesion. When there are multiple (suspicious) lesions, vulvar mapping should be performed to assess the size of the lesions and whether the lesion is uni- or multifocal (Figs. 58.3 and 58.4). For treatment purposes it is important to measure the diameter and invasion depth of the tumor, besides classifying the histological tumor type.

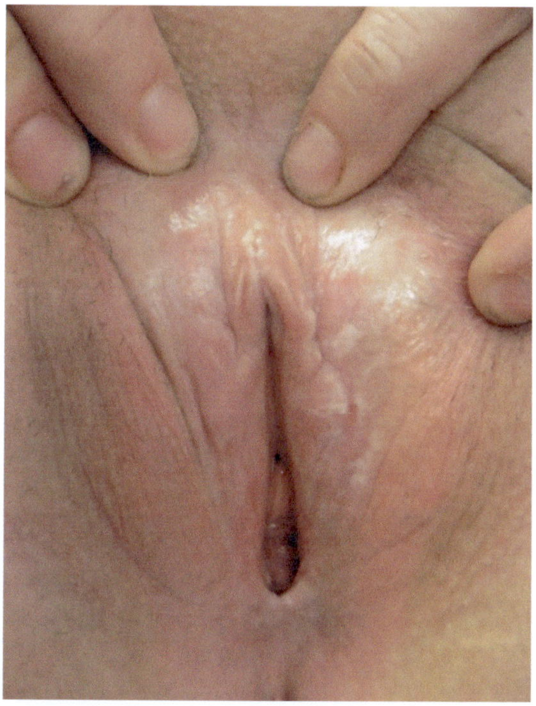

Fig. 58.4 Microinvasive squamous cell carcinoma on the left side in a patient with lichen sclerosus

Also a cervical smear is recommended because women with HPV-related VSCC have a higher risk for cervical cancer. Multicentric HPV infections affecting the cervix, vagina, and/or anus have been described; more than half of all vulvar HSIL patients have previous, concurrent, or subsequent premalignant lesions of the cervix, vagina, and/or anus or cervical cancer [5]. Further work-up (in case of suspicious groins and/or tumors >4 cm) should include computed tomography (CT) to exclude or diagnose bulky lymph nodes and/or distant metastases. In case of a suspicious lymph node, a fine needle aspiration can be performed for cytological examination. In patients eligible for the sentinel node procedure, imaging of the groins (ultrasound, CT, or MRI) is recommended to rule out gross nodal involvement.

58.4 Staging

The spread of VSCC may occur by three different routes. The initial spread occurs usually to the inguinofemoral lymph nodes. Even though the primary tumor is small, lymph node metastases can already be present. About 20–30% of the patients without suspicious lymph nodes at clinical examination appear to have lymph node metastases [6–8]. The inguinofemoral lymph nodes are the first lymph nodes to be affected and secondly the pelvic lymph nodes. Direct extension to adjacent structures and hematogenous dissemination can occur but is less frequent and generally presents in a more advanced-stage disease [9, 10]. VSCC is staged on tumor size, localization, stromal invasion, and the presence and number of lymph node metastases. These tumor characteristics are reflected in the surgicopathological staging according to the International Federation of Gynecology and Obstetrics (FIGO) (Table 58.1). In 2009, the FIGO stage was revised to ensure a better prognostic value and discrimination between stages and less disparity within stages [11].

58.5 Treatment

The method of treatment for VSCC depends on the extent of the disease. In general, surgery is the first choice of treatment in patients with primary VSCC. There is a limited role for primary radio- and/or chemotherapy. Despite the different pathogenesis of two different types of VSCC, treatment regimens are uniform.

The surgical treatment of VSCC has developed throughout the last decades; major changes were made to reduce morbidity without impairing the survival rates [3]. The classic radical vulvectomy with "en bloc" bilateral inguinofemoral lymphadenectomy (IFL) has been replaced by less radical treatment such as omission of pelvic lymphadenectomy, IFL by separate incisions, and radical local excision (RLE) of the tumor with a surgical tumor-free margin of at least 1–2 cm [12]. Furthermore, since the publication of two large trials, the sentinel node (SN) procedure has been integrated in the treatment in well-selected patients with early-stage VSCC [7, 13–19]. The SN procedure is a technique for determining the status of the regional lymph nodes with much less treatment-related morbidity: in case of a negative SN, IFL can be safely omitted.

Table 58.1 FIGO stage (2009) for carcinoma of the vulva

FIGO stage	Description
Stage I	Tumor confined to the vulva or perineum, no nodal metastases
IA	Lesions ≤2 cm with stromal invasion ≤1 mm[a]
IB	Lesions >2 cm in size or with stromal invasion >1 mm
Stage II	Tumor of any size with adjacent spread to the perineal structures (lower third urethra, lower third vagina, or the anus) and no nodal metastases
Stage III	Tumor of any size confined to vulva or with adjacent spread to the perineal structures (lower third urethra, lower third vagina, or the anus) with positive inguinofemoral lymph nodes
IIIA	(a) With 1 lymph node metastasis ≥5 mm (b) With 1 or 2 lymph node metastases <5 mm
IIIB	(a) With 2 or more lymph node metastases ≥5 mm, or (b) With 3 or more lymph node metastases <5 mm
IIIC	With positive lymph nodes with extracapsular spread
Stage IV	Tumor invades other regional (upper 2/3 urethra, upper 2/3 vagina) or distant structures
IVA	(a) Tumor with spread into upper urethra/vagina, bladder, rectal mucosa, bone or fixed to pelvic bone (b) Tumor with fixed or ulcerated inguinofemoral lymph nodes
IVB	Any distant metastases, including pelvic lymph nodes

Adapted from the FIGO classification from Pecorelli [11]
[a]The depth of invasion is defined as the measurement of the tumor from the epithelial stromal junction of the adjacent most superficial dermal papilla to the deepest point of invasion

Currently, standard treatment of a microinvasive tumor (depth of invasion ≤1 mm) measuring ≤2 cm entails a RLE only, because of the negligible chance of lymph node metastasis (<1%) [20, 21]. For a RLE, the incision on the vulva should be carried down to the inferior fascia of the urogenital diaphragm. It is recommended to obtain surgical tumor-free lateral margins of at least 1–2 cm [12] (Fig. 58.5a, b).

The standard treatment for a macro-invasive tumor (depth of invasion >1 mm) entails a RLE with surgical tumor-free margins of 1–2 cm, combined with a SN procedure and/or IFL. The GROINSS-V I is a large international observational study which showed that the SN procedure is safe in patients with a unifocal macro-invasive (>1 mm) vulvar tumor <4 cm without suspicious groin lymph nodes [19]. The SN procedure is performed by the combined technique in which a radioactive tracer and blue dye are used to identify the SN(s) [6]. Before surgery, the radioactive tracer is intracutaneously injected around the tumor, and after injection a lymphoscintigram is performed. Just prior to the surgery, blue dye is injected around the tumor, and guided by the radioactivity and the blue dye, the SN(s) is/are detected during the surgery and removed. The removed lymph nodes are sent in for pathological examination [22]. If the SN is negative on routine histopathologic examination, ultrastaging is performed [19]. Ultrastaging is a method to improve the detection of micrometastasis in the lymph node which is done by immunohistochemistry. In case of negative SN, patients will undergo close follow-up. If the SN is positive, complete IFL is indicated. Currently GROINSS-V II study is running to investigate the safety of radiotherapy instead of IFL in case of a micrometastasis (metastasis ≤ 2 mm) in the SN. Final results were expected in 2018.

In case of a tumor ≥4 cm in diameter and/or multifocal disease, RLE is combined with a uni- or bilateral IFL. For lateralized tumors (>1 cm from the midline), only an ipsilateral IFL is sufficient. For a tumor ≤1 cm from the midline, a tumor involving the midline structures, or multifocal disease, IFL should be performed bilaterally. For IFL, separate incisions parallel to the inguinal ligament are made, and the node-bearing fat pad is removed. The extent of the dissection is the inguinal ligament cephalad, the adductor longus muscle medially, and the sartorius muscle infero-laterally (the femoral triangle) with sparing of the saphenous vein if possible. After opening the cribriform fascia, all node-bearing fatty tissue medial from the femoral vein will be removed as well. A vacuum suction drain is placed in the groin postoperatively. Unfortunately, IFL has significant short- and long-term complications in up to 85% of the patients such as wound breakdown, wound infection, formation of lymphoceles,

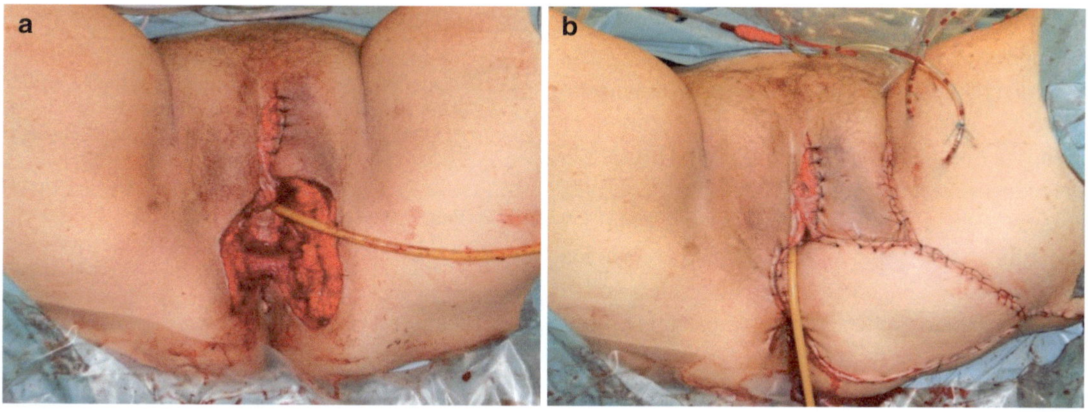

Fig. 58.5 (**a**, **b**) Radical local excision of a large recurrent vulvar squamous cell carcinoma with plastic reconstruction

development of lymphedema, and cellulitis/erysipelas [7, 18].

In case of more than one intranodal metastasis and/or extranodal growth, postoperative radiotherapy to the groin is indicated. In case of positive margins after surgery, local re-excision is advised. Only in cases where re-excision is not possible, radiotherapy can be an alternative. Currently, it is questionable if adjuvant treatment after surgery where the margin was close to the tumor (<8 mm after fixation) improves the prognosis of the patient. One might hypothesize that vulvar recurrences occurring short after primary treatment are real local recurrences due to close or positive margins. Vulvar cancer occurring more than 2 years after primary treatment is in fact a new primary lesion, arising in underlying vulvar disease such as lichen sclerosus or intraepithelial lesion such as dVIN or HSIL [5, 23, 24].

Around 10% of the patients are diagnosed with a FIGO stage III or IV disease [25]. Different, more individualized treatment regimens are used for these patients. When neighboring structures are involved and an exenteration and/or (partial) resection of affected bones or muscles would be necessary to remove the tumor with clear resection margins, VSCC is considered to be locally advanced, although a clear definition for "advanced disease" is lacking. Surgery is the first treatment option, but in initially unresectable locally advanced disease, other strategies must be considered such as radiotherapy combined with chemotherapy, followed by surgery (Fig. 58.6).

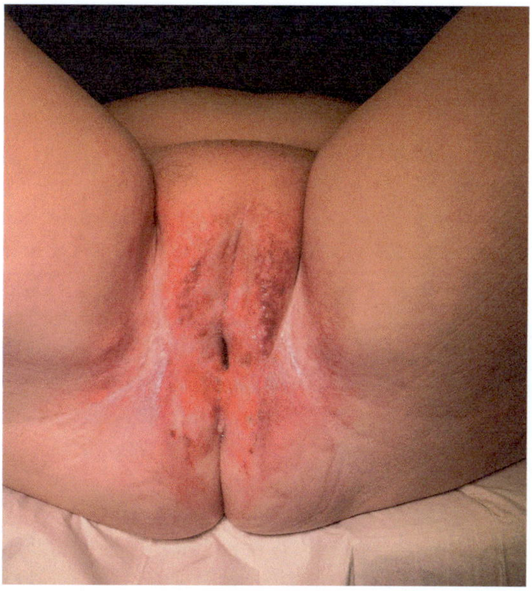

Fig. 58.6 Recurrent squamous cell carcinoma at different areas after chemoradiation

In case of distant metastases, treatment will be palliative. Chemotherapy can be considered with limited success.

58.6 Recurrences

Local recurrence of VSCC is reported in up to 40% of the patients [26]. Of the patients with a local recurrence, 49% develops a second local recurrence [26]. Treatment of a local recurrence consists of RLE. In case of no previously performed IFL and a macro-invasive tumor (depth of invasion of >1 mm), an IFL is indicated [27]. Limited data with divergent results is available on the diagnostic accuracy of the SN procedure in the treatment of recurrent disease [28–32]. Therefore the repeat SN procedure is controversial [33]. As a consequence, patients with a local recurrence after earlier SN procedure, undergoing an IFL, do not perceive the benefits of the SN procedure anymore, in terms of a reduction in morbidity. Further research is needed to validate the safety of a repeat SN procedure in case of a local recurrence of VSCC.

Groin and distant recurrences are less common in early-stage VSCC; groin recurrence rates are described in up to 18.5% and distant recurrences in 3–8% of the patients. They both occur mostly within 1 or 2 years after initial surgery [12, 34–37].

58.7 Prognosis

The inguinofemoral lymph node status at initial diagnosis (reflected in FIGO stage) is of critical prognostic importance for patients with VSCC [9, 10, 14, 34, 38]. Overall survival for early-stage VSCC patients is good with 75% at 5-year survival [26]. It has been shown that the disease-specific survival decreases significantly in case of a local recurrence. This finding was observed both in SN-positive as well as in SN-negative patients [26]. In patients suffering from a groin recurrence, prognosis is very poor with a 5-year survival rate of 0–15% [8, 34, 36].

Vulvar Carcinoma: Breaking the Myths

- Vulvar carcinoma is not a single entity. There are two etiopathologic types: HPV-associated and lichen sclerosus-associated.
- Despite the different etiopathologic types, treatment regimens of vulvar carcinoma are identical.
- If the sentinel lymph nodes are negative, there is still another level of examination: "ultrastaging," improving the detection of micrometastasis by immunohistochemistry.

References

1. Howlader N, Noone A, Krapcho M, Garshell J, Miller D, Altekruse S. 2016. SEER cancer statistics review, 1975–2012. [Online]. Available: http://seer.cancer.gov/csr/1975_2012.
2. Pleunis N, Schuurman MS, Van Rossum MM, Bulten J, Massuger LF, de Hullu JA, Van der Aa MA. Rare vulvar malignancies; incidence, treatment and survival in the Netherlands. Gynecol Oncol. 2016;142(3):440–5.
3. Schuurman MS, Van den Einden LC, Massuger LF, Kiemeney LA, Van der Aa MA, de Hullu JA. Trends in incidence and survival of Dutch women with vulvar squamous cell carcinoma. Eur J Cancer. 2013;49:3872–80.
4. Bornstein J, Bogliatto F, Haefner HK, Stockdale CK, Preti M, Bohl TG, Reutter J. The 2015 International Society for the Study of Vulvovaginal Disease (ISSVD) terminology of vulvar squamous intraepithelial lesions. Obstet Gynecol. 2016;127:264–8.
5. Van de Nieuwenhof HP, Van der Avoort IA, de Hullu JA. Review of squamous premalignant vulvar lesions. Crit Rev Oncol Hematol. 2008;68:131–56.
6. de Hullu JA, Hollema H, Piers DA, Verheijen RH, Van Diest PJ, Mourits MJ, Aalders JG, Van der Zee AG. Sentinel lymph node procedure is highly accurate in squamous cell carcinoma of the vulva. J Clin Oncol. 2000;18:2811–6.
7. Gaarenstroom KN, Kenter GG, Trimbos JB, Agous I, Amant F, Peters AA, Vergote I. Postoperative complications after vulvectomy and inguinofemoral lymphadenectomy using separate groin incisions. Int J Gynecol Cancer. 2003;13:522–7.
8. Oonk MH, Van Hemel BM, Hollema H, de Hullu JA, Ansink AC, Vergote I, Verheijen RH, Maggioni A, Gaarenstroom KN, Baldwin PJ, Van Dorst EB, Van der Velden J, Hermans RH, Van der Putten HW, Drouin P, Runnebaum IB, sluiter WJ, Van der Zee AG. Size of sentinel-node metastasis and chances of non-sentinel-node involvement and survival in early stage vulvar cancer: results from GROINSS-V, a multicentre observational study. Lancet Oncol. 2010;11:646–52.
9. Beller U, Quinn MA, Benedet JL, Creasman WT, Ngan HY, Maisonneuve P, Pecorelli S, Odicino F, Heintz AP. Carcinoma of the vulva. FIGO 26th annual report on the results of treatment in gynecological cancer. Int J Gynaecol Obstet. 2006;95(Suppl 1):S7–27.
10. Hacker NF, Berek JS, Lagasse LD, Leuchter RS, Moore JG. Management of regional lymph nodes and their prognostic influence in vulvar cancer. Obstet Gynecol. 1983a;61:408–12.
11. Pecorelli S. Revised FIGO staging for carcinoma of the vulva, cervix, and endometrium. Int J Gynaecol Obstet. 2009;105:103–4.
12. de Hullu JA, Hollema H, Lolkema S, Boezen M, Boonstra H, Burger MP, Aalders JG, Mourits MJ, Van der Zee AG. Vulvar carcinoma. The price of less radical surgery. Cancer. 2002;95:2331–8.

13. Hacker NF, Leuchter RS, Berek JS, Castaldo TW, Lagasse l D. Radical vulvectomy and bilateral inguinal lymphadenectomy through separate groin incisions. Obstet Gynecol. 1981;58:574–9.
14. Hacker NF, Nieberg RK, Berek JS, Leuchter RS, Lucas WE, Tamimi HK, Nolan JF, Moore JG, Lagasse LD. Superficially invasive vulvar cancer with nodal metastases. Gynecol Oncol. 1983b;15:65–77.
15. Hacker NF, Van der Velden J. Conservative management of early vulvar cancer. Cancer. 1993;71:1673–7.
16. Hopkins MP, Reid GC, Morley GW. Radical vulvectomy. The decision for the incision. Cancer. 1993;72:799–803.
17. Levenback CF, Ali S, Coleman RL, Gold MA, Fowler JM, Judson PL, Bell MC, de Geest K, Spirtos NM, Potkul RK, Leitao MM Jr, Bakkum-Gamez JN, Rossi EC, Lentz SS, Burke JJ 2nd, Van Le L, Trimble CL. Lymphatic mapping and sentinel lymph node biopsy in women with squamous cell carcinoma of the vulva: a gynecologic oncology group study. J Clin Oncol. 2012;30:3786–91.
18. Podratz KC, Symmonds RE, Taylor WF, Williams TJ. Carcinoma of the vulva: analysis of treatment and survival. Obstet Gynecol. 1983;61:63–74.
19. Van der Zee AG, Oonk MH, de Hullu JA, Ansink AC, Vergote I, Verheijen RH, Maggioni A, Gaarenstroom KN, Baldwin PJ, Van Dorst EB, Van der Velden J, Hermans RH, Van der Putten H, Drouin P, Schneider A, Sluiter WJ. Sentinel node dissection is safe in the treatment of early-stage vulvar cancer. J Clin Oncol. 2008;26:884–9.
20. Magrina JF, Gonzalez-Bosquet J, Weaver AL, Gaffey TA, Leslie KO, Webb MJ, Podratz KC. Squamous cell carcinoma of the vulva stage IA: long-term results. Gynecol Oncol. 2000;76:24–7.
21. Yoder BJ, Rufforny I, Massoll NA, Wilkinson EJ. Stage IA vulvar squamous cell carcinoma: an analysis of tumor invasive characteristics and risk. Am J Surg Pathol. 2008;32:765–72.
22. Oonk MH, Van der Zee AG. Sentinel node mapping and groin dissection. In: Abu-Rustum N, Barakat R, Levine D, editors. Atlas of procedures in gynecologic oncology. 3rd ed. Boca Raton: Tayler & Francis Group; 2013.
23. Nooij LS, Van der Slot MA, Dekkers OM, Stijnen T, Gaarenstroom KN, Creutzberg CL, Smit VT, Bosse T, van Poelgeest MI. Tumour-free margins in vulvar squamous cell carcinoma: does distance really matter? Eur J Cancer. 2016b;65:139–49.
24. Yap JK, Fox R, Leonard S, Ganesan R, Kehoe ST, Dawson CW, Woodman CB, Luesley DM. Adjacent lichen sclerosis predicts local recurrence and second field tumour in women with vulvar squamous cell carcinoma. Gynecol Oncol. 2016;42(3):420–6.
25. Stroup AM, Harlan LC, Trimble EL. Demographic, clinical, and treatment trends among women diagnosed with vulvar cancer in the United States. Gynecol Oncol. 2008;108:577–83.
26. Te Grootenhuis NC, Van der Zee AG, Van Doorn HC, Van der Velden J, Vergote I, Zanagnolo V, Baldwin PJ, Gaarenstroom KN, Van Dorst EB, Trum JW, Slangen BF, Runnebaum IB, Tamussino K, Hermans RH, Provencher DM, de Bock GH, de Hullu JA, Oonk MH. Sentinel nodes in vulvar cancer: long-term follow-up of the GROningen INternational Study on Sentinel nodes in Vulvar cancer (GROINSS-V) I. Gynecol Oncol. 2016;140:8–14.
27. Oonk MH, Hollema H, de Hullu JA, Van der Zee AG. Prediction of lymph node metastases in vulvar cancer: a review. Int J Gynecol Cancer. 2006;16:963–71.
28. de Hullu JA, Piers DA, Hollema H, Aalders JG, Van der Zee AG. Sentinel lymph node detection in locally recurrent carcinoma of the vulva. BJOG. 2001;108:766–8.
29. Ennik TA, Allen DG, Bekkers RL, Hyde SE, Grant PT. Effects of previous surgery on the detection of sentinel nodes in women with vulvar cancer. Int J Gynecol Cancer. 2011;21:1679–83.
30. Landkroon AP, de Hullu JA, Ansink AC. Repeat sentinel lymph node procedure in vulval carcinoma. BJOG. 2006;113:1333–6.
31. Van Doorn HC, Van Beekhuizen HJ, Gaarenstroom KN, Van der Velden J, Van der Zee AG, Oonk MH, de Hullu JA. Repeat sentinel lymph node procedure in patients with recurrent vulvar squamous cell carcinoma is feasible. Gynecol Oncol. 2016;140:415–9.
32. Woelber L, Grimm D, Vettorazzi E, Wisotzki C, Trillsch F, Jaenicke F, Schwarz J, Choschzick M, Mahner S. Secondary sentinel node biopsy after previous excision of the primary tumor in squamous cell carcinoma of the vulva. Ann Surg Oncol. 2013;20:1701–6.
33. Oonk MH, de Hullu JA, Van der Zee AJ. Letter to the editor on "the importance of performing a sentinel node biopsy in case of recurrent vulvar cancer". Int J Gynecol Cancer. 2014;24:1537.
34. Maggino T, Landoni F, Sartori E, Zola P, Gadducci A, Alessi C, Solda M, Coscio S, Spinetti G, Maneo A, Ferrero A, Konishi de Toffoli G. Patterns of recurrence in patients with squamous cell carcinoma of the vulva. A multicenter CTF study. Cancer. 2000;89:116–22.
35. Woolderink JM, de Bock GH, de Hullu JA, Davy MJ, Van der Zee AG, Mourits MJ. Patterns and frequency of recurrences of squamous cell carcinoma of the vulva. Gynecol Oncol. 2006;103:293–9.
36. Nooij LS, Brand FA, Gaarenstroom KN, Creutzberg CL, de Hullu JA, Van Poelgeest MI. Risk factors and treatment for recurrent vulvar squamous cell carcinoma. Crit Rev Oncol Hematol. 2016a;106:1–13.
37. Tantipalakorn C, Robertson G, Marsden DE, Gebski V, Hacker NF. Outcome and patterns of recurrence for International Federation of Gynecology and Obstetrics (FIGO) stages I and II squamous cell vulvar cancer. Obstet Gynecol. 2009;113:895–901.
38. Gadducci A, Tana R, Barsotti C, Guerrieri ME, Genazzani AR. Clinico-pathological and biological prognostic variables in squamous cell carcinoma of the vulva. Crit Rev Oncol Hematol. 2012;83:71–83.

59 Surgical Procedures of Preneoplastic and Neoplastic Conditions

Fabrizio Bogliatto and Jacob Bornstein

59.1 Background

Surgical management represents the cornerstone of treatment for most of the vulvar premalignant and malignant lesions. Particularly, during the years, treatment of early vulvar neoplasia has shifted from a radical surgical approach to tissue-sparing surgery and preservation of sexual function [1, 2]. Knowledge and consistent application of less invasive surgery concepts, along with experience integrating radiation and chemotherapy in the pre- or postoperative treatment strategy [3–5], is what defines the modern surgical approach to vulvar lesions. The recent principles of ontogenetic theory of local tumor spread, focusing on embryologically defined compartments and sub-compartments rather than organs and structures, have a considerable impact on oncologic vulvar surgery in terms of local failure rate and severe disturbance of the patients' body image.

F. Bogliatto (✉)
Department of Obstetrics and Gynaecology, Lower Female Anourogenital Tract Network, Chivasso Civic Hospital, Turin, Italy

J. Bornstein
Department of Obstetrics and Gynecology Galilee Medical Center, Bar-Ilan University Faculty of Medicine, Nahariya, Israel

59.2 Clinical Staging Implications

Superficially invasive vulvar squamous cancer, stage IA (Table 59.1) [6], has essentially no risk of nodal metastases. In contrast, with tumors

Table 59.1 FIGO staging of superficially invasive and invasive vulvar cancer after surgery

1	Tumor confined to the vulva
1a	Lesions ≤2 cm in size, confined to the vulva or perineum and with stromal invasion ≤1.0 mm
1b	Lesions >2 cm in size with stromal invasion >1.0 mm, confined to the vulva or perineum
2	Tumor of any size with extension to adjacent perineal structures (lower/distal 1/3 urethra, lower/distal 1/3 vagina, anal involvement)
3	Tumor of any size with or without extension to adjacent perineal structures (lower/distal 1/3 urethra, lower/distal 1/3 vagina, anal involvement) with positive inguino-femoral lymph nodes
3a	(1) 1 lymph node metastasis greater than or equal to 5 mm
	(2) 1–2 lymph node metastasis(es) of less than 5 mm
3b	(1) 2 or more lymph nodes metastases greater than or equal to 5 mm
	(2) 3 or more lymph nodes metastases less than 5 mm
3c	Positive node(s) with extracapsular spread
4a	Tumor of any size with extension to any of the following: upper/proximal 2/3 of urethra, upper/proximal 2/3 vagina, bladder mucosa, rectal mucosa, or fixed to pelvic bone
4b	Any distant metastases including pelvic lymph nodes

J. Bornstein (ed.), *Vulvar Disease*, https://doi.org/10.1007/978-3-319-61621-6_59

3 mm deep, the risk of nodal metastasis is approximately 12%. With a 5 mm depth of invasion, there is a reported risk of nodal metastases of approximately 15% [7].

Follow-up of women with vulvar superficially invasive carcinoma is essential. These women, although they have a relatively low risk of local recurrence, are at risk of having a "reoccurrence" of a new primary tumor or the vulva, independent of the original tumor site. Although this risk is low, awareness and observation, with biopsy when indicated, can reduce the risk of metastases or death from a recurrent or new "reoccurrent" vulvar carcinoma.

59.3 Vulvar Surgical Procedure Terminology

During the years, different terms were used to identify the various surgical procedures employable in vulvar treatment:

Wide local excision means excision of the skin affected by a vulvoscopically detected lesion.

Skinning vulvectomy means excision of the entire vulvar skin affected by the lesion. Although this seems to be an option for treating extensive VIN, this operation is rarely done.

In *simple vulvectomy* the entire vulva is removed. The procedure is performed for benign or premalignant conditions of the vulva that are extensive or multifocal and are not to be removed with local excision alone. The procedure is typically reserved for older patients in whom preservation of vulvar contour and sexual function is not paramount.

Radical vulvectomy can be complete (total) or partial, extended to perineal membrane in depth. This procedure is applied in invasive cancer only, not in VIN treatment. When part of the vulva, including the deep tissue, is removed, the operation is called a *partial radical vulvectomy*. In small lesions, a *local radical excision* may be considered, maintaining more than 1 cm tissue free margin and extending the excision to perineal membrane in depth. In a *complete (total) radical vulvectomy*, the entire vulva and deep tissues, including the clitoris, are removed. A complete radical vulvectomy is often not needed.

A large study which evaluates various treatments found no difference in rates of recurrence of VIN or progression to invasive disease after skinning vulvectomy, simple or partial vulvectomy, local excision, or laser vaporization procedures; free surgical margins did not reduce the risk of progression. This supports the general consensus that local excision is the best surgical method for treating VIN, as it limits iatrogenic morbidity.

59.4 Surgical Technique

Many procedures available for diagnosis and management of vulvar lesions are adequately and appropriately addressed in a clinic or ambulatory care setting. The choice of a hospital versus an ambulatory operating room facility is generally based on the degree of surgical dissection required, the availability of appropriate instrumentation, and the level of anesthesia necessary for adequate patient comfort.

There are no data regarding the risk of infection following conservative vulvar excision, but there is a potential for wound infection due to the presence of skin and vaginal pathogens. There are no guidelines regarding antibiotic prophylaxis of surgical site infection for these procedures, and prophylactic antibiotics for vulvar wide local excision are not recommended. Use of prophylactic antibiotics for simple or skinning vulvectomy is advisable, with cefazolin or amoxicillin.

Thromboprophylaxis for minor vulvar surgery in low-risk patients is not recommended. Women who undergo skinning or simple vulvectomy may require a period of postoperative bed rest or limited ambulation. In these cases, thromboprophylaxis with low-molecular-weight heparin (LMWH) for 3 weeks after surgery permits to reduce the risk of a deep vein thrombosis or pulmonary embolism.

Wide Local Excision (Fig. 59.1a–c) The vulvar skin is prepared with chlorhexidine 1% aqueous solution. The site of the incision is infiltrated with 1% lidocaine without epinephrine, in order to reduce late bleeding. The incision is made with a no. 15 or 22 blade, perpendicular to the skin's surface. Electrosurgery may be used with a 35 watts scalpel cutting power. The elliptical incision is ideal, since the shape provides generally an easy closure of the edges. A portion of subcutaneous tissue below the lesion should be included in the incision. Independently from the lesion shape, the incisions on the labia or lateral labial area have to be parallel to the labial axis. Incisions at the introitus should follow the physiological curvature, and incisions on the perineal body have to be usually horizontal. These attempts permit to reduce the tension on the incision line. A 5- to 10-mm border of surrounding normal tissue is recommended for most lesions. In doubt of invasive lesion, 20-mm border could be advisable. In this case, the depth of the incision should reach the perineal membrane. The defect is usually closed with continuous locked 3.0 absorbable suture with direct reapproximation of the skin edges. Subcutaneous diathermy of small vessels may be required.

Skinning Vulvectomy The vulvar skin is removed after incision made using a no. 15 or 22 blade, perpendicular to the skin's surface, or an electrosurgical blade. Removed tissue is usually replaced with a split-thickness skin graft. The procedure is performed through the partially avascular plane below the epidermis, while preserving the subcutaneous tissue. The surgical plane to be developed is located above the superficial fascia or Colles' fascia. This procedure preserves the contours of the vulva, which are derived from the underlying subcutaneous fat and fascia, to be preserved. The vulvar skin is removed and replaced with a split-thickness skin graft. The graft is taken from the inner thigh. It is important to obtain good hemostasis before the graft is applied. The undersurface of the graft is applied to the defect and the edges secured to the wound edges using 3-0 polyglactin (Vicryl™) suture.

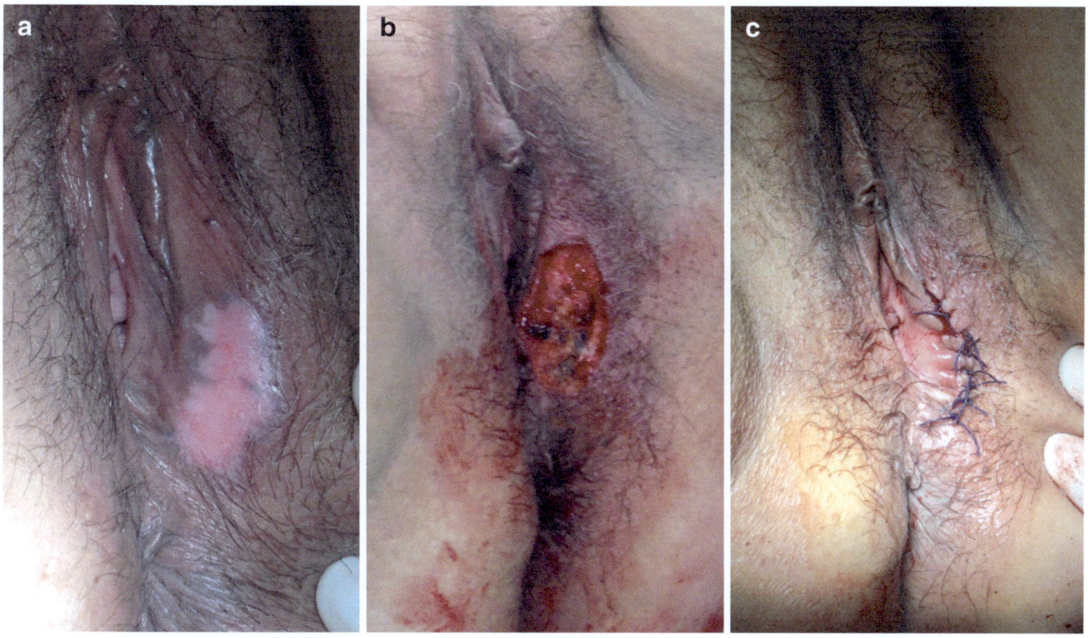

Fig. 59.1 (**a**) HSIL of the vulva, formerly VIN usual, in a young woman. The lesion covers a large cutaneous area, two-thirds of the left labius major in the hairless skin. (**b**) Wide local excision: Incision of the skin encompasses the entire lesion of HSIL with a lesion free margin of more than 8mm. The depth of the incision reaches the level of the deep dermis, just above the superficial or Colles fascia. (**c**) Wound suture with 30 absorbable sutures. A continuous suture may be applied. In this case the mobilization of the wound margins does not require transposition flaps

Simple Vulvectomy The entire vulva is removed using the same procedure of the skinning vulvectomy. The surgical plane to be developed is located beneath the superficial fascia or Colles' fascia. It is not necessary to reach the urogenital membrane or perineal fascia plane. The vulvar subcutaneous tissue is removed and the vessels require a good hemostasis by coagulation. Superficial perineal vessels should be isolated and secured. Clitoral body, cavernous body, and vestibule bulbs may be preserved. During closure, if it appears, the edges may be under too much tension; the lateral and posterior vagina and skin edges may be further undermined. Local skin flaps may be required. Care must be taken to leave sufficient subcutaneous tissue attached when undermining vulvar skin, in order to prevent devascularization. Small open areas may be allowed to granulate.

Radical Vulvectomy (Fig. 59.2a–c) The goal of radical vulvectomy is to remove the primary lesion to the depth of the perineal fascia with a 2-cm circumferential margin. The incision is performed as in simple vulvectomy, extended in depth to the plane of perineal fascia, which is to be left in situ. Tissue surrounding the urethra is to be preserved as much as possible, to facilitate closure and avoid distortion of the urethral meatus. The resection laterally depends upon the extent of disease but may include all of the labia majora. If possible the clitoris should be spared.

The incision is performed through the skin across the perineum at first and then laterally up to the level of the urethra. The posterior edge of the specimen is grasped with forceps. Dissection by finger and scissors is then used to separate the skin from the underlying perineal tissues to the level beyond the vaginal margin. Mobilization of the lower vagina helps the closure. Stretching the vulvar skin to create a flat surface facilitates the surgical dissection. Care must be taken to avoid damaging the rectum during dissection. Laterally, the dissection is performed by Mayo scissors or electrosurgical scalpel. Perineal vessels are to be dissected and secured. The specimen is then detached from the vagina laterally and posteriorly. Urethral meatus and surrounding tissue are to be preserved. Anteriorly, if excision of the clitoris is necessary, the suspensory ligament is divided and ligated. The body of clitoris is isolated and ligated. The incision continues above and laterally to the urethral meatus. The specimen is then completely detached and hemostasis is obtained with an electrosurgical instrument. Bleeding from venous sinuses around the urethra and vaginal margin may be controlled with a running 2-0 polyglactin suture. For periurethral lesions, the distal 1 cm of urethra should be excised if the urethral margin is less than 1 cm tissue free. This will cause no loss of urinary continence. Suture may be made using 2-0 polyglactin separate stitches. For perineal lesions, proximity to the anus may preclude adequate surgical margins, and consideration should be given to additional therapy.

Radical Local Vulvectomy (Figs. 59.3, 59.4, 59.5, 59.6, and 59.7) Includes the malignant tumor with adequate normal-looking margins of 2 cm. The depth of dissection is the same as with radical vulvectomy.

Postoperative Care The bladder catheter is left in place for 5–7 days. The patient should be out of bed and to move to a chair as soon as possible. Stair climbing and abduction of the legs are prohibited in the first 10 days, according to skin repair time. The sutures may be trimmed after 7 days, if they are causing irritation. Perineal hygiene with sitz baths and gentle cleansing with chlorhexidine 1% detergent are encouraged, usually followed by carefully drying the area with a dryer. Exposure to the air is helpful.

59.5 Management: Premalignant Condition or VIN (H-SIL of the Vulva and D-VIN)

Extensive surgery, such as vulvectomy, is no longer advisable for vulvar high-grade squamous intraepithelial lesion (VHSIL, usual VIN) (Fig. 59.1). Rather, standard therapy for patients with VIN consists of surgical removal of all visi-

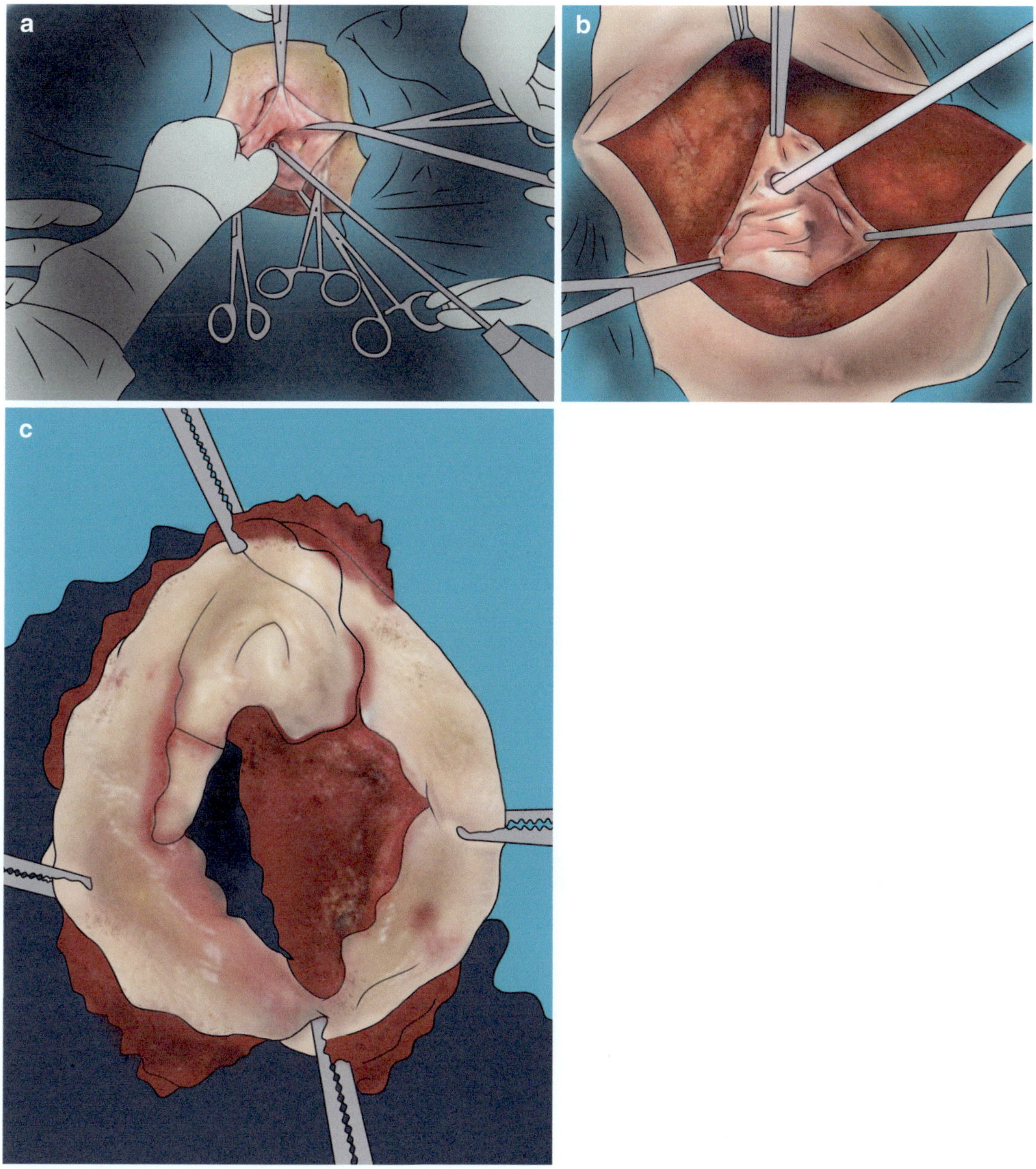

Fig. 59.2 (**a**) A drawing showing starting a radical total vulvectomy for invasive vulvar cancer. The depth of the procedure reaches the level of the perineal membrane. Clitoris and corpora cavernosa are removed. Vagina and urethral meatus are in situ. Reconstruction is made by separate stitches. (**b**) A drawing depicting the defect in the vulva after excision of the specimen in radical vulvectomy (**c**) A drawing of the surgical vulvar specimen of radical vulvectomy. Courtesy of Professor Jacob Bornstein

ble lesions to relieve symptoms and prevent development of invasive disease. In 1995, the importance of individualizing surgical treatment was outlined, with the goals of preserving normal anatomy and function of the vulva, while avoiding psychosexual distress due to extensive surgical mutilation. Surgical treatment can be performed using cold knife or CO2 laser vaporization as single techniques or in combination. When representative biopsies have been taken beforehand, vaporization may be considered an effective treatment especially in non-hair-bearing

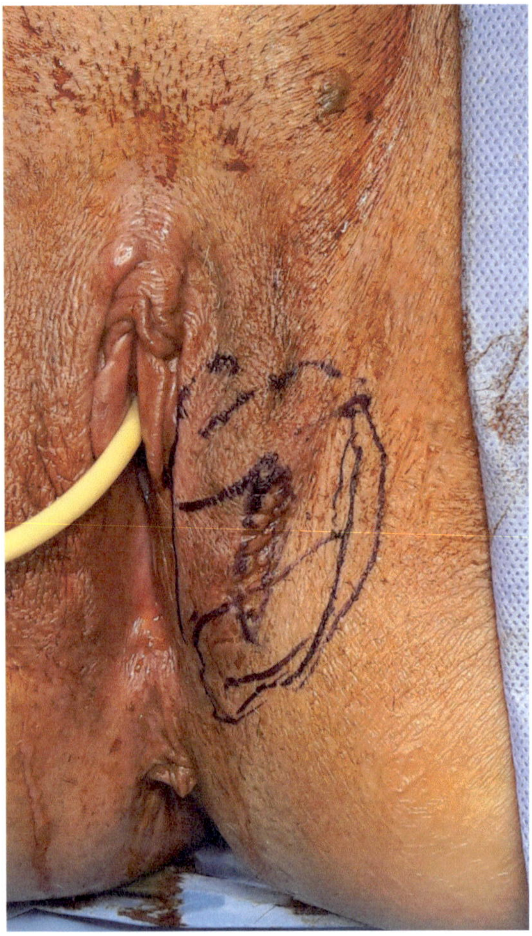

Fig. 59.3 A patient with Vulvar Carcinoma Stage 1b -measuring 3 cm. A marking pen was used to mark the excision area to include the lesion and an adequate normal looking borders.

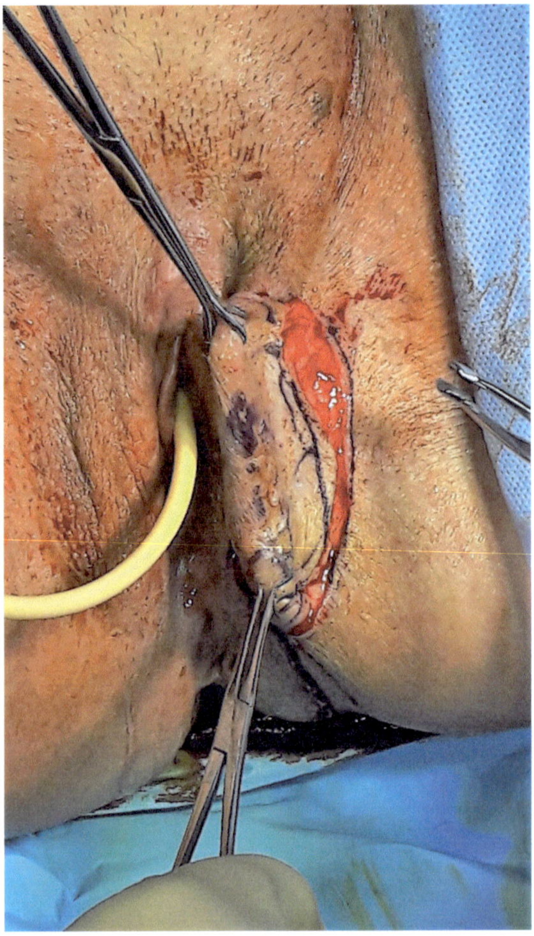

Fig. 59.4 Local Radical Excision: First incision is made on the patient shown in Fig. 3. The lesion is retracted by two Babcock's clamps to avoid damage to the lesion

areas. An excisional margin of 5–10 mm is desirable.

Margins Involvement A retrospective literature review found 66% of women treated with surgical excision had positive margins. Of those patients with positive margins, 46% suffered recurrence, compared to 17% with negative margins. Margin negativity conferred a 3 times lower risk of recurrence as well as a longer disease-free interval. An occult squamous cancer was found at the time of initial treatment in 22% of patients. These would have been missed had ablation been performed, which emphasizes caution in patient selection for ablative therapy. Skinning vulvectomy (removal of all vulvar skin) is rarely indicated, although it may be useful in cases of confluent multifocal lesions, which can occur in immunocompromised women.

Ablative Treatment A recent study quotes recurrence-free survival rates at 5 years among 50 women treated for VIN were 91.0% for surgery and 51.3% for the laser vaporization. This indicates recurrence after CO2 laser vaporization is more common and requires regular, close, and extended monitoring.

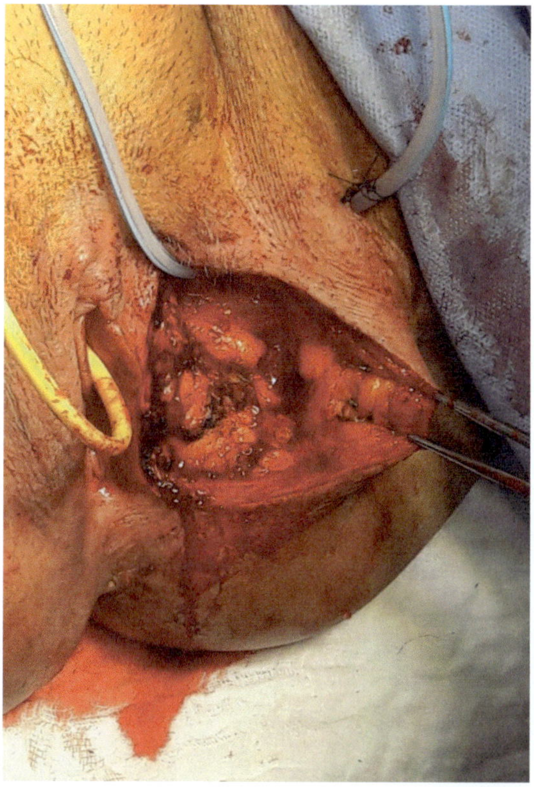

Fig. 59.5 Local Radical Excision - continued: The tumor has been excised. The surgical plane was developed to Colles' fascia

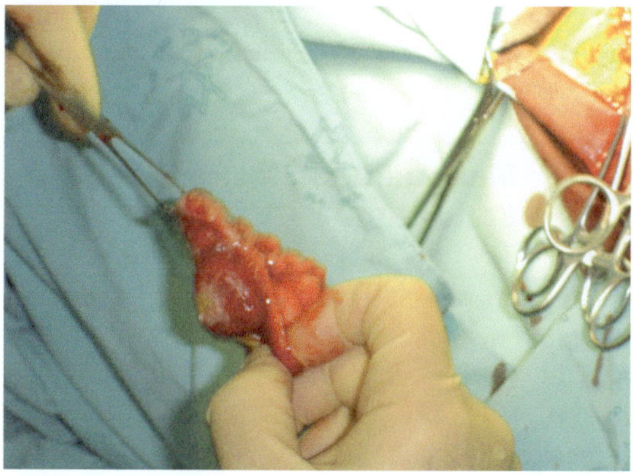

Fig. 59.6 Local Radical Excision: The specimen removed includes adequately normal-looking margins

In hair-bearing areas, laser procedures must ablate hair follicles, which can contain VIN and extend into the subcutaneous tissue for 3 mm or more. Therefore, in the case of large VIN lesions

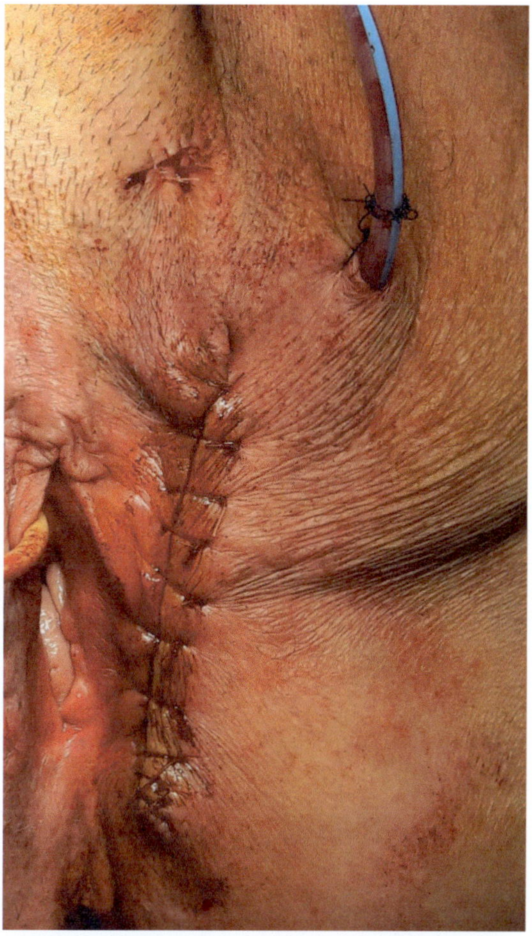

Fig. 59.7 Local Radical Excision: The skin has been primarily sutured. A drain has been left in place

over hair-bearing areas, other therapeutic modalities are preferred. Ablation for non-hair-bearing VIN should extend only through the dermis (up to 2 mm) to avoid skin retraction and hypertrophic scarring. A power setting of 750–1250 W/cm^2 is required to avoid deep coagulation injury.

59.5.1 Risk of Malignancy

HSIL of the vulva, VIN, usual type: 4–6% of these lesions shows a progression to invasive cancer.

D-VIN: The risk of malignancy is not well established, since this is an uncommon histologic type, and data are limited to a few small studies; however, the risk appears to be quite high (32%).

59.6 Vulvar Reconstruction After Premalignant Condition Surgery

Optimal esthetic and functional vulvar reconstruction is now considered an integral part of treatment of the premalignant vulvar condition as it may markedly improve the quality of life, self-esteem, and sexual rehabilitation of the patient with vulvar damage. The broad range of techniques employed for vulvar reconstruction implies that no one technique can address the requirements of such reconstruction in all patients. When primary closure does not suffice, split-thickness or full-thickness skin grafts may be used to cover vulvar excised area.

In some cases of large excision, the pudendal thigh or vulvoperineal flap anteriorly and the infragluteal flap posteriorly are to be used (Figs. 59.8, 59.9, and 59.10).

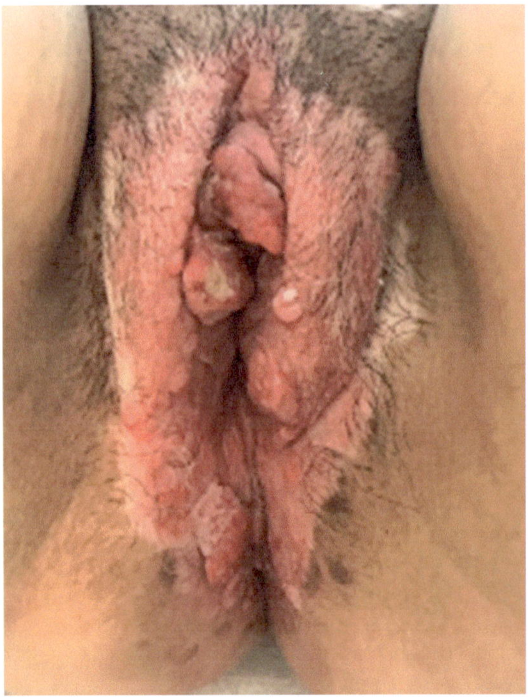

Fig. 59.8 A large vulvar lesion, composed mainly of VHSIL, but with multiple invasive foci

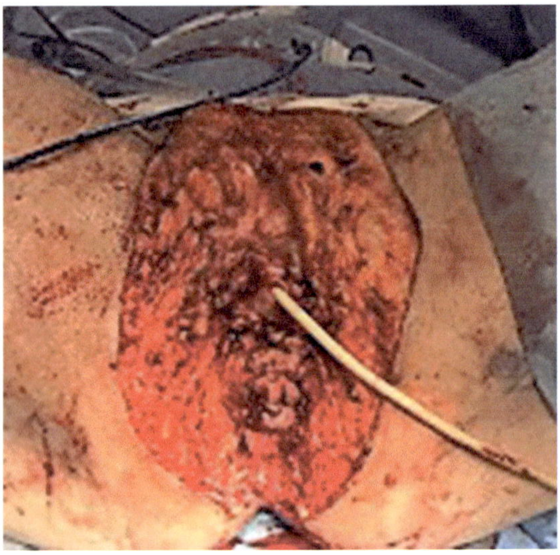

Fig. 59.9 Radical vulvectomy has been made, excising the lesion completely

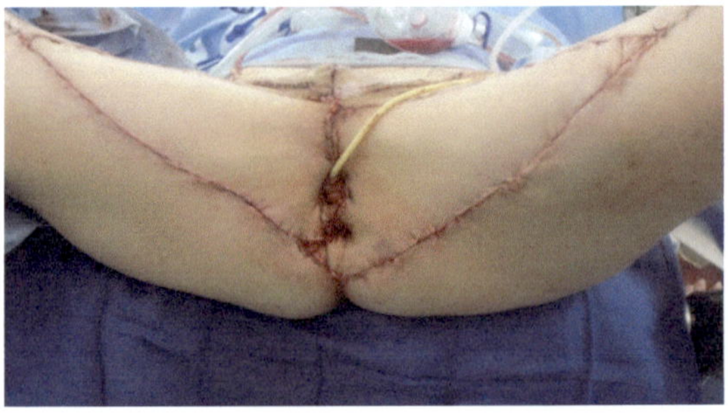

Fig. 59.10 Reconstruction of the vulva after radical vulvectomy

59.7 Management: Malignant Condition

Vulvar cancer is a rare malignancy (4% of all gynecological malignancies and 1% of all cancers in women) consisting principally in squamous cell cancer. The curability in early-stage disease is high and includes theoretically conservative and radical resection of the primary vulvar tumor and excision of local lymph nodes, which are major prognostic factors and drive adjuvant treatment.

This kind of treatment has undergone a major paradigm shift from a radical surgical approach to tissue-sparing surgery and preservation of sexual function. Stage I and II tumors represent two-thirds of the cases, and 5-year survival rates reach 80–90%. These tumors, with clinically negative nodes, do not require metastatic work-up, and the patients are submitted to surgery consisting in radical excision of the vulvar lesion, with inguinal lymphadenectomy.

Lymphadenectomy Technique (Figs. 59.11, 59.12, and 59.13) The routine pelvic lymphadenectomy is to be omitted. The use of separate groin incisions for the inguinal-femoral lymphadenectomy instead of en bloc resection has improved wound healing dramatically without compromising survival.

Unilateral rather than bilateral lymphadenectomy is performed whenever possible because it decreases postoperative morbidity. In lateral disease, unilateral lymphadenectomy is associated with a <3% risk of contralateral groin node metastases.

A unilateral lymphadenectomy is recommended for women with a lesion up to 4 cm diameter and >1 cm from the vulvar midline and no palpable inguinal nodes on examination or abnormal lymph nodes on ultrasound.

Lesions involving the anterior labia minora should have bilateral dissection because of the more frequent contralateral lymphatic drainage from this region.

Because properly planned radiation is capable of sterilizing micrometastases in lymph nodes, there is no need to do a complete groin dissection if frozen section confirms metastatic disease. In patients who have palpably enlarged groin nodes, a preoperative CT scan of the pelvis should be obtained to determine the presence or absence of enlarged pelvic nodes.

The traditional description of groin lymphadenectomy includes ligation of the saphenous vein during removal of the tissue containing superficial groin nodes. A review of 139 cases of groin node dissection demonstrated that when the saphenous vein is preserved, the incidence of wound cellulitis and acute and chronic lymphedema is significantly lower.

The groin lymphadenectomy should be performed with the preservation of the femoral fas-

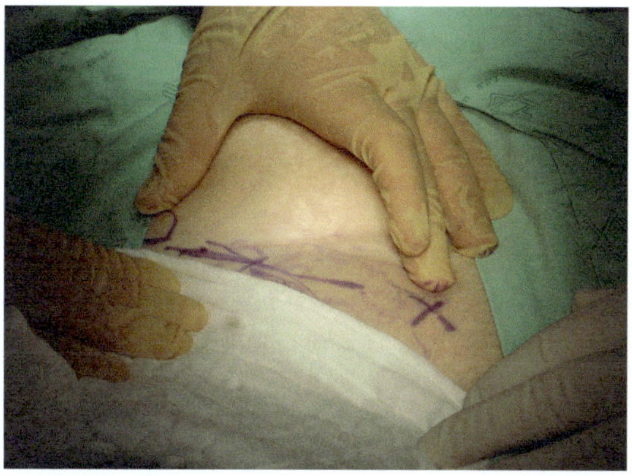

Fig. 59.11 Inguinal lymph node dissection in case of vulvar cancer stage 1b. The incision line is marked with a marking pen. It extends from the anterior superior iliac spine to the pubic tubercle, about 1 cm above and parallel to the groin fold

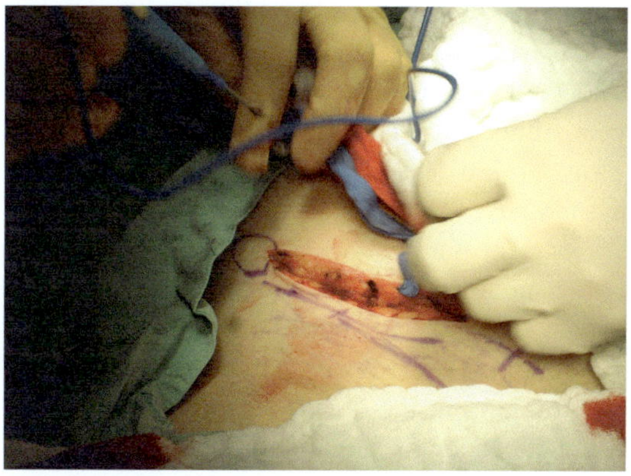

Fig. 59.12 The inguinal incision has been made, and dissection is begun

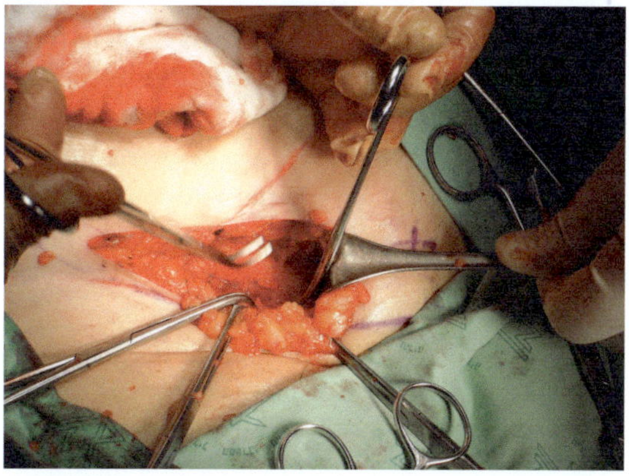

Fig. 59.13 Inguinal dissection including lymph nodes above and below the superficial facia

cia, removing the deep nodes located into the fossa ovalis medially to the femoral vein. This technique permits to avoid damage to femoral artery and nerve, limiting the dissection only to the tissue containing lymph nodes [8].

The skin incision is made along the medial four-fifths of a line drawn between the anterior superior iliac spine and the pubic tubercle, about 1 cm above and parallel to the groin fold. On the basis of embryological and anatomical studies, we have demonstrated that the superficial circumflex iliac vessels represent the lateral surgical landmark. The incision is carried through the subcutaneous tissues to the superficial fascia that is grasped with artery forceps to put it on traction, and the fatty tissue between it and the fascia lata is removed over the femoral triangle. The dissection is carried 2 cm above the inguinal ligament to include all the inguinal nodes. The saphenous vein is usually resected at the apex of the femoral triangle and at its point of entry into the femoral vein, although some surgeons preserve the vein. To avoid skin devascularization, all subcutaneous tissue above the superficial fascia must be preserved. The fatty tissue containing the femoral lymph nodes is removed from within the fossa ovalis. There are only one to three femoral lymph nodes, and they are always situated medial to the femoral vein in the opening of the fossa ovalis. Cloquet's node is not consistently present but should be checked for by retraction of the inguinal ligament cephalad over the femoral canal. At the conclusion of the dissection, a suction drain is placed in the groin. There are no standardized protocols for the duration of drainage, but in most cases the drains are left in situ for at least 5 days; the postoperative management is to remove the drains when the production has decreased under 50–100 ml/day. Skin is sutured with separate 3-0 polyglactin suture or staples.

Sentinel Lymph Node Evaluation of the lymph nodes using sentinel node mapping appears promising, in patients with a unifocal tumor <4 cm without abnormal groin nodes, is safe, and results in less than 2.5% groin recurrences after long-term follow-up. In 2012, the Gynecologic Oncology Group published the results of lymphatic mapping and sentinel lymph node biopsy (SLNB) in 452 women with squamous cell carcinoma of the vulva. There were 132 node-positive women, including 11 women (8.3%) with false-negative nodes, concluding that SLNB should be offered to well-selected patients, preferably to those patients with primary tumors smaller than 4 cm [9].

Deep Nodes The Taussig-Way's classic technique of total inguinal lymphadenectomy consists of removing several anatomical structures, including the sartorius muscle fascia, the fat lying lateral to the femoral artery, the femoral fascia from the sartorius to the adductor longus muscle, and the fascia of the latter. In addition, the sartorius muscle was detached at its origin at the anterior superior iliac spine and moved to cover the femoral vessels by suturing the free upper end to the inguinal ligament. This technique is accompanied by significant complications which lead many authors to propose modifications of the groin dissection ranging from omission to superficial groin dissection. Embryological studies have clarified some anatomical issues from a morphogenetic point of view, giving a more appropriate definition of groin landmarks with surgical relevance: (1) The femoral fascia does not divide into superficial and deep layers as reported in many anatomy textbooks. (2) The cribriform lamina covering the fossa ovalis is thickening of the connective tissue. (3) The deep inguinal lymph nodes originate directly and not independently from the superficial lymphatic tissue and are located just medially to the femoral vein. The Cloquet's node is a mythical one. No lymph nodes are present beneath the femoral fascia distal to the lower margin of the fossa ovalis.

Margins Involvement Although current guidelines recommend a surgical resection margin of at least 1 cm, there are several studies indicating that the extent of resection margins seems to be of minor importance. Some studies could demonstrate a higher risk for disease recurrence when the pathological tumor-free margin was less than 8 mm, while recent analyses failed to show any impact of the margin distance for prognosis.

59.8 The Minimally Invasive Groin Dissection (SAFE-MILND)

Recently, an operative intervention defined as minimally invasive inguinal lymphadenectomy (SAFE-MILND) is applied in groin dissection in obese patients. This procedure is a laparoscopic lymphadenectomy of the groin, to be used preferably in obese patients. This is a three-trocar technique to the inguinal dissection that respects the same anatomic boundaries as the conventional open procedure. The early experience shows that the introduction of the minimally invasive technique is possible in experienced centers with a well-organized training. Even in the early stages of adoption of this new technique, morbidity is already lower compared to open surgery, and the results are in line with the data.

59.8.1 The New Surgical Theory Approach

The ontogenetic compartment theory of local tumor spread by Hoeckel may be applied to vulvar cancer [10]. The revisitation of the anatomy under an embryonic development point of view maps morphogenetic units in the mature body in addition to the functional units, the subject of surgical anatomy. According to this observation, the tumor is confined for a relatively long phase into a morphogenetic compartment. The tumor spread follows an ontogenetic diffusion into a permissive compartment derived from a common primordium in embryonic development. Tumor permeation is isotropic within the permissive ontogenetic compartment, but it is suppressed at the compartment borders. Modulating surgery according to these borders, in a series of 54 consecutive patients with vulvar cancer, 46 tumors were locally confined to the ontogenetic compartment differentiated from the vulvar anlage. The eight tumors that transgressed into adjacent compartments exhibited signs of advanced malignant progression. Thirty-eight patients were treated based on the ontogenetic principles of cancer spread with compartment resection and anatomical reconstruction, and no local failures were found at a mean 19-month follow-up.

59.9 Practice Points

1. A lesion of the vulva that does not respond to a standard treatment, after 3–6 months should be biopsied.
2. Multiple biopsies should be taken to "map" all potential sites of vulvar pathology in multiple suspected areas occurring in a woman with a vulvar cancer.
3. FIGO stage 1a—vulvar superficially invasive cancer requires surgical resection of the primary lesion alone by wide local excision without inguinal-femoral lymphadenectomy.
4. A sentinel node (SN) procedure in patients with a unifocal tumor <4 cm without abnormal groin nodes is safe and results in less than 2.5% groin recurrences after long-term follow-up, and treatment-related morbidity is minimal.
5. Surgical margins should be 1–2 cm to prevent local recurrences.
6. For women with lateral lesions <4 cm without abnormal lymph nodes, a unilateral lymphadenectomy may be appropriate.
7. Lifelong follow-up is recommended in vulvar premalignant and malignant lesion.

Surgery: Breaking the Myths

- Not all cases of vulvar cancer are metastatic to lymph nodes—Superficially invasive vulvar squamous cancer, stage IA, has essentially no risk of nodal metastases
- In complete (total) radical vulvectomy, the entire vulva and deep tissues, including the clitoris, are removed. However, a complete radical vulvectomy is rarely needed.

References

1. Knol AC, Hage JJ. The infragluteal skin flap: a new option for reconstruction in the perineogenital area. Plast Reconstr Surg. 1997;99:1954–9.
2. De Hullu JA, Hollema H, Lolkema S, Boezen M, Boonstra H, Burger MP, Aalders JG, Mourits MJ, Van Der Zee AG. Vulvar carcinoma. The price of less radical surgery. Cancer. 2002;95:2331.
3. Van der Zee AGJ, Oonk MH, De Hullu JA, Ansink AC, Vergote I, Verheijen RH, et al. Sentinel node dissection is safe in the treatment of early-stage vulvar cancer. J Clin Oncol. 2008;26:884–9.
4. van der Velden J, Fons G, Lawrie TA. Primary groin irradiation versus primary groin surgery for early vulvar cancer. Cochrane Database Syst Rev. 2011;5:CD002224.
5. Wills A, Obermair A. A review of complications associated with the surgical treatment of vulvar cancer. Gynecol Oncol. 2013;131:467–79.
6. FIGO Committee on Gynecologic Oncology. FIGO staging for carcinoma of the vulva, cervix, and corpus uteri. Int J Gynaecol Obstet. 2014;125:97–8.
7. Lawrie TA, Patel A, Martin-Hirsch PPL, Bryant A, Ratnavelu NDG, Naik R, Ralte A. Sentinel node assessment for diagnosis of groin lymph node involvement in vulval cancer. Cochrane Database Syst Rev. 2014;6:CD010409.
8. Micheletti L, Preti M. Surgery of the vulva in vulvar cancer. Best Pract Res Clin Obstet Gynaecol. 2014;28:1074–87.
9. Covens A, Vella ET, Kennedy EB, Reade CJ, Jimenez W, Le T. Sentinel lymph node biopsy in vulvar cancer: systematic review, meta-analysis and guideline recommendations. Gynecol Oncol. 2015;137:351–61.
10. Höckel M, Schmidt K, Bornmann K, Horn LC, Dornhöfer N. Vulvar field resection: novel approach to the surgical treatment of vulvar cancer based on ontogenetic anatomy. Gynecol Oncol. 2010;119(1):106–13.

MIX
Papier aus verantwortungsvollen Quellen
Paper from responsible sources
FSC® C105338
www.fsc.org

If you have any concerns about our products,
you can contact us on
ProductSafety@springernature.com

In case Publisher is established outside the EU,
the EU authorized representative is:
Springer Nature Customer Service Center GmbH
Europaplatz 3, 69115 Heidelberg, Germany

Printed by Libri Plureos GmbH
in Hamburg, Germany